Essentials of Critical Care Pharmacology

Abridged from
*The Pharmacologic Approach
to the Critically
Ill Patient,*
Second Edition

Essentials of Critical Care Pharmacology

Abridged from
*The Pharmacologic Approach
to the Critically
Ill Patient,*
Second Edition

EDITOR

Bart Chernow,

M.D., F.A.C.P., F.C.C.P.

Associate Professor of Anaesthesia (Critical Care)
Harvard Medical School
Associate Director, Respiratory-Surgical Intensive Care Unit
Co-Director, Henry K. Beecher Anesthesia Research Laboratories
Massachusetts General Hospital
Boston, Massachusetts

Associate Editors:

John W. Holaday, Ph.D., Washington, D.C.
Gary P. Zaloga, M.D., Winston-Salem, North Carolina
Arno L. Zaritsky, M.D., Chapel Hill, North Carolina

Editorial Assistants:

Robert M. Burke
Donia M. Goss
Anne L. Macaulay

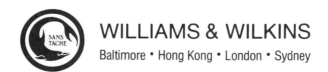

WILLIAMS & WILKINS
Baltimore • Hong Kong • London • Sydney

Editor: Susan M. Glover
Associate Editor: Marjorie Kidd Keating
Design: Dan Pfisterer
Illustration Planning: Wayne Hubbel
Production: Anne G. Seitz

Library of Congress Cataloging-in-Publication Data

Essentials of critical care pharmacology: abridged from The Pharmacologic approach to the critically ill patient, second edition/editor, Bart Chernow; associate editiors, John W. Holaday, Gary P. Zaloga, Arno L. Zaritsky; editorial assistants, Robert M. Burke, Donia M. Goss, Anne L. Macaulay.

    p. cm.
  Includes index.
  ISBN 0-683-01523-0
  1. Pharmacology. 2. Intensive care nursing. I. Chernow, Bart. II. Pharmacologic approach to the critically ill patient.
  [DNLM: 1. Critical Care . 2. Drug Therapy. 3. Pharmacology,
Clinical. QV 38 E775]
RM301.E865 1989
615.5'8--dc19
DNLM/DLC
for Library of Congress   89-5590
                                              CIP
                      89 90 91 92 93
         1 2 3 4 5 6 7 8 9 10

To my parents for all of their love, support, and encouragement.

Preface

The purpose of providing an abridged version of *The Pharmacologic Approach to the Critically Ill Patient, Second Edition,* is to make this information on critical care pharmacology available to a larger clinical audience. This abridged text, entitled *Essentials of Critical Care Pharmacology,* is for those who may have found the price of the unabridged version to be prohibitive.

The material for this book was selected because of its clinical relevance and scientific importance; much of the material is not easily found elsewhere. The book has been prepared with two groups in mind: critical care nurses (medical, surgical, and coronary care) and medical and surgical house officers. These individuals are important providers of critical care in most hospitals.

As with the unabridged version, I hope that all critical care practitioners find *Essentials of Critical Care Pharmacology* to be useful and informative.

Preface to *The Pharmacologic Approach to the Critically Ill Patient, Second Edition*

The responses of readers and reviewers of the first edition of this book were gratifying. This second edition is an attempt to extend and update knowledge available on the pharmacologic approach to critically ill patients. In order to achieve this goal, I have enlisted the help of three associate editors—Drs. John W. Holaday, Gary P. Zaloga, and Arno L. Zaritsky. Their expertise in experimental therapeutics, metabolism, and pediatric pharmacology, respectively, has been invaluable in organizing this text. I am greatly indebted to each of them and I am confident that readers will appreciate the improvements in this second edition.

In the five years since publication of the first edition of this book, many pharmacologic advances have been made. For this reason, *every* previously published chapter has been completely revised and updated. More importantly, new chapters on adjustment of medications in heart failure, adrenergic receptors, red cell substitutes, thrombolytic therapy, digitalis, glucocorticoids in sepsis, fibronectin, management of patients requiring bone marrow transplantation, special problems in pediatric pharmacotherapy, and calcium in shock states have been added.

All chapters have extensive bibliographies that permit the reader to investigate the basis for statements made in the text. Some "overlap" of topics exists so that the reader is provided with information about a medication from different viewpoints. For example, thrombolytic therapy is discussed as a therapeutic agent in one place, and then again in the chapter on anticoagulants. Similarly, catecholamines are reviewed under resuscitation pharmacology and in the chapter dedicated to the pharmacology of these agents. I have included an extensive index, so that clinicians at the bedside can find information rapidly.

In one of the journal reviews of the first edition, this book was called, "a scholarly work." If this adjective holds true for the second edition, it will be because the contributors whom my associates and I have enlisted as chapter authors are scholars. I am honored and grateful that so many experts were willing to give their time and energy to this book. I hope that the multidisciplinary nature of the contributors (anesthesiologists, internists, neurologists, pediatricians, pharmacists, pharmacologists, physiologists, and surgeons) helps to provide a balance in the suggestions for various pharmacologic approaches to critically ill patients.

Critical care medicine has evolved into a large and important subspecialty of anesthesiology, medicine, pediatrics, and surgery. With its growth, and the complexity of patient problems now seen in critical care units, reference sources have become essential. This book is written for all those who contribute to the care of critically ill patients. I sincerely hope that physicians, nurses, therapists, pharmacists, students, nutritionists, and physician assistants will find the book to be a valuable resource providing both clinically useful prescribing information, as well as basic science data and advanced pharmacokinetic principles, to enhance our care of critically ill patients.

Bart Chernow, M.D., F.A.C.P.

Contributors

Patricia A. Arns, M.D.
Research Fellow
Division of Clinical Pharmacology
Vanderbilt University School of Medicine
Nashville, Tennessee

Frank J. Balestrieri, D.D.S., M.D.
Assistant Professor of Anesthesia
George Washington University School
    of Medicine and
Bowman Gray School of Medicine
Staff Anesthetist
Fairfax Hospital
Falls Church, Virginia

Timothy P. Blair, M.D.
Assistant Professor of Medicine
Uniformed Services University of the Health
    Sciences
F. Edward Hebert School of Medicine
Director, Coronary Care Unit
Bethesda Naval Hospital
Bethesda, Maryland

Robert A. Branch, M.D.
Professor of Medicine and Pharmacology
Vanderbilt University School of Medicine
Nashville, Tennessee

D. Craig Brater, M.D.
Professor of Medicine
Indiana University School of Medicine
Director of Clinical Pharmacology
Wishard Memorial Hospital
Indianapolis, Indiana

Hugh J. Carroll, M.D.
Professor of Medicine
State University of New York
Health Science Center at Brooklyn
Director, Hypertension Division
Down State Medical Center
Brooklyn, New York

Edward L. Cattau, Jr., M.D.
Associate Professor of Medicine
Georgetown University School of Medicine
Chief, Clinical Endoscopy
Georgetown University Medical Center
Washington, D.C.

Bart Chernow, M.D.
Associate Professor of Anesthesia (Critical Care)
Harvard Medical School
Associate Director, Respiratory-
Surgical Intensive Care unit
Co-Director Henry K. Beecher Anesthesia
    Research Laboratories
Massachusetts General Hospital
Boston, Massachusetts

John P. DiMarco, M.D., Ph.D.
Associate Professor
University of Virginia School of Medicine
Director, Clinical Electrophysiology
    Laboratory
Department of Internal Medicine
Division of Cardiology
University of Virginia Medical Center
Charlottesville, Virginia

Paul R. Eisenberg, M.D., M.P.H.
Assistant Professor of Medicine
Cardiovascular Division
Washington University School of Medicine
Assistant Director, Cardiac Care Unit
Barnes Hospital
St. Louis, Missouri

James F. English, M.D.
Departments of Anesthesia and Critical Care
Bethesda Naval Hospital
Bethesda, Maryland

Glenn C. Freas, M.D.
Clinical Assistant Professor
Department of Military and Emergency
    Medicine

Uniformed Services University of the Health
 Sciences
F. Edward Hebert School of Medicine

Head, Emergency Medicine Department
Bethesda Naval Hospital
Bethesda, Maryland

John P. Grant, M.D.
Associate Professor of Surgery
Duke University School of Medicine

Director, Nutritional Support
Duke University Medical Center
Durham, North Carolina

Kathryn L. Hall-Boyer, M.D.
Lieutenant Commander, Medical Corps,
United States Navy

Chairman, Department of Emergency
 Medicine
Naval Hospital
Camp Pendleton, California

John M. Hallenbeck, M.D.
Acting Vice Chairman and Professor of
 Neurology and Physiology
Uniformed Services University of the Health
 Sciences
F. Edward Hebert School of Medicine

Chairman, Department of Neurology
Bethesda Naval Hospital
Bethesda, Maryland

Allan S. Jaffe, M.D.
Associate Professor of Medicine
Cardiovascular Division
Washington University School of Medicine

Director, Cardiac Care Unit
Barnes Hospital
St. Louis, Missouri

David A. Johnson, M.D.
Assistant Professor of Medicine
Uniformed Services University of the Health
 Sciences
F. Edward Hebert School of Medicine

Staff Gastroenterologist
Bethesda Naval Hospital
Bethesda, Maryland

John F. Maher, M.D.
Professor of Medicine
Uniformed Services University of the Health
 Sciences
F. Edward Hebert School of Medicine

Director, Nephrology Division
Bethesda Naval Hospital
Bethesda, Maryland

Henry Masur, M.D.
Professor of Medicine
George Washington University

Chief, Critical Care Medicine Department
Clinical Center
National Institutes of Health
Bethesda, Maryland

Joseph A. Miller, M.D.
Associate Professor of Neurology
Uniformed Services University of the Health
 Sciences
F. Edward Hebert School of Medicine

Director, EEG Laboratory
Staff Neurologist
Bethesda Naval Hospital
Bethesda, Maryland

Daniel A. Notterman, M.D.
Assistant Professor of Pediatrics, Pharma-
 cology, and Pediatrics in Surgery
Cornell University Medical College

Director, Division of Critical Care Pediatrics
Department of Pediatrics
The New York Hospital-Cornell Medical
 Center
New York, New York

Man S. Oh, M.D.
Associate Professor of Medicine
State University of New York
Health Science Center at Brooklyn
Brooklyn, New York

Joseph E. Parrillo, M.D.
Chief, Critical Care Medicine
National Institutes of Health
Bethesda, Maryland

Thomas G. Rainey, M.D.
Associate Professor of Medicine
Uniformed Services University of the Health
 Sciences
F. Edward Hebert School of Medicine

Head, Critical Care Medicine
Bethesda Naval Hospital
Bethesda, Maryland

Laurence H. Ross, M.D.
Staff Physician
Department of Surgery
Duke University School of Medicine
Durham, North Carolina

Rodney W. Savage, M.D.
Attending Physician
White House
Washington, D.C.

Marissa Seligman, Pharm.D.
Pharmacy Coordinator
Drug Information/Staff Development
Pharmacist, Respiratory/Surgical Intensive
 Care Unit
Massachusetts General Hospital
Boston, Massachusetts

Michael R. Vasko, Ph.D.
Assistant Professor of Pharmacology
The University of Texas Health Science
 Center at Dallas
Chief, Pharmacology Section
Veterans Administration Medical Center
Dallas, Texas

Peter J. Wedlund, Ph.D.
Assistant Professor
College of Pharmacy
University of Kentucky
Lexington, Kentucky

Gary P. Zaloga, M.D.
Associate Professor of Anesthesia and
 Medicine

Section on Critical Care
Bowman Gray School of Medicine
Wake Forest University
Staff Physician
North Carolina Baptist Hospital
Winston-Salem, North Carolina

Arno L. Zaritsky, M.D.
Assistant Professor of Pediatrics
University of North Carolina School
 of Medicine
Director, Pediatric Intensive Care Unit
North Carolina Memorial Hospital
Chapel Hill, North Carolina

Michael G. Ziegler, M.D.
Associate Professor of Medicine
University of California, San Diego, School
 of Medicine
Director, Hypertension Program
University of California, San Diego, Medical
 Center
San Diego, California

Contents

1

Drug Interactions

Michael R. Vasko, Ph.D.
D. Craig Brater, M.D.

In recent years, increasing emphasis has been placed on both the study and the clinical importance of drug interactions. Several books and reviews provide extensive listings of drug interactions, both observed and theoretical (128, 221, 272, 312, 328). These listings, although contributing valuable information, are often voluminous and include anecdotal case reports, extrapolations from animal data, and interactions of questionable clinical relevance. Literal use of these listings could, therefore, overcomplicate therapeutic decisions and hinder rather than assist the clinician. Since some drug interactions are critical for optimal patient care and since new interactions are routinely discovered, it is important for clinicians to be aware of various types of drug interactions and their mechanisms. This caveat is particularly true in critical care medicine in which multiple drugs with narrow therapeutic indices are frequently coadministered to severely ill patients. In such settings, the margin for error is small and a drug interaction can dictate the success or failure of therapy.

The purpose of this chapter is to illustrate pharmacologic principles that may be important in clinically relevant drug interactions. It is not the intent of this chapter to present comprehensive listings of drug interactions, but to use examples to illustrate the types of interactions that can occur. The reader should then be able to extrapolate these principles to individual patient situations (210).

GENERAL PRINCIPLES FOR DRUG INTERACTIONS

Pharmacokinetic Interactions

For the purpose of this chapter, pharmacokinetic drug interactions result from altered

Table 1.1
Types of Drug Interactions

Pharmacokinetic
  Absorption
    Physicochemical complexing
    Changes in pH
    Changes in gastrointestinal motility
  Distribution
    Protein binding
  Metabolism
    Induction
    Inhibition
    Excretion
Pharmacodynamic
  Receptor (pharmacologic)
  Physiologic
  Modification of conditions at the site of action
  Physicochemical complexing

absorption, distribution, metabolism or excretion of a drug (Table 1.1). Some of these interactions are beneficial to the patient, whereas most result in untoward effects.

Drug interactions at sites of absorption alter either the rate or extent of drug absorption. In general, the latter are more important clinically, since they can result in considerable reductions in steady state plasma drug concentrations. Absorption of a drug has multiple determinants, including physicochemical properties of the drug, gastric pH, site of absorption in the gastrointestinal tract, rate of gastric emptying, intestinal motility, surface area for absorption, mucosal function, and blood flow to the absorption site. When two or more drugs are coadministered, interactions involving any of these factors may occur, particularly in critically ill patients whose condition may independently affect these same parameters.

Drug interactions can also occur by alterations in the tissue distribution of drugs. Many drugs bind reversibly to plasma proteins and this binding limits the free drug concentration that is available to tissue sites of action. For example, a decrease from the normal 99% binding of coumarin to 96% may seem like a small decrement, but the concentration of free drug that is available to the site of action has quadrupled from 1 to 4%. In most instances, however, an increase in free drug concentration is transient and is rapidly compensated for by an increase in distribution of drug to nonpharmacologically active sites or an increase in metabolism and/or excretion of the free drug (207). If, however, the patient's disease or another drug interaction compromises drug elimination, the increased free concentration may be sustained and serious consequences may result.

The majority of pharmacokinetic drug interactions involve elimination of drug by either metabolism or excretion. Metabolic drug interactions can result in an increase or decrease in the clearance of drugs and can occur by multiple mechanisms including alterations in hepatic blood flow (affecting drugs for which the limiting step in metabolism is delivery to metabolic enzymes), competitive inhibition at sites of metabolism, or induction of liver microsomal enzymes. Because there are limited pathways for drug metabolism, many drugs are metabolized by similar pathways. Consequently, interactions involving competitive inhibition or induction of metabolic enzymes are common. It is important, therefore, for clinicians to be familiar with the metabolism of each drug administered to a patient to predict the possibility of an interaction.

Most drugs are metabolized by first order kinetics, i.e., the rate of metabolism is dependent on the drug concentration. Consequently, enzymatic sites of drug metabolism are not saturated and an increase in drug concentration does not alter the rate of metabolism. In some instances, however, drugs are metabolized by zero order kinetics, i.e., only a specific amount of drug is metabolized per unit time. In addition, drugs metabolized by first order kinetics are capable of saturating their metabolic sites and shifting to zero order kinetics. This phenomenon usually occurs only at high plasma concentrations. When two drugs are administered simultaneously, however, they may compete for the same metabolic sites, and lesser concentrations of each are needed to saturate the metabolic enzymes. Therefore, a drug interaction may result in a disproportional increase in the half-life and decreased clearance of drug if the interaction not only competes for metabolism but also causes a

change from a nonsaturated to a saturated state. One could speculate that this phenomenon is more likely to occur in critically ill patients in whom diminished hepatic perfusion or metabolic function would readily occur because of their primary disease.

Finally, pharmacokinetic drug interactions can occur at sites of drug excretion, mainly the kidney, by affecting blood flow to the kidneys, glomerular filtration rate, urine pH, and secretion or reabsorption of the drug. Drug interactions can occur via any of these possible mechanisms or their combination.

Pharmacodynamic Drug Interactions

Pharmacodynamic drug interactions result in an alteration in the biochemical or physiologic effects of a drug (Table 1.1). In general, interactions of this type can be divided into four classes: (a) interactions at the drug receptor (pharmacologic); (b) interactions due to different cellular mechanisms acting in concert or in opposition (physiologic); (c) interactions by one drug changing the cellular environment and thereby altering the actions of a second drug; and (d) chemical neutralization of drugs.

A majority of pharmacodynamic drug interactions involve drugs binding to the same receptor. To exert the desired effect, most drugs bind to specific receptor sites (affinity), which activates a biochemical event or series of events that result in the pharmacologic action (intrinsic activity). *Drugs that have both high affinity for the receptor site and intrinsic activity are called agonists; drugs that have high affinity for binding sites but little or no intrinsic activity are called antagonists; drugs with varying degrees of affinity and intrinsic activity are termed mixed agonist-antagonists.* The overall outcome of drug interactions at receptor sites is dependent on the varying affinities and intrinsic activities of the different agents involved.

In many instances, drug interactions between agonists and antagonists are clinically useful. For example, the specific narcotic antagonist, naloxone, attenuates the undesirable actions of opioids. β-adrenergic antagonists are used extensively to block the effects of both endogenous and exogenous catecholamines. In some instances, however, receptor interactions are deleterious to the patient. For example, congestive heart failure or chronic obstructive pulmonary disease may worsen with β-adrenergic receptor antagonists by their attenuating the beneficial effects of catecholamines.

Pharmacodynamic drug interactions of the physiologic type can also produce either an enhanced or attenuated response. The use of combinations of agents with different mechanisms of action to lower blood pressure is clearly beneficial to the patient. Conversely, indomethacin reduces the antihypertensive effects of captopril (221), β-adrenergic antagonists (86, 87, 88, 194), and hydralazine (65) and decreases the response to loop diuretics (42, 255), presumably by inhibiting prostaglandin synthesis.

The third type of pharmacodynamic interaction occurs when the action of one drug results in a change in the intracellular or extracellular environment that modifies the action of another drug. The best such example is the increased toxicity of cardiac glycosides when administered with drugs that cause potassium depletion (31, 48). Another example is the interaction between reserpine and indirectly acting sympathomimetic agents (37, 50). Since reserpine depletes norepinephrine in nerve terminals (50), there is less response to drugs that act primarily by releasing the neurotransmitter.

The final type of interaction involves chemical neutralization of one drug by another. Several interactions of this type occur in the gastrointestinal tract and are discussed in detail below ("Interactions Affecting Drug Absorption"). This type of interaction also occurs within the circulation and may be desirable, as is the case with the use of protamine to neutralize heparin, or deleterious, as is illustrated by the inactivation of gentamicin by ureidopenicillins in patients with end-stage renal disease (266, 332, 355).

SPECIFIC TYPES OF DRUG INTERACTIONS

Interactions Affecting Drug Absorption

In this chapter, we focus on drug interactions affecting oral absorption since a large majority of documented drug interactions occur in the gastrointestinal (GI) tract. The principles applied here are also applicable, however, to other sites of drug absorption. In addition, the discussion does not include drug-food interactions. For these interactions and for a more extensive discussion of interactions of specific drugs affecting absorption, the reader is referred to reviews on the subject (129, 227, 356).

Drug interactions at sites of absorption can alter the rate and/or extent of drug absorption. The rate determines how rapidly the drug enters the blood and when the peak plasma concentration is achieved. The extent of absorption affects the total amount of the drug systemically available. In general, drug interactions altering the extent of absorption are of greater clinical importance than those affecting rate. If the patient requires a known concentration of drug in a short time, as often occurs in critical care settings, then intravenous administration can be employed, thus obviating uncertainties about rate as well as extent of absorption. If one drug interferes with the total amount of another drug absorbed, then the relationship between dose and plasma concentrations achieved (and subsequently clinical effect) is altered and dosing adjustments are required. For the most part, drug interactions of this type result in a decrease in circulating drug concentrations, and if this decrease is substantial, the interaction can compromise therapy. Less frequently, the interaction can result in increased absorption and could subject the patient to drug toxicity.

Since oral absorption of drugs is dependent on many factors involving both the properties of the drug and the characteristics of the GI tract, it is not surprising that interactions involve a number of mechanisms. In general, a majority of drug interactions affecting absorption involve (a) formation of drug complexes due to absorption, chelation, or binding; (b) alterations in gastric pH that change the ionization of drugs; and (c) changes in GI motility that affect the transit time of drugs. Other interactions, such as alterations in the GI mucosa (function, area, blood flow, or metabolism) also occur, but their clinical importance is yet to be determined. Some of these drug interactions involve only one mechanism while others are multifactorial. Table 1.2 summarizes some of the major drug interactions occurring at sites of drug absorption.

Several drugs can alter absorption by forming complexes with other agents. These drugs include antacids, activated charcoal, kaolin-pectin, and the hypocholesterolemic agents, cholestyramine and colestipol (Table 1.2). In most instances, the complex formed between the drug and the ion is less soluble and thereby less absorbable, resulting in a decrease in the amount of drug absorbed. Compounds with reduced absorption include digoxin (46, 158),

Table 1.2
Drug Interactions at Sites of Absorption

Proposed Mechanism	Drug Affected	Drug Causing Effect	Results of Interaction	References
Formation of complexes, chelation, adsorption	Bishydroxycoumarin	Antacids	Increased absorption	8, 13
	Carbamazepine	Activated charcoal	Decreased absorption, increased elimination	229
	Cephalexin	Cholestyramine	Decreased absorption	254
	Chlorothiazide	Cholestyramine	Decreased absorption	154
	Chlorpromazine	Antacids	Decreased absorption	91, 267
	Diflunisal	Antacids	Decreased absorption	344
	Digitoxin	Cholestyramine	Decreased absorption, increased elimination	53, 56
	Digoxin	Activated charcoal	Decreased absorption	228
		Antacids	Decreased absorption	46, 158
		Cholestyramine	Decreased absorption	47
		Kaolin-pectin	Decreased absorption	9, 46
	Isoniazid	Antacids	Decreased absorption	141
	Penicillamine	Antacids	Decreased absorption	251
	Phenobarbital	Activated charcoal	Decreased absorption, increased elimination	27, 187, 229
	Phenytoin	Activated charcoal	Decreased absorption	228
	Propranolol	Antacids	Decreased absorption	83
		Cholestyramine	Decreased absorption	136
	Ranitidine	Antacids	Decreased absorption	211
	Tetracyclines	Antacids	Decreased absorption	20, 105
	Theophylline	Activated charcoal	Decreased absorption, increased elimination	29
	Tolbutamide	Activated charcoal	Decreased absorption	230
	Valproate	Activated charcoal	Decreased absorption	230
	Warfarin	Cholestyramine	Decreased absorption, increased elimination	144, 284
Alterations in gastric pH	Cimetidine	Antacids	Decreased absorption	122, 324
	Ketoconazole	Cimetidine	Decreased absorption	186
	Tetracyclines	Cimetidine	Decreased absorption	105
		Sodium bicarbonate	Decreased absorption	20
Alterations in gastric motility				
Increase in motility	Acetaminophen	Metoclopramide	Increased rate of absorption	237
	Chlorothiazide	Metoclopramide	Increased rate of absorption	252
	Cimetidine	Metoclopramide	Decreased absorption	122, 152
	Digoxin	Metoclopramide	Decreased absorption	202
	Ethanol	Metoclopramide	Increased rate of absorption	108
	Lithium	Metoclopramide	Increased rate of absorption	69
Decrease in motility	Acetaminophen	Narcotic analgesics	Decreased rate of absorption	238
		Propantheline	Decreased rate of absorption	237
	Benzodiazepines	Antacids	Decreased rate of absorption	116, 118
	Bishydroxycoumarin	Amitriptyline	Increased absorption	269
	Chlorothiazide	Propantheline	Decreased rate of absorption	252
	Digoxin	Propantheline	Increased absorption	202
	Ethanol	Propantheline	Decreased rate of absorption	108
	Isoniazid	Antacids	Decreased rate of absorption	141
	Lithium	Propantheline	Decreased rate of absorption	69
	Phenytoin	Antacids	Decreased rate of absorption	103, 171
	Propranolol	Antacids	Decreased rate of absorption	83
Effects on gastrointestinal mucosa	Aminoglycoside antibiotics	Ethanol	Increased absorption due to mucosal damage	161
	Digoxin	Neomycin	Decreased absorption	191
		Sulfasalazine	Decreased absorption	149
		Erythromycin	Increased absorption	192
	Furosemide	Phenytoin	Decreased absorption	96

chlorpromazine (91), quinine (140), penicillamine (251), tetracyclines (20, 105), isoniazid (141), propranolol (83), ranitidine (211), and diflunisal (344). The resultant decrease in absorption can be 10–80%, depending on the drug involved; consequently, the interaction may be clinically important. Rarely, the drug complexes formed by interaction with antacids are more soluble, and thus increased absorption of drug occurs. For example, bishydroxy-coumarin chelates with magnesium to form a more absorbable complex (8, 13). Thus, patients taking this anticoagulant with magnesium hydroxide antacids may develop higher serum drug concentrations and a greater anticoagulant effect. Interestingly, warfarin absorption does not appear to be affected by antacids (8, 284).

Both activated charcoal (227–229) and kaolin-pectin (9, 10, 46) adsorb many drugs in the GI tract. This adsorption can cause significant reductions in the amount of drug absorbed. For example, activated charcoal can reduce the bioavailability of tolbutamide and valproate by 90% and 65%, respectively (230). In addition, this adsorption can result in a significant increase in clearance of drug from the body. Many drugs are secreted into the gut, and then reabsorbed (so-called enterohepatic circulation). In the presence of charcoal, however, the secreted drugs are adsorbed, preventing their reabsorption into the body; thus, they are cleared more rapidly. This increased clearance of drugs has been observed for phenobarbital, carbamazepine, and theophylline (29, 229). This type of interaction could be of benefit in the acutely intoxicated patient, but it could prove harmful in therapeutic settings by reducing the steady state plasma concentration of drugs below the therapeutic range. In a similar manner, cholestyramine and colestipol bind bile acids, cholesterol, and many other drugs in the GI tract (47, 53, 144, 186, 284). This binding results in the decreased absorption of many drugs, including chlorothiazide (154), propranolol (136), cephalexin (254), cardiac glycosides (47, 53), and anticoagulants (144, 284). To avoid the interaction rather than compensate for it, patients requiring these drug combinations should be administered drug (digoxin, digitoxin, or warfarin) 1 hour before or 4 hours after ingesting cholestyramine or colestipol.

The interaction between digitoxin or warfarin and cholestyramine is used to clinical advantage in patients who are toxic or poisoned with either of these agents. Both agents undergo enterohepatic circulation. Administration of cholestyramine sequesters drug in the gut, resulting in less reabsorption and decreasing serum concentrations (53, 56, 144, 284).

As mentioned above, some drugs affect the absorption of others by multiple mechanisms. For example, antacids not only form complexes with other drugs, but also affect absorption by altering gastric pH. Drug absorption is dependent on both dissolution of drug and extent of ionization. In the acidic environment of the stomach, drugs that are weak acids are less ionized and more rapidly absorbed. The opposite is true for weak bases. Thus, alteration in gastric pH by antacids and/or histamine H_2-antagonists can affect drug absorption (186) (Table 1.2). Fortunately, this interaction is rarely of clinical importance since most drugs, whether weak acids or weak bases, are predominantly absorbed in the small intestine via pathways that are not pH sensitive.

Since most drugs are absorbed in the small intestine, changes in gastric emptying can alter delivery to absorption sites and, thereby, alter the rate of drug absorption. Thus, antacids (356), narcotic analgesics (238), and drugs with anticholinergic properties that slow emptying decrease the rate of absorption of benzodiazepines (118), isoniazid (141), phenytoin (103, 171), and propranolol (83). In addition, the anticholinergic, propantheline, reduces gastric emptying and delays the absorption of acetaminophen (237), ethanol (108), and lithium (69).

Drugs that alter intestinal transit time can also affect the extent of drug absorption. Propantheline not only reduces gastric emptying but decreases GI motility. This slowed transit time increases the absorption of poorly soluble drugs such as chlorothiazide (252) and older preparations of digoxin (202). Presumably, amitriptyline increases the absorption of bishydroxycoumarin by the same mechanism (269). Many other drugs, including phenothiazines, other tricyclic antidepressants, antihistamines, and narcotic analgesics, may also reduce GI transit time, thereby altering either rate or extent of drug absorption.

In general, drugs that increase GI motility have the opposite effect on rate and extent of absorption (129). Thus, metoclopramide increases the rate of absorption of many drugs (69, 108, 237), and decreases quantitative absorption of cimetidine and of older preparations of digoxin (148, 152, 202).

Drug interactions affecting absorption also

occur as a result of one drug affecting the intestinal metabolism and/or transport of another. Although there are only limited reports of these interactions, they are worth discussing since they involve drugs that may be used in critical care medicine. The antibiotics, neomycin and sulfasalazine, decrease the absorption and plasma concentrations of digoxin, presumably by affecting the integrity of the GI mucosa (149, 191). In contrast, erythromycin can increase digoxin absorption, the proposed mechanism being a decrease in flora that metabolize digoxin in the small intestine of approximately 10% of patients (192). The latter interaction can result in sufficient increases in serum digoxin concentrations to cause toxicity.

Interactions Affecting Drug Distribution

Once a drug is absorbed into the systemic circulation, it is distributed to various tissues, including the site of action. Many drugs bind extensively to plasma proteins whereas only unbound drug is free to enter tissue storage sites or sites of action, or to be metabolized or excreted. The concentration of unbound drug in the circulation can be affected by competition of other drugs for binding sites. Consequently, displacement of one bound drug by another constitutes a major source of drug interaction. Recently, however, the relative clinical importance of displacement interactions has been questioned (207, 302), and it appears that these types of interactions are often misinterpreted.

The importance and occurrence of displacement interactions are dependent on three factors: the concentration of drug in the plasma, the relative binding affinity of the drug, and the volume of distribution (V_d). A high concentration of one drug relative to another will shift the binding equilibrium. Thus, assuming equal affinities, addition of large concentrations of one drug to the blood will rapidly decrease plasma protein binding of a second. Relative binding affinity is the second important factor. In general, only drugs with high binding affinity displace other drugs. These include digitoxin, bishydroxycoumarin, warfarin, diazoxide, phenytoin, clofibrate, valproic acid, hydralazine, quinidine, sulfonamides, tolbutamide, and most nonsteroidal antiinflammatory drugs including salicylates. Finally, if a drug has a small V_d, more of the displaced drug can remain in the plasma and

be delivered to sites of action with a concomitant increase in the pharmacologic effect.

The clinical relevance of displacement interactions is dependent on the therapeutic index of the drugs involved, the availability of other distribution sites, and the rate of elimination of the displaced drug. If a drug has a wide therapeutic index, then displacement from binding that results in higher free concentrations is of little concern. In addition, increasing the free drug concentration is less important clinically when the free drug can be distributed to other tissue storage sites. This is the reason that clinically important interactions are less likely with drugs that have a large V_d. Finally, for most drugs, elimination occurs by first order kinetics. Thus, increasing the free concentration of drug is rapidly compensated for by an increase in metabolism or excretion (207, 302). With increased elimination, a new steady state is achieved with a free drug concentration similar to that before the interaction. However, if elimination is compromised by disease or other drug interactions, a higher concentration of free drug may be maintained, creating a greater risk of toxicity. This rule especially applies to drugs with a low V_d, since the increase in free drug does not redistribute to other tissue storage sites. Thus, in patients with compromised hepatic or renal function there is a greater potential that the displacement interaction will result in increased free drug concentration and increased pharmacologic effect.

Even though the effect of displacement interactions is usually transient, during the period of increased free drug concentration an increased pharmacologic response may occur. Consequently, clinicians should exercise caution in treating patients during this transitional period. For example, the most important drug interactions involving displacement from plasma protein binding sites occur with coumarin anticoagulants (6, 33, 197). The transient period of increased unbound anticoagulant can result in bleeding. It is therefore important to determine successive prothrombin times when a potential interaction is suspected. The patient may remain relatively stable during the critical time of the interaction and return to the same baseline level of anticoagulation in a few days, but then again, he or she may not.

In drug displacement interactions, after a new steady state has been attained, the resulting *total* plasma concentration of drug may be below the "normal" therapeutic range. One

Table 1.3
Drug Interactions Due to Displacement from Protein Binding Sites

Drug Displaced	Causative Agent	References
Coumarin anticoagulants	Chloral hydrate	305, 340
	Clofibrate	33
	Diazoxide	304
	Ethacrynic acid	304
	Mefenamic acid	304
	Nalidixic acid	304
	Phenylbutazone	6
	Phenytoin	126, 197
	Salicylates	197
Diazepam	Heparin	290
	Valproic acid	82
Phenytoin	Phenylbutazone	231
	Salicylates	98
	Tolbutamide	357
	Valproic acid	204, 262
Tolbutamide	Phenylbutazone	167, 268
	Salicylates	167, 362
Valproic acid	Salicylates	250

should not misinterpret such "subtherapeutic" values, for they do not adequately reflect the concentration of free drug. The clinician must be aware of the potentially altered "therapeutic range" of that patient and also rely on clinical assessment of the drug effect.

In some instances, drug toxicity originally attributed to a displacement interaction is the result of multiple interactions, e.g., displacement plus impairment of metabolism. Phenylbutazone displaces warfarin from binding sites on serum proteins but also inhibits metabolism (6). Thus, the increased concentration of free anticoagulant is not compensated for by increased metabolism, increasing the likelihood of bleeding. A similar mechanism accounts for the increased incidence of phenytoin toxicity when tolbutamide is coadministered with the anticonvulsant (357). In contrast, lessening of potential toxicity can also occur with multiple drug interactions. Phenytoin displaces dicumarol from serum protein (126), but this has little importance in patients to whom phenytoin is chronically administered, because of induction of metabolism that increases elimination of the free dicumarol.

As mentioned above, displacement interactions with anticoagulants appear to be the most important clinically (Table 1.3). Several drugs can displace coumarin anticoagulants from plasma protein binding sites, including the active metabolite of chloral hydrate (305, 399), clofibrate (33), phenylbutazone (6), salicylates (197), and phenytoin (126, 197). Displacement

interactions with other drugs may also have clinical importance (Table 1.3). For example, patients taking tolbutamide may experience a hypoglycemic episode when started on high doses of salicylates (167, 362) or when administered phenylbutazone (268). In addition, the therapeutic range for total phenytoin in the plasma may be reduced in patients taking valproic acid, salicylates, or tolbutamide since these drugs increase the free fraction of phenytoin (98, 204, 262, 357). In a similar manner, salicylates can transiently displace valproic acid from binding sites (250).

The clinical importance of many displacement interactions is currently being reassessed. Clinicians should, however, closely monitor patients given multiple drugs that have high plasma protein binding. This monitoring is especially important during the initial period after adding another drug to the patient's regimen or when the patient has compromised drug elimination, as may occur in critical care settings because of the influence of other drugs or the patient's primary disease.

Interactions Due to Altered Drug Metabolism

Drug interactions of metabolism are numerous and of varying clinical relevance. The vast majority of metabolic interactions occur with induction or inhibition of the hepatic microsomal P-450 system (51, 68, 107). Indeed, drugs as well as environmental chemicals that are metabolized by these mixed function oxidases can induce their own metabolism (autoinduction) and also affect the metabolism of other agents. In like manner, drugs that are metabolized by the same enzyme system can act as competitive inhibitors and decrease the biotransformation of other agents.

There is a great deal of individual variability in the metabolic capacity of the hepatic enzyme systems and the degree to which it may be induced or inhibited by drugs (51, 107). In addition, the time course of drug interaction varies with different drugs and with the patient's ability to metabolize them (i.e., disease, genetics, age, etc.). Thus it is difficult to predict a priori the extent of an interaction in an individual patient. Each patient must be followed closely with clinical evaluation of therapeutic and toxic endpoints and drug toxicity, and if possible, with measurement of serum drug concentrations to assess the clinical importance of a drug interaction.

DRUG INTERACTIONS RESULTING IN ENHANCED METABOLISM

Although a number of agents induce the metabolism of other drugs (Table 1.4), emphasis is placed on a few drugs that induce the metabolism of many others, including the barbiturates (especially phenobarbital), ethanol, rifampin, and the anticonvulsants, phenytoin and carbamazepine. All of these agents induce the metabolism of oral anticoagulants, thereby increasing the dosage required to achieve therapeutic prolongation of the prothrombin time (70, 126, 127, 153, 168, 197, 309). For example, coadministration of rifampin with warfarin for 5–7 days doubles warfarin clearance, requiring an approximate 2-fold increase in dosing to maintain therapeutic plasma concentrations of the anticoagulant (16, 245, 247, 287). This type of interaction is important not only during the time of induced metabolism, but also after the inducing agent is withdrawn (168). When the inducing stimulus is no longer present, the hepatic enzyme activity slowly decreases, increasing serum concentrations and resulting in increased anticoagulation with the possible consequence of disastrous bleeding. Consequently, after removal of an inducing agent, the dose of anticoagulant needs to be readjusted.

Phenobarbital is a potent inducer of hepatic microsomal enzymes, resulting in reduced plasma concentrations and increased elimi-

nation of many drugs (Table 1.4), including chloramphenicol (360), cimetidine (320), phenytoin (49, 70, 173), dicumarol (70, 168, 197), nortriptyline (39), theophylline (177), and warfarin (168, 197). In a similar manner, phenytoin induces the metabolism of a large number of drugs (Table 1.4). Phenobarbital combined with phenytoin doubles the clearance of quinidine in humans, with a concomitant decrease in the elimination half-life of approximately 50% (73), presumably due to enzyme induction. Similarly, this anticonvulsant combination results in a significant increase in steroid clearance in transplant patients (102, 264). Since many epileptic patients receive long-term therapy with either phenytoin or phenobarbital or both, caution must be exercised when the patients receive additional medication.

Rifampin is one of the most potent inducers of metabolizing enzymes, increasing the clearance of warfarin (245, 247), glucocorticoids (28), digitoxin (31, 316), chloramphenicol (274), hexobarbital (366), metoprolol (25) and dapsone (367). Rifampin therapy also decreases the half-life of tolbutamide (51, 366), oral contraceptives (17), and theophylline (38, 285). Rifampin has a 2-fold effect on quinidine handling, decreasing quinidine's elimination half-life with no change in the volume of distribution (338). From the data, one would predict an approximate 3-fold increase in clearance with an identical decrement in the steady state plasma concentration or area under the curve (AUC) of plasma concentration versus time. The observed change in AUC of quinidine in these subjects, however, was a 6-fold decrease (338). The probable explanation for this discrepancy is a concomitant decrease in the bioavailability of quinidine due to an enhanced first pass effect through an induced hepatic enzyme system. The net result is a "multiplier" effect on drug concentrations achieved in plasma.

Nonprescription drugs, ethanol, and cigarette smoking also induce the microsomal enzyme system. Indeed, the clinician is not always aware of the chronic use of ethanol or cigarettes, and may initiate therapy with "normal doses" of drugs, which may not achieve therapeutic plasma concentrations. Consequently, it is important to be aware of possible drug interactions with "recreational" drugs. As is evident in Table 1.4, chronic ethanol use can result in increased metabolism of several drugs. However, the acute use of ethanol often has opposite effects on drug metabolism, as

Table 1.4
Examples of Drugs That Induce the Metabolism of Other Drugs

Drug Induced	Inducing Agent	References
Acetaminophen	Oral contraceptives	219
Carbamazepine	Phenytoin	62, 261, 262
Chloramphenicol	Phenobarbital	360
	Rifampin	274
Chlorpromazine	Phenobarbital	51
Cimetidine	Phenobarbital	320
Clonazepam	Phenytoin	261, 262
Cyclosporin	Phenytoin	99
Dapsone	Rifampin	367
Diazepam	Phenytoin	261, 262
Digoxin	Rifampin	106
Digitoxin	Phenobarbital	31, 316
	Phenytoin	31, 316
	Rifampin	31, 316
Doxycycline	Phenytoin	259
Fludrocortisone	Phenytoin	156
Glucocorticoids	Phenytoin	102, 264
	Rifampin	28
Griseofulvin	Phenobarbital	51
Meprobamate	Chronic ethanol (prior to hepatic impairment)	193, 216, 301, 303
Methadone	Phenytoin	261, 262
Metoprolol	Rifampin	25
Mexiletine	Rifampin	258
Oral anticoagulants	Carbamazepine	127, 168, 197
	Chronic ethanol	153, 309
	Gluthethimide	168, 197
	Griseofulvin	168, 197
	Phenobarbital	168, 197, 309
	Phenytoin	126, 168, 197
	Rifampin	245, 247, 287
Pentobarbital	Chronic ethanol	193, 216, 301, 303
Phenylbutazone	Phenobarbital	51
Phenytoin	Carbamazepine	127, 261, 262
	Chronic ethanol	193, 296, 301
	Phenobarbital	49, 70, 173
	Rifampin	155
Quinidine	Phenytoin	73
	Rifampin	338
Theophylline	Cigarette smoking	120
	Phenobarbital	177
	Phenytoin	212
	Rifampin	38, 285
Tolbutamide	Chronic ethanol	153, 193, 301, 303
	Rifampin	51, 358
Valproic acid	Phenytoin	261, 262, 293

discussed in the next section. Thus acute ethanol use appears to inhibit metabolism, while chronic use (prior to onset of liver disease) can result in enhanced metabolism due to enzyme induction (178). Finally, induction of the hepatic microsomal enzyme system by cigarette smoking may explain the increase in theophylline clearance in chronic smokers (120).

Several points regarding enzyme induction are important (Table 1.5). First, drug interactions involving induction are slow in onset and offset. It takes days or weeks before the enzymes are induced; consequently, patients need to be monitored for extended periods when clinically important interactions are predicted. For example, Romankiewicz and Ehrman (287) showed that the onset and offset of the increase in warfarin clearance produced by rifampin was maximal 5–7 days after starting and stopping rifampin therapy. Conse-

Table 1.5
Important Considerations Concerning Enzyme Induction

1. Slow in onset and offset
2. Dosage adjustment and clinical monitoring are as important during offset as during onset
3. Induction may be specific or nonspecific
4. Clinical relevance is a function of the therapeutic index of the interacting drugs

quently, the critical period of this interaction occurs approximately 1 week after initiation of therapy and 1 week after discontinuing the inducing agent. Second, offset of the drug interaction is as clinically important as onset. If, for example, a dosage adjustment is made when a patient has been receiving rifampin and warfarin to compensate for the increased metabolism, then another adjustment is needed some days after the rifampin is discontinued to readjust for the decreased clearance and to prevent excessive bleeding. Third, the induction of the microsomal enzyme system may be specific for one isoenzyme (i.e., one pathway) or nonspecific. For example, rifampin administration appears to selectively induce certain pathways of antipyrine metabolism (337) but does not appear selective in theophylline metabolism (285). Another example of selective induction is seen with acetaminophen and oral contraceptives (219). Oral contraceptives appear to increase the clearance of acetaminophen by selectively increasing glucuronidation. Whether this selectivity can be exploited for clinical use in acetaminophen poisoning is yet to be determined. Finally, the overall clinical relevance of drug interactions involving induction is clearly dependent on the therapeutic index of the drug involved. Affected drugs with a narrow therapeutic range are more clinically important than those with a wide range.

DRUG INTERACTIONS DUE TO INHIBITION OF METABOLISM

In general, drugs discussed above that are susceptible to induction of metabolism are also subject to inhibition (Table 1.6). Inhibitors are capable of decreasing the metabolism of any drug that is metabolized by the same enzyme system. As with induction, the clinical importance of these interactions is largely a function of the therapeutic index of the drugs involved. Unlike induction interactions, however, the onset and offset of these interactions are fairly rapid.

Most drug interactions involving inhibition of metabolism occur in the liver, and are due to competitive inhibition of enzymes involved in drug biotransformation. For example, cimetidine inhibits the metabolism of many drugs (Table 1.6), presumably by inhibiting the hepatic cytochrome P-450 mixed function oxidases (164, 276, 322). This inhibition results in a decrease in elimination of many drugs and often requires a change in the dosing regimen (Table 1.6). Of most clinical importance, however, are interactions between cimetidine and theophylline, lidocaine, and oral anticoagulants, since these latter drugs have a narrow margin of safety and thus critical toxicity can occur. Cimetidine decreases theophylline clearance by approximately 50% with a corresponding doubling of the elimination half-life (54, 66, 143, 270, 278, 347). Volume of distribution does not change. The result, if a patient's dosing regimen were not modified, would be a doubling of the serum theophylline concentration. In a similar manner, cimetidine reduces the clearance of oral anticoagulants, potentiating their actions and requiring a decrease in dosage (168, 197, 244, 309, 318). Cimetidine also decreases the clearance of lidocaine by 25–42%, presumably because of a decrease in metabolism of the antiarrhythmic

Table 1.6
Examples of Drugs that Inhibit the Metabolism of Other Drugs

Drug Causing Inhibition	Drugs Inhibited	References
Allopurinol	6-Mercaptopurine	19, 226
	Flecainide	311
Amiodarone	Phenytoin	114, 208
	Procainamide	292
	Quinidine	292
	Warfarin	350
Bishydroxycoumarin	Tolbutamide	168, 197
Chloramphenicol	Carbamazepine	32, 63, 261
	Chlorpropamide	32, 63

Drug Causing Inhibition	Drugs Inhibited	References
Chloramphenicol (*continued*)	Oral anticoagulants	32, 63, 168, 197
	Phenobarbital	32, 63, 169
	Phenytoin	32, 63, 169, 261, 262
	Tolbutamide	32, 63, 272
Chlorpromazine	Phenytoin	261, 348
	Propranolol	346
Cimetidine	Amitriptyline	71
	Benzodiazepines	78, 115, 162, 241, 291, 318
	Carbamazepine	200, 261
	5-Fluorouracil	19, 130
	Imipramine	4, 133
	Lidocaine	22, 92, 361
	Meperidine	121
	Metoprolol	25
	Phenytoin	11, 135, 232, 294
	Propranolol	93, 318
	Theophylline	54, 66, 143, 270, 278
	Tolbutamide	58
	Triamterene	222
	Warfarin	168, 244
Diltiazem	Antipyrine	23, 55
	Carbamazepine	45
Disulfiram	Benzodiazepines	198
	Phenytoin	159, 243
	Warfarin	168, 197, 246
Ethanol (acute)	Diazepam	196
	Meprobamate	193, 301, 303
	Pentobarbital	193, 301, 303
	Phenytoin	193, 261, 301, 303
	Tolbutamide	57, 193, 272
	Warfarin	168, 193, 197
Erythromycin	Carbamazepine	363, 365
	Cyclosporine	203
	Theophylline	41, 206, 282, 283
Isoniazid	Carbamazepine	341, 364
	Phenytoin	174, 225, 261
Ketoconazole	Methylprednisolone	112
Methylphenidate	Phenobarbital	104, 261
	Phenytoin	104, 261
	Primidone	104, 261
Oral contraceptives	Diazepam	2
	Imipramine	3
	Metoprolol	25
	Oral anticoagulants	80, 168, 197
	Prednisolone	184
	Theophylline	336
Propoxyphene	Carbamazepine	72
	Doxepin	5
	Phenytoin	5, 261
Propranolol	Diazepam	242
	Lidocaine	40, 240
Quinidine	Digitoxin	170
Sulfinpyrazone	Warfarin	335
Sulfonamides	Carbamazepine	32, 150
	Phenytoin	32, 150, 195, 261
	Tolbutamide	32, 195, 257, 272
	Warfarin	32, 168, 195, 197
Thymidine	5-Fluorouracil	19
Verapamil	Antipyrine	23
	Carbamazepine	199

(22, 92, 361); however, this interaction increases the lidocaine serum concentration by 50% indicating a concomitant decrease in volume of distribution (approximately 10–20%) (92, 361). Consequently, when coadministering lidocaine and cimetidine, one should decrease both the loading and maintenance lidocaine doses. Cimetidine may also decrease lidocaine clearance by reducing hepatic blood flow (92), thereby decreasing lidocaine access to the liver (327, 333), although the occurrence of this reduction in hepatic blood flow by cimetidine is controversial (134, 142, 361).

Other drugs clearly alter hepatic blood flow, resulting in a reduced elimination of drugs whose metabolism is limited by availability of drug to liver enzymes (drugs with a high extraction ratio). For example, the β-adrenergic blocking agents, propranolol, nadolol, and metoprolol, decrease lidocaine clearance by 20–50% (25, 297). In addition, hydralazine increases the peak concentration and AUC of metoprolol and propranolol after oral administration, by diminishing hepatic blood flow (25, 298). Aspirin and indomethacin decrease clearance of indocyanine green without altering antipyrine clearance (94), suggesting that inhibition of prostaglandin synthesis may alter hepatic blood flow. These results imply that inhibitors of prostaglandin synthesis may have important interactions with drugs such as lidocaine and propranolol.

Many other drug interactions inhibiting metabolism are clinically relevant (Table 1.6). For example, acute administration of ethanol inhibits the metabolism of many drugs (178, 193, 301, 303), including chloral hydrate (306), some benzodiazepines (79, 307, 308), propranolol (85), tolbutamide (57), phenytoin (193, 301, 303), and warfarin (193, 301, 303). As discussed earlier, chronic ethanol has an opposite effect on the clearance of many of these drugs because of induction of drug metabolism (Table 1.4). Tolbutamide metabolism is reduced by the coadministration of several drugs (63, 301), which can result in long-lasting and profound hypoglycemia. Drug inhibition of phenytoin and carbamazepine metabolism has resulted in many incidences of toxicity with these agents (63, 125, 174, 195, 225, 261, 263). This toxicity, although usually not life threatening, causes considerable trauma to the patient and often requires prolonged hospitalization. The potential consequences of drug interactions that inhibit metabolism of oral anticoagulants are obvious (80, 131, 166, 168, 195, 235, 246, 248, 249, 335), and to avoid

potential toxicity, compensatory changes in dosing are necessary when therapy with an interacting drug is commenced or discontinued.

Interactions affecting drug metabolism can also occur with extrahepatic enzymes. As a major example, a number of drugs used clinically act by inhibiting monoamine oxidase (313). The significance of interactions with these drugs is only lessened by the appropriate infrequent use of these agents. However, procarbazine (81), a drug used in treating Hodgkin's disease, and isoniazid (185, 315) have monoamine oxidase inhibitory activity. Concomitant use of sympathomimetic agents with these drugs requires awareness of this potential effect. Monoamine oxidase metabolizes sympathetic neurotransmitters that are retaken up into the sympathetic nerve ending from the synaptic cleft. During inhibition of this enzyme, administration of catecholamines or agents that release catecholamines, such as tyramine, ephedrine, pseudoephedrine, and amphetamines, can cause potentially fatal hypertensive crisis since metabolism of these drugs and of endogenous catecholamine is inhibited. In addition, some antihypertensive agents such as reserpine, guanethidine, methyldopa, and clonidine may (rarely) acutely release endogenous catecholamine stores, paradoxically raising blood pressure to dangerous levels.

Several important points regarding drug interactions due to metabolic inhibition should be stressed (Table 1.7). First, as mentioned above, the onset of these interactions may be quite rapid. An effect can be seen with the first dose; the maximum effect is dependent on attainment of a new steady state drug concentration, and therefore requires four to five times the *new* half-life of the drug. Second, the interaction between two drugs may be dependent on the amount of the drug administered and the total duration of administration. For

Table 1.7
Important Considerations Concerning Enzyme Inhibition

1. Onset can occur quickly
2. Time to maximum effect depends on the new half-life of the drug
3. Whether an interaction occurs may be dose-dependent
4. The patient's primary disease may increase susceptibility
5. The interaction may involve one but not other stereoisomers

example, allopurinol at a dosage of 300 mg/ day for 7 days does not alter the metabolism of theophylline in normal individuals, yet if the dosage is increased to 300 mg every 12 hours for 14 days, the clearance of theophylline is reduced 21% while the half-life and AUC are significantly increased (201). Thus, physicians must be cautious not only when adding a new drug to the therapeutic regimen, but also when altering the dosage of a drug the patient is already taking. Third, other factors (i.e., liver function, genetics) affecting drug metabolism may influence the incidence of drug interactions. For example, Rollinghoff and Paumgartner (286) demonstrated that therapeutic doses of cimetidine reduced aminopyrine metabolism to a greater degree in patients with compromised liver function than in subjects with normal liver function. They concluded that patients with chronic liver disease may be at increased risk for drug interactions with drugs that compete for metabolism. Another factor involves the patient's inherited ability to metabolize drug. Genetic variability of drug metabolism is well documented (176, 345, 353). The acetylation of isoniazid, for example, is rapid in approximately half the population and slow in the other half (89). Slow acetylation appears to predispose patients to increased toxicity from drugs metabolized by microsomal enzymes. This fact may explain the increased incidence of phenytoin toxicity in slow acetylators of isoniazid as opposed to rapid acetylators (172). Phenytoin metabolism is also genetically controlled, certain individuals slowly metabolizing the drug (175, 343). This genetic variability may prove to be an additional, important determinant of susceptibility to drug interactions.

A fourth important point involves inhibition of drug metabolism that selectively affects one enantiomer of a racemic mixture of a drug. For example, warfarin used in therapy is a racemic mixture, the $S(-)$ enantiomer having the predominant anticoagulant effect. Several drugs, including metronidazole, (249), trimethoprim-sulfamethoxazole (248), and sulfinpyrazone (335), inhibit the metabolism of $S(-)$-warfarin. When the interaction between these drugs and racemic warfarin is assessed, significant changes are observed in prothrombin time, yet no consistent or significant changes are observed in the pharmacokinetics of warfarin. The lack of a pharmacokinetic interaction is probably due to a masking of the inhibition of $S(-)$-warfarin by $R(-)$-warfarin. Consequently, clinicians should be aware that observed, yet unex-

plained, pharmacodynamic drug interactions may in fact have a pharmacokinetic component.

Finally, although this discussion has stressed drug interactions of metabolism that have deleterious consequences, some interactions of this type may be beneficial. For example, cimetidine selectively inhibits the oxidative metabolism of acetaminophen in the liver (1, 220). Since the oxidative metabolites of acetaminophen are more toxic than the conjugated metabolites, cimetidine-induced inhibition is potentially beneficial in treating acetaminophen overdose.

Ideally, the clinician should be aware of the metabolic pathways for various drugs, be able to predict potential drug interactions, and compensate for them. It is also possible, in some instances, for the clinician to substitute one drug for another if drug interactions are anticipated. For example, cimetidine inhibits the metabolism of several benzodiazepines, including diazepam and chlordiazepoxide, by inhibiting the mixed function oxidases in the liver (78, 115, 162, 241, 291, 318). It does not, however, usually inhibit glucuronidation or sulfation. Consequently, if a benzodiazepine is needed in a patient receiving cimetidine, one can select oxazepam or lorazepam since cimetidine does not block glucuronidation of these drugs (256). If a drug is needed to decrease gastric acid secretion and the patient is receiving other drugs metabolized by the hepatic P-450 enzyme system, the clinician could select antacids, sucralfate, or ranitidine instead of cimetidine for therapy. Cimetidine (as discussed above) inhibits liver metabolism of many drugs whereas ranitidine, a structurally different H_2-receptor blocker, does not appear to affect the metabolism of antipyrine, theophylline, warfarin, diazepam, tolbutamide, phenytoin, or β-adrenergic receptor blockers (43, 58, 132, 157, 163, 244, 270, 279, 310, 321, 351). Thus, ranitidine has the clinical advantage of limited potential for metabolic drug interactions.

Interactions Affecting Drug Excretion

As noted previously, most drug excretion occurs in the kidney; consequently, emphasis is placed on drug interactions involving renal excretion of both parent drug and metabolites. Drugs can be excreted by filtration or active secretion and can be reabsorbed into the systemic circulation. Logically, all three functions are potential sites for drug interaction. The other major route of drug excretion involves biliary secretion into the intestinal tract. For such drugs, interactions can occur in the GI tract with other drugs that bind or adsorb the secreted drugs (see "Interactions Affecting Drug Absorption"). This phenomenon is analogous to drug interactions decreasing the extent of absorption, as previously discussed.

Many drugs are eliminated by glomerular filtration; clinically important examples are the aminoglycoside antibiotics and digoxin. Theoretically, changes in glomerular filtration rate (GFR) affect handling of these and other drugs. Few studies, however, have addressed this potentially important area of drug interactions. Evidence suggests that furosemide causes a fall in GFR consequent to volume depletion (180). Presumably, by decreasing GFR, furosemide can reduce the clearance of digoxin and gentamicin (180, 334). Whether this interaction has clinical significance is yet to be determined. Furthermore, furosemide is a poor pharmacologic tool for assessing potential effects of GFR since the effect is most likely dependent on the degree of volume loss or replacement. Other pharmacologic agents can increase renal perfusion directly. For example, in dogs, dopamine increases GFR and the elimination of tobramycin (160). Such effects need further study in humans. However, many patients in critical care settings receive vasoactive drugs that can affect GFR. Similarly, many receive drugs dependent on glomerular filtration for excretion. It is important, therefore, for critical care physicians to consider the potential for these types of interactions, despite the paucity of available information.

A large number of drugs and metabolites are eliminated from the body by active secretion at the pars recta (straight segment) of the proximal tubule. This secretion occurs via two non-specific transport systems, one for organic acids and one for bases. Since the transport is non-specific, drugs can compete for transport with one another and the resultant interactions can be clinically important (271, 280, 354). There is also a secretory pathway for digoxin, located in the distal tubule, which is a site for drug interactions affecting digoxin (109, 325).

Several drugs that are organic acids have clinically important renal secretion (Table 1.8). These include many diuretics, nonsteroidal antiinflammatory drugs (15), penicillins (151), cephalosporins (119), methotrexate (7, 19, 234), and sulfa compounds (260). Clearly, the different acids compete with each other for se-

Table 1.8
Organic Acids Actively Secreted by the Kidney[a]

Acetazolamide
p-Aminohippurate
Captopril
Cephalosporins (most)
Dyphylline
Heparin
Loop-acting diuretics
Methotrexate
Nonsteroidal antiinflammatory agents
Penicillins
Probenecid
Salicylates
Sulfonamides
Sulfonylureas
Thiazide diuretics

[a] Data from references 7, 15, 19, 119, 151, 205, 234, 260, 288, 289, 295, 330, 357.

cretion; however, it is difficult to predict a priori the degree of competition.

The interaction between methotrexate and probenecid illustrates the interaction between organic acids. When probenecid is administered to patients taking methotrexate, most clinicians decrease the dosage of the anticancer drug (7). Few physicians are aware, however, of a similar need to decrease the dose if other drugs secreted by the organic acid transport system are coadministered with methotrexate (19, 234). Indeed, the increased sensitivity to methotrexate seen in some patients may be due to coadministration of drugs that inhibit its active secretion.

In addition to exogenous organic acids, endogenous organic acids can also compete for the transport system. This mechanism may account for the large doses of organic acid diuretics, such as furosemide, that are required to cause diuresis in uremic patients (288, 289). The endogenous acids produced in uremia may compete with the diuretics for transport into the renal tubular lumen, i.e., to their site of action.

The active transport system for organic bases and its clinical importance are less well understood. Like organic acids, many bases undergo potentially important active secretion (Table 1.9). Of these, the only interactions studied clinically are those between the H_2-receptor antagonists, cimetidine and ranitidine, and the antiarrhythmic, procainamide (64, 317, 319). Coadministration to healthy volunteers of cimetidine with procainamide results in a significant increase in AUC for procainamide and a significant decrease in the renal clearance of

Table 1.9
Organic Bases Actively Secreted by the Kidney[a]

Amantadine
Amiloride
Cimetidine
Ethambutol
Mecamylamine
Mepacrine (quinacrine)
N-Methylnicotinamide
Procainamide
Pseudoephedrine
Ranitidine
Tetraethylammonium

[a] Data from references 64, 265, 281, 317, 319.

both procainamide and its major metabolite, N-acetylprocainamide (64, 319). Ranitidine produces similar effects, which are dependent on the plasma concentrations of the H_2-receptor antagonist (317). Whether other clinically significant interactions occur between organic bases is yet to be determined.

The decrease in secretion of digoxin caused by several drugs is one of the most important drug interactions affecting secretion (24, 30, 60, 84, 123, 139, 181–183, 223, 299, 326, 358). This phenomenon is reviewed in detail elsewhere (30). The interaction occurs in at least 90% of patients with coadministration of quinidine and digoxin, with, on the average, a doubling of the serum digoxin concentration. The magnitude of the effect appears to be dependent on the serum quinidine concentration. The predominant mechanism of the interaction is decreased tubular secretion of digoxin (109), resulting in decreased overall clearance and a need to halve the dose (on average) to maintain the same serum concentration of digoxin. In addition, approximately two-thirds of patients also demonstrate a 10% or more decrease in digoxin's volume of distribution. The mechanism of this effect is presumably the displacement of digoxin from muscle binding sites by quinidine (147, 299).

If displacement of digoxin from muscle occurs, does displacement occur from sites of action on cardiac muscle? If so, the increase in serum concentrations of digoxin would not result in an increased pharmacological effect on the heart but may affect other systems. Data addressing this issue are inconsistent (24, 84, 138, 183, 299, 326, 358). Some studies report a decreased cardiac digoxin concentration with an increased concentration in the brain after quinidine administration (30). Although controversial, observations suggest enhanced elec-

trophysiologic action on the heart (24, 183, 223) with a decrease in inotropism (81, 138, 299, 326, 358). The electrophysiologic actions may be due to enhanced central nervous system effects on atrioventricular nodal conduction. If these effects occur as a result of the interaction, one clearly needs to decrease the dosage of digoxin to maintain the "therapeutic range." This decrease may thereby compromise the inotropic actions of the drug. In fact, in those patients who do not require digoxin for effects on conduction, alternative therapy may be more appropriate.

This interaction with digoxin is not unique to quinidine. Amiodarone, quinine, spironolactone, verapamil, and flecainide also increase serum digoxin concentrations (95, 182, 189, 349, 352). Like quinidine, spironolactone affects both the volume of distribution and the clearance of digoxin (95, 349). On average, clearance decreases 26%; however, there is great variability among patients, with a range of 0–74%. Similarly, the effect on volume of distribution is highly variable. Therefore, some patients may require dose adjustment while others will not. In general, loading and maintenance doses of digoxin are decreased by one-third in patients receiving spironolactone; some patients may need subsequent upward titration.

Some drugs are reabsorbed in the nephron after having gained access to the tubular lumen by filtration or secretion. Reabsorption of drugs in the distal tubule and collecting duct is related to urinary flow rate and pH (214). High rates of urine flow induced by diuretics or fluid loading increase excretion of phenobarbital and theophylline, but these increased flow rates would have to be maintained for long periods of time before they became clinically important. In animal studies, digoxin clearly has a reabsorptive component, presumably in the proximal tubule (110). Consequently, renal excretion of digoxin involves filtration, proximal reabsorption, and secretion at more distal tubular sites. The mechanism of digoxin's reabsorption is unclear but appears to follow general reabsorptive activity of the proximal tubule. Administration of saline or mannitol decreases proximal tubular reabsorption of sodium and of digoxin, whereas agents acting more distally to increase sodium excretion and urinary volume do not affect digoxin excretion (110). Whether drug interactions occur in humans via this pathway is unclear. These interactions may, however, be particularly important in critical care settings in which fluctuations in volume status may have major effects on proximal tubule reabsorption. In such cases, digoxin handling should be followed closely.

Lithium is reabsorbed in the nephron in parallel with sodium, and changes in sodium homeostasis (particularly in the proximal tubule) can therefore alter renal excretion of lithium. The mild volume depletion attending chronic administration of thiazide diuretics causes increased proximal tubular reabsorption of sodium and concomitantly decreases lithium excretion (77, 137). Furosemide, on the other hand, appears to have little effect (146). Administration of indomethacin or diclofenac increases steady state serum lithium concentrations by approximately 30%, presumably by facilitating the reabsorption of lithium in the proximal tubule (100, 277). Other agents affecting proximal reabsorption of sodium might also affect handling of lithium.

Finally, altering the pH of the urine could alter passive transport of weak acids and bases. For example, administration of therapeutic doses of antacids may raise urinary pH sufficiently to change the excretion of some drugs in clinically important amounts (188).

Pharmacodynamic Drug Interactions

Many drug interactions do not involve changes in the absorption, distribution, or elimination of drugs, but involve modification of the biologic effect of the drugs. These interactions may involve drug receptor interactions, may involve different cellular mechanisms, may be due to alterations in cellular environment, or may result from chemical neutralization.

Drug interactions at receptor sites are widely known and often used to clinical advantage. Clearly, drug antagonists are synthesized specifically for their effects on receptors, as is illustrated by the substantial number of β-adrenergic receptor blockers that are available. There are numerous examples of agonist/antagonist drug interactions. Often, however, antagonists lack specificity with regard to their receptor blocking ability. For example, phenothiazines, tricyclic antidepressants, and butyrophenones have α-adrenergic antagonist properties, accounting for the enhanced activity of other α-adrenergic blockers used concomitantly. In addition, this antagonist activity accounts for the use of directly acting sympathomimetics to reverse toxic α-adrenergic blockade caused by these drugs.

In a similar manner, some tricyclic antidepressants have potent antimuscarinic effects (233, 239). Consequently, adverse drug interactions can occur when multiple drugs are administered that block similar receptor sites. The clinician, therefore, needs to be aware of possible multiple receptor effects of drugs, not just of the major classes of agonists or antagonists.

Unanticipated but predictable interactions may occur with use of agents that have multiple receptor effects. For example, epinephrine is both an α- and β-adrenergic agonist; the α effect predominates in most instances, causing arteriolar vasoconstriction. Concomitant use of an α-adrenergic antagonist not only attenuates the vasoconstriction, but also may unveil the vasodilation caused by the β effect. Similarly, the use of propranolol for the treatment of hypertension can, in rare instances, exacerbate the hypertension by blocking β-induced vasodilation and potentiate preexisting α-mediated vasoconstriction, especially in patients with a pheochromocytoma (209, 236, 273). By a similar mechanism, in patients treated with clonidine, withdrawal of the drug during continued administration of propranolol can cause accentuation of the α-adrenergic effect of endogenous catecholamines (18).

Pharmacodynamic drug interactions also occur when two drugs administered together have different cellular mechanisms that either enhance or diminish the physiologic response. For example, indomethacin administration decreases the antihypertensive effects of captopril (101, 221), hydralazine (65), and propranolol (21, 86, 87, 194). The effect of indomethacin, although not known, may be due to inhibition of synthesis of prostaglandins responsible for vasodilation. This hypothesis is controversial, since the attenuation of the antihypertensive effects does not seem to occur with other inhibitors of prostaglandin synthesis (88).

In a similar manner, indomethacin decreases the acute response to furosemide whereas aspirin has no effect in normal subjects (26, 42, 255, 340). The indomethacin effect is not a result of a change in the amount of furosemide reaching its intraluminal site of action (61). Whether this interaction is of clinical importance is unclear; patients chronically receiving both drugs show no effect on sodium excretion, although the antihypertensive effect of furosemide is blunted by indomethacin (255).

Tricyclic antidepressants and guanethidine block neuronal uptake of catecholamines at the synaptic cleft (36, 323). Because reuptake of catecholamines is the major mechanism of attenuation of their effect, the response to exogenously administered catecholamines may be increased if used with these agents (67). In studies of normal subjects given imipramine (25 mg three times daily) for 5 days, the pressor effect of phenylephrine was potentiated by two to three times, norepinephrine by four to eight times, and epinephrine by two to four times (35). In a similar study in subjects administered debrisoquine (a guanidinium antihypertensive agent that blocks the catecholamine reuptake system), the effects of phenylephrine were markedly potentiated and prolonged (12). Sympathomimetics that act indirectly would not be expected to have an enhanced effect with guanethidine-like drugs, and would more likely have a decreased effect, since guanethidine, debrisoquine, and bethanidine deplete endogenous catecholamines.

Another set of important drug interactions involving the catecholamine reuptake mechanism is that occurring between the guanidinium antihypertensives, guanethidine, bethanidine, and debrisoquine, and a number of psychoactive agents. The former guanethidine antihypertensives are taken into the nerve ending by the catecholamine reuptake system, where they cause release and depletion of endogenous catecholamine stores. Tricyclic antidepressants reverse the antihypertensive effects of these agents by inhibiting their uptake to this site of action (36, 113, 124, 217, 218, 314, 329). Doxepin has less tendency to produce this effect than other antidepressants (90). A similar reversal of effect that probably results from inhibition of uptake or displacement from the site of action also occurs with amphetamine, ephedrine, methylphenidate, phenothiazines, butyrophenones, thiothixene, and possibly reserpine (59, 75, 76, 145, 329). A similar interaction has been reported with use of a nasal decongestant containing chlorpheniramine, isopropamide, and phenylpropanolamine (215). This last interaction is probably not clinically important in most patients, but use of over-the-counter "cold" remedies should be avoided in patients receiving guanethidine-like drugs.

Reversal of the antihypertensive effect of clonidine by desipramine is well documented (44, 342), implying that caution should be used when other tricyclic antidepressants and psychoactive drugs are administered to patients receiving clonidine.

There are several other examples of pharmacodynamic drug interactions resulting from different drug mechanisms. Phenothiazines and tricyclic antidepressants can produce a quinidine-like decrease in cardiac conduction time, resulting in a prolonged QRS complex and arrhythmias (14, 74, 97, 359). Concomitant use of quinidine, procainamide, or similar agents with these drugs could therefore have additive effects. Treatment of arrhythmias caused by phenothiazines or tricyclic antidepressants therefore requires agents that will not further depress conduction; these include lidocaine, tocainide, mexiletine, phenytoin, and β-adrenergic receptor blockers.

Verapamil, the slow calcium channel antagonist, slows atrioventricular (A-V) nodal conduction by inhibition of calcium influx into the myocardial cells (190, 331). Both propranolol and digoxin can also slow A-V nodal conduction via other mechanisms. The concomitant administration of verapamil with either propranolol or digoxin could therefore result in additive suppression of A-V nodal conduction and cause bradycardia, A-V block, or ventricular asystole (253, 300). Thus although most patients can tolerate such combinations without difficulty, caution should be exercised when these drugs are given together.

The third type of pharmacodynamic drug interaction involves one drug changing the extracellular or cellular environment such that the action of a second drug is affected. Perhaps the best example of this is the changes in electrolyte status that affect the response to digitalis glycosides (31, 48). Many drugs, including diuretics (117, 165, 275), amphotericin B (213), ampicillin (111), carbenicillin (52), and lithium (224), can cause hypokalemia. Potassium depletion increases the risk of digoxin toxicity. This interaction is particularly easy to overlook because substantial decreases in intracellular potassium can occur with normokalemia. Hypercalcemia and hypomagnesemia similarly increase the sensitivity to digitalis.

Finally, drugs can neutralize each other by forming complexes either in solution or in situ. Perhaps the best example of this type of interaction in situ involves heparin and protamine. The administration of protamine to neutralize heparin is widely known and used to clinical advantage. Another important interaction of this type that can be critical to the patient's well-being is the neutralization of aminoglycoside antibiotics by certain penicillins in patients with renal disease (266, 332, 355). The penicillins, carbenicillin, ticarcillin, and piperacillin, complex with the aminoglycoside. The effect appears to be dependent on the patient's level of renal function (179) and is related to both concentration and time (34).

The preceding constitute but a few of the myriad pharmacodynamic drug interactions. It should be clear that anticipation of these interactions requires a collation of knowledge concerning the fundamental pharmacologic characteristics of the drugs administered to a patient and the pathophysiology of the patient's disease(s).

APPLICATIONS TO CRITICAL CARE PRACTITIONERS

Patients in critical care settings are particularly susceptible to drug interactions. They frequently receive multiple drugs that have narrow therapeutic indices and/or are frequently implicated in drug interactions. Antiarrhythmic agents, sympathomimetics, cardiac inotropes, and histamine H_2-receptor antagonists are but a few examples of drugs administered to many, if not most, patients in critical care medicine. To compound potential problems, the patient's primary disease can have great influence on drug disposition and response. For example, cardiovascular instability can affect hepatic and renal perfusion and thereby influence elimination of a number of drugs, especially those agents used in critical care settings. Examples include diminished hepatic elimination of lidocaine with congestive hepatopathy, diminished V_d of lidocaine in heart failure, and diminished renal excretion of digoxin or aminoglycoside antibiotics when renal perfusion is compromised. Not anticipating such effects can clearly lead to potentially disastrous drug-induced consequences. Unfortunately, critical care patients are often so sick that adverse drug effects can easily be misinterpreted as a manifestation of the patient's underlying condition. Because of this fact, and the great potential for drug interactions in this setting, the critical care practitioner must maintain a constant alert for drug interactions. So doing will allow one to avoid toxicity and maximize efficacy of the potent drugs at our disposal.

SUMMARY

In this chapter, drug interactions are discussed from a mechanistic point of view. We hope that the use of this approach provides a framework that assists clinicians in predicting potentially important drug interactions without memorizing extensive listings. Furthermore, as new drugs are introduced into clinical medicine, the principles discussed in this chapter can be applied to predict potential interactions prior to their documentation. For example, if aware that a new drug is metabolized by the liver microsomal enzyme system, the clinician is alerted to the potential for enzyme induction and/or inhibition by other agents handled in a similar manner. Conversely, knowing that a drug has a large V_d and is not extensively bound to plasma proteins, the clinician does not need to be concerned about displacement interactions.

With the increasing numbers of new drugs available to the clinician and with the use of multiple drugs in a given patient, it is essential to be aware of important drug interactions. By understanding basic pharmacokinetic principles and the characteristics of given drugs, the clinician can be alerted to potential drug interactions. The appropriate steps can then be taken: closely monitoring the patient, altering the dosing of one or both drugs, or changing one of the drugs to minimize the likelihood of an interaction.

References

1. Abernethy DR, Greenblatt DJ, Divoll M, Ameer B, Shader RI: Differential effect of cimetidine on drug oxidation (antipyrine and diazepam) vs. conjugation (acetaminophen and lorazepam): prevention of acetaminophen toxicity by cimetidine. *J Pharmacol Exp Ther* 224:508–515, 1982.
2. Abernethy DR, Greenblatt DJ, Divoll M, Arendt R, Ochs HR, Shader RI: Impairment of diazepam metabolism by low-dose estrogen-containing oral-contraceptive steroids. *N Engl J Med* 306:791–792, 1982.
3. Abernethy DR, Greenblatt DJ, Shader RI: Imipramine disposition in users of oral contraceptive steroids. *Clin Pharmacol Ther* 35:792–797, 1984.
4. Abernethy DR, Greenblatt DJ, Shader RI: Imipramine-cimetidine interaction: impairment of clearance and enhanced absolute bioavailability. *J Pharmacol Exp Ther* 229:702–705, 1984.
5. Abernethy DR, Greenblatt DJ, Steel K, Shader RI: Impairment of hepatic drug oxidation by propoxyphene. *Ann Intern Med* 97:223–224, 1982.
6. Aggeler PM, O'Reilly RA, Leong L: Potentiation of anticoagulant effect of warfarin by phenylbutazone. *N Engl J Med* 276:496–501, 1967.
7. Aherne GW, Piall E, Marks V, Mould G, White WF: Prolongation and enhancement of serum methotrexate concentrations by probenecid. *Br Med J* 1:1097–1099, 1978.
8. Akers MA, Lach JL, Fischer LJ: Alterations in the absorption of bishydroxycoumarin by various excipient materials. *J Pharm Sci* 62:391–395, 1973.

9. Albert KS, Ayres JW, DiSanto AR, Weidler DI, Sakmar E, Hallmark MR, Stoll RG, Desante KA, Wagner JG: Influence of kaolin-pectin suspension on digoxin bioavailability. *J Pharm Sci* 67:1582–1586, 1978.

10. Albert KS, DeSante KA, Welsh DD, DiSanto AR: Pharmacokinetic evaluation of a drug interaction between kaolin, pectin, and clindamycin. *J Pharm Sci* 67:1579–1582, 1978.

11. Algozzine GJ, Stewart RB, Springer PK: Decreased clearance of phenytoin with cimetidine (letter). *Ann Intern Med* 95:244–245, 1981.

12. Allum W, Aminu J, Bloomfield TH, Davies C, Scales AH, Vere DW: Interaction between debrisoquin and phenylephrine in man. *Br J Clin Pharmacol* 1:51–57, 1974.

13. Ambre JJ, Fisher LJ: Effect of coadministration of aluminum and magnesium hydroxides on absorption of anticoagulants in man. *Clin Pharmacol Ther* 14:231–238, 1973.

14. Arita M, Surawicz B: Electrophysiologic effects of phenothiazines on canine cardiac fibers. *J Pharmacol Exp Ther* 184:619–630, 1973.

15. Baber N, Halliday L, Sibeon R, Littler T, Orme ML'E: The interaction between indomethacin and probenecid. A clinical and pharmacokinetic study. *Clin Pharmacol Ther* 24:298–306, 1978.

16. Baciewicz AM, Self TH: Rifampin drug interactions. *Arch Intern Med* 144:1667–1671, 1984.

17. Back DJ, Breckenridge AM, Crawford FE: The effect of rifampin on the pharmacokinetics of ethynylestradiol in women. *Contraception* 21:135–143, 1980.

18. Bailey RR, Neale TJ: Rapid clonidine withdrawal with blood pressure overshoot exaggerated by beta blockade. *Br Med J* 1:942–943, 1976.

19. Balis FM: Pharmacokinetic drug interactions of commonly used anticancer drugs. *Clin Pharmacokinet* 11:223–235, 1986.

20. Barr WH, Adir J, Garrettson L: Decrease of tetracycline absorption in man by sodium bicarbonate. *Clin Pharmacol Ther* 12:779–784, 1971.

21. Barrientos A, Alcazar V, Ruilope L, Jarillo D, Rodio JL: Indomethacin and beta-blockers in hypertension. *Lancet* 1:227, 1978.

22. Bauer LA, Edwards AD, Randolph FP: Cimetidine-induced decrease in lidocaine metabolism. *Am Heart J* 108:413–414, 1984.

23. Bauer LA, Stenwall M, Horn JR, Davis R, Opheim K, Greene L: Changes in antipyrine and indocyanine green kinetics during nifedipine, verapamil, and diltiazem therapy. *Clin Pharmacol Ther* 40:239–242, 1986.

24. Belz GG, Doering W, Aust PE, Heinz M, Matthews J, Schneider B: Quinidine-digoxin interaction. Cardiac efficacy of elevated serum digoxin concentration. *Clin Pharmacol Ther* 31:548–554, 1982.

25. Benfield P, Clissold SP, Brogden RN: Metoprolol: An updated review of its pharmacodynamic and pharmacokinetic properties, and therapeutic efficacy, in hypertension, ischaemic heart disease and related cardiovascular disorders. *Drugs* 31:376–429, 1986.

26. Berg KJ: Acute effects of acetylsalicylic acid on renal function in normal man. *Eur J Clin Pharmacol* 11:117–123, 1977.

27. Berg MJ, Berlinger WG, Goldberg MJ, Spector R, Johnson GF: Acceleration of the body clearance of phenobarbital by oral activated charcoal. *N Engl J Med* 307:642–644, 1982.

28. Bergrem H, Refvem OK: Altered prednisolone pharmacokinetics in patients treated with rifampicin. *Acta Med Scand* 213:339–343, 1983.

29. Berlinger WG, Spector R, Goldberg MJ, Johnson GF, Quee CK, Berg MJ: Enhancement of theophylline clearance by oral activated charcoal. *Clin Pharmacol Ther* 33:351–354, 1983.

30. Bigger JT, Leahey EB: Quinidine and digoxin. An important interaction. *Drugs* 24:229–239, 1982.

31. Binnion PF: Drug interaction with digitalis glycosides. *Drugs* 15:369–380, 1978.

32. Bint AJ, Burtt I: Adverse antibiotic drug interaction. *Drugs* 20:57–68, 1980.

33. Bjornsson TD, Meffin PJ, Swezey S, Blaschke TF: Clofibrate displaces warfarin from plasma proteins in man: an example of a pure displacement interaction. *J Pharmacol Exp Ther* 210:316–321, 1979.

34. Blair DC, Duggan DO, Schroeder ET: Inactivation of amikacin and gentamicin by carbenicillin in patients with end-stage renal failure. *Antimicrob Agents Chemother* 22:376–379, 1982.

35. Boakes AJ, Laurence DR, Teoh PC, Barar FSK, Benedikter LT, Prichard BNC: Interactions between sympathomimetic amines and antidepressant agents in man. *Br Med J* 1:311–315, 1973.

36. Boulline DJ: The action of antidepressants on the effects of other drugs. *Primary Care* 2:669–688. 1975.

37. Boura ALA, Green AF: Adrenergic neurone blockade and other acute effects caused by N-benzyl-N'-N''-dimethylguanidine and its orthochloro derivative. *Br J Pharmacol* 20:36–55, 1963.

38. Boyce EG, Dukes GE, Rollins DE, Sudds TW: The effect of rifampin on theophylline kinetics. *J Clin Pharmacol* 26:696–699, 1986.

39. Braitwaite RA, Flanagan RJ, Richens A: Steady state plasma nortryptyline concentrations in epileptic patients. *Br J Clin Pharmacol* 2:469–471, 1975.

40. Branch RA, Shand DG, Wilkinson GR, Nies AS: The reduction of lidocaine clearance by dl-propranolol: An example of hemodynamic drug interaction. *J Pharmacol Exp Ther* 184:515–519, 1973.

41. Branigan TA, Robbin RA, Cady WJ, Nickols JG, Ueda CT: The effects of erythromycin on the absorption and disposition kinetics of theophylline. *Eur J Clin Pharmacol* 21:115–120, 1981.

42. Brater DC: Analysis of the effect of indomethacin on the response to furosemide in man. Effect of dose of furosemide. *J Pharmacol Exp Ther* 210:386–390, 1979.

43. Breen KJ, Bury R, Desmond PV, Mashford ML, Morphett B, Westwood B, Shaw RG: Effects of cimetidine and ranitidine on hepatic drug metabolism. *Clin Pharmacol Ther* 31:297–300, 1982.

44. Briant RH, Reid JL, Dollery CT: Interaction between clonidine and desipramine in man. *Br Med J* 1:522–523, 1973.

45. Brodie MJ, MacPhee GJA: Carbamazepine neurotoxicity precipitated by diltiazem. *Br Med J.* 292:1170–1171, 1986.

46. Brown DD, Juhl RP: Decreased bioavailability of digoxin due to antacids and kaolin pectin. *N Engl J Med* 295:1034–1037, 1976.

47. Brown DD, Juhl RP, Warner SL: Decreased bioavailability of digoxin due to hypocholesterolemia interventions. *Circulation* 58:164–172, 1978.

48. Brown DD, Spector R, Juhl RP: Drug interactions with digoxin. *Drugs* 20:198–206, 1980.

49. Buchanan RA, Heffelfinger JC, Weiss CF: The effect of phenobarbital on diphenylhydantoin metabolism in children. *Pediatrics* 43:114–116, 1969.

50. Burn JH, Rand MJ: The action of sympathomimetic amines in animals treated with reserpine. *J Physiol* 144:314–336, 1958.

51. Burns JJ, Conney AH: Enzyme stimulation and inhibition in the metabolism of drugs. *Proc R Soc Med* 58:955–960, 1965.

52. Cabizuca SV, Desser KB: Carbenicillin associated hypokalemic alkalosis. *JAMA* 236:956–957, 1976.

53. Caldwell JH, Greenberger NJ: Interruption of the enterohepatic circulation of digitoxin by cholestyramine. I. Protection against lethal digitoxin intoxication. *J Clin Invest* 50:2626–2637, 1971.

54. Campbell MA, Plachetka JR, Jackson JE, Moon JF, Finley PR: Cimetidine decreases theophylline clearance. *Ann Intern Med* 95:68–69, 1981.

55. Carrum G, Egan JM, Abernethy DR: Diltiazem treatment impairs hepatic drug oxidation: studies of antipyrine. Clin Pharmacol Ther 40:140–143, 1986.

56. Carruthers SG, Dujovne CA: Cholestyramine and spironolactone and their combination in digitoxin elimination. Clin Pharmacol Ther 27:184–187, 1980.

57. Carulli N, Manenti F, Gallo M, Salvioli GF: Alcohol-drugs interaction in man: alcohol and tolbutamide. Eur J Clin Invest 1:421–424, 1971.

58. Cate EW, Rogers JF, Powell JR: Inhibition of tolbutamide elimination by cimetidine but not ranitidine. J Clin Pharmacol 26:372–377, 1986.

59. Chang CC, Costa E, Brodie BB: Reserpine-induced release of drugs from sympathetic nerve endings. Life Sci 3:839–844, 1964.

60. Chen T-S, Friedman HS: Alteration of digoxin pharmacokinetics by a single dose of quinidine. JAMA 244:669–672, 1980.

61. Chennavasin P, Seiwell R, Brater DC: Pharmacokinetic-dynamic analysis of the indomethacin-furosemide interaction in man. J Pharmacol Exp Ther 215:77–81, 1980.

62. Christiansen J, Dam M: Influence of phenobarbital and diphenylhydantoin on plasma carbamazepine levels in patients with epilepsy. Acta Neurol Scand 49:543–546, 1973.

63. Christensen LK, Skovested L: Inhibition of drug metabolism by chloramphenicol. Lancet 2:1397–1399, 1969.

64. Christian CD, Meridith CG, Speeg KV: Cimetidine inhibits renal procainamide clearance. Clin Pharmacol Ther 36:221–227, 1984.

65. Cinquegrani MP, Liang C-S: Indomethacin attenuates the hypotensive action of hydralazine. Clin Pharmacol Ther 39:564–570, 1986.

66. Cluxton RJ, Rivera JO, Ritschel WA, Pesce AJ, Hanenson IB: Cimetidine-theophylline interaction (letter). Ann Intern Med 96:684, 1982.

67. Cocco G, Ague C: Interactions between cardioactive drugs and antidepressants. Eur J Clin Pharmacol 11:389–393, 1977.

68. Conney AH: Pharmacological implications of microsomal enzyme induction. Pharmacol Rev 19:317–366, 1967.

69. Cramer JL, Rosser RM, Crane G: Blood levels and management of lithium treatment. Br Med J 3:650–654, 1974.

70. Cucinell SA, Conney AH, Sansur M, Burns JJ: Drug interaction in man. I. Lowering effect of phenobarbital on plasma levels of bishydroxycoumarin (Dicumarol) and diphenylhydantoin (Dilantin). Clin Pharmacol Ther 6:420–429, 1965.

71. Curry SH, DeVane CL, Wolfe MM: Cimetidine interaction with amitriptyline. Eur J Clin Pharmacol 29:429–433, 1985.

72. Dam M, Kristensen B, Hansen BS, Christiansen J: Interaction between carbamazepine and propoxyphene in man. Acta Neurol Scand 56:602–607, 1977.

73. Data JL, Wilkinson GR, Nies AS: Interaction of quinidine with anticonvulsant drugs. N Engl J Med 294:699–702, 1976.

74. Davis JM, Bartlett E, Termini BS: Overdosage of psychotropic drugs. A review. Dis Nerv Syst 29:157–164, 246–256, 1986.

75. Day MD: Effect of sympathomimetic amines on the blocking action of guanethidine, bretylium, xylocholine. Br J Pharmacol 18:421–439, 1962.

76. Day MD, Rand MJ: Antagonism of guanethidine by dexamphetamine and other related sympathomimetic amines. J Pharm Sci 14:541–549, 1962.

77. Depaulo JR Jr, Correa EI, Sapir DG: Renal toxicity of lithium and its implications. Johns Hopkins Med J 149:15–21, 1981.

78. Desmond PV, Patwardhan RV, Schenker S, Speeg KV: Cimetidine impairs elimination of chlordiazepoxide

79. (Librium) in man. Ann Intern Med 93:266–268, 1980.

79. Desmond PV, Patwardhan RV, Schenker S, Speeg KV: Short term ethanol administration impairs the elimination of chlordiazepoxide in man. Eur J Clin Pharmacol 18:275–278, 1980.

80. DeTeresa E, Vera A, Ortigosa J, Pulpon LA, Arus AP, DeArtaza M: Interaction between anticoagulants and contraceptives: an unsuspected finding. Br Med J 2:1260–1261, 1979.

81. DeVita VT, Hahn MA, Oliverio VT: Monoamine oxidase inhibition by a new carcinostatic agent, N-isopropyl-α-(2-methyl-hydrazino)-p-toluamide (MIH). Proc Soc Exp Biol Med 120:561–565, 1965.

82. Dhillon S, Richens A: Serum protein binding of diazepam and its displacement by valproic acid in vitro. Br J Clin Pharmacol 12:591–592, 1981.

83. Dobbs JH, Skoutakis VA, Acchardio SR, Dobbs BR: Effects of aluminum hydroxide on the absorption of propranolol. Curr Ther Res 21:877–892, 1977.

84. Doering W: Quinidine-digoxin interaction. Pharmacokinetics, underlying mechanism and clinical implications. N Engl J Med 301:400–404, 1979.

85. Dorian P, Sellers EM, Carruthers G, Hamilton C, Fan T: Propranolol-ethanol pharmacokinetic interaction. Clin Pharmacol Ther 31:219, 1982.

86. Durao B, Rico JMGT: Modification by indomethacin of the blood pressure lowering effect of pindolol and propranolol in conscious rabbits. Eur J Pharmacol 43:377–381, 1977.

87. Durao V, Prata MM, Gonclaves LMP: Modifications of antihypertensive effect of β-adrenoceptor-blocking agents by inhibition of endogenous prostaglandin synthesis. Lancet 2:1005–1007, 1977.

88. Easton PA, Koval A: Hypertensive reaction with sulindac. Can Med Assoc J 122:1273–1274, 1980.

89. Evans DAA, Mantey KA, McKusick VA: Genetic control of isoniazid metabolism in man. Br Med J 2:485–491, 1960.

90. Fann WE, Cavanaugh JH, Kaufmann JS: Doxepin: effects of transport of biogenic amines in man. Psychopharmacologia 22:111–125, 1972.

91. Fann WE, Davis JM, Janowsky DS, Sekerke WJ, Schmidt DM: Chlorpromazine: effects of antacids on its gastrointestinal absorption. J Clin Pharmacol 13:388–390, 1973.

92. Feely J, Wilkinson GR, McAllister CB, Wood AJJ: Increased toxicity and reduced clearance of lidocaine by cimetidine. Ann Intern Med 96:592–594, 1982.

93. Feely I, Wilkinson GR, Wood AJJ: Reduction of liver blood flow and propranolol metabolism by cimetidine. N Engl J Med 304:692–695, 1981.

94. Feely J, Wood AJJ: Effect of inhibitors of prostaglandin synthesis on hepatic drug clearance. Br J Clin Pharmacol 15:109–111, 1983.

95. Fenster PE, Hager WD, Goodman MM: Digoxin-quinidine-spironolactone interaction. Clin Pharmacol Ther 36:70–73, 1984.

96. Fine A, Henderson IS, Morgan DR, Wilstone WJ: Malabsorption of furosemide caused by phenytoin. Br Med J 2:1061–1062, 1977.

97. Fowler NO, McCall D, Chou T, Holmes JC, Hanenson IB: Electrocardiographic changes and cardiac arrhythmias in patients receiving psychotropic drugs. Am J Cardiol 37:223–230, 1976.

98. Fraser DG, Ludden TM, Evans RP, Sutherland EW: Displacement of phenytoin from plasma binding sites by salicylate. Clin Pharmacol Ther 27:165–169, 1980.

99. Freeman DJ, Laupacis A, Keown PA, Stiller CR, Carruthers SC: Evaluation of cyclosporin-phenytoin interaction with observations on cyclosporin metabolites. Br J Clin Pharmacol 18:887-893, 1984.

100. Frolich JC, Leftwich R, Ragheb M, Oates JA, Reimann I, Buchanan D: Indomethacin increases plasma lithium. Br Med J 1:1115–1116, 1979.

101. Fujita T, Yamashita N, Yamashita K: Effect of indo-

methacin on antihypertensive action of captopril in hypertension patients. *Clin Exp Hypertension* 3:939–952, 1981.

102. Gambertoglio JH, Holford NHG, Kapusnik JE, Nishikawa R, Saltiel M, Stanik-Lizak P, Birnbaum JL, Hau T, Amend WJC Jr: Disposition of total and unbound prednisolone in renal transplant patients receiving anticonvulsants. *Kidney Int* 25:119–123, 1984.

103. Garnett WR, Carter BL, Bellock JM: Bioavailability of phenytoin administered with antacids. *Ther Drug Monitoring* 1:435–437, 1979.

104. Garrettson LK, Perel JM, Dayton PG: Methylphenidate interaction with both anticonvulsants and ethyl discoumacetate. *JAMA* 207:2053–2056, 1969.

105. Garty M, Hurwitz A: Effect of cimetidine and antacids on intestinal absorption of tetracycline. *Clin Pharmacol Ther* 28:203–207, 1980.

106. Gault H, Longerich L, Dawe M, Fine A: Digoxin-rifampin interaction. *Clin Pharmacol Ther* 35:750–754, 1984.

107. Geleherter TD: Enzyme induction. *N Engl J Med* 294:522–526, 589–595, 646–651, 1976.

108. Gibbons DO, Lant AF: Effects of intravenous and oral propantheline and metoclopramide on ethanol absorption. *Clin Pharmacol Ther* 17:578–584, 1975.

109. Gibson TP, Quintanilla AP: Effect of quinidine on the renal handling of digoxin. *J Lab Clin Med* 96:1062–1070, 1980.

110. Gibson TP, Quintanilla AP: Effect of volume expansion and furosemide diuresis on the renal clearance of digoxin. *J Pharmacol Exp Ther* 219:54–59, 1981.

111. Gill MA, DuBe JE, Young WW: Hypokalemic, metabolic alkalosis induced by high-dose ampicillin sodium. *Am J Hosp Pharm* 34:528–531, 1977.

112. Glynn AM, Slaughter RL, Brass C, D'Ambrosio R, Jusko WJ: Effects of ketoconazole on methylprednisolone pharmacokinetics and cortisol secretion. *Clin Pharmacol Ther* 39:654–659, 1986.

113. Gokhale SD, Gulati OD, Udwadia BP: Antagonism of the adrenergic neurone blocking action of guanethidine by certain antidepressant and antihistamine drugs. *Arch Int Pharmacodyn* 160:321–329, 1966.

114. Gore JM, Haffajee CI, Alpert JS: Interaction of amiodarone and diphenylhydantoin. *Am J Cardiol* 54:1145, 1984.

115. Greenblatt DJ, Abernethy DR, Morse DS, Harmatz JS, Shader RI: Clinical importance of the interaction of diazepam and cimetidine. *N Engl J Med* 310:1639–1643, 1984.

116. Greenblatt DH, Allen DA, Maclaughlin DS, Harmatz JS, Shader RJ: Diazepam absorption: effect of antacids and food. *Clin Pharmacol Ther* 24:600–609, 1978.

117. Greenblatt DJ, Duhme DW, Allen MD, Koch-Weser J: Clinical toxicity of furosemide in hospitalized patients. *Am Heart J* 94:6–13, 1977.

118. Greenblatt DJ, Shader RI, Harmatz JS, Franke K, Koch-Weser J: Influence of magnesium and aluminum hydroxide mixture on chlordiazepoxide absorption. *Clin Pharmacol Ther* 19:234–239, 1976.

119. Griffith RS, Black HR, Brier GL, Wolny JD: Effect of probenecid on the blood levels and urinary excretion of cefamandole. *Antimicrob Agents Chemother* 11:809–812, 1977.

120. Grygiel JJ, Brikett DJ: Cigarette smoking and theophylline clearance and metabolism. *Clin Pharmacol Ther* 30:491–496, 1981.

121. Guay DRP, Meatherall RC, Chalmers JL, Grahame GR: Cimetidine alters pethidine disposition in man. *Br J Clin Pharmacol* 18:907–914, 1984.

122. Gugler R, Brand M, Somogyi A: Impaired cimetidine absorption by antacids and metoclopramide. *Eur J Clin Pharmacol* 20:225–228, 1981.

123. Hager WD, Fenster P, Mayersohn M, Perrier D, Graves P, Marcus FI, Goldman S: Digoxin-quinidine interaction. Pharmacokinetic evaluation. *N Engl J Med* 300:1238–1241, 1979.

124. Hanahoe THP, Ireson JD, Large BJ: Interactions between guanethidine and inhibitors of noradrenaline uptake. *Arch Int Pharmacodyn* 182:349–353, 1969.

125. Hansen JM, Kristensen M, Skovsted L: Sulthiame (Opsollot[R]) an inhibitor of diphenylhydantoin metabolism. *Epilepsia* 9:17–22, 1968.

126. Hansen JM, Siersbaek-Nielsen K, Kristensen M, Skovsted L, Christensen LK: Effects of diphenylhydantoin on the metabolism of dicoumarol in man. *Acta Med Scand* 189:15–19, 1971.

127. Hansen JM, Siersbaek-Nielsen K, Skovsted L: Carbamazepine-induced acceleration of diphenylhydantoin and warfarin metabolism in man. *Clin Pharmacol Ther* 12:539–543, 1971.

128. Hansen PD: *Drug Interactions.* Philadelphia, Lea & Febiger, 1985.

129. Harrington RA, Hamilton CW, Brogden RN, Linkewich JA, Romankiewicz JA, Heel RC: Metoclopramide: an updated review of its pharmacological properties and clinical use. *Drugs* 25:451–494, 1983.

130. Harvey VJ, Slevin ML, Dilloway MR, Clark PI, Johnston A, Lant AF: The influence of cimetidine on the pharmacokinetics of 5-fluorouracil. *Br J Clin Pharmacol* 18:421–430, 1984.

131. Haworth E, Burroughs AK: Disopyramide and warfarin interaction. *Br Med J* 2:866–867, 1977.

132. Heagerty AM, Castleden CM, Patel I: Failure of ranitidine to interact with propranolol. *Br Med J* 284:1304, 1982.

133. Henaver SA, Hollister LE: Cimetidine interaction with imipramine and nortriptyline. *Clin Pharmacol Ther* 35:183–187, 1984.

134. Henderson JM, Ibrahim SZ, Millikan WJ Jr, Santi M, Warren WD: Cimetidine does not reduce liver blood flow in cirrhosis. *Hepatology* 3:919–922, 1983.

135. Hetzel DJ, Bochner F, Hallpike F, Shearman DJC, Hann CS: Cimetidine interaction with phenytoin. *Br Med J* 282:1512, 1981.

136. Hibbard DM, Peters JR, Hunninghake DB: Effects of cholestyramine and colestipol on the plasma concentrations of propranolol. *Br J Clin Pharmacol* 18:337–342, 1984.

137. Himmelhoch JM, Poust RI, Mallinger AG: Adjustment of lithium dose during lithium-chlorothiazide therapy. *Clin Pharmacol Ther* 22:225–227, 1977.

138. Hirsh PD, Weiner HJ, North RL: Further insights into digoxin-quinidine interaction: lack of correlation between serum digoxin concentration and inotropic state of the heart. *Am J Cardiol* 46:863–867, 1980.

139. Holt DW, Hayler AM, Edmonds ME, Ashford RF: Clinically significant interaction between digoxin and quinidine. *Br Med J* 2:1401, 1979.

140. Hurwitz A: The effects of antacids on gastrointestinal drug absorption II. Effect on sulfadiazine and quinine. *J Pharmacol Exp Ther* 179:485–490, 1971.

141. Hurwitz A, Schlozman DL: Effects of antacids on gastrointestinal absorption of isoniazid in rat and man. *Am Rev Respir Dis* 109:41–47, 1974.

142. Jackson JE: Reduction of liver blood flow by cimetidine (letter). *N Engl J Med* 305:99–100, 1981.

143. Jackson JE, Powell JR, Wandell M, Bentley J, Dorr R: Cimetidine decreases theophylline clearance. *Am Rev Respir Dis* 123:615–617, 1981.

144. Jahnchen E, Meinertz T, Gilfrich H-J, Kersting F, Groth V: Enhanced elimination of warfarin during treatment with cholestyramine. *Br J Clin Pharmacol* 5:437–440, 1978.

145. Janowsky DS, El-Yousef MK, Davis JM, Fann WE: Antagonism of guanethidine by chlorpromazine. *Am J Psychiatry* 130:808–812, 1973.

146. Jefferson JW, Kalin NH: Serum lithium levels and long-term diuretic use. *JAMA* 241:1134–1136, 1979.

147. Jogestrand T, Schenck-Gustafsson K, Nordlander R, Dahlqvist R: Quinidine-induced changes in serum and skeletal muscle digoxin concentration; evidence of

saturable binding of digoxin to skeletal muscle. *Eur J Clin Pharmacol* 27:571–575, 1984.

148. Johnson BF, Bustrack JA, Urbach DR, Hull JH, Marwaha R: Effect of metoclopramide on digoxin absorption from tablets and capsules. *Clin Pharmacol Ther* 36:724–730, 1984.

149. Juhl RP, Summers RW, Guillory JK, Blang SM, Cheng RH, Brown DD: Effect of sulfasalazine on digoxin bioavailability. *Clin Pharmacol Ther* 20:387–394, 1976.

150. Kabins SA: Interactions among antibiotics and other drugs. *JAMA* 219:206–212, 1972.

151. Kampmann J, Hansen JM, Siersbaek-Nielsen K, Laursen H: Effect of some drugs on penicillin half-life in blood. *Clin Pharmacol Ther* 13:516–519, 1972.

152. Kanto J, Allonen HJ, Jalonen H, Mantyla R: The effect of metoclopramide and propantheline on the gastrointestinal absorption of cimetidine. *Br J Pharmacol* 11:527–530, 1981.

153. Kater RMH, Roggin G, Tobon F, Zieve P, Iber FL: Increased rate of clearance of drugs from the circulation of alcoholics. *Am J Med Sci* 258:35–39, 1969.

154. Kauffman RE, Azarnoff DL: Effect of colestipol on gastrointestinal absorption of chlorothiazide in man. *Clin Pharmacol Ther* 14:886–889, 1973.

155. Kay L, Kampmann JP, Svendsen TL, Vergman B, Hansen JE, Skovsted L, Kristensen M: Influence of rifampicin and isoniazid on the kinetics of phenytoin. *Br J Clin Pharmacol* 20:323–326, 1985.

156. Keilholz U, Guthrie GP Jr: Case Report: adverse effect of phenytoin on mineralocorticoid replacement with fludrocortisone in adrenal insufficiency. *Am J Med Sci* 291:280–283, 1986.

157. Kelly HW, Powell JR, Donohue JF: Ranitidine at very large doses does not inhibit theophylline elimination. *Clin Pharmacol Ther* 39:577–581, 1986.

158. Khalil SAH: Bioavailability of digoxin in presence of antacids. *J Pharm Sci* 63:1641–1642, 1974 (letter).

159. Kiorboe E: Phenytoin intoxication during treatment with Antabuse[R] (disulfiram). *Epilepsia* 7:246–249, 1966.

160. Kirby MG, Dasta JF, Armstrong DK, Tallman R Jr: Effect of low-dose dopamine on the pharmacokinetics of tobramycin in dogs. *Antimicrob Agents Chemother* 29:168–170, 1986.

161. Kitto W: Antibiotics and the ingestion of alcohol. *JAMA* 193:411, 1965.

162. Klotz U, Reimann IW: Delayed clearance of diazepam due to cimetidine. *N Engl J Med* 304:1012–1014, 1980.

163. Klotz V, Reimann IW, Ohnhaus EE: Effect of ranitidine on the steady state pharmacokinetics of diazepam. *Eur J Clin Pharmacol* 24:357–360, 1983.

164. Knodell RG, Holtzman JL, Crankshaw DL, Steele NM, Stanley LN: Drug metabolism by rat and human hepatic microsomes in response to interaction with H₂-receptor antagonist. *Gastroenterology* 82:84–88, 1982.

165. Kochar MS, Itskovitz HD: Effects of hydrochlorothiazide in hypertensive patients and the need for potassium supplementation. *Curr Ther Res* 15:298–304, 1973.

166. Koch-Weser J: Drug interactions in cardiovascular therapy. *Am Heart J* 90:93–116, 1975.

167. Koch-Weser J, Sellers EM: Binding of drugs to serum albumin. *N Engl J Med* 294:311–316, 526–531, 1976.

168. Koch-Weser J, Sellers EM: Drug interactions with coumarin anticoagulants. *N Engl J Med* 285:487–498, 547–558, 1971.

169. Koup JR, Gilbaldi M, McNamara P, Hilligoss DM, Colburn WA, Bruck E: Interaction of chloramphenicol with phenytoin and phenobarbital. *Clin Pharmacol Ther* 24:571–575, 1978.

170. Kuhlmann J, Dohrmann M, Marcin S: Effects of quinidine on pharmacokinetics and pharmacodynamics of digitoxin achieving steady-state conditions. *Clin Pharmacol Ther* 39:288–294, 1986.

171. Kulshrestha VK, Thomas M, Wadsworth J, Richens A: Interaction of phenytoin and antacids. *Br J Clin Pharmacol* 6:177–179, 1978.

172. Kutt H, Brennan R, Dehejia H, Verebely K: Diphenylhydantoin intoxication. A complication of isoniazid therapy. *Am Rev Resp Dis* 101:377–384, 1970.

173. Kutt H, Haynes J, Verebely K, McDowell F: The effect of phenobarbital on plasma diphenylhydantoin level and metabolism in man and in rat liver microsomes. *Neurology* 19:611–616, 1969.

174. Kutt H, Verebely K, McDowell F: Inhibition of diphenylhydantoin metabolism in rats and in rat liver microsomes by antitubercular drugs. *Neurology* 18:706–710, 1968.

175. Kutt H, Wolk M, Scherman R, McDowell F: Insufficient para-hydroxylation as a cause of diphenylhydantoin toxicity. *Neurology* 14:542–548, 1964.

176. LaDu BN: Pharmacogenetics. *Med Clin North Am* 53:839–85, 1969.

177. Landay RA, Gonzalez MA, Taylor JC: Effect of phenobarbital on theophylline disposition. *J Allerg Clin Immunol* 62:27–29, 1978.

178. Lane EA, Guthrie S, Linnoila M: Effects of ethanol on drug and metabolite pharmacokinetics. *Clin Pharmacokinet* 10:228–247, 1985.

179. Lau A, Lee M, Flascha S, Prasad R, Sharifi R: Effect of piperacillin on tobramycin pharmacokinetics in patients with normal renal function. *Antimicrob Agents Chemother* 24:533–537, 1983.

180. Lawson DH, Tilstone WJ, Gray JMB, Srivastava PK: Effect of furosemide on the pharmacokinetics of gentamicin in patients. *J Clin Pharmacol* 22:254–258, 1982.

181. Leahey EB, Rieffel JA, Drusin RE, Heissenbuttel RH, Lovejoy WP, Bigger JT: Interaction between quinidine and digoxin. *JAMA* 240:533–534, 1978.

182. Leahey EB, Reiffel JA, Giardina E-GV, Bigger JT: The effect of quinidine and other oral antiarrhythmic drugs on serum digoxin. *Ann Intern Med* 92:605–608, 1980.

183. Leahey EB, Reiffel JA, Heissenbuttel RH, Drusin RE, Lovejoy WP, Bigger JT: Enhanced cardiac effect of digoxin during quinidine treatment. *Arch Intern Med* 139:519–521, 1979.

184. Legler UF, Benet LZ: Marked alterations in dose-dependent prednisolone kinetics in women taking oral contraceptives. *Clin Pharmacol Ther* 39:425–429, 1986.

185. Lejonc JL, Gusmini D, Brochard P: Isoniazid and reaction to cheese (letter). *Ann Intern Med* 91:793, 1979.

186. Levine RR: Factors affecting gastrointestinal absorption of drugs. *Am J Digest Dis* 15:171–188, 1970.

187. Levy G: Gastrointestinal clearance of drugs with activated treated charcoal (editorial). *N Engl J Med* 307:676–678, 1982.

188. Levy G, Lampman T, Kamath BL, Garrettson LK: Decreased serum salicylate concentration in children with rheumatic fever treated with antacid. *N Engl J Med* 293:323–325, 1975.

189. Lewis GP, Holtzman JL: Interaction of flecainide with digoxin and propranolol. *Am J Cardiol* 53:52B–57B, 1984.

190. Lewis JG: Adverse reactions to calcium antagonists. *Drugs* 25:196–222, 1983.

191. Lindenbaum J, Maulitz RM, Butler VP: Inhibition of digoxin absorption by neomycin. *Gastroenterology* 71:399–404, 1976.

192. Lindenbaum J, Rund DH, Butler VP, Tse-Eng D, Saha JR: Inactivation of digoxin by the gut flora: reversal by antibiotic therapy. *N Engl J Med* 305:789–794, 1981.

193. Linnoila M, Mattila MJ, Kitchell BS: Drug interactions with alcohol. *Drugs* 18:229–311, 1979.

194. Lopez-Ovejero JA, Weber MA, Drayer JIM, Sealey JE, Laragh JH: Effects of indomethacin alone and during diuretic or β-adrenoreceptor-blockade therapy on blood pressure and the renin system in essential hypertension. *Clin Sci Mol Med* 55:203–205, 1978.

195. Lumholtz B, Siersbaek-Nielsen K, Skovsted L, Kampmann J, Hensen JM: Sulfamethizole-induced inhibition of diphenylhydantoin, tolbutamide, and warfarin

metabolism. *Clin Pharmacol Ther* 17:731–734, 1975.

196. MacLeod SM, Giles HG, Patzalek G, Thiessen JJ, Sellers EM: Diazepam actions and plasma concentrations following ethanol ingestion. *Eur J Clin Pharmacol* 11:346–349, 1977.

197. MacLeod SM, Sellers EM: Pharmacodynamic and pharmacokinetic drug interactions with coumarin anticoagulants. *Drugs* 11:461–470, 1976.

198. MacLeod SM, Sellers EM, Giles HG, Billings BJ, Martin PR, Greenblatt DJ, Marshman JA: Interaction of disulfiram with benzodiazepines. *Clin Pharmacol Ther* 24:583–589, 1978.

199. Macphee GJA, Thompson GG, McInnes GT, Brodie MJ: Verapamil potentiates carbamazepine neurotoxicity: a clinically important inhibitory interaction. *Lancet* 1:700–703, 1986.

200. Macphee GJA, Thompson GG, Scobie G, Agnew E, Park BK, Murray T, McColl KEL, Brodie MJ: Effects of cimetidine on carbamazepine auto- and hetero-induction in man. *Br J Clin Pharmacol* 18:411–419, 1984.

201. Manfred RL, Vesell ES: Inhibition of theophylline metabolism by long-term allopurinol administration. *Clin Pharmacol Ther* 29:224–229, 1981.

202. Manninen V, Apajalahti A, Simonen H, Reissel P: Effect of propantheline and metoclopramide on absorption of digoxin. *Lancet* 1:398, 1973.

203. Martell R, Heinrichs D, Stiller CR, Jenner M, Keown PA, Dupre J: The effects of erythromycin in patients treated with cyclosporine. *Ann Intern Med* 104:660–661, 1986.

204. Mattson RH, Cramer JA, Williamson PC, Novelly RA: Valproic acid in epilepsy: clinical and pharmacological effects. *Ann Neurol* 3:20–25, 1978.

205. May CD, Jarboe CH: Inhibition of clearance of dyphylline by probenecid (letter). *N Engl J Med* 304:791, 1981.

206. May DC, Jarboe CH, Ellenburg DT, Roe EJ, Karibo J: The effects of erythromycin on theophylline elimination in normal males. *J Clin Pharmacol* 22:125–130, 1982.

207. McElnay JC, D'Arcy PF: Protein binding displacement interactions and their clinical importance. *Drugs* 25:495–513, 1983.

208. McGovern B, Geer VR, LaRaia PJ, Garan H, Ruskin JN: Possible interaction between amiodarone and phenytoin. *Ann Intern Med* 101:650–651, 1984.

209. McMurty RJ: Propranolol, hypoglycemia, and hypertensive crisis. *Ann Intern Med* 80:669–670, 1974.

210. Melmon KL, Nierenberg DW: Drug interactions and the prepared observer (editorial). *N Engl J Med* 304:723–724, 1981.

211. Mihaly GW, Marino AT, Webster LK, Jones DB, Louis WJ, Smallwood RA: High dose of antacid (Mylanta II) reduces bioavailability of ranitidine. *Br Med J* 285:998–999, 1982.

212. Miller M, Cosgriff J, Kwong T, Morken DA: Influence of phenytoin on theophylline clearance. *Clin Pharmacol Ther* 35:666–669, 1984.

213. Miller RP, Bates JH: Amphotericin B toxicity. A follow-up report of 53 patients. *Ann Intern Med* 71:1089–1095, 1969.

214. Milne MD, Scribner BH, Crawford MA: Non-ionic diffusion and the excretion of weak acids and bases. *Am J Med* 24:709–729, 1958.

215. Misage JR, McDonald RH: Antagonism of hypotensive action of bethanidine by "common cold" remedy. *Br Med J* 4:347, 1976.

216. Misra PS, Leferve A, Ishii H, Rubin E, Lieber CS: Increase of ethanol, mebrobamate and pentobarbital metabolism after chronic ethanol administration in man and rats. *Am J Med* 51:346–351, 1971.

217. Mitchell JR, Arias L, Oates JA: Antagonism of the antihypertensive action of guanethidine sulfate by desipramine hydrochloride. *JAMA* 202:973–976, 1967.

218. Mitchell JR, Cavanaugh JH, Arias L, Oates JA: Guanethidine and related agents. III. Antagonism by drugs which inhibit the norepinephrine pump in man. *J Clin Invest* 49:1596–1604, 1970.

219. Mitchell MC, Hanew T, Meredith CG, Schenker S: Effects of oral contraceptive steroids on acetaminophen metabolism and elimination. *Clin Pharmacol Ther* 34:48–53, 1983.

220. Mitchell MC, Schnecker S, Speeg KV: Selective inhibition of acetaminophen oxidation and toxicity by cimetidine and other histamine H_2 receptor antagonists *in vivo* and *in vitro* in the rat and in man. *J Clin Invest* 73:383–391, 1984.

221. Moore TJ, Crantz TR, Hollenberg NK, Koletsky RJ, Leboff MS, Swartz SL, Levine L, Podolsky S, Dluhy RG, Williams GH: Contribution of prostaglandins to the antihypertensive action of captopril in essential hypertension. *Hypertension* 3:168–173, 1981.

222. Muirhead MR, Somogyi AA, Rolan PE, Bochner F: Effect of cimetidine on renal and hepatic drug elimination: studies with triamterene. *Clin Pharmacol Ther* 40:400–407, 1986.

223. Mungall DR, Robichaux RP, Perry W, Scott JW, Robinson A, Burelle T, Hurst D: Effects of quinidine on serum digoxin concentration. *Ann Intern Med* 93:689–693, 1980.

224. Murphy DL, Bunney WE, Jr: Total body potassium changes during lithium administration. *J Nerv Ment Dis* 152:381–389, 1971.

225. Murray FJ: Outbreak of unexpected reactions among epileptics taking isoniazid. *Am Rev Respir Dis* 86:729–732, 1962.

226. Murrell GAC, Rapeport WG: Clinical pharmacokinetics of allopurinol. *Clin Pharmacokinet* 11:343–353, 1986.

227. Neuvonen PJ: Clinical pharmacokinetics of oral activated charcoal in acute intoxication. *Clin Pharmacokinet* 7:465–489, 1982.

228. Neuvonen PJ, Elfring SM, Elonen E: Reduction of absorption of digoxin, phenytoin and aspirin by activated charcoal in man. *Eur J Clin Pharmacol* 13:213–218, 1978.

229. Neuvonen PJ, Elonen E: Effect of activated charcoal on absorption and elimination of phenobarbitone, carbamazepine, and phenylbutazone in man. *Eur J Clin Pharmacol* 17:51–57, 1980.

230. Neuvonen PJ, Kannisto H, Hirvisalo EL: Effect of activated charcoal on absorption of tolbutamide and valproate in man. *Eur J Clin Pharmacol* 24:243–246, 1983.

231. Neuvonen PJ, Lehtovaara R, Bardy A, Elonen E: Antipyrine analgesics in patients on antiepileptic drug therapy. *Eur J Clin Pharmacol* 15:263–268, 1979.

232. Neuvonen PJ, Tokola RA, Kaste M: Cimetidine-phenytoin interactions: effect on serum phenytoin concentration and antipyrine test in man. *Eur J Clin Pharmacol* 21:215–220, 1981.

233. Newton RW: Physostigmine salicylate in the treatment of tricyclic antidepressant overdosage. *JAMA* 231:941–944, 1974.

234. Nierenberg DW: Competitive inhibition of methotrexate in kidney slices by nonsteroidal anti-inflammatory drugs. *J Pharmacol Exp Ther* 226:1–6, 1983.

235. Nies AS: Adverse reactions and interactions limiting the use of antihypertensive drugs. *Am J Med* 58:495–503, 1975.

236. Nies AS, Shand DG: Hypertensive response to propranolol in a patient treated with methyl dopa—a proposed mechanism. *Clin Pharmacol Ther* 14:823–826, 1973.

237. Nimmo WS, Heading RC, Tothill P, Prescott LF: Pharmacological evaluation of gastric emptying: effect of propantheline and metoclopramide on paracetamol absorption. *Br Med J* 1:587–589, 1973.

238. Nimmo WS, Heading RC, Wilson J, Tothill P, Prescott LF: Inhibition of gastric emptying and drug absorption

by narcotic analgesics. *Br J Clin Pharmacol* 2:502–513, 1975.

239. Noble J, Matthew H: Acute poisoning by antidepressants: clinical features and management of 100 patients. *Clin Toxicol* 2:403–421, 1969.

240. Ochs HR, Carstens G, Greenblatt DJ: Reduction in lidocaine clearance during continuous infusion and by coadministration of propranolol. *N Engl J Med* 303:373–377, 1980.

241. Ochs HR, Greenblatt DJ, Gugler R: Cimetidine impairs nitrazepam clearance. *Clin Pharmacol Ther* 34:227–230, 1983.

242. Ochs HR, Greenblatt DJ, Verburg-Ochs B: Propranolol interactions with diazepam, lorazepam, and alprazolam. *Clin Pharmacol Ther* 36:451–455, 1984.

243. Olesen OV: Disulfiram (Antabuse^R) as inhibitor of phenytoin metabolism. *Acta Pharmacol Toxicol* 24:317–322, 1966.

244. O'Reilly RA: Comparative interaction of cimetidine and ranitidine with racemic warfarin in man. *Arch Intern Med* 144:989–991, 1984.

245. O'Reilly RA: Interaction of chronic daily warfarin therapy and rifampin. *Ann Intern Med* 83:506–508, 1975.

246. O'Reilly RA: Interaction of sodium warfarin and disulfiram (Antabuse^R) in man. *Ann Intern Med* 78:73–76, 1973.

247. O'Reilly RA: Interaction of sodium warfarin and rifampin. *Ann Intern Med* 81:337–340, 1974.

248. O'Reilly RA: Stereoselective interaction of trimethoprim-sulfamethoxazole with the separated enantiomers of racemic warfarin in man. *N Engl J Med* 302:33–35, 1980.

249. O'Reilly RA: The stereoselective interaction of warfarin and metronidazole in man. *N Engl J Med* 295:354–357, 1976.

250. Orr JM, Abott FS, Farrell K, Ferguson S, Sheppard L, Godolphin W: Interaction between valproic acid and aspirin in epileptic children: serum protein binding and metabolic effects. *Clin Pharmacol Ther* 31:642–649, 1982.

251. Osman MA, Patel RB, Schuna A, Sundstrom WR, Welling PG: Reduction in oral penicillamine absorption by food, antacid and ferrous sulfate. *Clin Pharmacol Ther* 33:465–470, 1983.

252. Osman MA, Welling PG: Influence of propantheline and metaclopramide on the bioavailability of chlorothiazide. *Curr Ther Res* 34:404–408, 1983.

253. Packer M, Meller J, Medina N, Yushak M, Smith H, Holt J, Guererro J, Todd GD, McAllister RG, Gorlin R: Hemodynamic consequences of combined beta-adrenergic and slow calcium channel blockade in man. *Circulation* 65:660–668, 1982.

254. Parsons, RL, Paddock GM: Absorption of two antibacterial drugs, cephalexin and co-trimoxazole in malabsorption syndromes. *J Antimicrob Chemother* 1(suppl):59–67, 1975.

255. Patak RV, Mookerjee BK, Bentzel CJ, Hysert PE, Babej M, Lee JB: Antagonism of the effects of furosemide by indomethacin in normal and hypertensive man. *Prostaglandins* 10:649–659, 1980.

256. Patwardhan RV, Yarborough GW, Desmond PV, Johnson RF, Schenker S, Speeg KV: Cimetidine spares the glucuronidation of lorazepam and oxazepam. *Gastroenterology* 79:912–916, 1980.

257. Pedersen AK, Jackobsen P, Kampmann JP, Hansen JM: Clinical pharmacokinetics and potentially important drug interactions of sulphinpyrazone. *Clin Pharmacokinet* 7:42–56, 1982.

258. Pentikainen PJ, Koivula IH, Hiltunen HA: Effect of rifampicin treatment on the kinetics of mexiletine. *Eur J Clin Pharmacol* 23:261–266, 1982.

259. Penttila O, Neuvonen PJ, Aho K, Lehtovarra R: Interaction between doxycycline and some antiepileptic drugs. *Br Med J* 2:470–472, 1974.

260. Perel JM, Dayton PG, Snell MM, Yu TF, Gutman AB: Studies of interactions among drugs in man at the renal level: probenecid and sulfinpyrazone. *Clin Pharmacol Ther* 10:834–840, 1969.

261. Perucca E: Pharmacokinetic interactions with antiepileptic drugs. *Clin Pharmacokinet* 7:57–84, 1982.

262. Perucca E, Hebdige S, Gatti G, Leccini S, Frigo BM, Crema A: Interaction between phenytoin and valproic acid: plasma protein binding and metabolic effects. *Clin Pharmacol Ther* 28:779–789, 1980.

263. Perucca E, Richens A: Drug interactions with phenytoin. *Drugs* 21:120–137, 1981.

264. Petereit LB, Meikle AW: Effectiveness of prednisolone during phenytoin therapy. *Clin Pharmacol Ther* 22:912–916, 1977.

265. Peters L: Renal tubular excretion of organic bases. *Pharmacol Rev* 12:1–35, 1960.

266. Pickering IK, Rutherford I: Effect of concentration and time upon inactivation of tobramycin, gentamicin, netilmicin and amikacin by azlocillin carbenicillin, mecillinam, mezlocillin and piperacillin. *J Pharmacol Exp Ther* 217:345–349, 1981.

267. Pinell OC, Fenimore DC, Davis GM, Fann WE: Drug-drug interactions of chlorpromazine and antacids (abstract). *Clin Pharmacol Ther* 23:125, 1978.

268. Pond SM, Birkett DJ, Wade DN: Mechanisms of inhibition of tolbutamide metabolism: phenylbutazone, oxyphenbutazone, sulfaphenazole. *Clin Pharmacol Ther* 22:573–579, 1978.

269. Pond SM, Graham GG, Birkett DJ, Wade DN: Effects of tricyclic antidepressants on drug metabolism. *Clin Pharmacol Ther* 18:191–199, 1975.

270. Powell JR, Rogers JF, Wargin WA, Cross RE, Eshelman FN: Inhibition of theophylline clearance by cimetidine but not ranitidine. *Arch Intern Med* 144:484–486, 1984.

271. Prescott LF: Mechanisms of renal excretion of drugs. *Br J Anaesth* 44:246–251, 1972.

272. Prescott LF: Pharmacokinetic drug interactions. *Lancet* 2:1239–1243, 1969.

273. Prichard BNC, Ross EJ: Use of propranolol in conjunction with alpha receptor blocking drugs in pheochromocytoma. *Am J Cardiol* 18:394–398, 1966.

274. Prober CG: Effect of rifampin on chloramphenicol levels. *N Engl J Med* 312:788–789, 1985.

275. Puschett JB, Rastegar A: Comparative study of the effects of metolazone and other diuretics on potassium excretion. *Clin Pharmacol Ther* 15:397–405, 1974.

276. Puurunen J, Solaniemi E, Pelkonen O: Effect of cimetidine on microsomal drug metabolism in man. *Eur J Clin Pharmacol* 18:185–187, 1980.

277. Reimann IW, Frolich JC: Effects of diclofenac on lithium kinetics. *Clin Pharmacol Ther* 30:348–352, 1981.

278. Reitberg DP, Bernhard H, Schentag JJ: Alteration of theophylline clearance and half-life by cimetidine in normal volunteers. *Ann Intern Med* 95:582–586, 1981.

279. Rendic S, Alebic-Kolbah T, Kajfez F: Interaction of ranitidine with liver microsomes. *Xenobiotica* 12:9–17, 1982.

280. Rennick BR: Renal excretion of drugs: tubular transport and metabolism. *Annu Rev Pharmacol* 12:141–156, 1972.

281. Rennick BR: Renal tubule transport of organic cations. *Am J Physiol* 240:F83–F89, 1981.

282. Renton KW, Gray JD, Hung OR: Depression of theophylline elimination by erythromycin. *Clin Pharmacol Ther* 30:422–426, 1981.

283. Richer C, Mathieu M, Bah H, Thuillex C, Duroux P, Giudicelli J-F: Theophylline kinetics and ventilatory flow in bronchial asthma and chronic airflow obstruction: influence of erythromycin. *Clin Pharmacol Ther* 31:579–586, 1982.

284. Robinson DS, Benjamin DM, McCormack JJ: Interaction of warfarin and nonsystemic gastrointestinal drugs. *Clin Pharmacol Ther* 12:491–495, 1971.

285. Robson RA, Miners JO, Wing LMH, Birkett DJ: Theophylline-rifampin interaction: non-selective induc-

tion of theophylline metabolic pathways. *Br J Clin Pharmacol* 18:445–448, 1984.

286. Rollinghoff W, Paumgartner G: Inhibition of drug metabolism by cimetidine in man: dependence on pretreatment microsomal liver function. *Eur J Clin Invest* 12:429–434, 1982.

287. Romankiewicz JA, Ehrman M: Rifampin and warfarin: a drug interaction. *Ann Intern Med* 82:224–225, 1975.

288. Rose HJ, Pruitt AW, Dayton PG, McNay JL: Relationship of urinary furosemide excretion rate to natriuretic effect in experimental azotemia. *J Pharmacol Exp Ther* 199:490–497, 1976.

289. Rose HJ, Pruitt AW, McNay J: Effect of experimental azotemia on renal clearance of furosemide in the dog. *J Pharmacol Exp Ther* 196:238–247, 1976.

290. Routledge PA, Kitchell BB, Bjornsson TD, Skinner T, Linnoila M, Shand DG: Diazepam and N-desmethyldiazepam redistribution after heparin. *Clin Pharmacol Ther* 27:528–532, 1980.

291. Ruffalo RL, Thompson JF, Segal JL: Diazepam-cimetidine drug interaction: a clinically significant effect. *South Med J* 74:1075–1078, 1981.

292. Saal AK, Werner JA, Greene HL, Sears GK, Graham EL: Effect of amiodarone on serum quinidine and procainamide levels. *Am J Cardiol* 53:1264–1267, 1984.

293. Sackellares JC, Sato S, Dreifuss FE, Penry JK: Reduction of steady state valproate levels by other antiepileptic drugs. *Epilepsia* 22:437–441, 1981.

294. Salem RB, Breland BD, Mishra SK, Jordan JE: Effect of cimetidine on phenytoin serum levels. *Epilepsia* 24:284–288, 1983.

295. Sanchez G: Enhancement of heparin effect by probenecid (letter). *N Engl J Med* 292:48, 1975.

296. Sandor P, Sellers EM, Dumbrell M, Klouw V: Effect of short and long term alcohol use on phenytoin kinetics in chronic alcoholics. *Clin Pharmacol Ther* 30:390–397, 1981.

297. Schneck DW, Luderer JR, Davis D, Vary JE: Effects of nadolol and propranolol on plasma lidocaine clearance. *Clin Pharmacol Ther* 36:584–587, 1984.

298. Schneck DW, Vary JE: Mechanism by which hydralazine increases propranolol bioavailability. *Clin Pharmacol Ther* 35:447–453, 1984.

299. Schenck-Gustafsson K, Jogestrand T, Nordlander R, Dahlqvist R: Effect of quinidine on digoxin concentration in skeletal muscle and serum in patients with atrial fibrillation. Evidence for reduced binding of digoxin in muscle. *N Engl J Med* 305:209–211, 1981.

300. Schwartz JB, Keefe D, Kates RE, Kirsten E, Harrison DC: Acute and chronic pharmacodynamic interaction of verapamil and digoxin in atrial fibrillation. *Circulation* 65:1163–1170, 1982.

301. Seixas FA: Alcohol and its drug interactions. *Ann Intern Med* 83:86–92, 1975.

302. Sellers EM: Plasma protein displacement interactions are rarely of clinical significance. *Pharmacology* 18:225–227, 1979.

303. Sellers EM, Holloway MR: Drug kinetics and alcohol ingestion. *Clin Pharmacokinet* 3:440–452, 1978.

304. Sellers EM, Koch-Weser J: Displacement of warfarin from human albumin by diazoxide and ethacrynic, mefenamic, and nalidixic acids. *Clin Pharmacol Ther* 11:524–529, 1970.

305. Sellers EM, Koch-Weser J: Potentiation of warfarin-induced hypoprothrombinemia by chloral hydrate. *N Engl J Med* 283:827–831, 1970.

306. Sellers EM, Lang M, Koch-Weser J, LeBlanc E, Kalant H: Interaction of chloral hydrate and ethanol in man. I. Metabolism. *Clin Pharmacol Ther* 13:37–49, 1972.

307. Sellers EM, Naranjo CA, Giles HG, Frecker RC, Beeching M: Intravenous diazepam and oral ethanol interaction. *Clin Pharmacol Ther* 28:638–645, 1980.

308. Sellman F, Kanto J, Raijola E, Pekkarinen A: Human and animal study on elimination from plasma and metabolism of diazepam after chronic alcohol intake. *Acta Pharmacol Toxicol* 36:33–38, 1975.

309. Serlin MJ, Breckenridge AM: Drug interactions with warfarin. *Drugs* 25:610–620, 1983.

310. Serlin MJ, Sibeon RG, Breckenridge AM: Lack of effect of ranitidine on warfarin action. *Br J Clin Pharmacol* 12:791–794, 1981.

311. Shea P, Lal R, Kim SS, Schechtman K, Ruffy R: Flecainide and amiodarone interaction. *J Am Coll Cardiol* 7:1127–1130, 1986.

312. Shinn AF, Shrewsbury RP: *Evaluation of Drug Interactions.* St. Louis, CV Mosby, 1985.

313. Sjoqvist F: Psychotropic drugs (2). Interaction between monoamine oxidase (MAO) inhibitors and other substances. *Proc R Soc Med* 58:967–977, 1965.

314. Skinner C, Coull DC, Johnston AW: Antagonism of the hypotensive action of bethanidine and debrisoquin by tricyclic antidepressants. *Lancet* 2:564–566, 1969.

315. Smith CK, Durack DT: Isoniazid and reaction to cheese. *Ann Intern Med* 88:520–521, 1978.

316. Solomon HM, Abrams WB: Interactions between digitoxin and other drugs in man. *Am Heart J* 83:277–280, 1972.

317. Somogyi A, Bochner F: Dose and concentration dependent effect of ranitidine on procainamide disposition and renal clearance in man. *Br J Clin Pharmacol* 18:175–181, 1984.

318. Somogyi A, Gugler R: Drug interactions with cimetidine. *Clin Pharmacokinet* 7:23–41, 1982.

319. Somogyi A, McLean A, Heinzow B: Cimetidine-procainamide pharmacokinetic interaction in man: evidence of competition for tubular secretion of basic drugs. *Eur J Clin Pharmacol* 25:339–345, 1983.

320. Somogyi A, Theilscher S, Gugler R: Influence of phenobarbital treatment on cimetidine kinetics. *Eur J Clin Pharmacol* 19:343–347, 1981.

321. Spahn H, Mutschler E, Kirch W, Ohnhaus EE, Janisch HD: Influence of ranitidine on plasma metoprolol and atenolol concentrations. *Br Med J* 286:1546–1547, 1983.

322. Speeg KV, Patwardham RV, Avant GR, Mitchell MC, Schenker S: Inhibition of microsomal drug metabolism by histamine H_2-receptor antagonist studied *in vivo* and *in vitro* in rodents. *Gastroenterology* 82:89–96, 1982.

323. Stafford JR, Fann WE: Drug interactions with guanidinium antihypertensives. *Drugs* 13:57–64, 1977.

324. Steinberg WM, Lewis JH, Katz DM: Antacids inhibit absorption of cimetidine. *N Engl J Med* 307:400–404, 1982.

325. Steiness E: Renal tubular secretion of digoxin. *Circulation* 50:103–107, 1974.

326. Steiness E, Waldorff S, Hansen PB, Kjaergard H, Buch J, Egeblad H: Reduction of digoxin-induced inotropism during quinidine administration. *Clin Pharmacol Ther* 27:791–795, 1980.

327. Stenson RE, Constantino RT, Harrison DC: Interrelationships of hepatic blood flow, cardiac output, and blood levels of lidocaine in man. *Circulation* 43:205–211, 1971.

328. Stockley I: *Drug Interactions.* Oxford, Blackwell Scientific Publications, 1981.

329. Stone CA, Porter CC, Stavorski JM, Ludden CT, Totaro JA: Antagonism of catecholamine-depleting agents by antidepressant and related drugs. *J Pharmacol* 144:196–204, 1964.

330. Sweeney KR, Chapron DJ, Brandt JL, Gomolin IH, Feig PU, Kramer PA: Toxic interaction between acetazolamide and salicylate: case reports and a pharmacokinetic explanation. *Clin Pharmacol Ther* 40:518–524, 1986.

331. Talbert RL, Bussey HI: Update on calcium-channel blocking agents. *Clin Pharm* 2:403–416, 1983.

332. Thompson MJB, Russo ME, Saxon BJ, Atkinthor E, Matsem JM: Gentamicin inactivation by piperacillin or carbenicillin in patients with end stage renal dis-

ease. *Antimicrob Agents Chemother* 21:268–273, 1982.

333. Thompson PD, Melmon KL, Richardson JA, Cohn K, Steinbrunn W, Cudihee R, Rowland M: Lidocaine pharmacokinetics in advanced heart failure, liver disease, and renal failure in humans. *Ann Intern Med* 78:499–508, 1973.

334. Tilstone WJ, Semple PF, Lawson DH, Boyle JA: Effects of furosemide on glomerular filtration rate and clearance of practolol, digoxin, cephaloridine, and gentamicin. *Clin Pharmacol Ther* 22:289–294, 1977.

335. Toon S, Low LK, Gibaldi M, Trager WF, O'Reilly RA, Motley CH, Goulart DA: The warfarin-sulfinpyrazone interaction: stereochemical considerations. *Clin Pharmacol Ther* 39:15–24, 1986.

336. Tornatore KM, Kanarkowski R, McCarthy TL, Gardner MJ, Yurchak AM, Jusko WJ: Effect of chronic oral contraceptive steroids on theophylline disposition. *Eur J Clin Pharmacol* 23:129–134, 1982.

337. Touerud EL, Boobis AR, Brodie MJ, Murray S, Bennett PN, Whitmarsh V, Davies DS: Differential induction of antipyrine metabolism by rifampicin. *Eur J Clin Pharmacol* 21:155–160, 1981.

338. Twun-Barima Y, Carruthers SG: Quinidine-rifampin interaction. *N Engl J Med* 304:1466–1469, 1981.

339. Udall JA: Warfarin-chloral hydrate interaction. Pharmacological activity and clinical significance. *Ann Intern Med* 81:341–344, 1974.

340. Valette H, Apoil E: Interaction between salicylate and two loop diuretics. *Br J Clin Pharmacol* 8:592–594, 1979.

341. Valsalan VC, Cooper GL: Carbamazepine intoxication caused by interaction with isoniazid. *Br Med J* 285:261–262, 1982.

342. VanZwieten PA: The reversal of clonidine-induced hypotension by protryptyline and desipramine. *Pharmacology* 14:227–231, 1976.

343. Vasko MR, Bell RD, Daly DD, Pippenger CE: Inheritance of phenytoin hypometabolism: a kinetic study of one family. *Clin Pharmacol Ther* 27:96–103, 1980.

344. Verbeeck R, Tjandramaga TB, Mullie A: Effect of aluminum hydroxide on diflunisal absorption. *Br J Clin Pharmacol* 13:519–522, 1979.

345. Vessell E: Introduction: genetic and environment factors affecting drug response in man. *Fed Proc* 31:1253–1269, 1972.

346. Vestal RE, Kornhauser DM, Hollifield JW, Shand DG: Inhibition of propranolol metabolism by chlorpromazine. *Clin Pharmacol Ther* 25:19–24, 1979.

347. Vestal RE, Thummel KE, Musser B, Mercer GD: Cimetidine inhibits theophylline clearance in patients with chronic obstructive pulmonary disease: a study using stable isotope methodology during multiple oral dose administration. *Br J Clin Pharmacol* 15:411–418, 1983.

348. Vincent FM: Phenothiazine-induced phenytoin intoxication (letter). *Ann Intern Med* 93:56–57, 1980.

349. Waldorff S, Andersen JD, Heeboll-Nielson N, Nielsen OG, Moltke E, Sorensen U, Steiness E: Spironolactone-induced changes in digoxin kinetics. *Clin Pharmacol Ther* 24:162–167, 1978.

350. Watt AH, Stephens MR, Buss DC, Routledge PA: Amiodarone reduces plasma warfarin clearance in man. *Br J Clin Pharmacol* 20:707–709, 1985.

351. Watts RW, Hetzel DJ, Bochner F, Hallpike JF, Hann CS, Shearman DJC: Lack of interaction between ranitidine and phenytoin. *Br J Clin Pharmacol* 15:499–500, 1983.

352. Weeks CE, Conard GJ, Kvam DC, Fox JM, Chang SF, Paone RP, Lewis GP: The effect of flecainide acetate, a new antiarrhythmic, on plasma digoxin levels. *J Clin Pharmacol* 26:27–31, 1986.

353. Weber WW: The relationship of genetic factors to drug reactions. In Heyler L, Peck NM (eds): *Drug-Induced Diseases*. Amsterdam, Excerpta Medica, vol 4, 1972.

354. Weiner IM, Mudge GJ: Renal tubular mechanisms for excretion of organic acids and bases. *Am J Med* 36:743–762, 1964.

355. Weibert R, Keane W, Shapiro F: Carbenicillin inactivation of aminoglycosides in patients with severe renal failure. *Trans Am Soc Artif Intern Organs* 22:439–443, 1976.

356. Welling PG: Interactions affecting drug absorption. *Clin Pharmacokinet* 9:404–434, 1984.

357. Wesseling H, Mols-Thurkow I: Interaction of diphenylhydantoin (DPH) and tolbutamide in man. *Eur J Clin Pharmacol* 8:75–78, 1975.

358. Williams JF, Mathew B: Effect of quinidine on positive inotropic action of digoxin. *Am J Cardiol* 47:1052–1055, 1981.

359. Williams RB, Sherter C: Cardiac complications of tricyclic antidepressant therapy. *Ann Intern Med* 74:395–398, 1971.

360. Windorfer A Jr, Pringshein W: Studies on the concentration of chloramphenicol in the serum and cerebrospinal fluid of neonates, infants and small children. Reciprocal reactions between chloramphenicol, penicillin and phenobarbitone. *Eur J Pediatr* 124:129–138, 1977.

361. Wing LMH, Miners JO, Birkett DJ, Fornander T, Lillywhite K, Wanwimolruk S: Lidocaine disposition—sex differences and effects of cimetidine. *Clin Pharmacol Ther* 35:695–701, 1984.

362. Wishinsky N, Glasser EJ, Peakal S: Protein interactions of sulfonylurea compounds. *Diabetes* 2(suppl):18–25, 1962.

363. Wong YY, Ludden TM, Bell RD: Effect of erythromycin on carbamazepine kinetics. *Clin Pharmacol Ther* 33:460–464, 1983.

364. Wright JM, Stokes EF, Sweeny VP: Isoniazid-induced carbamazepine toxicity and vice versa: a double drug interaction. *N Engl J Med* 307:1325–1327, 1982.

365. Wroblewski BA, Singer WD, Whyte J: Carbamazepine-erythromycin interaction. *JAMA* 255:1165–1167, 1986.

366. Zilly W, Breimer DD, Richter E: Induction of drug metabolism in man after rifampin treatment measured by increased hexobarbital and tolbutamide clearance. *Eur J Clin Pharmacol* 9:219–227, 1975.

367. Zuidema J, Hilbers-Modderman ESM, Merkus FWHM: Clinical pharmacokinetics of dapsone. *Clin Pharmacokinet* 11:299–315, 1986.

2

Pharmacokinetic Alterations with Renal Failure and Dialysis[a]

John F. Maher, M.D.

GENERAL CONSIDERATIONS

With few exceptions, patients with acute renal failure tolerate the usual dose of a drug, *once*. The major pharmacologic problem in such patients is how much to give as a maintenance dose and at what intervals. Although impaired drug elimination predominates, pharmacokinetics are more complex than simple dose adjustment based on the fractional reduction in glomerular filtration rate. Nevertheless, restricting the use of drugs in patients with renal failure to those unequivocally necessary, reducing doses according to established guidelines, limiting the duration of therapy, measuring blood levels where available, and careful clinical monitoring for signs of toxicity would eliminate most toxicologic problems encountered. Several reviews provide detailed information and abundant references about pharmacokinetic abnormalities in renal failure (1, 5, 9, 10, 44, 70, 90, 91, 92, 112, 140).

The effectiveness and safety of drugs in renal failure depend on bioavailability, the route of elimination, the activity of metabolites, the severity of the consequences of drug or metabolite retention, alterations in the substrate and target organs, metabolic loads presented by drugs, renal adaptive changes to nephron loss, the margin of safety of the drug, and the capability of removing excesses by dialysis or hemoperfusion.

Bioavailability

Clinicians knew several decades ago that mercurial diuretics injected into the edematous lower extremities were absorbed slowly and were not as effective as when given intramuscularly or subcutaneously in the arm. Renal failure can affect gastrointestinal absorption because of higher gastric pH due to ammonia buffering, impaired transport secondary to vitamin D deficiency, or binding, for example to antacids. First pass metabolism during absorptive transit through the liver can eliminate a high fraction of absorbed drug (5). Indeed, hepatic metabolism of cancer chemotherapeutics administered intraperitoneally can prevent toxic drugs from reaching the systemic circulation allowing localized treatment. The liver is generally not overtly impaired functionally in uremic patients, but hepatic drug metabolism is often submaximal. When acute renal failure follows ischemia, hepatic perfusion may also be subnormal, limiting metabolic disposition of drugs. Concurrent drug therapy may induce cytochrome P-450 or other enzymes augmenting biotransformation, so the amount of a given drug reaching the systemic circulation is poorly predictable. When in doubt, only a modest reduction of the loading dose (10–20%) is warranted and clinical assessment can be used before commencing maintenance therapy.

The peak plasma drug concentration relates directly to the absorbed dose and inversely to the distribution space. After a bolus injection, a high drug concentration decreases rapidly as the drug distributes. Distribution occurs predominantly by diffusion, and if the rate deviates in uremic patients, it may be faster be-

[a]The opinions and assertions contained herein are those of the author and are not to be construed as official or as representing those of the Uniformed Services University of the Health Sciences or the Department of Defense.

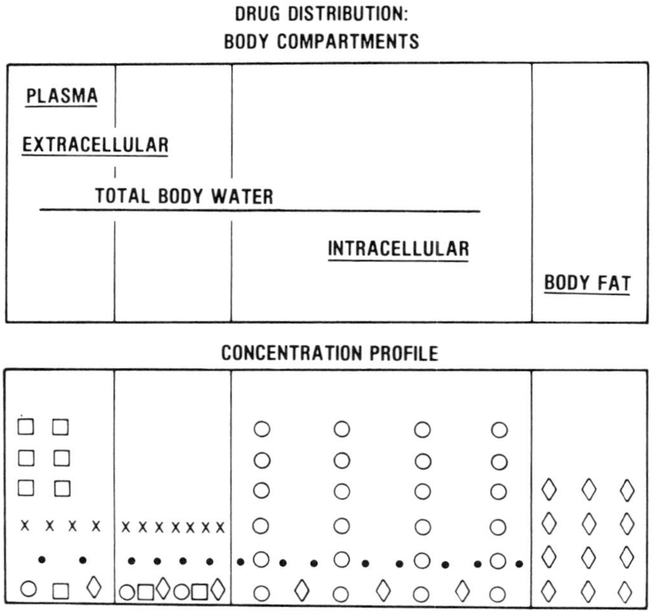

DRUG DISTRIBUTION:
BODY COMPARTMENTS

CONCENTRATION PROFILE

Figure 2.1. Illustration of potential distribution volumes of drugs and their impact on plasma concentrations. □, plasma protein bound; x, extracellular fluid; •, total body water; ○, cellular protein bound; ◇, sequestered in fat.

cause of increased capillary permeability. Following the rapid decline there is a slower (β phase) decrease in concentration that correlates with the elimination rate. Using this exponential decay curve, a theoretical peak concentration at time zero can be calculated assuming instantaneous distribution. From this value the distribution space can be calculated as volume = dose/concentration.

Distribution Space

Each solute has a characteristic distribution space (Fig. 2.1). For some solutes this approximates total body water (e.g., antipyrine). Body water is ordinarily a higher fraction of body mass in uremic patients, so peak concentration at a given dose should be lower. Other drugs (e.g., bromide) distribute in extracellular fluid, which often is increased in uremic patients. Some drugs bind to plasma proteins (e.g., phenytoin), reducing the amount available for distribution into extravascular and plasma water, the concentration with which pharmacologic and toxic effects correlate best and from which elimination occurs directly. Uremia reduces fractional plasma protein binding of many drugs. Corollaries of such reduced binding are lower plasma concentrations, higher distribu-

tion volumes, and higher plasma water concentrations, and so potentially more pharmacologic activity and toxicity and more rapid hepatic elimination. Thus, the dosing interval may need to be shortened. For drugs eliminated by the kidney, the decreased elimination rate overrides the increased availability for elimination. Some drugs are bound by cellular proteins (e.g., digoxin). Such drugs have large apparent volumes of distribution, often exceeding body mass, and low plasma concentrations. Despite high clearances these drugs are eliminated slowly because the reservoir is so large. Uremia decreases intracellular binding of digoxin, raising plasma concentrations but lowering the fraction in muscle such as myocardium. Other drugs sequester preferentially in body fat (e.g., phenothiazines). These drugs also have large apparent distribution volumes that prolong their effects. Although chronic uremia often decreases body fat, it is doubtful that such drugs distribute abnormally in acute renal failure.

Metabolic Loads Induced by Drugs

Although the drug itself may be innocuous in renal failure, it may provide an intolerable metabolic load (Table 2.1). The most quoted

Table 2.1
Metabolic Effects of Drugs

Effect	Example
Potassium excess	Penicillin
Sodium load	Kayexalate
Magnesium load	Laxatives
Calcium load	Vitamin D
Acidosis	Phenformin
Alkalosis	Carbenicillin
Nitrogen load	Tetracycline
Water retention	Morphine
Dehydration	Lithium
Cation depletion	Cis-platinum

example is hyperkalemia due to the potassium content of penicillin. Metabolic effects of drugs include depletion as well as solute excess. For example, a cation must be excreted with carbenicillin. When sodium intake is limited and homeostatic mechanisms promote sodium conservation, potassium or hydrogen ion must be excreted with carbenicillin, potentially causing hypokalemic alkalosis.

Alterations in Substrate and Target Organs

Gastrointestinal irritability in uremic patients increases the likelihood that vomiting will complicate the use of mucosal irritants. The resultant extracellular fluid volume depletion can adversely affect vital organ perfusion. Myocardial irritability also increases in uremic patients. Hence, arrhythmia is a more frequent drug complication than occurs when renal function is normal. The action of central nervous system depressants is augmented, not immediately after binephrectomy, but once azotemia has occurred. Regrettably, drug-induced sedation continues to occur in such patients and is often misinterpreted as uremia.

Many adverse drug effects in uremic patients present as dermal reactions. These may be misinterpreted as uremic dermatitis, may exaggerate uremic pruritus, and often lead to excoriation and hemorrhage.

Renal failure itself connotes the inability to achieve high renal or urinary concentrations of drugs except at the expense of high plasma levels. Thus, adequate urinary levels of antimicrobials cannot be achieved without the use of toxic doses, and often diuretics are minimally effective despite doses that cause a high incidence of toxic effects such as deafness.

Drug Elimination

Drugs are eliminated only via a few routes. Although some are eliminated by the lung (e.g., paraldehyde), and losses through the skin, gastrointestinal tract, and drainage fluids can sometimes be substantial, the kidney and the liver are the major organs of drug elimination. Artificial methods such as dialysis often add substantially to drug elimination. Hepatic elimination is usually a biotransformation process. The drug metabolite ordinarily depends on renal elimination. Such biotransformed drugs may be inactive, but active metabolites can be retained in uremia (e.g., N-acetylprocainamide) or toxic metabolites may persist (e.g., normeperidine). Thus, hepatic elimination of a drug does not assure freedom from "retention" toxicity in patients with acute renal failure.

It is a common misconception that the renal clearance of drugs decreases comparably with the decline in glomerular filtration rate. Few drugs are handled exclusively by glomerular filtration. Many undergo tubular secretion, the rate of decrement of which may differ from the fall in filtration rate. Other drugs are filtered and reabsorbed. Fractional reabsorption of many solutes decreases as renal failure progresses, maintaining excretion rates relatively well compared to glomerular filtration rate. These concepts are appreciated by recalling that potassium and phosphate excretion do not decrease as much as creatinine excretion, and without a change in production rates these solutes do not accumulate in plasma to the same extent as creatinine. Of course, in the anuric patient such compensatory mechanisms do not apply. Elimination rates are dose dependent when excretion involves a rate-limited transport mechanism for tubular secretion or reabsorption. Moreover, when drugs accumulate in uremic patients, metabolic clearance rates may decline because of enzyme saturation.

Elimination Rate, Half-life

The rate of elimination of a drug can be quantified as a clearance, expressed in units of volume/time. Conventionally, creatinine clearance is expressed in milliliters per minute, but drug clearances are often expressed as liters per kilogram per hour. The clearance indicates functional efficiency of the pertinent organ of elimination, but as an isolated parameter does not guide drug therapy. When a given clearance, e.g., 100 ml/min, removes a drug from a large distribution volume, e.g., 400 liters, the drug disappears slowly. In contrast, the same clearance value removing a drug from a 15-liter space would cause a rapid decrement in concentration. Hence, it may be preferable to express the elimination rate as a coefficient that defines the fractional removal of a drug in a given time, e.g., in 1 hour.

When half of the total quantity of the drug is removed in 1 hour and the plasma concentration (equilibrated with extravascular concentrations) decreases by 50%, the half-life of the drug is defined. The half-life is an inverse function of the removal rate and is calculated as $t_{1/2} = 0.7 \ V_d/Cl$, where V_d equals the distribution volume and Cl equals the clearance. Total body clearance cannot be measured as readily as renal clearance, which derives from the Fick principle. When neither arteriovenous difference nor the quantity excreted is available, half-life is estimated by plotting the decay slope of plasma concentrations determined serially.

Following a bolus injection, the rapid decrease in peak plasma concentration (α phase) does not represent elimination, but rather drug distribution. Unless serial sampling is done in the postdistributive phase, a falsely short half-life is estimated, a frequent error. The half-life of a drug in plasma is the major determinant of the appropriate interval for maintenance doses.

Because of their inverse relationship, halving the clearance doubles the half-life, a decrease in the clearance to one-tenth of normal causes a 10-fold increase in the half-life, and so forth. Because the margin of safety of most drugs is not very narrow (cardiac glycosides and aminoglycosides are notable exceptions), drug accumulation is only important clinically when the organ of elimination is severely impaired. When two organs contribute importantly to elimination, functional loss of one is usually insufficient to affect the half-life substantially. However, enzyme saturation kinetics or other transport ceilings may limit the adaptive increase in elimination by the healthy organ.

Dosage Adjustment in Renal Failure

Usually, maintenance doses are 50–100% of the loading dose given after one to several half-life intervals have elapsed. Administration of half the loading dose at intervals of one half-life should allow plasma concentrations to vary approximately from the peak to half that level. When the half-life is prolonged but the usual dosing interval is used, the drug accumulates in plasma, equilibrating after about six half-lives at a concentration about as many-fold increased as the extent of prolongation of the half-life.

Either the dose should be reduced or the dosing interval prolonged to adjust for impaired elimination. Because it is difficult to fractionate pills accurately, it is customary to prolong the dosing interval. Moreover, by administering a small dose, for example after the plasma level has decreased to only 90% of the peak level, the mean concentration is higher than if a 50% repletion is given after one half-life. This higher mean concentration can increase toxicity, whereas for many drugs an intermittent peak concentration achieves the desired therapeutic effect.

Drug clearance is ordinarily not measured clinically. When available, sequential plasma drug concentrations can be used to monitor therapy. Attention should be paid to the trough (predose) level, and also to the rate of decrease in concentration, a reflection of elimination efficiency. Often, dosing must be guided by a measure of organ function such as creatinine clearance. The plasma level of the endogenous metabolite, creatinine, which relates inversely to the elimination rate, is often used but is not a good estimate of renal function in patients with acute renal failure because equilibrium has not been reached. Indeed, under any circumstance of rapidly changing renal function the plasma creatinine concentration lags behind the increase or decrease in clearance. With stable chronic renal failure the plasma creatinine concentration correlates directly with the prolongation of the half-life and inversely with the elimination rate of many drugs. Because creatinine production also determines the concentration, it is not as high as anticipated for the severity of functional loss in the elderly or those with malnutrition and muscle wasting. Nevertheless, it is customary to prolong the dosing interval according to the level of plasma creatinine. For example, multiplying the serum creatinine concentration by four approximates the appropriate dosing interval in hours for gentamicin. However, it may be inadvisable to prolong the interval between doses of antibiotics more than 24 hours because of the loss of antibacterial activity. A combination of dosage reduction and interval prolongation is preferable.

Removal of Drugs and Poisons by Dialysis

The dialysis of drugs can also be considered kinetically. Solute (drug) removal rates or clearances are determined by concentration gradients and are inversely proportional to molecular mass. Blood flow rate, dialysis fluid flow rate, membrane area, and permeability determine the transfer rate of a given solute. Because of higher flow rates, hemodialysis is much more efficient than peritoneal dialysis despite a less permeable membrane. With intermittent peritoneal dialysis the urea clearance should be about 20 ml/min. For an unbound solute of undetermined transport properties, the clearance can be estimated by multiplying urea clearance by the ratio of the square root of the weight of urea to the square root of the other solute's weight. For example, a drug with a molecular mass of 400 daltons has an expected clearance of $20 \times \sqrt{60}/\sqrt{400}$ ($20 \times 7.75/20$) or 7.75 (76). Clearances by continuous ambulatory peritoneal dialysis are lower and never exceed the dialysate exchange rate, maximally 8.0 ml/min. The urea clearance with hemodialysis is usually about 150 ml/min and the decrease in clearance that occurs as solute size increases is estimated more closely as (mass urea/mass larger solute) × urea clearance than by a ratio of mass roots. With either technique, large drugs such as vancomycin and polymyxin are cleared slowly.

Protein binding limits the transport rate of many drugs (111). To adjust for binding, the clearance (estimated by solute size) should be reduced by multiplying by the ratio of unbound to total plasma drug concentration. The considerable difference in barbiturate clearances by dialysis correlates with the extent of protein binding, not the small difference in molecular mass. For drugs such as cloxacillin and furosemide that are more than 90% protein bound in plasma, removal by dialysis is negligible. This observation does not apply to reverse dialysis; rapid absorption from dialysate is not impeded by binding. There is also considerable difference in efficiency of various hemodialyzers and techniques.

Hemoperfusion is not limited appreciably by membrane transport resistance or by protein binding. Thus, when a procedure is specifically indicated for drug removal, hemoperfusion is often preferred; however, it does not correct urea retention, fluid and electrolyte abnormalities, or acid-base imbalance. Hence, dialysis continues to be preferred for some intoxications such as salicylism.

Hemofiltration clears solutes, without discrimination by size, until membrane sieving occurs as the solute size approaches that of the membrane pore. It is an effective method of removing large solutes, but not as efficient as hemodialysis in clearing small solutes. Continuous arteriovenous hemofiltration clears most drugs at a rate close to the ultrafiltration rate multiplied by the unbound fraction.

Dialysis has little impact on the course of some intoxications, not because the drug is impermeable, but rather because the distribution volume is so large. In general, this guideline is more likely to apply to those drugs eliminated by the liver; digoxin, excreted by the kidney from a very large distribution volume, is a notable exception, however. Only a small fraction of the drug circulates at any given time and is available for removal by the dialyzer.

For some drugs, removal by dialysis or hemoperfusion is faster than the intercompartmental transfer rate. This fast removal rate causes a rapid decrease in concentration within a small compartment, followed by a rebound increase as reequilibration occurs. During the procedure the quantity removed may be overestimated. Intoxicated patients often show marked clinical improvement, albeit temporary, when plasma concentrations decrease appreciably; there is little evidence to suggest that toxins sequestered in body fat stores contribute directly to toxicity.

The role of dialysis and hemoperfusion in removing poisons must also be considered in relation to pharmacodynamics (140). Intoxication by those drugs having an immediate action that does not persist (so-called hit-and-run toxins) does not respond to removal after the fact. Toxicity must be concentration dependent and sufficiently gradual to allow successful intervention.

Removal by dialysis must add significantly to the usual mode of elimination under the circumstances encountered. Aminoglycoside removal from the anuric patient by dialysis is much faster than endogenous elimination. The same removal rate has much less of an impact on the half-life of the acutely (single dose) overdosed patient who still has normal renal function. Similarly, the very slow removal rate of heavy metals by dialysis may contribute appreciably to the overall elimination rate in the anuric patient. In contrast, very rapid removal of bromide by hemodialysis is usually not necessary, since forced diuresis corrects bromism rapidly enough in most patients. In general, removal of 25% of the body burden of a drug is considered clinically significant.

PHARMACOKINETICS OF INDIVIDUAL DRUGS

The generalizations outlined above indicate that the data shown here must be interpreted thoughtfully. In the individual patient, physiologic derangements may cause deviations from the anticipated pharmacokinetics. Clinical judgment must supersede specific guidelines. The pharmacokinetic parameters listed are only approximations based on available published values. Tables 2.2 to 2.8 list data for patients with normal elimination kinetics, those with anuria, and those undergoing dialysis. For patients with renal failure and some residual function, values may be interpolated between those for anephric and normal subjects for approximations.

Penicillins (Table 2.2)

The major side effect of penicillins, hypersensitivity, is not dose dependent and may involve the kidney as an acute interstitial nephritis. Massive dosage of penicillins in patients with renal failure (or when tubular secretion is blocked, e.g., by probenecid) causes neurotoxicity with myoclonic seizures and coma. Hepatotoxicity and coagulation abnormalities are less frequent. Potassium (1.7 mEq/million units of penicillin) accumulation can also occur. Synthetic penicillins contain as much sodium as 5 mEq/g, contributing to sodium retention or inducing hypokalemic alkalosis.

The molecular mass of the penicillins ranges from about 350 to 470 daltons. Their relatively slow removal by dialysis results more from 18–95% protein binding in plasma, however. The distribution volume of the penicillins ranges from 0.13 to 0.33 liters/kg and most are eliminated predominantly by the kidney. Fortunately, there is a wide margin of safety for these very useful drugs. Knowledge of the pharmacokinetic data of penicillins (Table 2.2) may help guide therapy. Penicillin clearance is reduced considerably by acute renal failure, prolonging the half-life appreciably. Clearance by hemodialysis is somewhat more than ex-

Table 2.2
Penicillin Pharmacokinetics[a,b]

Drug	Clearance (ml/min)		Half-life (hr)				Dose (% N)[c]
	N	A	N	A	H	P	A
Penicillin	420	36	0.5	1.2	4.0	11	15
Ampicillin	270	30	1.3	14	5.0	12	50
Amoxicillin	310	40	1.2	12	3.0	10	50
Methicillin	425	50	0.6	4.0	—	—	30
Nafcillin	410	200	0.8	2.0	2.0	2.0	100
Oxacillin	400	200	0.5	1.5	1.4	—	100
Cloxacillin	150	—	0.5	1.5	—	—	75
Carbenicillin	100	11	1.2	20	8.0	14	20
Ticarcillin	120	16	1.2	14	3.5	8.8	25
Azlocillin	180	60	1.1	5.0	2.8	—	40
Piperacillin	260	60	1.2	3.5	1.9	—	75
Mecillinam	380	70	1.0	4.0	2.4	3.7	30
Temocillin	44	10	4.5	24	8.3	—	50
Mezlocillin	450	50	0.9	6.0	2.1	5.5	30

[a] Data from references 1, 2, 9, 10, 14, 18, 26, 28, 57, 68, 82, 90, 99, 115.
[b] N, normal values; A, values in anephric patients; H, values with hemodialysis; P, values with peritoneal dialysis. Interpolate values for renal failure with some residual function. For example, with 10% function add 10% of elimination rate (for penicillin $(420 - 36) = 384 \times 0.1 = 38$). This doubles clearance, decreases half-life to 6 hours, and should allow dosing at 30% of normal.
[c] Dose = percentage of normal 24-hour total dose for anephric patients.

trarenal clearance, and the combination reduces the half-life by more than 50%, but not to normal values. Penicillin toxicity may occur despite regular dialysis, and more rapid removal of this protein-bound antibiotic occurs with hemoperfusion.

The phenoxymethyl derivative, penicillin V, is absorbed better, but elimination kinetics are similar to those of penicillin G. Hetacillin, pivampicillin, bacampicillin, talampicillin, cyclacillin, and epicillin have pharmacokinetics similar to those of ampicillin (68). The isoxazolyl penicillins, oxacillin, dicloxacillin, and floxacillin, have pharmacokinetics (Table 2.2) similar to those for cloxacillin (99). Little, if any, dosage modification of these drugs is required in acute renal failure or during dialysis treatment. Ticarcillin, azlocillin, and mezlocillin have pharmacokinetics similar to those of carbenicillin (82). Clavulanic acid, an adjunct to penicillin therapy, is retained in renal failure, prolonging the half-life from 1.0

to 4.0 hours, but hemodialysis restores the elimination rate to normal (26, 57).

Cephalosporins (Table 2.3)

The cephalosporins are chemically similar to the penicillins, are excreted predominantly by the kidney by filtration and secretion, and have a broad antibacterial spectrum. Hypersensitivity reactions to cephalosporins are similar to those of penicillins, and neurotoxicity can occur with excessive accumulation. Coagulopathy correlates with a cephalosporin side chain that accumulates in uremic patients. Nephrotoxicity occurs with some congeners, especially when the drugs accumulate or there is concurrent exposure to other nephrotoxins or potent diuretics. Cephaloridine nephrotoxicity is sufficiently frequent to recommend its abandonment.

The cephalosporins have molecular masses

Table 2.3
Cephalosporin Pharmacokinetics[a]

Drug	Clearance (ml/min) N	Clearance (ml/min) A	Half-life (hr) N	Half-life (hr) A	Half-life (hr) H	Half-life (hr) P	Dose (% N) A
Cephalothin	450	30	0.6	12	3.0	5.1	30
Cefaclor	240	90	0.8	2.6	1.7	2.4	50
Cefadroxil	170	12	1.4	24	3.2	17	25
Cefamandole	320	20	1.0	12	5.5	10	25
Cefazolin	70	5.0	2.0	35	9.0	30	20
Cefixime	165	40	3.2	14.9	8.2	—	50
Cefmetazole	110	—	0.8	15	—	—	20
Cefonicid	23	2.0	5.5	65	65	—	25
Cefoperazone	80	64	2.0	2.6	2.1	2.4	80
Ceforanide	46	6.0	3.0	24	12	22	30
Cefotetan	40	16	3.6	30	6.5	16	20
Cefotiam	300	—	0.6	8.0	—	—	30
Cefotaxime	230	85	1.1	3.5	1.8	3.0	50
Cefoxitin	350	15	0.8	18	4.0	14	25
Cefroxadine	200	5.0	0.9	32	3.4	20	15
Cefsulodin	120	15	1.9	12	1.9	10	30
Ceftazidime	125	11	1.8	32	3.6	8.7	30
Ceftezole	220	—	0.6	11	—	—	30
Ceftizoxime	160	12	1.6	28	—	12	20
Ceftriaxone	15	8.0	7.0	15	10	12	80
Cefuroxime	165	10	1.4	17	3.3	12	25
Cephacetrile	330	—	1.4	25	2.0	—	20
Cephalexin	250	17	0.9	28	5.2	8.5	15
Cephapirin	270	70	0.8	2.4	1.8	2.3	80
Cephradine	360	25	1.0	15	—	13	20
Cefmenoxime	232	21	0.8	7.6	4.2	—	30
Aztreonam	90	24	1.7	8.0	2.7	7.1	50
Moxalactam	90	12	2.6	19	3.2	16	25

[a] Data from references 1, 2, 6, 9, 10, 22, 24, 25, 38, 40, 50, 59, 61, 63, 64, 70, 74, 77, 90, 97, 100, 142. See footnotes *b* and *c* of Table 2.2.

that range from about 350 to 500 daltons. Protein binding of cephalosporins in plasma, ranges from 10% to 90%, and distribution volumes are between 0.13 and 0.33 liters/kg. Renal excretion of these drugs represents 50–96% of total elimination (Table 2.3).

Peritoneal dialysis removes cephalosporins at less than half the rate of hemodialysis, so the supplemental dose should be no more than half of that following hemodialysis. Hemoperfusion clears cephalosporins much faster. Cephradine is only minimally bound to plasma proteins, so it should be removed rapidly by dialysis. Cephaloglycin, ceftotetan, and cephanone are retained in uremic patients and require dosage reduction, as do most cephalosporins. Cephoperazone and cefotaxime have the lowest fractional elimination by the kidney and are least affected by dialysis. All other cephalosporins require major dose reduction when renal failure has occurred, and an appreciable supplemental dose should be given after hemodialysis. The deacetyl metabolite of cefotaxime is active and retained in renal failure. Cephaloridine should be avoided because of the high incidence of nephrotoxicity.

Aminoglycosides (Table 2.4)

The aminoglycosides are very effective antibiotics, the use of which is limited by dose-dependent ototoxicity, nephrotoxicity, and neuromuscular blockade. Aminoglycoside nephrotoxicity is more likely with some congeners (e.g., neomycin), advancing age, prior renal dysfunction, exposure to other nephro-

toxins, or prior extracellular volume depletion. Nephrotoxicity follows renal cortical accumulation of the aminoglycosides of which the half-life is usually several days (4, 60, 69, 116). The introduction of slightly less nephrotoxic aminoglycoside congeners has not lowered the incidence of acute renal failure because of somewhat more liberal dosing of these drugs. High dosage for 1 or 2 days is not likely to cause toxicity; it is persistent administration and drug accumulation between the 10th and 20th day of treatment that usually precedes overt toxicity.

Most aminoglycosides are poorly absorbed from the gastrointestinal tract, are negligibly bound to plasma proteins (except streptomycin, which is about 30% bound), and distribute in volumes of 0.2–0.28 liters/kg. Molecular mass ranges from about 440 to 620 daltons, and excretion of aminoglycosides is more than 90% renal.

Table 2.4 lists pharmacokinetic data for most of the aminoglycosides. As a guideline, the 24-hour maintenance dose for anuric patients should be about 10% of that recommended for those with normal renal function and an additional 20% or 25% should be given after hemodialysis. Intermittent peritoneal dialysis achieves clearances of about 8 ml/min and reduces the half-life in anuric patients to about 20 hours; thus supplemental dosage, if any, should be less than half of that after hemodialysis. Continuous ambulatory peritoneal dialysis clears aminoglycosides at about 4 ml/min, so the half-life is about 30 hours. Hemoperfusion removes aminoglycosides somewhat faster than hemodialysis, but the supplemental

Table 2.4
Aminoglycoside Pharmacokinetics[a]

| Drug | Clearance (ml/min) | | Half-life (hr) | | | | Dose (% N) |
	N	A	N	A	H	P	A
Amikacin	85	1.6	2.0	60	5.0	30	15
Gentamicin	90	2.0	2.2	50	7.0	36	8
Kanamycin	78	4.0	2.4	55	6.0	30	10
Netilmicin	70	5.0	2.5	45	6.0	22	8
Streptomycin	80	2.0	2.3	70	5.0	30	10
Tobramycin	79	4.0	2.2	55	5.0	35	10
Dibekacin	96	4.3	2.3	42	3.7	—	—
Sisomicin	—	—	2.7	50	—	—	—
Lividomycin	—	—	2.0	44	—	—	—
Paromomycin[b]	—	—	2.0	40	—	—	—
Neomycin[b]	—	—	2.0	24	9.0	—	—

[a] Data from references 1, 9, 10, 23, 27, 88, 90, 102, 110, 116. See footnotes b and c of Table 2.2.
[b] Restricted to oral use.

Table 2.5
Half-lives of Miscellaneous Antibiotics and Antimicrobials[a]

Drug	Half-life (hr)			Dose (% N)
	N	A	H	A
Tetracycline	8.0	70	>30	10
Chlortetracycline	6.0	8.0	—	60
Demeclocycline	13	70	>30	15
Doxycycline	18	21	—	80
Minocycline	16	24	—	80
Oxytetracycline	9.0	60	>30	15
Colistimethate	4.0	15	14	20
Polymyxin B	4.0	36	35	10
Sulfisoxazole	6.0	12	6.0	50
Sulfamethoxazole	11	25	12	40
Sulfadiazine	10	22	11	50
Trimethoprim	12	27	25	50
Chloramphenicol	3.0	4.5	4.2	80
Clindamycin	3.0	3.2	3.2	100
Lincomycin	4.5	12	10	60
Vancomycin	6.0	200	120	10
Erythromycin	1.6	5.0	4.5	80
Imipenem	1.0	3.7	2.5	30
Fosfomycin	1.5	15	3.0	25
Ciprofloxacin	4.5	11	3.2	50
Ethambutol	3.0	10	5.0	30
Isoniazid[b]	1.0, 3.5	5.0, 12	1.5, 5.0	60
Rifampin	3.5	4.0	4.0	100
p-Aminosalicylate	1.0	20	18	10
Amphotericin B	24	24	24	90
Flucytosine	4.0	120	10	10
Ketoconazole	2.4	2.1	—	100
Miconazole	22	22	—	100
Acyclovir	2.4	20	5.5	20
Amantadine	12	200	—	10
Metronidazole	7.0	9.0	3.0	80
Ornidazole	12	11	6.0	100
Tinidazole	13	14	4.3	100

[a] Data from references, 1, 9, 10, 15, 19, 23, 33, 40, 42, 45, 49, 52, 54, 56, 65, 69, 77, 84, 90, 95, 96, 103, 112, 113, 123, 127, 137. See footnotes b and c of Table 2.2.
[b] Data are given for rapid and slow isoniazid acetylators.

dose can be the same after this briefer procedure. Despite dosage adjustment there is an appreciable incidence of nephrotoxicity, but it is usually milder. Netilmicin appears to be the safest drug for uremic patients.

Other Antibiotics (Table 2.5)

The tetracyclines should be avoided, if possible, in patients with renal failure (124). Doxycycline is the least likely to aggravate azotemia. Molecular masses of tetracyclines average about 450 daltons. Most are more than 60% bound in plasma, predicting low clearances by dialysis. Distribution volumes of tetracyclines are high (1.0–1.9 liters/kg), and renal excretion varies from 10% to 50% of the total elimination

rate (54). Demeclocycline inhibits renal tubular free water reabsorption, potentially causing dehydration or removing retained water in patients with inappropriate antidiuretic hormone secretion. Hemoperfusion can remove toxic accumulations of tetracyclines.

Renal and neural toxicity are major drawbacks to therapy with the polymyxins, a group of polypeptides of which colistimethate and polymyxin B are the least toxic (56). Dosage should be kept below 2.0 mg/kg/day in anuric patients. Because of their large molecular size, these drugs are removed slowly by dialysis.

Most sulfonamides are well absorbed from the gastrointestinal tract, bind highly to proteins in plasma (50–90%), and distribute in volumes that can range from 0.15 to 0.60 liters/kg. Elimination of both free and acetylated sulfonamides is predominantly renal, so half-lives are prolonged in uremic patients (137). Alkalinization of the urine increases the renal clearance and decreases the likelihood of nephrotoxicity due to crystalline precipitates. Sulfonamides and their numerous chemical derivatives are important causes of acute interstitial nephritis. Uremia decreases protein binding of sulfonamides, hence hemodialyzer clearance in patients with renal failure decreases the half-life appreciably.

Chloramphenicol is eliminated predominantly by hepatic conjugation. The glucuronide conjugate persists in renal failure with a half-life of about 100 hours but is not considered toxic to the bone marrow. Protein binding in plasma (55%), albeit decreased in uremia, inhibits removal by dialysis (127). Chloramphenicol distributes in a volume of 0.9 liters/kg. The dose must be reduced substantially with hepatic failure.

Clindamycin is about 95% bound in plasma and distributes in 0.7 liters/kg from which it is rapidly cleared, mostly by the liver. Neither renal failure nor dialysis affects the half-life appreciably (103). The clearance by hemoperfusion may exceed 100 ml/min. Lincomycin has similar pharmacokinetics.

Imipenim accumulates in renal failure and is rapidly removed by dialysis (42). Cilastin, which inhibits the enzymatic catabolism of imipenim, is even more dependent on renal elimination and readily dialyzed.

Vancomycin, a large solute (molecular mass about 1800 daltons), is about 10% bound in plasma and distributes slowly into a volume of about 0.6 liters/kg. Elimination is almost exclusively renal, and the dose should be decreased in anuric patients from 1.0 g every 12 hours to 1.0 g every 7 days to avoid nephrotoxicity (84). Dialysis removes vancomycin very slowly.

Erythromycin (734 daltons) is moderately absorbed when given orally, distributes in 0.7 liters/kg, and is 70% bound in plasma. Elimination is mostly hepatic and neither renal failure nor dialysis should affect pharmacokinetics appreciably; ototoxicity correlates with modest accumulation (96).

Novobiocin pharmacokinetics are not changed substantially by renal failure or dialysis. Fosfomycin is retained in renal failure but removed by dialysis. The dose in anuric patients should be reduced (113). Bacitracin is too nephrotoxic for systemic use. When absorbed, it is cleared mostly by the kidney and is poorly dialyzable.

Long-term use of tuberculostatic drugs can be complicated in renal failure. Isoniazid is biotransformed by acetylation, and elimination is only modestly affected by renal failure (45). Hemodialysis doubles the elimination rate, so a supplement is required thereafter. Rifampin is highly protein bound and distributes in a large volume. Neither renal failure nor dialysis affects elimination kinetics sufficiently to warrant dosage modification (112). Ethambutol distributes in a large volume, is minimally bound in plasma, and is rapidly excreted by the kidney. The dose should be reduced when renal failure occurs, and a supplemental dose given after dialysis. Cycloserine is excreted by the kidney and removed by dialysis. P-Aminosalicylate should be avoided in anuric patients; it is retained in uremic patients and removed by dialysis. Both pyrazinamide and viomycin depend on renal elimination whereas ethionamide does not.

In general, urinary antiseptics should be avoided in patients with advanced renal failure. Nitrofurantoin accumulates in uremic patients and can cause peripheral neuropathy (32). Methenamine mandelate, nalidixic acid, norfloxacin, pipemidic acid, and ascorbic acid are each retained somewhat with renal failure and exaggerate metabolic acidosis. Phenazopyridine is potentially nephrotoxic and depends on renal elimination. Elimination of cinoxacin is delayed in patients with renal failure, decreasing efficacy and potentially causing toxicity.

Miscellaneous Antimicrobials (Table 2.5)

The fungicide, amphotericin B, causes dose-dependent nephrotoxicity but does not depend on the kidney for elimination. Dose reduction is not required with preexistent renal failure, but often the dose is somewhat limited because there is no leeway for a further renal functional loss. The development or progression of azotemia warrants dose reduction or cessation if possible. Because acute renal failure induced by amphotericin B can be irreversible, the drug should be continued only for serious fungal infection once renal failure occurs. The normal half-life is several days and negligible amounts of amphotericin are removed by dialysis.

Renal failure prolongs the half-life of 5-fluorocytosine from 5 to 100 hours, so the maintenance dose in anuric patients should be curtailed sharply. Because dialysis removes this drug rapidly, a supplement of about 15% of the usual daily maintenance dose should be given thereafter (13). Miconazole is eliminated mainly by the liver and is about 90% bound in plasma (130). Neither renal failure nor dialysis appreciably alters the pharmacokinetics of miconazole or ketoconazole.

Chloroquine normally has a long half-life and is eliminated predominantly by the liver, but somewhat slower in uremic patients (112). Modest dosage reduction is required with severe renal failure. The elimination of chloroguanide is delayed somewhat in uremic patients. Primaquine is rapidly biotransformed but the metabolite is active. Guidelines for dosage reduction are not established. Pyrimethamine has a long half-life and may be retained in anuric patients. The half-life of trimethoprim increases in uremic patients, and modest dosage reduction is advisable (10). The liver hydroxylates quinine and the 6-hour half-life is not prolonged in uremic patients. Hemodialysis improves quinine intoxication (34).

Dapsone and other sulfones used for leprosy are excreted mostly by the kidney, so dosage reduction is advisable (1). Clofazimine (another antileprosy agent) has a large distribution volume and a long half-life minimally affected by renal failure.

Pentamidine distributes rapidly into tissues, where it persists for months (10). Chronic use should be at a lower dosage in uremic patients but short-term therapy is probably unaffected by renal failure.

Amantidine, an antiviral agent, accumulates in uremic patients and can induce arrhythmias and neuropsychiatric toxicity (143). Hemodialysis reduces the half-life toward normal. Acyclovir is excreted in the urine, retained in uremia, and rapidly removed by dialysis (123).

Thiabendazole (used for strongyloidiasis) and mebendazole (for echinococcosis) are eliminated mainly by the liver. Neither renal failure nor dialysis affects their pharmacokinetics appreciably (118).

Sedatives, Tranquilizers, and Psychotherapeutic Drugs (Table 2.6)

The long-acting barbiturates are excreted by the kidney and rapidly cleared by hemodialysis. Barbital accumulates in uremic patients, distributes into a small volume, binds minimally in plasma, and is removed rapidly by hemodialysis. Renal excretion of phenobarbital is increased by alkaline diuresis and ac-

Table 2.6
Half-lives of Sedatives and Analgesics[a]

Drug	Half-life (hr)		
	N	A	H
Phenobarbital	80	110	9
Secobarbital	25	30	18
Pentobarbital	30	35	18
Chloral hydrate[b]	30/7	—	4
Chlordiazepoxide	10	12	11
Diazepam	40	65	60
Oxazepam	10	25	24
Nortriptyline	23	25	23
Metoclopramide	4.2	14	13.6
Bromide	24	—	2
Lithium	22	50	4
Salicylate	12	—	4
Acetaminophen	2.5	2.5	1.6
Ibuprofen	2	2	2
Naproxen	17	17	17
Phenylbutazone	80	60	—
Piroxicam	45	44	—
Sulfinpyrazone	25	95	—
Propoxyphene	12	12	11
Morphine	2.0	1.8	—

[a] Data from references 3, 7, 8, 9, 10, 17, 39, 40, 55, 90, 117, 120, 140, 141. See footnotes b and c of Table 2.2.
[b] Trichlorethanol, the active metabolite of chloral hydrate, has a 7-hour half-life.

counts for about 25% of total elimination. The dosage of phenobarbital should be limited with renal failure. Intoxication can mimic uremic coma and responds to hemodialysis or more slowly to peritoneal dialysis (120). Elimination is impeded by 20% protein binding and a distribution volume of 0.9 liters/kg. Secobarbital and pentobarbital (preferentially distributed in body fat and about 35% bound in plasma) are short-acting and eliminated predominantly by hepatic biotransformation, but can aggravate uremic lethargy and coma. Removal by either forced diuresis or dialysis is relatively slow. Thiopental, which is ultrashort-acting, rapidly distributes in body fat. Although eliminated by metabolism, thiopental narcosis is prolonged by uremia, and protein binding decreases. Amobarbital and butabarbital are intermediate in their elimination rates by dialysis, protein binding, lipid partition, and duration of action. Lipid-soluble, protein-bound barbiturates are cleared faster by hemoperfusion through resin or charcoal columns (140). Decreased protein binding, saturation of metabolic biotransformation processes, and retention of conjugates argue for some dosage reduction of all barbiturates in uremic patients, and careful observation for signs of oversedation.

The benzodiazepines are all highly bound to proteins in plasma and undergo hepatic biotransformation. Although the metabolites have long half-lives and depend on renal elimination, most of these drugs are well tolerated by uremic patients (112). Chlordiazepoxide, diazepam, and flurazepam have active metabolites whereas the metabolites of lorazepam and oxazepam are inactive. Multiple dosing prolongs the half-life of benzodiazepines. Uremia decreases protein binding of benzodiazepines, and may increase the large distribution volumes and impair the rate of hepatic biotransformation. Although dosage does not usually have to be restricted, the patients should be observed for signs of metabolic encephalopathy. Hemoperfusion should remove the benzodiazepines at clearances of 100–150 ml/min, which is faster than achieved by hemodialysis, 5–60 ml/min.

Chloral hydrate circulates about 50% bound to plasma proteins and is biotransformed to trichlorethanol, an active metabolite eliminated by the liver and the kidney (17). Hemodialysis rapidly clears both chloral hydrate and trichlorethanol.

Glutethimide is about 50% bound in plasma, distributes into a large volume (about 3 liters/kg), and is eliminated mainly by saturable hepatic metabolism (89). Hemodialysis decreases the half-life appreciably but hemoperfusion clears glutethimide more rapidly (140). Neither forced diuresis nor peritoneal dialysis affects pharmacokinetics appreciably.

Ethchlorvynol, about 40% bound in plasma and distributed in a volume of 4 liters/kg, is also eliminated mainly by hepatic metabolism. Removal by hemodialysis or peritoneal dialysis can decrease the normal 25-hour half-life, but hemoperfusion clears it even faster (132, 140).

Meprobamate is only about 20% bound in plasma, and has a distribution volume approximating total body water and a half-life of about 10 hours. About 20% is excreted unchanged by the liver, while the remainder is biotransformed. Modest reduction of dosage is warranted with renal failure, and overdosage responds to dialysis or hemoperfusion (85, 140).

Methyprylon undergoes predominantly extrarenal elimination, so dosage reduction is not required in uremic patients. Intoxication responds to either dialysis or hemoperfusion (101).

Methaqualone intoxication responds well to hemoperfusion. Clearances by dialysis are considerably lower because 80% is bound in plasma (140). Elimination is hepatic from a volume of about 6 liters/kg with a 25-hour half-life.

Uremia increases susceptibility to paraldehyde acidosis, but elimination is mostly hepatic and some unchanged drug is expired (51). Paraldehyde intoxication responds to dialysis.

The phenothiazines, such as chlorpromazine, avidly bind to plasma and tissue proteins and are highly lipophilic. Elimination is slow by hepatic metabolism (9). Uremic patients have increased susceptibility to extrapyramidal myoclonus and toxic psychosis from these drugs. Because distribution volumes may be as high as 20 liters/kg, neither dialysis nor hemoperfusion removes appreciable quantities of phenothiazines.

Amitriptyline, nortriptyline, imipramine, and their congeners also avidly bind to plasma proteins, are highly lipophilic, and distribute in volumes of about 10 liters/kg. Elimination of the tricyclic antidepressants is by hepatic metabolism and only a small fraction is removed by dialysis of hemoperfusion, although transient clinical improvement may occur (9). Active conjugated hydroxymetabolites are retained in uremic patients (83).

The pharmacologic effects of monoamine oxidase inhibitors such as phenelzine persist after the drugs or their active metabolites are eliminated. These drugs are not retained in uremic patients. Although clinical improvement has occurred with dialysis, there is no pharmacokinetic rationale for such treatment (140).

The central dopaminergic antagonist, metoclopramide, is an antiemetic that is retained in renal failure because of decreased renal and nonrenal clearance. Haloperidol (another dopaminergic antagonist) has a long half-life that depends only moderately on renal function.

Sodium bromide is eliminated from extracellular fluid by the kidney at a clearance below 2 ml/min. It accumulates in patients retaining salt, e.g., in heart failure, cirrhosis, or nephrotic syndrome, and is eliminated faster in salt-losing nephritis, with diuretics, and possibly in patients with polyuric renal failure. When administered to anuric patients it accumulates and can cause psychosis, and is rapidly removed by dialysis (117).

Lithium salts accumulate in renal failure and are eliminated rapidly by forced diuresis or dialysis. Toxicity correlates with total body lithium, not with the plasma concentration, and includes neuromuscular irritability and nephrogenic diabetes insipidus with distal tubular necrosis. With chronic excess, the distribution volume expands and reequilibrates slowly with plasma as dialysis rapidly lowers concentrations (62).

Analgesics (Table 2.6)

Salicylates are small solutes, distributed in a volume of 15% of body weight and as much as 50% bound in plasma (9). Their pharmacokinetics are complex. The kidney excretes salicylate and several metabolites and accumulation can occur with renal failure, causing such problems as prolonged bleeding. Dialysis removes salicylates rapidly and corrects the metabolic abnormalities of salicylism. The half-life of salsalate, a salicylate precursor, increases from 1.2 to 2.1 hours with renal failure. Diflunisal, a difluorophenyl salicylate, is more than 99% bound in plasma and thus is poorly filtrable and not dialyzable. Its metabolite is unstable and depends on renal elimination.

Phenacetin and its major metabolite, acetaminophen, are biotransformed by the liver, but the conjugates accumulate in uremic plasma (44). Hemodialysis and hemoperfusion remove these drugs rapidly, but not as fast as hepatic clearance (139). Acute overdosage should be treated by N-acetylcysteine infusion to prevent hepatic necrosis.

Most nonsteroidal antiinflammatory drugs are highly bound to plasma proteins, do not depend on renal elimination, and have inactive metabolites. With renal failure, fractional protein binding may decrease, raising the metabolic clearance and shortening the half-life. Toxic renal syndromes include acute renal ischemia, hyperkalemic acute interstitial nephritis, nephrotic syndrome, tubular necrosis, and papillary necrosis (21). Inhibition of prostaglandin synthetase and hypersensitivity contribute to these lesions. Indomethacin has biphasic elimination with half-lives of 1–9 hours, unaffected by renal failure. Tolmetin, ibuprofen, fenoprofen, and mefenamic acid have short half-lives negligibly influenced by renal failure or dialysis. Naproxen, piroxicam, and phenylbutazone have long half-lives that decrease somewhat with renal failure. Sulfinpyrazone is excreted by the kidney and accumulates in patients with renal failure.

Propoxyphene is eliminated by the liver and dosage adjustment is not necessary in uremic patients. The distribution volume is large (10–25 liters/kg). Dialysis and hemoperfusion remove some propoxyphene, but hepatic metabolism is faster (39).

The half-life of antipyrine is shorter in uremic patients than in normal subjects, a paradox attributed to hepatic microsomal induction since the distribution volume does not change.

Pentazocine is oxidized and conjugated in the liver. Uremic patients do not require dosage modification.

The opiates rapidly distribute into a large volume and are eliminated by hepatic biotransformation (136). Although opiates are not retained in uremic patients, increased sensitivity to standard dosage often occurs. Morphine intolerance relates to a decreased distribution volume raising plasma levels and to retention of active glucuronide metabolites (141). Morphine is partially removed by dialysis. Methadone is used in uremic patients without complications since it is about 85% bound in plasma and eliminated by the liver. Caution is advised with codeine since standard doses can cause narcosis in patients with renal failure. About 10% of meperidine is excreted by the kidney, while most of the drug degrades rapidly in the liver to normeperidine, which accumulates in uremic patients and induces convulsions (131).

Cardiovascular Drugs (Table 2.7)

Digitalis toxicity is a frequent, serious problem in patients with renal failure. Emphasis should be on control of salt and water intake in patients with renal failure rather than on liberal use of digitalis.

Ouabain is rapidly excreted by the kidney and accumulates in uremic patients (119). Plasma protein binding is negligible and the large distribution space decreases with uremia. Dialysis removes a modest fraction of ouabain. Digitalis is excreted more slowly from a large volume and accumulates in uremic patients.

Digoxin is well absorbed, is about 25% bound in plasma, and distributes in a volume of 9 liters/kg. Absorption is slower and delayed by aluminum hydroxide in uremic patients, but peak concentrations are higher because the distribution space is about 50% smaller. The number of binding sites and their affinity for digoxin are decreased in patients with renal failure. Excretion is predominantly renal and the maintenance dose should be decreased in uremic patients to 20–35% of the usual. Digoxin dosage based on formulas depending on

Table 2.7
Half-lives of Cardiovascular Drugs[a]

Drug	Half-life (hr)		
	N	A	H
Ouabain	16	60	45
Digoxin	40	120	100
Digitoxin	155	165	160
Hydralazine	4.0	11	10
Methyldopa	6.0	15.6	9.5
Clonidine	12	40	24
Minoxidil	4	4	—
Propranolol	3.9	3.6	3.6
Nadolol	19	45	28
Sotalol	7	50	8
Practolol	9	60	14
Atenolol	6	60	6
Metoprolol	3.5	3.5	2.5
Labetalol	4.5	5.5	5.0
Lidocaine	1.7	2.0	—
Procainamide	3	13	6
Quinidine	7	10	9.0
Disopyramide	7	18	13
Bretylium	8	32	13
Thiazides	1.5	5.0	—
Furosemide	0.7	3.0	2.3
Amiloride	6.0	80	—
Diltiazem	5.0	3.4	3.4
Nifedipine	2.5	2.6	2.6
Verapamil	5.0	3.7	3.7

[a] Data from references 9, 10, 31, 36, 41, 48, 58, 63, 71, 73, 90, 93, 107, 119, 122, 134. See footnote b of Table 2.2.

creatinine clearance, body weight, and distribution volume are not fully reliable, so therapy should be guided by plasma level determinations (36). Toxicity is frequent at concentrations about 3.0 ng/ml, or lower if hypercalcemia or hypokalemia is present. Removal by dialysis is too slow to improve intoxication, but hemoperfusion can be useful (43). (Dialysis may precipitate digitalis intoxication by correcting protective metabolic abnormalities.)

Digitoxin is extensively metabolized by hepatic microsomal enzymes, the kidney excreting mostly inactive metabolites. It is highly bound in plasma and normally has a long half-life that is affected only slightly by renal failure or dialysis (63). Hemoperfusion removes appreciable amounts of digitoxin (121).

ANTIHYPERTENSIVE AGENTS

Uremic patients often require antihypertensive agents despite control of salt and water balance by limiting intake and by ultrafiltration. The blood pressure response is generally the best guide to dosage of antihypertensives, but complications may accompany accumulation of drugs or metabolites.

Reserpine distributes in a large volume and is eliminated partly unchanged by the kidney and partly after metabolic hydrolysis. The long half-life (80 hours) doubles in renal failure but dialysis has little effect (144). Reserpine toxicity can mimic uremia.

Hydralazine is about 85% bound in plasma, distributes in a volume of 1.6 liters/kg, and is eliminated mainly by hepatic acetylation (9). Increased concentrations in uremic patients may represent a retained metabolite. The effect of dialysis appears to be minimal.

Prazosin distributes in a volume of 1.6 liters/kg and protein binding in plasma exceeds 90%. The half-life of about 3 hours increases modestly with renal failure and should not be influenced by dialysis, but the blood pressure response may be increased in uremic patients (87).

Methyldopa undergoes hepatic conjugation, and the metabolite is eliminated by the kidney (98). This biphasic elimination occurs with half-lives of 2 hours and 6 hours. In uremic patients, the metabolite is retained but hepatic biotransformation accelerates. Dialysis removes 30–40% of an administered dose, decreasing the half-life appreciably.

Clonidine distributes in a volume of about 3.0 liters/kg and is about 30% bound in plasma. Elimination is predominantly renal, but usually only modest dosage reduction to 25–50% of normal is necessary in patients with renal failure (58).

Guanfacine has properties similar to clonidine, but is biotransformed and does not accumulate in uremic patients. The half-life is about 15 hours in normal subjects and in uremic patients. The hemodialyzer clearance of 53 ml/min adds only 15% of the elimination rate (72).

Guanethidine distributes into a large space from which it is slowly removed by both hepatic metabolism and renal excretion. The normal half-life of several days is prolonged in anuric patients. The effects of renal failure and dialysis require further quantification.

The ganglionic blockers, hexamethonium, mecamylamine, and tetraethylammonium, depend primarily on the kidney for elimination. Blood pressure reduction should be titrated using lower doses than usual when patients have renal failure.

Minoxidil is cleared from a distribution volume approaching 3 liters/kg by hepatic conjugation, with a half-life of 3–4 hours (48). Accumulation is not expected in uremic patients and the effects of dialysis are unknown. Minoxidil is often effective for patients with renal failure who have resistant hypertension.

Diazoxide effectiveness correlates with the level of the unbound drug. Protein binding occurs rapidly and normally exceeds 90%, a value that decreases in uremic patients. Renal failure, however, does not appreciably change the long half-life in plasma, but dialysis may decrease it (106).

Nitroprusside is rapidly metabolized to thiocyanate, which depends on renal elimination, can cause psychosis and hypothyroidism, and is eliminated rapidly by dialysis.

Captopril is eliminated by the liver and the kidney with a half-life of about 2 hours, which increases appreciably with renal failure, prolonging the antihypertensive effect (29). Hemodialysis decreases the half-life to 4 hours. Captopril may decrease renal blood flow, aggravating uremia and hyperkalemia. The half-life of enalapril is normally 8.4 hours and increases to 10.9 hours in renal failure (125). Its antihypertensive effects are comparable with those of captopril but it has a more salutary effect on renal blood flow. Saralasin has a very short half-life since it is metabolized by aminopeptidases. The α-adrenergic blockers, phentolamine and phenoxybenzamine, depend on both hepatic and renal elimination. Doxazosin has a half-life of 9.5 hours, minimally prolonged by renal failure and uninfluenced by dialysis (20).

The β-adrenergic blockers do not have uniform pharmacokinetics (31, 73, 134). Propranolol is more than 90% bound in plasma, distributes in a large volume, and is eliminated by hepatic metabolism. In uremic patients the half-life is slightly shorter because of a decreased distribution volume, but active hydroxy-metabolites persist in plasma and are cleared rapidly by dialysis. Nadolol is removed by the kidney and by dialysis. The dose for anuric patients is 25% of the normal. Pindolol, only partially eliminated by the kidney with a 3.5-hour half-life, does not accumulate in uremic patients. Sotalol accumulates in patients with renal failure but is removed rapidly by dialysis. Atenolol also depends on renal elimination; it accumulates in uremic patients, mandating a dose reduction to 25% of normal, and is cleared rapidly by hemodialysis. Practolol has similar pharmacokinetics. Acebutolol and metoprolol are eliminated by hepatic bio-

transformation, but their metabolites accumulate in uremic patients and are removed by dialysis. Labetolol is rapidly biotransformed by the liver. The elimination half-lives of several other β-blockers (alprenolol, bufuralol, mepindolol, terazosin, timolol, and tolamolol) are not prolonged by renal failure.

ANTIARRHYTHMIC AGENTS

The antiarrhythmic, lidocaine, is eliminated from a large distribution volume almost entirely by the liver. Its half-life is not appreciably affected by uremia or dialysis (133). Tocainamide, a longer acting lidocaine analogue, is retained somewhat in renal failure and is cleared by dialysis (138). Lorcainide does not accumulate in uremic patients.

Procainamide is eliminated by both hepatic acetylation and renal excretion. The half-life is prolonged with renal failure and the active N-acetyl metabolite is retained as well, so the dose should be reduced to about 20% of the normal, or the drug avoided (41). A small supplement is warranted after dialysis. N-Acetyl procainamide may accumulate despite modest removal by hemodialysis, and hemoperfusion can be required to treat toxicity.

Quinidine distributes in a large space and is about 75% bound in plasma. Hepatic elimination is not delayed in uremic patients, but metabolites accumulate (71). Hemodialysis clears quinidine slowly, but has induced improvement in intoxicated patients.

Disopyramide, about 30% bound in plasma and distributed in a volume approaching 1.0 liter/kg, is partly eliminated by the kidney, accumulates with renal failure, and is modestly affected by dialysis (66). Bretylium depends mostly on renal excretion. It has a low molecular weight, is minimally bound, and is rapidly removed by dialysis (67). Mexiletine elimination is mostly independent of renal function. The half-life increases from about 11 to 15 hours with renal failure and is not reduced by dialysis because of 70% plasma protein binding and a large distribution volume. The half-life of cibenzoline is approximately doubled with renal failure, whereas amiodarone elimination is not affected by uremia or by dialysis.

The calcium channel blocking agents, diltiazem, nifedipine, and verapamil, are all highly protein bound in plasma, distribute in large volumes, and are rapidly metabolized by the liver. Dialysis does not remove these drugs or their metabolites appreciably.

DIURETICS

As renal failure progresses, diuretics become less effective but tend to be given in higher doses, causing more toxicity. Mannitol accumulates in uremic patients and can precipitate circulatory congestion with pulmonary edema, hyperosmolality, hypernatremia, and intracellular dehydration. Organic mercurials depend on renal elimination and are contraindicated in patients with renal failure. Acetazolamide is tightly bound to carbonic anhydrase in tissues and is excreted by the kidney (112). It is retained in uremic patients and may aggravate metabolic acidosis. Thiazides are not effective when renal failure is moderate or severe and are eliminated by the kidney (9). Chlorthalidone has a long half-life and is eliminated by both renal and nonrenal mechanisms. Ethacrynic acid may induce saluresis but often only after high doses with the risk of ototoxicity (81). Elimination is partly hepatic and partly renal. Like other loop diuretics, ethacrynic acid is highly protein bound. Furosemide can also induce a clinically effective diuresis, despite renal failure and potential ototoxicity (81). It accumulates in patients with renal failure or cirrhosis and is not readily removed by dialysis because of high fractional protein binding, which is reduced somewhat by uremia. Piretanide is eliminated in part by the kidney; the half-life is prolonged from 0.7 to 2.8 hours with renal failure (11). Bumetanide accumulation is minimal in renal failure, however, because decreased protein binding accelerates nonrenal clearance (104). Torazemide is not retained in renal failure or removed by dialysis (86). The major problem with these potent diuretics is their overzealous use in an attempt to achieve diuresis in depleted patients who instead should be repleted. Spironolactone is less effective in patients with renal failure, but the risk of hyperkalemia is increased (1). It is rapidly biotransformed by the liver to active metabolites that may accumulate in uremic patients. Triamterene also is a less effective saluretic in uremic patients but may cause hyperkalemia. Elimination is predominantly hepatic but hydroxy-metabolites accumulate and may be pharmacologically active. Amiloride depends on renal elimination and accumulates in uremic patients (37). Protein binding limits the removal of most diuretics by dialysis.

Table 2.8
Half-lives of Miscellaneous Drugs[a]

Drug	Half-life (hr)		
	N	A	H
Theophylline	6.2	7.3	2.6
Dyphylline	2.0	11.9	5.5
Cortisone	1.3	3.5	3.4
Prednisolone	3.2	4.2	4.2
Cyclophosphamide	6.0	7.0	2.5
Bleomycin	3.0	22	—
Tolbutamide	5.0	5.0	5.0
Chlorpropamide	30	200	150
Phenytoin	16	8.0	7.6
Valproic acid	12	10	8.3
Propylthiouracil	17	50	—
Methimazole	2.0	9.0	—
Organic iodides	1.0	30	4.2
Cimetidine	1.9	4.3	2.5
Ranitidine	2.0	7.0	4.3
Clofibrate	17	100	—
Gallamine	2.2	12.5	6.0
Atracurium	0.3	0.4	—
Vecuronium	1.3	1.6	—
Pancuronium	2.2	4.3	—
Metocurine	6.0	11.4	—

[a] Data from references 1, 9, 12, 16, 44, 53, 78, 79, 90, 105, 114, 135. See footnote b Table 2.2.

Miscellaneous Drugs (Table 2.8)

Theophylline is eliminated mainly by the liver and does not accumulate with renal failure. Despite appreciable protein binding it is rapidly removed by hemodialysis, which doubles the elimination rate, and by peritoneal dialysis. Hemoperfusion clears theophylline even faster than dialysis. Dyphylline has a high renal clearance, accumulates in uremic patients, and is rapidly cleared by dialysis (79). Terbutaline is metabolized by the liver with a normal half-life of about 1.2 hours.

Allopurinol is rapidly metabolized to oxipurinol, which inhibits xanthine oxidase. Oxipurinol is slowly excreted by the kidney and accumulates in uremic patients, so the allopurinol dose should not exceed 300 mg/day (30). Oxipurinol is readily dialyzable. Colchicine is very rapidly eliminated even in uremic patients. Probenecid is more slowly eliminated. Although it is metabolized before excretion, this drug should be avoided in uremic patients.

Adrenal corticosteroids are removed metabolically and dosage does not have to be restricted in uremic patients, although azotemia is aggravated by inhibition of anabolism by these drugs.

Cyclophosphamide is mostly biotransformed in the liver, yet with renal failure its half-life increases slightly. Dosage reduction is usually required because of the potential severity of toxicity and because of active metabolites rather than concern for retention of the parent compound (135). Cyclophosphamide is cleared rapidly by dialysis. Other alkylating agents, such as chlorambucil, mechlorethamine, melphalan, and busulfan, are metabolized and uninfluenced by renal failure or dialysis.

Azathioprine is rapidly cleaved nonenzymatically to 6-mercaptopurine and oxidized (44). Although not retained in patients with renal failure, other considerations often warrant dosage reduction in uremic patients. Dialysis increases azathioprine elimination minimally.

Methotrexate is eliminated mainly by renal excretion (9, 44). This drug accumulates in renal failure, and binding in plasma decreases. Hence, both peak and trough concentrations increase, so the dose must be decreased and the dosing interval prolonged. Methotrexate is not effectively removed by dialysis, but hemoperfusion rapidly lowers plasma levels. The nitrosoureas, carmustine, lomustine, and streptozocin, can be nephrotoxic. Their elimination is hepatic but active metabolites can be retained in uremic patients. The pyrimidine analogues, 5-fluorouracil and cytosine arabinoside, are rapidly metabolized. Renal failure does not delay elimination and the large distribution spaces limit removal by dialysis. Bleomycin accumulates in uremic patients, causing increased cutaneous and gastrointestinal toxicity (105). It is not removed by dialysis. Doxorubicin and daunorubicin are eliminated by the liver, do not accumulate in uremic patients, but can cause renal injury (44). Mithramycin is eliminated by the kidney and can be nephrotoxic.

Cyclosporine is a large, highly bound solute that distributes into body fat. Renal elimination is minimal and removal by dialysis is insignificant (109). The normal half-life is 7 hours. Bredinin is another new immunosuppressive drug used for transplants, which depends on renal elimination and is rapidly removed by dialysis.

Many organic compounds of heavy metals accumulate in patients with renal functional impairment and cause further renal injury. Such compounds include arsenicals, antimonials, gold compounds, bismuth preparations, iron-dextran, and cis-platinum. Chelates accelerate removal of some of these metals, which are normally highly bound in plasma and tissue (91, 108). Chelates can accumulate and can also be nephrotoxic.

Uremic patients have delayed elimination of insulin and peripheral resistance to its action (35). They have increased sensitivity to the oral hypoglycemic agents. Tolbutamide is the preferred oral hypoglycemic agent because it does not depend on renal elimination and is not removed appreciably by dialysis (128). The metabolites of tolazamide and acetohexamide cause hypoglycemia and depend on renal elimination. Chlorpropamide, about 90% bound in plasma, accumulates in uremic patients causing recurrent hypoglycemia and is not removed appreciably by dialysis (128). The biguanides, phenformin and buformin, are rapidly excreted by the kidney. Phenformin is no longer recommended because it causes lactic acidosis.

Phenytoin is eliminated by oxidation, conjugation, and renal excretion of the metabolite. Uremia decreases protein binding, reducing the distribution space and accelerating elimination. Phenytoin is well tolerated in uremic patients, and usually no dosage adjustment is required. Excessive phenytoin can be slowly removed by dialysis since binding is decreased. This slow removal helps clinically, because saturation kinetics limit metabolic removal at high concentrations (16).

Trimethadione and paramethadione are eliminated by the liver. Valproic acid undergoes β oxidation. Dosage modification is not required for any of these drugs. Carbamazepine is normally eliminated slowly, and hemodialyzer clearance exceeds the endogenous removal rate (80). Ethosuximide has similar pharmacokinetics, including a relatively high clearance by dialysis.

Neither heparin nor the oral anticoagulants, bishydroxycoumarin, warfarin, or phenindione, depends on renal elimination; dialysis does not augment their elimination (9, 44). Caution is advised with anticoagulant use, not because of abnormal pharmacokinetics, but because of the bleeding diathesis and lesions of uremia. Dipyridamole elimination is not influenced by uremia or dialysis. Thrombolytic agents are inactivated in circulation and are not known to be affected by uremia.

Propylthiouracil is excreted in part by the kidney and accumulates in uremic patients, hence dosage reduction is warranted (1). Methimazole is also retained in the plasma of uremic patients. The effect of dialysis on these antithyroid drugs is unknown.

Iodide is excreted by the kidney in competition with thyroidal uptake. Povidone-iodine absorbed locally can contribute to iodine retention. Iodinated radiographic contrast media accumulate in patients with renal failure, can accelerate renal functional loss, and can be removed by dialysis (53).

Cimetidine is eliminated mostly by the kidney, excretion correlating with creatinine clearance. In patients with severe renal failure, the dose must be reduced by 50% to prevent toxic symptoms that mimic uremic encephalopathy (75). Hemodialysis removes cimetidine (and its sulphoxide metabolite) rapidly, but hemoperfusion clears it even faster, while peritoneal clearance does not accelerate elimination appreciably. Cimetidine inhibits renal secretion of creatinine, raising plasma levels acutely. Ranitidine has similar pharmacokinetics (114). The dose of either histamine blocker should be reduced about 50% with renal failure.

Clofibrate is excreted by the kidney partly unchanged and partly after hepatic conjugation. Dosage reduction is mandatory in uremic patients, and removal by dialysis is slow because of extensive protein binding (46). Bezafibrate and fenofibrate are new hypolipemic drugs that are retained in patients with renal failure and are highly protein bound, preventing removal by dialysis.

Preexisting renal functional impairment predisposes to further nephron injury by the fluorinated anesthetics, enflurane and methoxyflurane (126). Atropine also depends in part on renal elimination, and caution is advised in prescribing it to uremic patients (47). Dialysis has negligible effects on its elimination kinetics.

The neuromuscular relaxant, gallamine, depends on renal excretion; it accumulates in renal failure, prolonging neuromuscular blockade, and can be removed by dialysis. Vecuronium and atracurium have short half-lives that are not prolonged with renal failure (12). Laudanosine, a metabolite of atracurium, accumulates in uremic patients, however, and stimulates the central nervous system. Pancuronium and metocurine accumulate to a moderate extent with renal failure. D-Tubocurarine also depends on renal elimination. Fazadinium and norcuron are metabolized.

Pyridostigmine depends on renal excretion. The metabolites of neostigmine and of succinylcholine are active and accumulate in patients with renal failure.

Even vitamins must be considered pharmacokinetically in uremic patients (94, 129). Vitamin C depletion can occur with renal failure, and losses are accelerated by dialysis. However, excessive supplementation of ascorbic acid leads to accumulation and metabolic breakdown that can contribute to the oxalosis of uremia. The B vitamins are water soluble and removed by dialysis. Only modest reduction in plasma concentrations occur (5–30%) with hemodialysis, and because of its large molecular size vitamin B_{12} traverses dialysis membranes slowly. Pyridoxine is the only B vitamin that requires supplementation in nourished uremic patients, the need arising from incomplete activation or a retained inhibitor. Folic acid is low in plasma but usually normal in erythrocytes, and plasma riboflavin levels are variably low. Chronic uremia often requires 1,25-dihydroxycholecalciferol supplements because of inadequate renal metabolic activation of vitamin D. Toxicity can ensue from excessive supplements. Vitamin A supplements can also cause toxicity, although much of the increment in measured levels represents retinol-binding protein.

CONCLUSIONS

When selecting a drug for the uremic patient, it is preferable to choose an agent that does not depend mainly on renal excretion, is minimally affected by changes in protein binding, distribution volume, or receptor sensitivity, and does not have active or toxic metabolites.

Critically ill patients often have hemodynamic abnormalities that impair metabolic clearance, as well as renal excretion. Accordingly, in these patients drug use should be restricted to definite indications, dosing must be monitored carefully following pharmacokinetic principles, and patients must be monitored carefully for drug toxicity, which must be considered whenever unexplained abnormalities occur. Those who rely blindly on nomograms and "cookbook" guidelines for dosing have no business administering potentially toxic drugs to patients with abnormal elimination mechanisms.

References

1. Anderson RJ, Bennett WM, Gambertoglio JG, Schrier RW: Fate of drugs in renal failure. In Brenner BM, Rector FC Jr (eds): *The Kidney*. Philadelphia, WB Saunders, 1981, pp 2659–2708.

2. Andrassy K, Ritz E: Antimicrobial therapy in dialysis patients. I. Penicillins and cephalosporins. *Blood Purif* 3:94–103, 1985.
3. Anttila M, Haataja M, Kasanen A: Pharmacokinetics of naproxen in subjects with normal and impaired renal function. *Eur J Clin Pharmacol* 18:263–268, 1980.
4. Appel GV, Neu HC: The nephrotoxicity of antimicrobial agents. *N Engl J Med* 296:663–670, 722–728, 784–787, 1977.
5. Atkinson AJ Jr, Kushner W: Clinical pharmacokinetics. *Annu Rev Pharmacol Toxicol* 19:105–127, 1979.
6. Balant L, Dayer P, Rudhardt M, Allaz AF, Fabre J: Cefoperazone: pharmacokinetics in humans with normal and impaired renal function and pharmacokinetics in rats. *Clin Ther* 3:50–59, 1980.
7. Balogh A, Funfstuck R, Demme U, Kangas L, Sperschneider H, Traeger A, Stein G, Pekkarinen A: Dialysability of benzodiazepines of haemodialysis and controlled sequential ultrafiltration (CSU) in vitro. *Arch Pharmacol Toxicol* 49:174–180, 1981.
8. Bateman DN, Gokal R, Dodd TRP, Blain PG: The pharmacokinetics of single doses of metoclopramide in renal failure. *Eur J Clin Pharmacol* 19:437–441, 1981.
9. Benet LZ, Sheiner LB: Design and optimization of dosage regimens; pharmacokinetic data. In Gilman AG, Goodman LS, Rall TW, Murad F (eds): *Goodman and Gilman's The Pharmacological Basis of Therapeutics*, ed 7. New York, MacMillan, 1985, pp 1663–1733.
10. Bennett WM, Muther RS, Parker RA, Feig P, Morrison G, Golper TA, Singer I: Drug therapy in renal failure: dosing guidelines for adults. *Ann Intern Med* 93:62–89, 286–325, 1980.
11. Berg KH, Walstad RA, Bergh K: The pharmacokinetics and diuretic effects of piretanide in chronic renal insufficiency. *Br J Clin Pharmacol* 15:347–353, 1983.
12. Bevan DR, Donati F, Gyasi H, Williams A: Vecuronium in renal failure. *Can Anaesth Soc J* 31:491–496, 1984.
13. Block ER, Bennett JE, Levoti LG, Klein WJ, MacGregor RR, Henderson L: Flucytosine and amphotericin B: hemodialysis effects on the plasma concentration and clearance. *Ann Intern Med* 80:613–617, 1974.
14. Boelaert J, Daneels R, Schurgers M, Mellows G, Suaisland AJ, Lambert AM, Van Landuyt HW: Effects of renal functions and dialysis on temocillin pharmacokinetics. *Drugs* 29(suppl 5):109–113, 1985.
15. Boelaert J, Valcke Y, Schurgers M, Daneels R, Rosseel MT, Bogaert MG: The pharmacokinetics of ciprofloxacin in patients with impaired renal function. *J Antimicrob Chemother* 16:87–93, 1985.
16. Borgå O, Hoppel C, Odar-Cederlof I, Garle M: Plasma levels and renal excretion of phenytoin and its metabolites in patients with renal failure. *Clin Pharmacol Ther* 26:306–314, 1979.
17. Breimer DD: Clinical pharmacokinetics of hypnotics. *Clin Pharmacokinet* 2:93–109, 1977.
18. Brogard JM, Comte F, Spach MO, Lavillaureix J: Pharmacokinetics of mezlocillin in patients with kidney failure: special reference to hemodialysis and dosage adjustments in relation to renal function. *Chemotherapy* 29:318–326, 1982.
19. Bunke CM, Aronoff GR, Brier ME, Sloan RS, Luft FC: Vancomycin kinetics during continuous ambulatory peritoneal dialysis. *Clin Pharmacol Ther* 334:631–637, 1983.
20. Carlson RV, Bailey RR, Begg EJ, Cowlishaw MG, Sharman JR: Pharmacokinetics and effect on blood pressure of doxazosin in patients with renal failure. *Clin Pharmacol Ther* 40:561–566, 1986.
21. Carmichael J, Shankel SW: Effects of nonsteroidal antiinflammatory drugs on prostaglandins and renal function. *Am J Med* 78:992–1000, 1985.
22. Chodos J, Francke EL, Saltzman M, Neu HC: Pharmacokinetics of intravenous cefotaxime in patients undergoing chronic hemodialysis. *Ther Drug Monitor* 3:71–74, 1981.
23. Christopher TG, Blair AD, Forrey AW, Cutler RE: Hemodialyzer clearances of gentamicin, kanamycin, tobramycin, amikacin, ethambutol, procainamide, and flucytosine with a technique for planning therapy. *J Pharmacokinet Biopharm* 4:427–441, 1976.
24. Cohen D, Appel GB, Scully B, Neu HC: Pharmacokinetics of ceftriaxone in patients with renal failure and in those undergoing hemodialysis. *Antimicrob Agents Chemother* 24:529–432, 1983.
25. Craig WA, Welling PG, Jackson TC, Kunin CM: Pharmacology of cephazolin and other cephalosporins in patients with renal insufficiency. *J Infect Dis* 128:S347–S353, 1973.
26. Dalet F, Amado E, Cabrera E, Donate T, del Rio G: Pharmacokinetics of the combination of ticarcillin with clavulanic acid in renal insufficiency. *J Antimicrob Chemother* 17(suppl C):57–64, 1986.
27. Danish M, Schultz R, Jusko WJ: Pharmacokinetics of gentamicin and kanamycin during hemodialysis. *Antimicrob Agents Chemother* 6:841–847, 1974.
28. De Schepper PJ, Tjandramaga TB, Mullie A, Verbesselt R, van Hecken A, Verbeckmoes R, Verbist L: Comparative pharmacokinetics of piperacillin in normals and in patients with renal failure. *J Antimicrob Chemother* 9(suppl B):49–57, 1982.
29. Duchin KL, Pierides AM, Heald A, Singhvi SM, Rommel AJ: Elimination kinetics of captopril in patients with renal failure. *Kidney Int* 25:942–947, 1984.
30. Elion GB, Benezra FM, Beardmore TD, Kelley WN: Studies with allopurinol in patients with impaired renal function. *Adv Exp Med Biol* 122A:263–267, 1980.
31. Fabre J, Fox HM, Dayer P, Balant L: Differences in kinetic properties of drugs: implications as to the selection of a particular drug for use in patients with renal failure with special emphasis on antibiotics and β-adrenoceptor blocking agents. *Clin Pharmacokinet* 5:441–464, 1980.
32. Felts JH, Hayes DM, Gergen JA, Toole JF: Neural, hematologic and bacteriologic effects of nitrofurantoin in renal insufficiency. *Am J Med* 51:331–339, 1971.
33. Flouvat BL, Imbert C, Dubois DM, Temperville BP, Roux AF, Chevalier GC, Humbert G: Pharmacokinetics of tinidazole in chronic renal failure and in patients on haemodialysis. *Br J Clin Pharmacol* 15:735–741, 1983.
34. Floyd M, Hill AVL, Ormston BJ, Menzies R, Porter R: Quinine amblyopia treated by hemodialysis. *Clin Nephrol* 2:44–46, 1974.
35. Fuss M, Bergans A, Brauman H, Toussaint C, Vereerstraeten P, Franckson M, Corvilain J: ^{125}I-insulin metabolism in chronic renal failure treated by renal transplantation. *Kidney Int* 5:372–377, 1974.
36. Gault MH, Jeffrey JR, Chiruto E, Ward LL: Studies of digoxin dosage, kinetics and serum concentrations in renal failure and review of the literature. *Nephron* 17:161–187, 1976.
37. George CF: Amiloride handling in renal failure. *Br J Clin Pharmacol* 9:94–95, 1980.
38. Gerig JS, Bolton N, Swabb EA, Scheld WM, Bolton WK: Effect of hemodialysis and peritoneal dialysis on aztreonam pharmacokinetics. *Kidney Int* 26:308–318, 1984.
39. Giacomini KM, Gibson TP, Levy G: Effect of hemodialysis on propoxyphene and norpropoxyphene concentrations in blood of anephric patients. *Clin Pharmacol Ther* 27:508–514, 1980.
40. Gibson TP: Renal disease and drug metabolism: an overview. *Am J Kidney Dis* 8:7–17, 1986.
41. Gibson TP, Atkinson AJ Jr, Matusik E, Nelson LD, Briggs WA: Kinetics of procainamide and N-acetylprocainamide in renal failure. *Kidney Int* 12:422–429, 1977.
42. Gibson TP, Demetriades JL, Bland JA: Imipenem/cilastin pharmacokinetic profile in renal insufficiency. *Am J Med* 78(suppl 6A):54–61, 1985.

43. Gibson TP, Lucas SV, Nelson HA, Atkinson AJ Jr, Okita GR, Ivanovich P: Hemoperfusion removal of digoxin from dogs. *J Lab Clin Med* 91:673–682, 1978.

44. Gibson TP, Nelson HA: Drug kinetics and artificial kidneys. *Clin Pharmacokinet* 2:403–426, 1977.

45. Gold CH, Buchanan N, Tringham V, Viljoen M, Strickwold B, Moodley GP: Isoniazid pharmacokinetics in patients in chronic renal failure. *Clin Nephrol* 6:365–369, 1976.

46. Goldberg AP, Sherrard DJ, Haas LB, Brunzell JD: Control of clofibrate toxicity in uremic hypertriglyceridemia. *Clin Pharmacol Ther* 21:317–325, 1977.

47. Gosselin RE, Gabourel JD, Wills JH: Fate of atropine in man. *Clin Pharmacol Ther* 1:597–603, 1960.

48. Gotlieb TB, Thomas RC, Chidsey CA: Pharmacokinetic studies of minoxidil. *Clin Pharmacol Ther* 13:436–441, 1972.

49. Guay DR, Meatherall RC, Baxter H, Jacyk WR, Penner B: Pharmacokinetics of metronidazole in patients undergoing continuous ambulatory peritoneal dialysis. *Antimicrob Agents Chemother* 25:306–310, 1984.

50. Guay DRP, Meatherall RC, Harding GK, Brown GR: Pharmacokinetics of cefixime (CL 284, 635; FK 027) in healthy subjects and patients with renal insufficiency. *Antimicrob Agents Chemother* 30:485–490, 1986.

51. Gutman RA, Burnell MJ, Solak F: Paraldehyde acidosis. *Am J Med* 42:440–455, 1967.

52. Halstenson CE, Blevins RB, Salem NG, Matzke GR: Trimethoprim-sulfamethoxazole pharmacokinetics during continuous ambulatory peritoneal dialysis. *Clin Nephrol* 22:239–243, 1984.

53. Hansson R, Lindholm T: Elimination of hypaque (sodium 3,5 diacetamido-2,4,6 triiodobenzoate) and the effect of hemodialysis in anuria. A clinical study and an experimental investigation on rabbits. *Acta Med Scand* 174:611–626, 1963.

54. Heaney D, Eknoyan G: Minocycline and doxycycline kinetics in renal failure. *Clin Pharmacol Ther* 24:233–239, 1978.

55. Held H, Enderle C: Elimination and serum protein binding of phenylbutazone in patients with renal insufficiency. *Clin Nephrol* 6:388–393, 1976.

56. Hoeprich PD: The polymyxins. *Med Clin North Am* 54:1257–1265, 1970.

57. Horber FF, Frey FJ, Descoludres C, Murray AT, Reubi FC: Differential effects of impaired renal function on the kinetics of clavulanic acid and amoxicillin. *Antimicrob Agents Chemother* 29:614–619, 1986.

58. Hulter HN, Licht JH, Ilnicki LP, Singh S: Clinical efficacy and pharmacokinetics of clonidine in hemodialysis and renal insufficiency. *J Lab Clin Med* 94:223–231, 1979.

59. Humbert G, Fillastre JP, Leroy A, Godin M, Van Winzum C: Pharmacokinetics of cefoxitin in normal subjects and in patients with renal insufficiency. *Rev Infect Dis* 1:118–126, 1979.

60. Humes HD, Weinberg JM, Knauss TC: Clinical and physiologic aspects of aminoglycoside toxicity. *Am J Kidney Dis* 2:5–29, 1982.

61. Jacobson EJ, Zahrowski JJ, Nissenson AR: Moxalactam kinetics in hemodialysis. *Clin Pharmacol Ther* 30:487–490, 1981.

62. Jaeger A, Sauder P, Kopferschmitt J, Jaegle ML: Toxicokinetics of lithium intoxication treated by hemodialysis. *J Toxicol Clin Toxicol* 23:501–517, 1986.

63. Jeliffe RW, Buell J, Kalaba R, Sridhar R, Rockwell R, Wagner JG: An improved method of digitoxin therapy. *Ann Intern Med* 72:453–464, 1970.

64. Johnson CA, Zimmerman SW, Rogge M: The pharmacokinetics of antibiotics used to treat peritoneal dialysis-associated peritonitis. *Am J Kidney Dis* 4:3–17, 1984.

65. Johnson RJ, Blair AD, Ahmad S: Ketoconazole kinetics in chronic peritoneal dialysis. *Clin Pharmacol Ther* 37:325–329, 1985.

66. Johnston A, Henry JA, Warrington SJ, Hamer NAJ: Pharmacokinetics of oral disopyramide phosphate in patients with renal impairment. *Br J Clin Pharmacol* 10:245–248, 1980.

67. Josselson J, Narang PK, Adir J, Yacobi A, Sadler JH: Bretylium kinetics in renal insufficiency. *Clin Pharmacol Ther* 33:144–150, 1983.

68. Jusko WJ, Lewis GP, Schmitt GW: Ampicillin and hetacillin pharmacokinetics in normal and anephric subjects. *Clin Pharmacol Ther* 14:90–99, 1973.

69. Keller F, Lode H, Offerman G: Antimicrobial therapy in dialysis patients. II. Remaining antibiotics and antimicrobial agents. *Blood Purif* 3:104–108, 1985.

70. Keller F, Offerman G, Lode H: Supplementary dose after hemodialysis. *Nephron* 30:220–227, 1982.

71. Kessler KM, Lowenthal DT, Warner H, Gibson T, Briggs W, Reidenberg MM: Quinidine elimination in patients with congestive heart failure or poor renal function. *N Engl J Med* 290:706–709, 1974.

72. Kirch W, Kohler H, Axthelm T: Pharmacokinetics of guanfacine in patients undergoing haemodialysis. *Eur J Drug Metab Pharmacokinet* 7:277–280, 1982.

73. Klooker P, Bommer J, Ritz E: Treatment of hypertension in dialysis patients. *Blood Purif* 3:15–26, 1985.

74. Konishi K: Pharmacokinetics of cefmenoxime in patients with impaired renal function and in those undergoing hemodialysis. *Antimicrob Agents Chemother* 30:901–905, 1986.

75. Larsson R, Erlanson P, Bodemar G, Walan A, Bertler A, Fransson L, Norlander B: The pharmacokinetics of cimetidine and its sulphoxide metabolites in patients with normal and impaired renal function. *Br J Clin Pharmacol* 13:163–170, 1982.

76. Lasrich M, Maher JM, Hirszel P, Maher JF: Correlation of peritoneal transport rates with molecular weight: a method for predicting clearances. *asaio J* 2:107–113, 1979.

77. Lee CS, Marbury TC: Drug therapy in patients undergoing haemodialysis. Clinical pharmacokinetic considerations. *Clin Pharmacokinet* 9:42–66, 1984.

78. Lee CS, Peterson JC, Marbury TC: Comparative pharmacokinetics of theophylline in peritoneal dialysis and hemodialysis. *J Clin Pharmacol* 23:274–280, 1983.

79. Lee CS, Wang LH, Majeske BL, Marbury TC: Pharmacokinetics of dyphylline elimination by uremic patients. *J Pharmacol Exp Ther* 217:340–344, 1981.

80. Lee CS, Wang LH, Marbury TC, Bruni J, Perchalski RJ: Hemodialysis clearance and total body elimination of carbamazepine during chronic hemodialysis. *Clin Toxicol* 17:429–438, 1980.

81. Levin NW: Furosemide and ethacrynic acid in renal insufficiency. *Med Clin North Am* 55:107–119, 1971.

82. Libke RD, Clarke JT, Ralph ED, Luthy RP, Kirby WMM: Ticarcillin vs carbenicillin: clinical pharmacokinetics. *Clin Pharmacol Ther* 17:441–446, 1975.

83. Lieberman JA, Cooper TB, Suckow RF, Steinberg H, Borenstein M, Brenner R, Kane JM: Tricyclic antidepressant and metabolite levels in chronic renal failure. *Clin Pharmacol Ther* 37:301–307, 1985.

84. Lindholm DD, Murray JS: Persistence of vancomycin in the blood during renal failure and its treatment by hemodialysis. *N Engl J Med* 274:1047–1051, 1966.

85. Lobo PI, Spyler D, Surratt P, Westervelt FB Jr: Use of hemodialysis in meprobamate overdosage. *Clin Nephrol* 7:73–75, 1977.

86. Loute G, Adam A, Ers P, Heremans C, Willems B: The influence of haemodialysis and haemofiltration on the clearance of torazemide in renal failure. *Eur J Clin Pharmacol* 31(suppl):53–55, 1986.

87. Lowenthal DT, Hobbs D, Affrime MB, Twomey TM, Martinez EW, Onesti G: Prazosin kinetics and effectiveness in renal failure. *Clin Pharmacol Ther* 27:779–783, 1980.

88. Luft FC, Brannon DR, Stropes LL, Costello RJ, Sloan RS, Maxwell DR: Pharmacokinetics of netilmicin in patients with renal impairment and in patients on dialysis. *Antimicrob Agents Chemother* 14:403–407, 1978.

89. Maher JF: Determinants of serum half life of gluteth-imide in intoxicated patients. *J Pharmacol Exp Therap* 174:450–455, 1970.

90. Maher JF: Pharmacological aspects of renal failure and dialysis. In Drukker W, Parsons FM, Maher JF (eds): *Replacement of Renal Function by Dialysis*. The Hague, Martinus Nijhoff, 1983, pp 749–797.

91. Maher JF: Toxic and irradiation nephropathies. In Earley LE, Gottschalk CW (eds): *Strauss and Welt's Diseases of the Kidney*. Boston, Little, Brown & Co, 1979, pp 1431–1474.

92. Manuel MA, Paton TW, Cornish WR: Drugs and peritoneal dialysis. *Peritoneal Dial Bull* 3:117–125, 1983.

93. Martre H, Sari R, Taburet AM, Jacobs C, Singlas E: Haemodialysis does not affect the pharmacokinetics of nifedipine. *Br J Clin Pharmacol* 20:115–158, 1985.

94. Marumo F, Kamata K, Okubo M: Deranged concentrations of water-soluble vitamins in the blood of undialyzed and dialyzed patients with chronic renal failure. *Int J Artif Intern Organs* 9:17–24, 1986.

95. Merdjan H, Baumelou A, Diquet B, Chick O, Singlas E: Pharmacokinetics of ornidazole in patients with renal insufficiency; influence of haemodialysis and peritoneal dialysis. *Br J Clin Pharmacol* 19:211–217, 1985.

96. Mery A, Kanfer A: Ototoxicity of erythromycin in patients with renal insufficiency. *N Engl J Med* 301:944, 1979.

97. Moellering RC Jr, Swartz MN: The newer cephalosporins. *N Engl J Med* 294:24–28, 1976.

98. Myhre E, Rugstad HE, Arnold E, Stenback O, Hansen T: Pharmacokinetics of methyldopa in renal failure and bilaterally nephrectomized patients. *Scand J Urol Nephrol* 16:257–263, 1982.

99. Nauta EH, Mattie H: Dicloxacillin and cloxacillin pharmacokinetics in healthy and hemodialysis subjects. *Clin Pharmacol Ther* 20:98–108, 1976.

100. Ohkawa M, Kuroda K: Pharmacokinetics of ceftezole in patients with normal and impaired renal function. *Chemotherapy* 26:242–247, 1980.

101. Pancorbo AS, Palagi PA, Piecoro JJ, Wilson HD: Hemodialysis in methyprylon overdose; some pharmacokinetic considerations. *JAMA* 237:470–471, 1977.

102. Pechere J, Dugal R: Pharmacokinetics of intravenously administered tobramycin in normal volunteers and in renal-impaired and hemodialyzed patients. *J Infect Dis* 134:S118–S124, 1976.

103. Peddie BA, Dann E, Bailey RR: The effect of impairment of renal function and dialysis on the serum and urine levels of clindamycin. *Aust NZ J Med* 5:198–202, 1975.

104. Pentikäinen PJ, Pasternak A, Lampainen E, Neuvonen PJ, Penttila A: Bumetanide kinetics in renal failure. *Clin Pharmacol Ther* 37:582–588, 1985.

105. Pitrilli ES, Castaldo TW, Matutat RJ, Ballon SC, Gutierrez ML: Bleomycin pharmacology in relation to adverse effects and renal function in cervical cancer patients. *Gynecol Oncol* 14:350–354, 1982.

106. Pohl JEF, Thurston H: Use of diazoxide in hypertension with renal failure. *Br Med J* 4:142–145, 1971.

107. Pozet N, Brazier JL, Hadj Aissa A, Khenfer D, Faucon G, Apoil E, Traeger J: Pharmacokinetics of diltiazem in severe renal failure. *Eur J Clin Pharmacol* 24:635–638, 1983.

108. Prestayko AW, Luft FC, Einhorn L, Crooke ST: Cisplatin pharmacokinetics in a patient with renal dysfunction. *Med Pediatr Oncol* 5:183–188, 1978.

109. Ptachcinski RJ, Venkataramanan R, Burckart GJ: Clinical pharmacokinetics of cyclosporin. *Clin Pharmacokinet* 11:107–132, 1986.

110. Regeur L, Golding H, Jensen H, Kaupmann JP: Pharmacokinetics of amikacin during hemodialysis and peritoneal dialysis. *Antimicrob Agents Chemother* 11:214–218, 1977.

111. Reidenberg MM: The binding of drugs to plasma proteins and the interpretation of measurements of plasma concentrations of drugs in patients with poor renal function. *Am J Med* 62:467–474, 1977.

112. Reidenberg MM: *Renal Function and Drug Action.* Philadelphia, WB Saunders, 1971, p 113.

113. Revert L, Lopez J, Pons J, Olag T: Fosfomycin in patients subjected to periodic hemodialysis. *Chemotherapy* 23(suppl 1):204–209, 1977.

114. Roberts AP, Harrison C, Dixon GT, Curtis JR: Plasma ranitidine concentrations after intravenous administration in normal volunteers and haemodialysis patients. *Postgrad Med J* 59:25–27, 1983.

115. Schapira A: Single dose kinetics and dosage of mecillinam in renal failure and haemodialysis. *Clin Pharmacokinet* 9:364–370, 1984.

116. Schentag JJ, Cerra FB, Plaut ME: Clinical and pharmacokinetic characteristics of aminoglycoside toxicity in 201 critically ill patients. *Antimicrob Agents Chemother* 21:721–726, 1982.

117. Schmitt GW, Maher JF, Schreiner GE: Ethacrynic acid enhanced bromuresis. A comparison with peritoneal and hemodialysis. *J Lab Clin Med* 68:913–922, 1966.

118. Schumaker JD, Band JD, Lensmeyer GL, Craig WA: Thiabendazole treatment of severe strongyloidiasis in a hemodialyzed patient. *Ann Intern Med* 89:644–645, 1978.

119. Selden R, Haynie G: Ouabain plasma level kinetics and removal by dialysis in chronic renal failure. A study in fourteen patients. *Ann Intern Med* 83:15–19, 1975.

120. Setter JG, Freeman RB, Maher JF, Schreiner GE: Factors influencing the dialysis of barbiturates. *Trans Am Soc Artif Intern Organs* 10:340–344, 1964.

121. Shah G, Nelson HA, Atkinson AJ Jr, Okita GT, Ivanovich P, Gibson TP: Effect of hemoperfusion on the pharmacokinetics of digitoxin in dogs. *J Lab Clin Med* 93:370–380, 1979.

122. Shah GM, Winer RL: Verapamil kinetics during maintenance hemodialysis. *Am J Nephrol* 5:338–341, 1985.

123. Shah GM, Winer RL, Krasny HC: Acyclovir pharmacokinetics in a patient on continuous ambulatory peritoneal dialysis. *Am J Kidney Dis* 7:507–510, 1986.

124. Shils ME: Renal disease and the metabolic effects of tetracycline. *Ann Intern Med* 58:389–408, 1963.

125. Shionoiri H, Miyazaki N, Yasuda G, Sugimoto K, Uneda S, Kaneko Y: Blood concentration and urinary excretion of enalapril in patients with chronic renal failure. *Nippon Jinzo Gakkai Shi* 27:1291–1297, 1985.

126. Sievenpiper TS, Rice SA, McClendon F, Kosek JC, Mazze RI: Renal effects of enflurane anesthesia in Fischer rats with preexisting renal insufficiency. *J Pharmacol Exp Ther* 211:36–41, 1979.

127. Slaughter RL, Cerra FB, Koup JR: Effect of hemodialysis on total body clearance of chloramphenicol. *Am J Hosp Pharm* 37:1083–1086, 1980.

128. Smith DL, Vecchio TI, Forist AA: Metabolism of antidiabetic sulfonylureas in man. *Metabolism* 14:229–240, 1965.

129. Stein G, Sperschneider H, Koppe S: Vitamin levels in chronic renal failure and need for supplementation. *Blood Purif* 33:52–62, 1985.

130. Stevens DA, Levine HB, Deresinski SC: Miconazole in coccidioidomycosis. II. Therapeutic and pharmacologic studies in man. *Am J Med* 60:191–202, 1976.

131. Szeto HH, Inturrisi CE, Houde R, Saal S, Cheigh J, Reidenberg MM: Accumulation of normeperidine, an active metabolite of meperidine in patients with renal failure or cancer. *Ann Intern Med* 86:738–741, 1977.

132. Teehan BP, Maher JF, Carey JJH, Flynn PD, Schreiner

GE: Acute ethchlorvynol (Placidyl^R) intoxication. *Ann Intern Med* 72:875–882, 1970.

133. Thomson PD, Melmon KL, Richardson JA, Cohn K, Steinbrunn W, Cudihee R, Rowland M: Lidocaine pharmacokinetics in advanced heart failure, liver disease and renal failure in humans. *Ann Intern Med* 78:499–508, 1973.

134. Tjandramaga TB: Altered pharmacokinetics of β-adrenoreceptor blocking drugs in patients with renal insufficiency. *Arch Int Pharmacodyn Ther* 248(suppl):38–53, 1980.

135. Wang LH, Lee CS, Majeske BL, Barbury TC: Clearance and recovery calculations in hemodialysis: application to plasma, red blood cell and dialysate measurements for cyclophosphamide. *Clin Pharmacol Ther* 29:365–372, 1981.

136. Wang T, Wuellner D, Woosley RL, Stone WJ: Pharmacokinetics and nondialyzability of mexilitine in renal failure. *Clin Pharmacol Ther* 37:649–653, 1985.

137. Weinstein L, Madoff MA, Samet CM: The sulfonamides. *N Engl J Med* 263:793–800, 842–849, 1960.

138. Wiegers U, Hanrath P, Kuck KH, Pottage A, Graffner C, Augustin J, Runge M: Pharmacokinetics of tocainide

in patients with renal dysfunction and during haemodialysis. *Eur J Clin Pharmacol* 24:503–507, 1983.

139. Winchester JR, Gelfand MC, Helliwell M, Vale JA, Goulding R, Schreiner GE: Extracorporeal treatment of salicylate or acetaminophen poisoning—is there a role? *Arch Intern Med* 141:370–374, 1981.

140. Winchester JF, Gelfand MC, Knepshield JH, Schreiner GE: Dialysis and hemoperfusion of poisons and drugs update. *Trans Am Soc Artif Intern Organs* 23:762–842, 1977.

141. Woolner DF, Winter D, Frendin TJ, Begg EJ, Lynn KL, Wright GJ: Renal failure does not impair the metabolism of morphine. *Br J Clin Pharmacol* 22:55–59, 1986.

142. Wright N, Wise R, Hegarty T: Ceftotetan elimination in patients with varying degrees of renal dysfunction. *J Antimicrob Chemother* 11(suppl A):213–216, 1983.

143. Wu MJ, Ing TS, Soung LS, Daugirdas JT, Hano JE, Gandhi VC: Amantidine pharmacokinetics in patients with impaired renal function. *Clin Nephrol* 17:19–23, 1982.

144. Zsoter TT, Johnson GE, DeVeber GA, Paul H: Excretion and metabolism of reserpine in renal failure. *Clin Pharmacol Ther* 14:325–330, 1973.

3

Alterations in Pharmacology Caused by Congestive Heart Failure in the Critically Ill Patient

Rodney W. Savage, M.D., F.A.C.C.
Timothy P. Blair, M.D., F.A.C.C., F.A.C.P.

GENERAL CONSIDERATIONS

Heart failure may lead to important alterations in drug absorption, distribution, biotransformation, action, interaction, and excretion in the critically ill patient. Unfortunately, systematic study of many of the pharmacologic alterations remains incomplete. In this chapter, we discuss a variety of pharmacotherapeutic considerations that are pertinent in patients with heart failure.

Pathophysiology and Etiologies of Congestive Heart Failure

Congestive heart failure in the critically ill patient results from several pathophysiologic states. Arterial hypertension causes pressure overload with resulting left ventricular hypertrophy, decreased diastolic compliance, and increased left ventricular end diastolic pressure. Later, left ventricular dilatation with decreased ejection fraction and increased wall stress may occur. Coarctation of the aorta and aortic stenosis lead to a similar response by the left ventricle. Mitral stenosis causes increased left atrial pressure leading to pulmonary hypertension and right heart failure. Other causes of pulmonary hypertension include (a) left-sided heart failure (the most common situation); (b) chronic obstructive, restrictive, or interstitial lung disease; (c) recurrent pulmonary emboli; (d) primary pulmonary hypertension; and (e) obliterative pulmonary vascular disease from congenital heart disease (Eisenmenger's syndrome). The right ventricle responds to pressure overload in the same fashion as the left ventricle. The acute onset of pulmonary hypertension to pressures greater than 50 mm Hg, however, is poorly tolerated by the less muscular normal right ventricle and may precipitate acute right-sided failure (53).

Volume overload commonly results from regurgitant valvular lesions such as aortic insufficiency and mitral regurgitation. When acute and severe, pulmonary edema and low output shock rapidly ensue. Emergency valve repair or replacement is required. Chronic volume overload, on the other hand, may be surprisingly well tolerated until the patient suffers progressive dilatation of the left ventricle resulting in reduced contractility. In addition, the physiologic stress of another illness may precipitate left ventricular failure in previously compensated situations. Although clinically less common, pulmonary insufficiency and tricuspid regurgitation may lead to similar difficulties in the right heart. These lesions are often well tolerated, but may lead to a low output state, hepatic congestion, ascites, and malnutrition due to malabsorption from bowel edema. High output states represent a type of volume overload that may also precipitate congestive heart failure in a previously compensated, diseased heart. When severe (acute or chronic), high output states may lead to heart failure even with an otherwise previously normal heart (114).

Decreased contractility may result from damage imposed by chronic pressure or volume overload, as discussed above. It may also result from primary muscle loss or dysfunction as seen in dilated cardiomyopathies. Finally, ischemia leads to a reduction in ventricular function (29). Myocardial infarction results in scar and the potential for aneurysm formation, increased wall stress of remaining muscle, and decreased ventricular compliance. Cardiogenic shock results when more than 40% of the left ventricular myocardium is lost (113).

Restricted filling leads to increased filling pressure and limited, then reduced, cardiac output. Pericardial tamponade from a variety of causes must be considered in the critically ill patient with elevated right-sided filling pressures. Ventricular hypertrophy with decreased diastolic compliance is a more frequent cause of restricted filling (102). Although usually secondary to arterial hypertension, left ventricular hypertrophy may also be due to aortic stenosis, idiopathic hypertrophic cardiomyopathy, or infiltrative disease such as amyloidosis. Endomyocardial fibrosis is a rare cause of restrictive cardiomyopathy.

Profound bradyarrhythmias can lead to a low cardiac output, pulmonary congestion, and systemic venous congestion—even in the presence of an otherwise normal heart. Tachyarrhythmias from atrial fibrillation, atrial flutter, paroxysmal supraventricular tachycardia, and ventricular tachycardia can also lead to congestive heart failure. Although sinus tachycardia is usually compensatory, in the face of a reduced stroke volume it may occasionally represent an overcompensation, and clinical improvement may occur following careful use of β blockade (136).

Hemodynamic Alterations and Effects on the Periphery

Heart failure is defined as "the pathophysiological state in which an abnormality of cardiac function is responsible for the failure of the heart to pump blood at a rate commensurate with the requirements of the metabolizing tissues" (21). Restated, this definition implies a relative mismatch between the metabolic needs of the periphery and the heart's ability to deliver nourishing blood flow. Although cardiac output is often reduced in absolute terms, it may be reduced in only relative terms. This reduction results in clinical fatigue and frequently leads to prerenal azotemia. Plasma levels of norepinephrine and vasopressin increase (47, 52). The renin-angiotensin-aldos-

terone axis is activated (3). Ultimately, the tissues shift to anaerobic metabolism with the production of lactic acid. These changes may occur with or without hypotension and with increased, normal, or decreased systemic vascular resistance. In the usual case, left ventricular end diastolic pressure increases lead to pulmonary congestion, which may dominate the clinical picture. Secondary pulmonary hypertension may or may not occur. In its presence, right heart failure may develop with increased central venous pressure, hepatic congestion, and edema. Primary right heart failure may occur in certain disease states with "right-sided" changes occurring earlier in the clinical presentation and followed by signs of decreased output as left-sided filling limitations occur. In all of the above situations, an increase in the basal heart rate is common, perhaps representing a maladaptive overcompensation in some cases (3).

Alterations in the Periphery and Pharmacologic Effects

Heart failure alters both pharmacokinetics and pharmacodynamics. Furthermore, with the use of multiple drugs, drug interactions demand the clinician's constant attention. The disturbances in normal drug metabolism, however, can be quite complex since the physiology of congestive heart failure may vary considerably from patient to patient. The clinician, then, must consider not only the drug, but also how the specific peripheral effects of congestive heart failure alter that drug by affecting its absorption, distribution, biotransformation, actions, interactions, and excretion.

Increased central venous pressure causing gut edema may cause decreased gastrointestinal absorption of medications as demonstrated with quinidine sulfate (35). Drug absorption improves with diuretic therapy, necessitating both clinical monitoring and drug level reevaluation with clinical improvement. The transcutaneous route of administration becomes less efficient with decreased skin blood supply, which often accompanies the increased systemic vascular resistance of congestive heart failure. Studies using transdermal nitroglycerin in heart failure patients show a significant but variable reduction in absorption (56, 105). For similar reasons, intramuscular absorption of lidocaine is also reduced in heart failure (91). Although sublingual and pulmonary absorption probably remain rapid, these routes of administration have not, to our knowledge, been systematically studied in any of the various pathophysiologic subtypes of congestive heart failure. The same may be said for the rectal and subcutaneous routes of drug administration. The intravenous route, of course, circumvents these difficulties of absorption and remains the most direct and reliable pathway for drug administration.

Drug distribution to various body compartments also changes with congestive heart failure. Total body water increases in congestive heart failure, resulting in an increased volume of distribution for highly water-soluble medications. Similarly, lowering the extracellular fluid pH causes an increase in the intracellular concentration of weak acids and a decrease in that of weak bases, provided that intracellular pH also does not change (14). Altered binding of acidic drugs to albumin and basic drugs to α-1-acid-glycoprotein may also alter drug distribution. Delivery of nonpolar drugs to fat stores may be reduced as a result of shunting of blood away from such areas in severe congestive heart failure.

As a general rule, weak organic acids or bases that are lipid soluble are not easily eliminated until biotransformed. Most such reactions occur in the liver via microsomal and nonmicrosomal enzyme systems (68, 83). Other tissues active in this process include plasma, kidney, lung, and gastrointestinal tract. Decreased hepatic blood flow may significantly reduce the rate of metabolism of drugs cleared by the liver, such as lidocaine, leading to overt clinical toxicity at relatively normal clinical doses (38). Furthermore, a reduced capacity to eliminate drugs in congestive heart failure may not be accompanied by abnormalities in routine liver function tests. The aminopyrine breath test has been found to be helpful in such cases, but is not readily available to the clinician (62). β-Blockers can cause a decrease in hepatic blood flow, especially when given during congestive heart failure (110). Competitive inhibition between most substrates for microsomal enzymes usually does not occur since most agents are inactivated by exponential (first order) rather than linear (zero order) kinetics. Some drugs, however, normally exhibit saturable inactivation in the presence of another drug. For example, dicumerol inhibits the metabolism of phenytoin (14), an inhibition possibly exaggerated by decreased hepatic blood flow and hepatic congestion.

Heart failure alters drug excretion by reducing renal blood flow, altering the acid-base balance, and increasing extravascular volume. Renal clearance of digoxin decreases dramatically as glomerular filtration rate falls (42, 106), predisposing to drug-induced toxicity. If liver dysfunction coexists, however, digoxin-like immunoreactive substance may be measured with the same digoxin assay (107). Quinidine, highly protein bound and largely metabolized by the liver, is also excreted by the kidneys (20% of administered drug) and may well exhibit decreased excretion in congestive heart failure secondary to either hepatic or renal function alterations (31, 75). Renal excretion of this weak base is enhanced by an acidic urine.

Changes in drug action in congestive heart failure may occur because of alterations in number or affinity of drug receptors. Acidosis, for example, can blunt the effectiveness of various sympathomimetic amines (145). In chronic congestive heart failure, decreased β-adrenergic receptor number and affinity occur as a result of increased levels of norepinephrine (22, 138), leading to decreased effect for any dose of drug. Furosemide also shows decreased effectiveness for any given dose as a result of decreases in glomerular filtration rate and tubular blood flow induced by heart failure (127).

Finally, the clinician must always consider drug interactions. These are made more likely by the many drugs often required by critically ill patients and are potentially accentuated by altered renal clearance, decreased hepatic function, and altered electrolyte or acid-base status.

SPECIFIC DRUGS

Unfortunately, many of the drugs used in treating critically ill patients have not been well studied in terms of their effects in patients with congestive heart failure. The clinician must apply available knowledge to the specific hemodynamic situation of each patient, anticipating possible alterations in drug metabolism. The patient should be observed carefully using bedside, electrocardiographic, hemodynamic, and laboratory methods. Circulating drug levels can be followed as the state of heart failure changes, in an effort to minimize drug-induced toxicity and optimize drug effectiveness. In the following sections we shall explore what is known about the metabolism of a number of drugs commonly used in critically ill patients with congestive heart failure.

Digoxin

Digoxin is widely used for rate control of atrial fibrillation and as a weak inotrope in chronic congestive heart failure. Oral administration of the tablet form results in 60–75% absorption from the gastrointestinal tract (70). A new capsule formulation is approximately 20% more bioavailable (17). A peak serum concentration in either case is reached 45–60 minutes after ingestion. Elimination, mostly by renal excretion of unconjugated drug, leads to a half-life of 31.3 hours (41). Normal absorption may be distorted in critically ill patients due to ileus, gut edema, decreased perfusion, changes in bowel flora, and the presence of other drugs. These changes remain difficult to quantitate from patient to patient, but seem less dramatic with the capsule preparation. Intravenous administration, of course, avoids these vagaries and achieves tissue distribution and binding in 30 minutes (41).

Once absorbed, digoxin is only 20–25% protein bound (95), allowing for excellent glomerular filtration of the predominantly unmetabolized, polar drug. Hyperkalemia and hyponatremia may reduce myocardial binding. Hypomagnesemia increases the risk of toxicity (43). Reduced digoxin excretion occurs in renal failure. Glomerular filtration plays the predominant role in excretion, but tubular secretion is also involved. Sodium depletion, however, results in increased reabsorption of sodium in the proximal tubule causing a decrease in digoxin clearance even in the presence of a stable creatinine clearance (55). To further complicate the picture, plasma digoxin levels may be falsely elevated in congestive heart failure patients with severe renal dysfunction because of the presence of digoxin-like immunoreactive substance (107).

With or without congestive heart failure, digoxin has many drug interactions. The quinidine-digoxin interaction reduces the volume of distribution of digoxin by 30–40% and reduces renal clearance by 30–50% (24). The increased rate of digoxin absorption with concomitant quinidine therapy is too small to be of clinical importance. Reduced nonrenal clearance also produces only minimal changes in circulating digoxin levels. Recent work shows a near doubling of serum digoxin concentrations five weeks after starting amiodarone, an increase due to a change in volume of distribution since urinary digoxin clearance was unchanged (122). Verapamil may cause a 70% increase in serum digoxin concentration. This increase is dose-dependent and thought to occur secondary to reduced renal excretion without a reduction in glomerular filtration (77). As renal secretion of digoxin declines with hypokalemia (134), any diuretic that causes kaliuresis would be expected to increase digoxin levels. This rule holds true with furosemide but not bumetanide (60). Triamterene (115) and spironolactone (133) both cause decreased renal tubular secretion of digoxin. Amiloride, in contrast, increases tubular secretion of digoxin, but decreases extrarenal clearance, yielding only a slight decline in total body clearance (142). Antacids and kaolin-pectin each reduce peak serum digoxin concentrations, but not the time to peak concentration or completeness of absorption (5). Digoxin tablet absorption is increased by propantheline, which reduces gut motility (98). Finally, in approximately 10% of patients, antibiotic therapy changes gut flora and may result in a doubling of serum digoxin concentrations (92). Other interactions certainly exist, some of which are indirect. For example, rifampin increases the elimination of quinidine, which in turn may lead to a reduction of serum digoxin (4).

Dobutamine and Dopamine

Dobutamine and dopamine are rapidly metabolized, titratable intravenous sympathomimetic inotropes that are frequently used in critically ill patients. Dobutamine differs from dopamine in that it has less chronotropic effect and is devoid of dopaminergic renal vasodilation and peripheral vasoconstriction. Both drugs are rapidly distributed and metabolized by monoamine oxidase and catechol-O-methyltransferase in the periphery (88). This metabolism is not apparently altered in congestive heart failure, although the volume of distribution increases with edema (73). Sequestration of β-adrenergic receptors occurs rapidly in congestive heart failure (97), causing down regulation of β-receptors and diminished β-adrenergic effects (129). Dobutamine and dopamine may improve hemodynamics in congestive heart failure (93) and alter the pharmacokinetics of other agents. Dobutamine infusion, in addition, may lead to statistically significant reductions in serum potassium and magnesium concentrations (51).

Nitroprusside

Nitroprusside, a balanced arteriolar and venous vasodilator, possesses a rapid intravenous onset of action and is rapidly metabolized and excreted. It is used to lower systemic resistance in the setting of arterial hypertension, dissection of the aorta, and congestive heart failure. The pharmacokinetics and pharmacodynamics of the agent have not been studied in normal subjects versus congestive heart failure patients. However, these parameters are probably minimally affected, except for the occurrence of reduced thiocyanate excretion when prerenal azotemia complicates the clinical picture. Initial decomposition of nitroprusside involves the nonenzymatic conversion to cyanide, which is then rapidly converted by mitochondrial rhodanese to thiocyanate, a reaction requiring a sulfur donor (29). This enzyme is thought to be deficient in patients with tobacco amblyopia or Leber's optic atrophy (147). Dosages considerably above 3 μg/min may lead to toxicity, especially when used for longer than 3 days. In this situation, free cyanide ion combines with cytochromes, leading to anaerobic metabolism and lactate production. Such metabolic acidosis is followed by confusion, hyperreflexia, and coma. Toxicity from nitroprusside can be minimized by monitoring blood thiocyanate levels, with concentrations of less than 10 mg/dl considered safe (29). Also, prophylactic infusion of hydroxycobalamin, which reacts with cyanide to form cyanocobalamin, may avoid toxicity (32). Other than discontinuation of the infusion and dialysis, toxicity may be treated with the administration of thiosulfate (a sulfur donor) and sodium nitrate (which induces methemoglobin to combine with cyanide forming cyanomethemoglobin). Finally, variable hypoxemia secondary to increased pulmonary shunting may occur with nitroprusside administration.

Nitrates

The nitrates show great flexibility in routes of administration—topical, sublingual, buccal, oral, and intravenous. Mucosal absorption of nitroglycerin is excellent. Transdermal absorption varies with dose, vehicle, and place of application. Once absorbed, the drug is rapidly distributed, bound, and metabolized in the periphery to 1,2- and 1,3-glyceryl dinitrate and subsequently excreted in the urine. Isosorbide dinitrate tablets are more slowly absorbed via the oral mucosa or gastrointestinal tract; this drug exhibits a high level of first pass hepatic metabolism (20–25% bioavailability) by glutathione organic reductase to 2- and 5-isosorbide mononitrate, both active metabolites. All related compounds are excreted in the urine. The mechanism of action of nitroglycerin and isosorbide dinitrate remains unknown, but resides in the vascular smooth muscle (i.e., does not involve the neuroendocrine system) (2). Veins show greater avidity for nitrates than arteries, and veins dilate at lower nitroglycerin doses (67). Tolerance to nitrate therapy is more common with sustained blood levels and frequently repeated large doses (1). Nitrate-free periods restore normal responsiveness (112), but are difficult to employ in the critically ill patient. No significant alteration in nitrate pharmacokinetics occurs in patients with congestive heart failure (48).

Furosemide

Furosemide continues to fill a vital role in the treatment of congestive heart failure. Its immediate effect is to increase venous capacitance, which is followed by a brisk diuresis (39). The potential side effects of such therapy are hypokalemia, hypomagnesemia, metabolic alkalosis, and hypovolemia. Serum digoxin levels are increased with furosemide therapy (42, 106, 134). Time to peak serum concentration is increased and peak serum concentrations are reduced with oral furosemide in decompensated congestive heart failure compared with the compensated state. The total amount of furosemide absorbed, however, does not differ between the two states (11). Furosemide is less excreted by the kidneys, is less effective, and has a longer half-life in patients with renal insufficiency (141). The drug is secreted into the proximal tubule and initiates a diuresis from the luminal side of the ascending loop of Henle (23). Since patients with heart failure often have reduced renal blood flow, it is not surprising that less drug is delivered to its site of action and results in diminished diuresis. Hydralazine (an arteriolar vasodilator) increases both urinary sodium excretion and furosemide excretion in this setting (108). Whether other vasodilators show similar effects is unknown.

Bumetanide

Bumetanide demonstrates much greater potency than furosemide in heart failure. Drug absorption is more rapid and bioavailability improved. Although quantitative absorption is not affected by congestive heart failure, time of peak concentration is increased and peak concentration is diminished through undetermined mechanisms (20). The diuretic action of bumetanide is diminished with renal insufficiency (15). The drug's activity results from effects on both the blood and luminal sides of the nephron, instead of solely on the luminal side, as with furosemide (19).

Lidocaine

Lidocaine was originally synthesized in 1943 and was utilized for two decades as a local anesthetic (135). Its antiarrhythmic properties were noted in the 1960s, and it quickly became the primary therapy for treatment and prophylaxis of ventricular rhythm disturbances in intensive care units (59). Lidocaine is a class I drug and acts by shortening duration of the action potential, shortening the effective refractory period, and decreasing automaticity (148). When administered by a continuous infusion, it requires several hours before a steady state is achieved; therefore, lidocaine is usually administered as a bolus of 50–100 mg followed by a continuous infusion at 1–4 mg/min. Serum therapeutic levels are considered to be 2–6 μg/ml. Toxic side effects include paresthesis, slurred speech, somnolence, psychosis, apnea, and convulsions, and occur frequently when serum levels are above 9 μg/ml (150).

Lidocaine disposition after an intravenous bolus is described by a two-compartment model with a fast distribution phase (half-life, 8 minutes) and a slower distribution phase (half-life, 100 minutes). Seventy percent of lidocaine clearance is by hepatic metabolism and its clearance varies directly with hepatic blood flow (135, 139). The site of the remainder of lidocaine metabolism has not been identified (139), but less than 5% is excreted in the urine.

The rate of lidocaine metabolism is extensively altered in congestive heart failure. Thomson and associates (139) noted a decreased volume of distribution and a 37% decrease in plasma lidocaine clearance in patients with heart failure. Plasma clearance of lidocaine was also reduced in patients with liver disease. Patients receiving dialysis did not have abnormalities in lidocaine clearance. However, metabolites that undergo renal clearance might accumulate with prolonged infusion. It takes 5–8 hours to reach a new steady state in normal subjects following a change in lidocaine infusion rate. This time is prolonged in patients with heart failure.

The elimination phase for lidocaine may be considerably longer when the infusion is continued beyond 12 hours and in patients with acute myocardial infarction. Le Lorier and associates (89) found a mean half-life of 3.2 hours in patients with acute myocardial infarction. Furthermore, the patients had a serum lidocaine level of more than twice the predicted level. Prescott and colleagues (119) found the clearance half-life of lidocaine to be increased from 1.4 hours in normal volunteers to 4.3 hours in patients with uncomplicated acute myocardial infarction and 10.2 hours in heart failure. One patient in cardiogenic shock demonstrated no fall in serum lidocaine levels over 8 hours. The authors postulated a decrease in hepatic blood flow and other contributory factors, such as stress, hypoxia, hepatic venous congestion, competitive inhibition caused by accumulation of lidocaine metabolites, and administration of other drugs, as the cause for the decreased drug metabolism. They recommended limiting lidocaine infusions, after a loading bolus, to 2 mg/min unless persistent arrhythmias occur.

Zito and associates (151) studied the effects of a 1 mg/kg bolus of lidocaine followed by a constant infusion of 35 μg/kg/min. Both normal volunteers and patients with coronary artery disease (without heart failure) developed an early dip in plasma lidocaine levels, which fell below a therapeutic level of 2.4 μg/ml and lasted for 90 minutes. However, in patients with chronic heart failure (New York heart class IV), or acute myocardial infarction (Killip class II or III), the dip did not occur. The authors hypothesized that the higher plasma lidocaine levels resulted from decreased hepatic extraction.

Zito and Reid (150) subsequently extended their observations by showing that the clearance of lidocaine was directly proportional to the clearance of indocyanine green dye. Nineteen percent of their patients had toxic levels; all of these patients had heart failure and 15% had clinical evidence of toxicity. The authors recommended a lidocaine infusion rate of 35–38 µg/kg/min for New York class I failure, 12–35 µg/kg/min for class II, and 5–12 µg/kg/min for class III–IV. They also found that lidocaine infusion rates could be calculated from the indocyanine green clearance as follows: lidocaine rate = 0.3 + 1.07 (indocyanine green clearance) × desired lidocaine level.

Although Bax and colleagues (9) did not find a linear correlation between indocyanine clearance and lidocaine clearance, Lopez and associates (94) compared the dosage recommended by Zito and Reid (150) in New York heart class I–II heart failure with a control group that received a bolus followed by a 1–4 mg/min infusion. In the control group, 30% of the drug levels were in the toxic range and 12% were subtherapeutic. In the group that received the dose recommended by Zito and Reid, 81% of the drug levels were in the therapeutic range and none were in the toxic range.

These data indicate that adjustments in lidocaine administration must be made in patients with acute myocardial infarction, heart failure, or hepatic disease. Furthermore, constant adjustments in lidocaine infusions must be made as the hemodynamic status of the patient fluctuates.

Procainamide

Procainamide is a class I drug with properties similar to quinidine, and has been in clinical use since 1950. It is a second-line drug for treatment of ventricular rhythm disturbances (130).

Therapeutic plasma concentrations range from 4 to 8 mg/liter. Toxicity is frequently seen with serum levels above 8 mg/liter and almost universal toxicity occurs above 16 mg/liter (80).

Gastrointestinal absorption of procainamide ranges from 72 to 94% (83). Peak serum levels occur in 1–2 hours. The mean circulating half-life is 3.5 hours and does not change with prolonged administration, suggesting that there is no induction of metabolizing enzymes. About 48% of procainamide is excreted unchanged in the urine. The renal clearance ranges from 179 to 309 ml/min, whereas plasma clearance is 396–680 ml/min; therefore, active renal secretion occurs.

A major metabolite is N-acetylprocainamide (NAPA), which also possesses antiarrhythmic properties. Impaired renal function due to either primary renal disease or low cardiac output states results in a marked rise in serum NAPA levels (81). The dosage of procainamide should be adjusted based on serum procainamide and NAPA levels.

In acute myocardial infarction, the time of absorption after an oral dose of procainamide can vary greatly: only four of 15 patients had peak levels at 1 hour, and in six, levels were still rising at 3 hours (80). The delay in procainamide absorption may be secondary to delayed gastric emptying, decreased intestinal motility, food, altered gastric pH, or decreased splanchnic blood flow. Since plasma concentrations after oral administration are unpredictable, a parenteral route of administration should be used in the first hours after myocardial infarction.

Early work suggested that procainamide had a reduced volume of distribution and prolonged half-life during congestive heart failure. This finding has been recently challenged. Kessler and associates (74) assessed procainamide kinetics in controls, patients with acute myocardial infarction, and patients with congestive heart failure. They found no difference in half-life, volume of distribution, peak NAPA levels, or percentage of unbound procainamide in the various groups. Patients with acute infarction had lower thresholds for suppression of premature ventricular contractions. The investigators thought this difference in response to procainamide was due to variation in the electrophysiologic properties of the heart during acute infarction. Administration of procainamide does not alter serum digoxin levels.

Quinidine

Quinidine is a membrane stabilizing drug. Peak levels occur 2 hours after oral administration, and the circulating half-life is 6.5–7.0 hours (35, 75). Side effects include diarrhea, nausea, vomiting, and prolongation of the QRS and QT intervals.

In congestive heart failure, the absorption of quinidine after oral administration is slower and results in peak plasma quinidine levels at 4 hours after dosing (12). Compared with normal subjects, only half as much orally administered quinidine is absorbed from the gut. A decreased volume of distribution is suggested in heart failure patients by the finding that plasma levels were 41% higher than in controls (12, 35). The circulating half-life is only slightly increased to 8.2 hours in heart failure (75). However, in patients with renal failure, quinidine's half-life after oral administration is 11.7 hours (12, 75). Quinidine may be given by the intramuscular route (75); however, the very slow absorption makes this route a poor choice.

The risk of adverse effects from quinidine is increased in the setting of hypokalemia (126, 149). Roden and coworkers (126) examined 22 patients with quinidine-induced torsade de pointes and found that 80% were taking diuretics. Hypokalemia was present in six patients, and 12 had serum potassium levels in the low-normal range (3.5–3.9 μg/liter). The investigators recommended maintaining the serum potassium level above 4 mEq/liter before initiating quinidine therapy.

Although intravenous quinidine, in experimental animals, decreases heart rate and blood pressure, the effect on left ventricular contractility is variable. Echocardiographic study of patients with cardiomyopathy did not reveal any change of left ventricular function as measured by end diastolic dimension, percentage fractional shortening, or posterior wall velocity (34). The same study could not eliminate the possibility that quinidine may have a mild depressant effect in normal subjects that is masked by its vagolytic effects.

The addition of quinidine may result in elevated serum digoxin concentrations (40, 54) and clinical toxicity (64, 86). Garty and associates (50) reported that quinidine produced a 63% reduction in total body digitoxin clearance without causing a change in the apparent volume of distribution of the central compartment. These quinidine-induced changes resulted in a 2.5-fold increase in the digitoxin elimination half-life.

Disopyramide

Disopyramide is a class I antiarrhythmic agent with electrophysiologic properties similar to those of quinidine (decreased rate of phase IV diastolic depolarization, decreased upstroke velocity of phase 0, and increased action potential duration) (79, 117). It is generally regarded to be as effective as quinidine, with fewer side affects. It has little effect on PR, QRS, and QT intervals in normal therapeutic doses (79). The major side effects of disopyramide are due to its anticholinergic effects and are manifested by dry mouth, blurred vision,

and urinary retention. It is almost completely absorbed from the gastrointestinal tract. Excretion is predominantly by glomerular filtration: 55% as the unchanged drug; 15–25% as the N-monodealkylated metabolite, which has weak antiarrhythmic properties; and 10% as minor metabolites (79, 85). The normal circulating half-life of disopyramide is 4.4–7.0 hours (79). In congestive heart failure, the rate of absorption is slower than normal, but the peak serum concentration is higher than in normal subjects, probably because of decreased volume of distribution (79). There is no change in serum digoxin levels when disopyramide is initiated.

Intravenous disopyramide has prominent negative inotropic effects (100, 146). Cardiac output is decreased 10% by an intravenous infusion of 1–2 mg/kg, 22% by 5 mg/kg, and 49% by 10 mg/kg (146). The basis for the cardiac depression is not known. Chronic therapy with oral disopyramide also possesses negative inotropic properties. Podrid and coworkers (117) noted the development of congestive heart failure in patients given disopyramide. Most patients were also taking digitalis and diuretics. These investigators employed a loading dose of 300 mg and maintenance doses of 300–800 mg/day, which would now be considered large. Sixteen percent of their patients developed heart failure: a minority of these (19%) had the onset of heart failure within 48 hours of initiation of therapy; the remainder developed failure during longer therapy (up to 9 months). In the absence of a history of cardiac failure, the chance of developing heart failure was less than 5%. Although effective in suppressing arrhythmias, this medication should be avoided if there is a history of heart failure.

Tocainide

Tocainide is a primary amine analogue of lidocaine. It produces shortening of both the action potential duration and the effective refractory periods and depresses the maximal upstroke phase 0 (96). It has relatively low hepatic extraction and may be administered orally (96). Therapeutic plasma concentrations (compared with 2–6 μg/ml for lidocaine) range from 3 to 4 μg/ml (96, 125). The clearance half-life is 11 hours in normal subjects. About 38–50% of the drug is excreted unchanged by the kidneys and the remainder undergoes hepatic glucuronidation before renal excretion (44, 78).

The mean renal clearance rate of tocainide is 104–154 ml/min. Side effects are similar to those of lidocaine and occur in 38% of patients. These include nausea, vomiting, dizziness, tremor, confusion, and psychosis (44, 78). It is not possible to predict which patients will develop tocainide-induced side effects. Side effects cannot be predicted from serum plasma values; however, central nervous system and gastrointestinal side effects can be decreased by reducing dosage (77). Tocainide is as effective as quinidine (143) or disopyramide (101) in its antiarrhythmic effects and suppresses premature ventricular contractions in about 65% of patients (125, 143).

There are no reports of tocainide interactions with other drugs, in particular, digoxin (125). Tocainide may work synergistically with quinidine (65).

Exacerbation of congestive heart failure is very uncommon with oral tocainide (65). Some investigators have found no differences in elimination half-life, volume of distribution, or total body clearance of tocainide when comparing normal volunteers with patients with acute myocardial infarction. (104) However, intravenous tocainide caused a small decrease in cardiac output and an increase in systemic vascular resistance in patients with heart failure secondary to myocardial infarction (109). Another study of patients with acute myocardial infarction and failure, but not pulmonary edema, found an increase in plasma clearance half-life to 15.6 hours after intravenous administration of 250 mg of tocainide (96). Mean plasma tocainide levels 5 minutes after the infusion were 2.95 μg/ml. The mean cardiac index initially was 2.4 liters/min/m^2. It decreased to 2.07 liters/min/m^2 5 minutes after completion of the infusion, returned to baseline by 90 minutes, and increased to 2.49 liters/min/m^2 at 24 hours. There was no change in heart rate, blood pressure, or pulmonary artery pressure. Since the negative inotropic effects were seen at levels well below the therapeutic range, the authors urged caution in employing higher doses of the drug in patients with left ventricular dysfunction after acute myocardial infarction.

In renal insufficiency, the clearance of tocainide is markedly reduced to 35–94 ml/min and the elimination half-life prolonged to a mean of 22 hours (144). Therefore, a decrease in dosage or an increase in administration intervals, or both, should be employed in renal failure.

In the setting of concomitant hepatic and renal disease, the reduction of tocainide clearance appears to be largely attributable to renal dysfunction (111). No study of tocainide kinetics in isolated hepatic dysfunction has been performed (44).

Flecainide

Flecainide acetate is a class IC agent that markedly depresses the maximum upstroke of phase 0 of the action potential (33, 84). It shortens the duration of the action potential and effective refractory period in canine Purkinje fibers and prolongs them in ventricular muscle. The PR and QRS intervals are routinely prolonged (124). Twenty-seven percent of the drug is excreted unchanged in the urine by both filtration and active secretion. The remainder undergoes biotransformation to two major metabolites with less antiarrhythmic efficacy. The normal plasma half-life of flecainide is 14 hours; however, it increases by 20% to 19 hours in patients with congestive heart failure (124). In severe renal failure, the clearance of flecainide may be reduced 40% and the half-life increased to 58 hours (124). The decreased clearances of the drug and the increased plasma levels may result in serious cardiac toxicity (30, 46). Therefore, in the setting of cardiac and/or renal insufficiency, flecainide should be administered in lower doses and at longer intervals. Increases in dosage should be made no more often than every 4 days (124).

Flecainide also has multiple drug interactions. The clearance is decreased and prolonged by 13–27% with cimetidine (140). Flecainide interacts with propranolol to raise each drug's plasma concentration and results in additive negative inotropic effects (90). The simultaneous administration of amiodarone results in raised flecainide levels.

Flecainide is effective in the suppression of ventricular ectopy (63), more so than quinidine (45) or disopyramide (76). In one study, flecainide was 92% successful in suppressing premature ventricular contractions whereas disopyramide was only 39% successful (76).

Flecainide's major side effect has been exacerbation of congestive heart failure. In one study, 16% of patients with heart failure had exacerbation of symptoms with flecainide therapy (71). In another study of 32 patients who had nonsustained ventricular tachycardia and had failed previous antiarrhythmic therapy, three patients with left ventricular ejection fractions of 23–36% developed heart failure (84). This adverse effect could be controlled by increasing the dose of diuretics. Proarrhythmic effects occurred in one patient. The authors recommended initiating flecainide therapy with 200 mg/day, increasing dosages every 4 days, avoiding dosages greater than 400 mg/day, and maintaining plasma levels 1 μg/ml or less. Furthermore, caution should be employed in utilizing the drug in patients with severely depressed left ventricular function and in those whose depressed cardiac output results in variations in renal elimination.

In patients with an ejection fraction measured by radionuclide angiography of greater than 45%, an intravenous infusion of flecainide results in an 11% reduction in ejection fraction (72). A 21% ejection fraction reduction occurred in the group with ejection fractions of less than 45%. Furthermore, for the entire group, there was an 8% reduction in cardiac index and an 8% increase in systemic vascular resistance.

In summary, although flecainide has excellent antiarrhythmic properties, it should be used with extreme caution in settings of compromised ventricular function.

Mexiletine

Mexiletine is a lidocaine congener. It is well absorbed after oral administration, although absorption may be impaired in acute myocardial infarction (120).

Mexiletine, like lidocaine, mainly undergoes hepatic metabolism (10). In patients with hepatic or renal disease, mexiletine may accumulate (131). Patients with cirrhosis may have particularly marked prolongation of mexiletene clearance. One study found persistent levels of the drug in the serum of patients with cirrhosis 3 days after administration, but in none of the controls (131). Intravenous mexiletene does not produce myocardial depression at therapeutic levels; however, at toxic levels, myocardial depression has been noted (26).

Orally administered mexiletine does not appear to cause clinically important cardiac depression. Stein and associates (132) evaluated 10 patients with symptomatic ventricular tachycardia or fibrillation who also had ejection fractions of less than 50% by radionuclide angiography. In their 72-hour study of orally administered mexiletine, no change occurred in the mean left ventricular ejection fraction

(28% versus 27%) following the institution of therapy. There was a statistically insignificant fall in right ventricular ejection fraction from 46% to 41%. Mexiletine was effective in suppressing ventricular ectopy in 60% of patients at rest and 80% during exercise. No changes were observed in resting heart rate, exercise duration, or peak exercise heart rate.

The therapeutic effects of mexiletine can be enhanced by quinidine, permitting lower doses of mexiletine to be used and avoiding side effects (128). There is no change in serum digoxin level when mexiletine is initiated.

Another study evaluated mexiletine in patients with congestive heart failure who had no intrinsic hepatic or renal disease after acute myocardial infarction (87). The circulating half-life of the drug was 8.1 hours and the peak serum level occurred 3.2 hours after an oral dose. The renal elimination was 8%, which was not significantly different from normal.

Encainide

Encainide resembles procainamide but differs in having a p-substituted aromatic ring that is bridged to a tertiary amine by an amide (123). Encainide, like lidocaine, shortens the duration of the action potential. However, it also prolongs the effective refractory period. There is a dose-related prolongation of the PR and QRS intervals on the electrocardiogram. It has the advantage of being very effective in nanogram plasma concentrations, with minimal side effects (123). The half-life of encainide is 3–4 hours in normal subjects under steady state conditions. Furthermore, it does not alter radionuclide ejection fractions.

Encainide was evaluated in 19 patients with depressed left ventricular function (36). All patients had ejection fractions of less than 45%, and 63% had congestive heart failure. The mean ejection fraction was 22% before encainide and did not change with encainide therapy. The heart rate, blood pressure, stroke volume, and end diastolic volume did not change. However, a marked variability in plasma encainide levels was observed. Encainide does not alter digoxin levels.

Bretylium Tosylate

Bretylium acts by increasing the ventricular threshold (8). It is useful for treatment of refractory ventricular tachycardia or fibrillation. It is approved only for intramuscular or intravenous injection.

Approximately 70–80% of the drug is excreted unchanged in the urine (82). The half-life is 6–10 hours and increases in renal insufficiency (61). Although bretylium does not decrease myocardial contractility (61), it must be used with caution in critically ill patients since it may cause hypotension, even in the supine position (27). No evaluation of this drug in heart failure has been made. However, if renal function is compromised, the level of administration should probably be decreased.

Amiodarone

Amiodarone is a unique antiarrhythmic agent with excellent therapeutic efficacy for ventricular and supraventricular arrhythmias. Its therapeutic efficacy is offset by pulmonary, hepatic, thyroidal, ocular, and cutaneous toxicity. Amiodarone is predominantly metabolized by the liver and excreted in the bile. It undergoes enterohepatic recirculation (7). If hepatic insufficiency occurs because of heart failure or other etiology, the dosage should be reduced. Amiodarone is neither excreted by the kidney (6, 7, 121) nor removed by hemodialysis (18, 58).

Amiodarone interacts with numerous medications. It may elevate serum levels of the following drugs if administered to patients with previously achieved stable levels: aprindine, digoxin, flecainide, phenytoin, procainamide, quinidine, and warfarin (99). The amiodarone-induced elevations may result in undesirable clinical events, and it is recommended that the dosage of these drugs be decreased and their serum values monitored when amiodarone is initiated. Furthermore, since it may take many days or weeks before a stable state is established after initiation of amiodarone, the serum levels should be measured serially.

Although oral amiodarone is generally well tolerated in congestive heart failure, a study in patients with chagasic cardiomyopathy showed decreases in heart rate and cardiac index, and elevations of right atrial pressure, left ventricular end diastolic pressure, pulmonary artery pressure, and systemic vascular resistance during the 1st hour of intravenous amiodarone infusion. These parameters returned to baseline by 24 hours (13). Careful monitoring of bolus therapy is required when amiodarone is administered to patients with compensated heart failure.

Theophylline

Theophylline is widely used in the intensive care unit in patients with chronic obstructive pulmonary disease, bronchospasm, and occasionally, pulmonary edema. Its beneficial effects are mediated through bronchodilation, augmented diaphragmatic contraction, increased cardiac inotropy, arteriolar vasodilation, and increased venous capacitance. Therapeutic serum theophylline concentrations range from 10 to 20 μg/ml. Theophylline is eliminated by hepatic metabolism and follows first order kinetics. It is not affected by the dose or rate of administration (103). Although beneficial, theophylline is associated with cardiac and neurologic toxicity. Sixty percent of drug-related deaths in one intensive care unit were attributed to theophylline (25). Furthermore, patients with congestive heart failure or hepatic dysfunction are especially prone to seizures while receiving theophylline (152).

Administration of theophylline results in marked variability in serum levels in patients with heart failure. The volume of distribution is not significantly different from that in the normal control group, and the peak theophylline levels are similar after a single dose in patients with heart failure (116). However, patients with heart failure have markedly prolonged plasma half-lives. There is a 20-fold variation in these parameters in patients with pulmonary edema compared with a 4-fold variation in normal patients.

Serum levels may fluctuate during the course of heart failure. Jenne and coworkers (69) reported such an instance in a patient with chronic bronchitis who had near cessation of theophylline clearance when he developed severe heart failure. Following improvement in the heart failure, a marked increase in theophylline removal was observed. A bromosulphalein test also showed marked improvement with resolution of heart failure, suggesting that decreased liver blood flow or hypoxic liver dysfunction, or both, had resulted in decreased hepatic theophylline metabolism.

Marked individual variability in the rate of hepatic metabolism occurs, depending on the degree of pulmonary, hepatic, or cardiac disease. Powell and associates (118) established a standard clearance of 40.9 ml/hr/kg in normal controls. In smokers, theophylline clearance increased by a factor of 1.57 (57%). However, clearance was decreased to 43% of standard in congestive heart failure, to 37% by pneumonia, and to 84% by severe bronchial obstruction. Therefore, an estimate of theophylline clearance would rise to 64.1 ml/hr/kg for a smoker, but fall to 17.6 ml/hr/kg for a patient in heart failure. Furthermore, the logarithmic nature of the regression model makes the effect of multiple variables on theophylline clearance multiplicative rather than additive. In a patient who both smokes and has heart failure, the standard clearance of 40.9 ml/hr/kg is multiplied by both 1.57 and 0.43, resulting in a clearance rate of 27.6 ml/hr/kg, or 68% of standard. This value is close to the mean clearance found in patients with heart failure who also smoke.

Powell and associates (118) have developed a formula to guide infusions of theophylline. They recommend a loading dose of 6 mg/kg, to be infused at a rate of 0.2 mg/kg/min. A maintenance infusion is infused at 0.5 mg/kg/hr. If the patient is a smoker, the rate of infusion should be 0.8 mg/kg/hr; in heart failure and pneumonia, 0.2 mg/kg/hr; and if severe pulmonary obstruction is present, 0.4 mg/kg/hr.

Angiographic Contrast Agents

Critically ill patients frequently undergo angiographic evaluation. Administration of radiographic contrast agents is responsible for 10% of hospital-acquired acute renal failure and follows renal hypoperfusion states and major surgery as the third most common etiology (66). Ninety percent of patients who have acute renal dysfunction after receiving radiocontrast agents have preexisting renal insufficiency (57).

Taliercio and colleagues (137) evaluated 139 patients who underwent cardiac angiography and had a preprocedure serum creatinine of greater than 2 mg/dl. Thirty-two patients developed contrast nephropathy; 13 patients had oliguria or anuria and two patients required dialysis. The mean increment in serum creatinine was 2.6 mg/dl and the peak serum creatinine level occurred 2.8 days after angiography. Renal function returned to baseline in 25 patients. Cardiac events resulted in mortality in six patients 3–7 days after angiography. The most significant variable associated with the occurrence of contrast nephropathy was congestive heart failure. Contrast nephropathy developed in 25% of patients with New York heart class IV heart failure who did not have low cardiac output. However, in patients with New York heart class IV failure and low cardiac output who required continuous intravenous inotropic or vasodilator therapy or an intraaortic balloon pump, the incidence of contrast nephropathy was 71%. Other risk factors included multiple contrast studies within 72 hours, insulin-dependent diabetes mellitus, and radiocontrast dosage of more than 125 ml/study.

In addition to avoiding unnecessary procedures, a reduction in dye load may be achieved by using ultrasonic, nuclear imaging, or digital subtraction angiography when possible. The use of nonionic agents has not been associated with less nephrotoxicity (49).

An infusion of mannitol and furosemide has been utilized when performing angiographic studies (16) in patients with renal insufficiency to decrease the development of contrast-induced nephropathy. An effective regimen is to use a solution of 500 ml of 20% mannitol and add furosemide at a dose of 100 mg for each milligram per deciliter of serum creatinine. One hour before the administration of contrast, the infusion is started at a rate of 20 ml/hr and continued through the procedure and for 6 hours afterward. Urine output is replaced with a solution of 5% dextrose in 0.45% saline with 30 mg of potassium chloride added per liter (16).

SUMMARY

The clinician should use drugs sparingly in patients with heart failure and use clearly defined pharmacologic goals. When possible, an intravenous route of administration is preferable. Titratable drugs with short half-lives, which can be rapidly metabolized and excreted, offer many advantages. Renal function, acid-base balance, and hepatic function should be monitored. It must be remembered, however, that reduced hepatic enzymatic function often exists without abnormalities in standard liver enzyme determinations. The enlightened use of blood drug level determinations often helps avoid significant drug toxicity. Finally, hemodynamic changes mandate reevaluation of drug therapy.

Acknowledgments

Appreciation is expressed to Peter Marghella and Ron Landers for their assistance in preparation of this manuscript.

References

1. Abrams J: The brief saga of transdermal nitroglycerin discs: Paradise lost? Am J Cardiol 54:220–224, 1984.
2. Abrams J: Pharmacology of nitroglycerin and long-acting nitrates. Am J Cardiol 56:12A–18A, 1985.
3. Ader R, Chatterjee K, Ports T, Brundage B, Hiramatsu B, Parmley WW: Immediate and sustained hemodynamic and clinical improvement in chronic heart failure by an oral angiotensin converting enzyme inhibitor. Circulation 61:931–937, 1980.
4. Ahmad P, Mathur P, Ahuja S, Henderson R, Carruthers G: Rifampicin-quinidine interaction. Br J Dis Chest 73:409–411, 1979.
5. Allen MD, Greenblatt DJ, Harmatz JS, Smith TW: Effect of magnesium-aluminum hydroxide and kaolin-pectin on absorption of digoxin from tablets and capsules. J Clin Pharmacol 21:26–30, 1981.
6. Anastasion-Nana M, Levis GM, Moulopoulos S: Pharmacokinetics of amiodarone after intravenous and oral administration. Int J Pharmacol Ther Toxicol 20:524–529, 1982.
7. Andreason F, Agerback H, Bjerregaard P, Gotzsche H: Pharmacokinetics of amiodarone after intravenous and oral administration. J Clin Pharmacol 19:293–299, 1981.
8. Bacaner MB: Treatment of ventricular fibrillation and other acute arrhythmias with bretylium tosylate. Am J Cardiol 21:530–543, 1968.
9. Bax NDS, Tucker GT, Woods HF: Does indocyanine green predict lidocaine requirements? N Engl J Med 299:662–663, 1978.
10. Beckett AH, Chidomere EC: The distribution, metabolism, and excretion of mexiletene in man. Postgrad Med J 53(suppl I):60, 1977.
11. Beerman B, Dalen E, Lindstrom B: Elimination of furosemide in healthy subjects and in those with renal failure. Clin Pharmacol Ther 22:70–78, 1977.
12. Bellet S, Roman LR, Boza A: Relation between serum quinidine levels and renal function. Am J Cardiol 27:368–371, 1971.
13. Bellotti G, Silra LA, Filho AE, Rati M, De Moraes AV, Ramires JAF, da Luz P, Pileggi F: Hemodynamic effects of intravenous administration of amiodarone in congestive heart failure from chronic Chagas' disease. Am J Cardiol 52:1046–1049, 1983.
14. Benet LZ, Scheiner LB: Pharmacokinetics: the dynamics of drug absorption, distribution, and elimination. In Gilman AG, Goodman LS, Rall TW, Murad F, (eds): Goodman and Gilman's The Pharmacological Basis of Therapeutics, ed 7. New York, Macmillan, 1985, p 11.
15. Berg KJ, Tromsdal A, Wideroe TE: Diuretic action of bumetanide in advanced chronic renal insufficiency. Eur J Clin Pharmacol 9:265–275, 1976.
16. Berkseth RO, Kjellstrand CM: Radiologic contrast-induced nephropathy. Med Clin North Am 68:351–370, 1984.
17. Binnion PF: A comparison of digoxin bioavailability in capsule, tablet, and solution taken orally with I.V. digoxin. J Clin Pharmacol 16:461–467, 1976.
18. Bonati M, Galletti F, Volpi A, Cunnetti C, Rumolo R, Tognoni G: Amiodarone in patients on long-term dialysis. N Engl J Med 308:906, 1983.
19. Brater DC: Disposition and response to bumetanide and furosemide. Am J Cardiol 57:20A–25A, 1986.
20. Brater DC, Day B, Burdette A, Anderson S: Bumetanide and furosemide in heart failure. Kidney Int 26:183–189, 1984.
21. Braunwald E: Pathophysiology of heart failure. In Braunwald E (ed): Heart Disease, ed 2. Philadelphia, WB Saunders, 1984, p 447.
22. Bristow MR, Ginsburg R, Minobe W, Cubicciotti R, Sageman WS, Lurie K, Billingham ME, Harrison PC, Stinson EB: Decreased catecholamine sensitivity and β-adrenergic-receptor density in failing human hearts. N Engl J Med 307:205–211, 1982.
23. Burg M, Stoner L, Cardinal J, Green N: Furosemide effect in isolated perfused tubules. Am J Physiol 225:119–124, 1973.
24. Bussey HI: The influence of quinidine and other agents on digitalis glycosides. Am Heart J 104:289–302, 1982.
25. Camarata SJ, Weil MH, Harashiro PK, Shubin H: Cardiac arrest in the critically ill. I: A study of predisposing causes in 132 patients. Circulation 44:688–695, 1971.
26. Carlier J: Hemodynamic, electrocardiographic, and toxic effects of the intravenous administration of increasing doses of mexiletene in the dog: comparison with similar effects produced by other antiarrhythmics. Acta Cardiol [Suppl] (Brux) 25:81–100, 1980.
27. Chatterjee K, Mandel WJ, Vyden JK, Parmley WW, Forrester JS: Cardiovascular effects of bretylium tosylate in acute myocardial infarction. JAMA 223:757–760, 1973.
28. Chatterjee K, Swan HJC, Parmley WW, Sustaita H, Marcus H, Matloff J: Depression of left ventricular function due to acute myocardial ischemia and its reversal following aortocoronary saphenous vein bypass. N Engl J Med 286:1117–1122, 1972.
29. Cohn JN, Burke LP: Nitroprusside. Ann Intern Med 91:752–757, 1979.
30. Conrad GJ, Oler RE: Metabolism of flecainide. Am J Cardiol 53:41B–51B, 1984.
31. Conrad KA, Molk BL, Chidsey CA: Pharmacokinetic studies of quinidine in patients with arrhythmias. Circulation 55:1–7, 1977.
32. Cottrell JE, Casthely P, Brodie JO, Patel K, Klein A, Turndorf H: Prevention of nitroprusside-induced cyanide toxicity with hydroxycobalamin. N Engl J Med 298:809–811, 1978.
33. Cowan CJC, Williams EMV: Characterization of new oral anti-arrhythmic drug, flecainide (R-818). Eur J Pharmacol 73:333–342, 1981.
34. Crawford MH, White DH, O'Rourke RA: Effects of oral quinidine on left ventricular performance in normal subjects and patients with congestive cardiomyopathy. Am J Cardiol 44: 714–718, 1979.
35. Crouthamel WG: The effect of congestive heart failure on quinidine pharmacokinetics. Am Heart J 90:335–339, 1975.
36. Dami M, Derbekyan VA, Lisbona R: Hemodynamic effects of encainide in patients with ventricular arrhythmia and poor ventricular function. Am J Cardiol 52:507–511, 1983.
37. Darbey JT, Thompson KA, Echt DS, Woosley RL, Roder DM: Combination of low dose quinidine and tocainide in the treatment of ventricular arrhythmias in man (abstract). J Am Coll Cardiol 7:108–121, 1986.
38. Davison R, Parker M, Atkinson AJ: Excessive serum lidocaine levels during maintenance infusions: mechanisms and prevention. Am Heart J 104:203–208, 1982.
39. Dikshit K, Byden JK, Forrester JS, Chatterjee K, Prakosh R, Swan HJC: Renal and extrarenal hemodynamic effects of furosemide in congestive heart failure after acute myocardial infarction. N Engl J Med 288:1087–1090, 1973.
40. Doering W: Quinidine-digoxin interaction: pharmacokinetics, underlying mechanism and clinical implications. N Engl J Med 301:400–404, 1979.

41. Doherty JE, Perkins WH, Mitchell GK: Tritiated digoxin studies in human subjects. *Arch Intern Med* 108:531–539, 1961.

42. Doherty JE, Perkins WH, Wilson MC: Studies with tritiated digoxin in renal failure. *Am J Med* 37:536–544, 1964.

43. Dyckner T, Webster PO: Ventricular extrasystoles and intracellular electrolytes before and after potassium and magnesium infusions in patients on diuretic treatments. *Am Heart J* 97:12–18, 1979.

44. Elvin At, Keenaghan JB, Byrnes EW: Tocainide conjugation in humans: novel biotransformation pathway for a primary amine. *J Pharmacol Ther* 69:47–49, 1980.

45. Flecainide-Quinidine Research Group: Flecainide versus quinidine for treatment of chronic ventricular arrhythmias: a multicenter clinical trial. *Circulation* 67:1117–1123, 1983.

46. Franciosa JA, Wilen M, Weeks CE, Tanenbaum R, Kuan DC, Miller AM: Pharmacokinetics and hemodynamic effects of flecainide in patients with chronic low output heart failure. *J Am Coll Cardiol* 1:699, 1983.

47. Francis GS, Goldsmith SR, Cohn JN: Relationship of exercise capacity to resting left ventricular performance and basal plasma norepinephrine levels in patients with congestive heart failure. *Am Heart J* 104:725–731, 1982.

48. Fung HL, Ruggirello D, Stone JA, Parker JO: Effects of disease, route of administration, cigarette smoking, and food intake on the pharmacokinetics and circulating effects of isosorbide dinitrate. *Z Kardiol* 72(suppl 3):5–10, 1983.

49. Gale ME, Robbins AH, Hamberger I, Widrich WC: Renal toxicity of contrast agents: iopamidol, iothalamate, diatrizoate. *AJR* 142:333–335, 1984.

50. Garty M, Sood P, Rollins D: Digitoxin elimination reduced during quinidine therapy. *Ann Intern Med* 94:35–37, 1981.

51. Goldenberg IF, Low BT, Olivari MJ, Daniel JA, Nelson RR, VanTassel RA, Ochi R, Levine TB, Cohn JN: Effect of dobutamine infusion on serum electrolytes and arterial oxygenation in congestive heart failure. *J Am Coll Cardiol* 9:34A, 1987.

52. Goldsmith SR, Francis GS, Crawley AW, Levine TB, Cohn JN: Increased plasma arginine vasopressin in patients with congestive heart failure. *J Am Coll Cardiol* 1:1385–1390, 1983.

53. Grossman W, Alpert JJ, Braunwald E: Pulmonary hypertension. In Braunwald E (ed): *Heart Disease*, ed 2. Philadelphia, WB Saunders, 1984, p 827.

54. Hager WD, Fenstar P, Mayersohn M, Perrier D, Graves P, Marcus FI, Goldman S: Digitoxin-quinidine interaction: pharmacokinetic evaluation. *N Engl J Med* 300:1238–1241, 1979.

55. Halkin H, Sheiner LB, Peck CC, Melmon KH: Determinants of the renal clearance of digoxin. *Clin Pharmacol Ther* 17:385–394, 1975.

56. Hansen MS, Woods SL, Willis RE: Relative effectiveness of nitroglycerin ointment according to site of application. *Heart Lung* 8:716–720, 1979.

57. Harkonen S, Kjellstrand CM: Contrast nephropathy. *Am J Nephrol* 1:69–77, 1981.

58. Harris L, Hird CRK, McKenna WJ: Renal elimination of amiodarone and its desethyl metabolite. *Postgrad Med J* 59:440–442, 1983.

59. Harrison DC, Sprous J, Morrow AG: Antiarrhythmic properties of lidocaine and procainamide: clinical and physiological studies on their cardiovascular effects in man. *Circulation* 28:486–491, 1963.

60. Hayes AH Jr, Shiroff RA, Limjuco RA, Schuech DW: Effect of bumetanide on the renal excretion of digoxin (abstract). *Clin Pharmacol Ther* 25:228, 1979.

61. Heissenbuttel RH, Ryger JT Jr: Bretylium tosylate, a newly available drug for ventricular arrhythmias. *Ann Intern Med* 91:229–238, 1979.

62. Hepner GW, Vesell ES, Tantum KR: Reduced drug elimination in congestive heart failure. *Am J Med* 65:271–276, 1978.

63. Hodges M, Haugland JM, Grarud G, Conard GJ, Asinger RW, Mikell FL, Krejci JA: Suppression of ventricular ectopic depolarization by flecainide acetate, a new antiarrhythmic agent. *Circulation* 65:879–885, 1982.

64. Hooymans PM, Merkus FWHM: Effect of quinidine on plasma concentrations (letter). *Br Med J* 2:1022, 1978.

65. Horn HR, Hadidan Z, Johnson JL, Vassallo HG, Williams JH, Young MD: Safety evaluation of tocainide in American Emergency Use Program. *Am Heart J* 100:1037–1040, 1980.

66. Hou SH, Bushinsky DA, Wish JB, Cohen JJ, Harrington JT: Hospital-acquired renal insufficiency: a prospective study. *Am J Med* 74:243–248, 1983.

67. Imhof PR, Ott B, Frankhausser P, Chu LC, Hodler J: Difference in nitroglycerin dose-response in the venous and arterial beds. *Eur J Clin Pharmacol* 18:455–460, 1980.

68. Jeaner P, Testa B (eds): *Concepts in Drug Metabolism, Drugs and the Pharmaceutical Sciences Series*, New York, Marcel Decker, 1981, vol 10, part B.

69. Jenne JW, Chick TW, Miller BA, Strickland RD: Apparent theophylline half-life fluctuations during treatment of acute left ventricular failure. *Am J Hosp Pharm* 34:408–409, 1977.

70. Johnson BF, Grear H, McCreavie J, Fowle A: Rate of dissolution of digoxin tablets as a predictor of absorption. *Lancet* 1:1473–1475, 1973.

71. Josephson MA, Ikeda N, Singh BN: Effects of flecainide on ventricular function: clinical and experimental correlations. *Am J Cardiol* 53:95B–100B, 1984.

72. Josephson MA, Kaul S, Hopkins J, Kra D, Singh BN: Hemodynamic effects of intravenous flecainide relative to the level of ventricular function in patients with coronary artery disease. *Am Heart J* 109:41–45, 1985.

73. Kates RE, Leier CV: Dobutamine pharmacokinetics in severe heart failure. *Clin Pharmacol Ther* 24:537–541, 1978.

74. Kessler KM, Kayder DS, Estes D, Kozlosskis P, Sequira R, Myerbraid RJ: Procainamide pharmacokinetics/pharmacodynamics in acute myocardial infarction or congestive heart failure (abstract). *Circulation* 70(suppl 2):446, 1984.

75. Kessler KM, Lowenthal DT, Warner H, Gibson T, Briggs W, Reidenberg MM: Quinidine elimination in patients with congestive heart failure or poor renal function. *N Engl J Med* 290:706–709, 1974.

76. Kjekshus J, Bathen J, Orning OM, Storsteiin L: A double-blind crossover comparison of flecainide acetate and disopyramide phosphate in the treatment of ventricular premature complexes. *Am J Cardiol* 53:72B–78B, 1984.

77. Klein HO, Long R, Weiss E, DiSegni E, Libhaber C, Guerrero J, Kaplinsky E: The influence of verapamil on serum digoxin concentration. *Circulation* 65:998–1003, 1982.

78. Klein MD, Leveine PA, Ryan TJ: Antiarrhythmic efficacy, pharmacokinetics, and clinical safety of tocainide in convalescent myocardial infarction patients. *Chest* 77:726–730, 1980.

79. Koch-Weser J: Disopyramide. *N Engl J Med* 300:957–962, 1979.

80. Koch-Weser J: Pharmacokinetics of procainamide in man. *Ann NY Acad Sci* 179:370–382, 1971.

81. Koch-Weser J, Klein SW: Procainamide dosage schedules, plasma concentrations, and clinical effects. *JAMA* 214:1454–1460, 1971.

82. Kuntzman R, Tsai I, Chang R, Conney AH: Disposition of bretylium in man and rat. *Clin Pharmacol Ther* 11:829–837, 1970.

83. LaDu BN, Mandel HG, Way EL (eds): *Fundamentals*

of Drug Metabolism and Drug Disposition Baltimore, Williams & Wilkins, 1971.

84. Lal R, Chapman PD, Naccarelli GV, Schectman KB, Rinkerberger RL, Troup PJ, Kim SS, Dougherty AH: Flecainide in the treatment of nonsustained ventricular tachycardia. *Ann Intern Med* 105:493–498, 1986.

85. Landmark K, Bredesen JE, Thaulow E, Simons S, Amlie JP: Pharmacokinetics of disopyramide in patients with imminent to moderate cardiac failure. *Eur J Clin Pharmacol* 19:187–192, 1981.

86. Leahey EB, Reiffel JA, Giardina EGV, Bigger JT: The effect of quinidine and other oral antiarrhythmic drugs on serum digoxin: a prospective study. *Ann Intern Med* 94:34–37, 1981.

87. Leahey GB, Giardina EGU, Bigger JT: Effect of ventricular failure on stady state kinetics of mexiletine (abstract). *Clin Res* 26:239, 1980.

88. Leier CV, Unverferth DV: Dobutamine. *Ann Intern Med* 99:490–496, 1983.

89. Le Lorier J, Grenor D, Latour Y, Caille G, Dumont G, Brosseau A, Solignac A: Pharmacokinetics of lidocaine after prolonged intravenous infusions in uncomplicated myocardial infarction. *Ann Intern Med* 87:700–702, 1977.

90. Lewis GP, Haltzman JL: Interaction of flecainide with digoxin and propranolol. *Am J Cardiol* 53:52B–57B, 1984.

91. Lie KI, Liem KL, Louridtz WJ, Janse MJ, Willebrands AF, Durrer: Efficacy of lidocaine in preventing primary ventricular fibrillation within one hour after a 300 mg intramuscular injection. *Am J Cardiol* 42: 486–488, 1978.

92. Lindenbaum J, Rund DG, Butler VP Jr, Tse-Eng D, Saha JR: Inactivation of digoxin by gut flora: reversal by antibiotic therapy. *N Engl J Med* 305:789–794, 1981.

93. Loeb HS, Bredakis J, Gunnar RM: Superiority of dobutamine over dopamine for augmentation of cardiac output in patients with chronic low output cardiac failure. *Circulation* 55:375–381, 1977.

94. Lopez I, Mehta JL, Robinson JD, Roberts RJ: Optimal lidocaine dosing in patients with myocardial infarction. *Ther Drug Monit* 4:271–276, 1982.

95. Lukas DS, DeMartino AG: Binding of digitoxin and some related corderolides to human plasma protein. *J Clin Invest* 48:1041–1053, 1969.

96. MacMahon B, Bakshi M, Braragan P, Kelly JG, Wash MJ: Pharmacokinetics and hemodynamic effects of tocainide in patients with acute myocardial infarction complicated by left ventricular failure. *Br J Clin Pharmacol* 19:429–434, 1985.

97. Maisel AS, Motulsky JH, Isnel PA: Sequestration of beta-adrenergic receptors in acute heart failure: comparison of lymphocytes and heart (abstract). *Circulation* 74(suppl II):81, 1986.

98. Manninen V, Melin J, Apajalahti A, Karesoja M: Altered absorption of digoxin in patients given propantheline and metoclopramide *Lancet* 1:398–399, 1973.

99. Mason JW: Amiodarone. *N Engl J Med* 316:455–466, 1987.

100. Mathur PP: Cardiovascular effects of a new antiarrhythmic agent: disopyramide phosphate. *Am Heart J* 84:764–770, 1972.

101. McLaren CJ, Hassack KF, Mielson GH, Seskied V: Oral tocainide versus disopyramide: a double blind, randomized, cross-over study of outpatients with stable ventricular premature beats. *J Cardiovasc Pharmacol* 6:657–662, 1984.

102. Mirsky I, Parmley WW: Assessment of passive elastic stiffness for isolated muscle and the intact heart. *Circ Res* 33:233–243, 1973.

103. Mitenko PA, Ogilvie RI: Rational intravenous doses of theophylline. *N Engl J Med* 289:600–603, 1973.

104. Mohiuddin SM, Esterbrooks D, Hilleman DE, Aronow WS, Patterson AJ, Mooss AN, Hee TT, Reich JW: Tocainide kinetics in congestive heart failure. *Clin Pharmacol Ther* 34:596–603, 1983.

105. Muller P, Imhoff PR, Burkart F, Chu LC, Gerodin A: Human pharmacological studies of a new transdermal system containing nitroglycerin. *Eur J Pharmacol* 22:473–480, 1982.

106. Naafs MAB, Vanderltoek C, vanDuin S, Koorevaar G, Schoman W, Silberbusch J: Decreased renal clearance of digoxin in chronic congestive heart failure. *Eur J Clin Pharmacol* 29:249–252, 1985.

107. Nanj AA, Greenway DC: Widely differing plasma digoxin levels in patients with congestive heart failure and severe liver dysfunction. *Arch Pathol Lab Med* 110:75–76, 1986.

108. Nomura A, Yasuda H, Minami M, Akimoto T, Miyazuki K, Arita T: Effect of furosemide in congestive heart failure. *Clin Pharmacol Ther* 30:177–182, 1981.

109. Nyquist O, Forssell G, Nordlarder R, Schenck-Gustafson K: Hemodynamic and antiarrhythmic effects of tocainide in patients with acute myocardial infarction. *Am Heart J* 100:1000–1005, 1980.

110. Ochs HR, Carstens G, Greenblatt DJ: Reduction in lidocaine clearance during continuous infusion and by coadministration of propranolol. *N Engl J Med* 303:333–377, 1980.

111. Oltmans D: Pharmacokinetics of tocainamide in patients with chronic liver disease (abstract). *Naunyn Schmiedebergs Arch Pharmacol* 321(suppl):R49, 1982.

112. Packer M, Kessler PD, Lee WH, Medina N, Yushak M, Gottlieb SS: Does the intermittent administration of nitroglycerin prevent the development of hemodynamic tolerance in patients with severe heart failure? *J Am Coll Cardiol* 9:103A, 1987.

113. Page DL, Caufield JB, Kastor JA, DeSanctis RW, Sardeus CA: Myocardial changes associated with cardiogenic shock. *N Engl J Med* 285:133–137, 1971.

114. Parmley WW: Pathophysiology of congestive heart failure. *Am J Cardiol* 55:9A–14A, 1985.

115. Pederson KE, Hastrup J, Hvidt S: The effect of quinidine on digoxin kinetics in cardiac patients. *Acta Med Scand* 207:291–295, 1980.

116. Piafsky KM, Sitar OS, Rangno RE, Ogilvie RI: Theophylline kinetics in acute pulmonary edema. *Clin Pharmacol Ther* 21:310–316, 1977.

117. Podrid PJ, Schoeneberger A, Lown B: Congestive heart failure caused by oral disopyramide. *N Engl J Med* 302:614–617, 1980.

118. Powell JR, Vozeh S, Hopewell P, Costello J, Scheiner LB, Reigelman S: Theophylline disposition in acutely ill hospitalized patients: the effect of smoking, heart failure, severe airway obstruction, and pneumonia. *Am Rev Respir Dis* 118:229–238, 1978.

119. Prescott LF, Adjepon-Yamoah KK, Talbot RG: Impaired lignocaine metabolism in patients with myocardial infarction and cardiac failure. *Br Med J* 1:939–941, 1976.

120. Prescott LF, Pottage A, Clements JA: Absorption, distribution, and elimination of mexiletene. *Postgrad Med* 53(suppl 1):50–55, 1977.

121. Riva E, Gerna M, Zatini R, Giani P, Volpi A, Magzioni A: Pharmacokinetics of amiodarone in man. *J Cardiovasc Pharmacol* 4:264–269, 1982.

122. Robinson KC, Walter S, Johnston A, Mulraw JP, McKenna WJ, Holt DW: The digoxin-amiodarone interaction (abstract). *Circulation* 74(suppl II):225, 1986.

123. Roden DM, Reele SB, Higgins SB, Mayol RF, Gammans RE, Oates JA, Woosley RL: Total suppression of ventricular arrhythmias by encainide: pharmacokinetics and electrocardiographic characteristics. *N Engl J Med* 302:877–882, 1980.

124. Roden DM, Woosley RL: Flecainide. *N Engl J Med* 315:36–41, 1986.

125. Roden DM, Woosley RL: Tocainide. *N Engl J Med* 315:41–45, 1986.

126. Roden DM, Woosley RL, Bortick D, Bernard Y, Primm RK: Quinidine-induced long QT syndrome; incidence and presenting features (abstract). *Circulation* 68(suppl 3):267, 1983.

127. Rose JH, Pruitt AW, Dayton PG, McNay JL: Relationship of urinary furosemide excretion rate to natriuretic effect in experimental azoteuria. *J Pharmacol Exp Ther* 199:490–497, 1976.

128. Ruff HJ, Roden D, Primm RK, Oates JA, Woosley RL: Mexiletine in the treatment of resistant ventricular arrhythmias: enhancement of efficacy and reduction of dose-related side effects by combination with quinidine. *Circulation* 67:1124–1128, 1983.

129. Ruffolo RR Jr, Kopia GA: Importance of receptor regulation in the pathophysiology and therapy of contive heart failure. *Am J Med* 80(suppl 2B):67–72, 1986.

130. Schneeweiss A: *Drug Therapy in Cardiovascular Disease.* Philadelphia, Lea & Febiger: 1984, p 521.

131. Shelly JH: Harmony and discord; a review of interactions with mexiletine. In Sandoe E et al (eds): *Management of Ventricular Tachycardia: Role of Mexiletine.* Amsterdam, Excerpta Medica, 1978, p 841.

132. Stein J, Podrid P, Lawn B: Effects of oral mexiletine on left and right ventricular function. *Am J Cardiol* 54:575–578, 1984.

133. Steiness E: Renal tubular secretion of digoxin. *Circulation* 50:103–107, 1974.

134. Steiness E: Suppression of renal excretion of digoxin in hypokalemic patients. *Clin Pharmacol Ther* 23:511–514, 1978.

135. Stenson RE, Constantino RT, Harrison DC: Interrelationship of hepatic blood flow, cardiac output, and blood levels of lidocaine in man. *Circulation* 43:205–211, 1971.

136. Swedberg K, Hjalmarsan A, Waagstein F, Wallentin I: Beneficial effects of long-term beta blockade in congestive cardiomyopathy. *Br Heart J* 44:117–133, 1980.

137. Taliercio CP, Vliestra RE, Fisher LP, Burnett JC: Risks for renal dysfunction with cardiac angiography. *Ann Intern Med* 104:501–504, 1986.

138. Thomas JA, Markis BH: Plasma norepinephrine in congestive heart failure. *Am J Cardiol* 41:233–243, 1978.

139. Thomson PP, Melmon KI, Richardson JA, Cohn K, Steinbrunn W, Cudihee R, Rowland M: Lidocaine pharmacokinetics in advanced heart failure, liver disease, and renal failure in humans. *Ann Intern Med* 78:499–508, 1973.

140. Tjarda Maga B, Verbesselt R, Van Hecken Aa, Van Hecken A, Van Melle P, De Schepper PJ: Oral flecainide elimination kinetics: effects of cimetidine (abstract). *Circulation* 68(suppl 3):416, 1983.

141. Vasko MR, Brown-Cartwright D, Knochel JP, Nixon JV, Brater DC: Furosemide absorption altered in decompensated congestive heart failure. *Ann Intern Med* 102:314–318, 1985.

142. Waldorff S, Hansen PB, Kjaergard H, Bach J, Egeblad H, Steiness E: Amiloride-induced changes in digoxin dynamics and kinetics: abolition of digoxin-induced ionotropism with amiloride. *Clin Pharmacol Ther* 30:172–176, 1981.

143. Wasermiller JT, Aronow WS: Effects of tocainide and quinidine on premature ventricular contractions. *Clin Pharmacol Ther* 28:431–435, 1980.

144. Wiegers U, Hanrath P, Kuck KH, Pottage A, Craffner C, Augustin J, Runge M: Pharmacokinetics of tocainide in patients with renal dysfunction and during hemodialysis. *Eur J Clin Pharmacol* 24:503–507, 1983.

145. Williamson JR, Schaffer DW, Ford C, et al: Contribution of tissue acidosis to ischemic injury in the perfused rat heart. *Circulation* 53(suppl I):3–14, 1976.

146. Willis PW, III: The hemodynamic effects of norpace (Part II). *Angiology* 26(suppl 1):102–110, 1975.

147. Wilson J: Leber's hereditary optic atrophy: a possible defect of cyanide metabolism. *Clin Sci* 29:505–515, 1965.

148. Wittig J, Harrison LA, Wallace AG: Electrophysiological effects of lidocaine on distal Purkinje fibers (abstract). *Circulation* 46(suppl II):39, 1972.

149. Woosley RL, Echt DS, Roden DM: Treatment of ventricular arrhythmias in the failing heart: pharmacologic and clinical considerations. *Drug Ther* 19(10):1–7, 1985.

150. Zito RA, Reid PR: Lidocaine kinetics predicted by indocyanine clearance. *N Engl J Med* 299:662–663, 1978.

151. Zito RA, Reid PR, Longstreth JA: Variability of early lidocaine levels in patients. *Am Heart J* 94:292–296, 1977.

152. Zwillich CW, Sutton FD, Neff TA, Cohn WM, Matthay RA, Weinberger MM: Theophylline-induced seizures in adults: correlation with serum concentrations. *Ann Intern Med* 82:784–787, 1975.

4

Adjustment of Medications in Liver Failure

Patricia A. Arns, M.D.
Peter J. Wedlund, Ph.D.
Robert A. Branch, M.D.

Patients with liver disease are commonly treated with one or more different drugs in an effort to alleviate the numerous pathologic changes often associated with this and/or other concurrent disease processes. Commonly used drugs include diuretics, antibiotics, sedatives, and antiinflammatory, cardiovascular, and cancer chemotherapeutic agents. This use of potent and often multidrug therapy is generally considered to be a contributing factor to the frequent and sometimes fatal drug reactions that occur in this patient population (121). Of equal importance are the effects of liver disease on the absorption, distribution, elimination, and pharmacologic response to these drugs. Such changes may require reductions in drug dosage in order to avoid drug toxicity. The understanding of how liver disease can influence drug disposition and dosage requirements entails appreciation for:

1. The various types of functions that the liver performs;
2. The pathologic changes produced by liver disease and how these changes alter hepatic function; and
3. The parameters that influence drug disposition and how they are affected by liver disease.

LIVER FUNCTION IN HEALTH AND DISEASE: IMPLICATIONS FOR DRUG DISPOSITION

Hepatic Function

The strategic location of the liver between the splanchnic and systemic circulations is well suited for the large number of functions that this organ carries out. Included in this list of functions are *(a)* the synthesis of most plasma proteins (e.g., albumin, transport proteins, α-1-acid glycoproteins, lipoproteins, and clotting factors); *(b)* the regulation and synthesis of glucose, amino acids, fatty acids, and cholesterol; *(c)* the removal of ammonia, endotoxins, bilirubin, lactic acid, endogenous hormones, toxic substances, and waste products from the blood; and *(d)* the synthesis of bile and urea. Although this is a short list of the more than 1500 known functions carried out by the liver, it indicates the diversity and importance of this organ in maintaining homeostasis in the body.

The liver also plays an important role in the metabolism and elimination of drugs that may be too lipophilic to be efficiently removed by the kidneys. This function is carried out by a number of different enzymes located in liver cells. For example, one group of isoenzymes, referred to collectively as the cytochromes P-450, is important for carrying out many of the mixed function oxidative reactions that convert lipophilic compounds into more water-soluble products. Other enzymes in the liver may further transform these metabolites (or other drugs) by conjugating them with sugars, amino acids, sulfates, or acetate to form products that can be more readily eliminated in the bile or removed by the kidney. Still other liver enzymes (i.e., esterases, deaminases, hydrolases, and reductases) are important for the metabolic transformation and elimination of certain drugs and endogenous chemicals.

Many of these homeostatic and metabolic functions are compromised when the liver is damaged by different etiologic agents such as chemicals (including drugs) and diseases. The actual degree of damage to liver hemoperfusion, biliary excretion, and synthetic and metabolic functions in the liver can vary widely and therefore lead to variable changes in drug disposition. Such changes in drug disposition

65

reflect, to some extent, the degree to which the liver is impaired. For example, alcoholic liver disease can range from fatty liver, with little or no change in the disposition of most drugs, to severe cirrhosis, with major changes in the disposition of certain classes of drugs. Hepatic neoplasms also show great variability in the effect on drug disposition, depending on type (primary versus secondary), size, invasiveness, and vascularity of tumor mass. Moreover, certain acute injuries to the liver, as seen in viral hepatitis, may affect the disposition of some drugs, but this effect may be reversible as the injury subsides.

Hepatic reserves may help to maintain liver functions, and changes in drug metabolism may be slight since few if any liver functions are performed at 100% of their capacity. For example, under normal conditions, urea formation from ammonia and amino acids occurs at 60% of capacity. Glucose maintenance requires only 20% of liver function. Bilirubin elimination must fall below 10% of normal before jaundice develops, and albumin and clotting factors are synthesized by only a small percentage of the total liver cells at any one time. Furthermore, these and other liver processes may be increased when there is increased demand. As a result, it is often difficult to determine the extent of liver damage caused by an agent because reserve and repair mechanisms tend to maintain hepatic function.

Such reserve and recuperative properties are obviously advantageous for the liver. This regenerative capability allows the liver to recover completely following acute liver insult. Even when the damage is extensive, if the causative agent is removed, the liver is capable of full recovery. However, if the etiologic agent is not removed so that the liver becomes exposed to chronic damage, then hepatic reserves may become seriously depleted. A limited repertoire of liver responses to such chronic damage will result in a characteristic pathophysiologic state of cirrhosis. Under such circumstances, significant changes in drug disposition may occur. The level of cytochrome P-450 enzymes in the liver, for example, may decline (38, 171, 188) and this change can seriously impair the liver's ability to metabolize endogenous products and drugs (33, 188). Deterioration in other liver functions (i.e., the removal of bilirubin and fatty acids and synthesis of plasma proteins) may lead to further alterations in drug disposition by influencing drug binding and distribution in the body (15, 20, 88, 170, 205).

Architecture and Blood Flow in Cirrhosis

The development of cirrhosis begins with initial hepatocellular damage producing inflammation, followed by phagocytic removal of dead or necrotic cells. This damage stimulates the secretion of collagen by fibroblasts to help maintain the integrity of the liver architecture while the damaged and dead cells are repaired or replaced. As the damage continues, collagen secretion may be further stimulated resulting in its accumulation in liver sinusoidal spaces. This accumulation of collagen in the sinusoids leads to the formation of bands of connective scar tissue characteristic of cirrhosis. In compensation for hepatocellular damage, hepatocyte regeneration may lead to the clustered formation of new hepatocytes, which later form liver nodules. These nodules may increase in size and further distort the normal liver architecture.

As the liver architecture becomes distorted, the resistance to the flow of blood through the liver is increased. This increase in turn causes the portal venous pressure to rise. To alleviate an elevated pressure, portal venous blood is shunted around the liver through collateral channels directly into the systemic circulation. The development of these collateral channels for shunting the portal venous blood occurs primarily where tributaries of the portal venous system lie in close proximity to those of the systemic circulation (i.e., submucosa of the esophagus, stomach, rectum, left renal vein, and abdomen). The increased blood flow and pressure in gastroesophageal varices predispose cirrhotic patients to an increased risk of gastrointestinal hemorrhage; a major cause of death in these patients (45).

The development of collateral channels for shunting of portal venous blood around the liver can alter the effective hepatic blood flow and the amount of drug reaching the systemic circulation after oral administration (60, 143, 150, 184). These and other changes in drug disposition may require the dosage of some drugs to be reduced.

In addition, recent studies have shown that hepatic disease may also alter the microcirculation of the liver. Sinusoidal plasma in the healthy liver has direct access to the hepatocyte. Although the sinusoid is lined by endothelial cells, this is not a continuous layer; there is an incomplete basal lamina, and endothelial cells contain multiple fenestrations.

Between the sinusoidal endothelium and the hepatocyte is the space of Disse, which contains the microvilli of hepatic cells, reticular fibers, and fat storage cells. Alcoholic liver disease is associated with an increase in type III collagen in the space of Disse, formation of a basal lamina, and a decrease in the number of fenestrations and porosity of the endothelial cell as seen with scanning electron microscopy (63, 99, 137, 187). This endothelialization transforms sinusoids into capillary-like channels and limits the access of sinusoidal blood to the hepatocyte. Studies using multiple indicator dilution techniques support the concept that conversion of loose interendothelial cell junctions to tight endothelial cell junctions may provide a barrier to the movement of molecules into the proximity of the hepatocyte (65–67). This could be of importance in the diffusion of albumin and other large molecules, including protein-bound substances such as drugs, which may result in decreased ability for drug metabolism by the liver.

Renal Function

Hemodynamic changes may also be present in the kidneys of patients with liver disease. Renal blood flow has been shown to be decreased in cirrhosis without laboratory evidence of decreased renal function or the development of edema or ascites (159–161). Glomerular filtration rate is variable in early cirrhosis (83), but is usually decreased when ascites develops. Moreover, the handling of electrolytes by the kidneys is disturbed in patients with cirrhosis. Renal sodium retention is a well-known phenomenon associated with this disease and is an important factor in the development of ascites. With progression of liver disease, a number of these factors will further depress kidney function to the point of renal failure (175). It follows that drugs having a major renal route of elimination may have an altered disposition in patients with liver disease, because of the secondary development of functional renal failure.

Ascites Formation and Albumin Concentration

Increased sodium and fluid retention by the kidneys and increased production of lymph both contribute to the formation of ascites. The increased production of lymph is associated with increases in blood pressure in the sinusoidal spaces of the liver. Lymph production in the liver is particularly sensitive to changes in blood pressure because of the very "leaky" extravascular spaces that separate the hepatocytes from the sinusoidal blood. As the production of lymph within the liver is increased, lymph channels enlarge to accommodate the increased production. Unfortunately, these channels have a limited capacity to handle the increased production and may become blocked or overwhelmed. When lymph formation exceeds the ability of lymph channels to return it to the systemic circulation, lymph may weep from the liver into the peritoneal cavity contributing to the formation of ascites.

This lymph carries with it albumin and other plasma proteins, often at a time when the synthesis of new albumin and other proteins by the liver is depressed. In response to both these factors, total serum protein and albumin levels may fall. With the fall in serum protein levels, the binding and retention of drugs within the vascular compartment may decline. These changes may modify drug distribution and/or pharmacologic response by allowing drug to pass from the blood into other tissue compartments of the body.

CHARACTERISTICS OF DRUG DISPOSITION

Whether pathologic changes associated with liver disease require an alteration in a normal drug regimen is determined by the dispositional characteristics of the drug and the biological determinants of the system. Drug disposition, which includes both the distribution and elimination of drug, is determined in part by the physical properties of the drug. Important characteristics include molecular size, charge, pK_a, and lipid solubility. These factors will determine distribution as well as the route of elimination. In general, water-soluble drugs have a small volume of distribution and can be eliminated unchanged in urine, and lipid-soluble drugs have a large volume of distribution and require metabolism to more water-soluble moieties. Depending on the physical characteristics of any given drug, the balance of physiologic factors influencing that drug's disposition will vary. These physiologic factors have the potential to be altered by disease states. Thus, the influence of any one disease process can be complex; it can be mediated by a variety of factors and can influence the disposition of different drugs to a variable extent.

Distribution

The major aspects of distribution affected by liver disease are volume of distribution (V_d) and plasma protein binding. Conceptually, the apparent volume of distribution is the volume into which a drug distributes in the body when it is at equilibrium and is related to the pool from which the drug concentration is measured. It is a theoretical concept and reflects the partitioning of drug between the fluid compartments in the body, e.g., plasma, interstitial fluid, and intracellular fluid. It is calculated by:

$$V_d = \frac{D}{Cp} \tag{1}$$

where D represents the fraction of the dose absorbed and Cp is drug concentration at equilibrium. One way that liver disease can affect the V_d is by the production of ascites, which may produce an increase in the body's total fluid compartment. For example, propranolol has been shown to exhibit a 2-fold increase in V_d in patients with ascites, regardless of the extent of protein binding (18).

Most drugs in plasma are reversibly bound to proteins, such as albumin, globulin, α-1-acid glycoprotein, lipoproteins, ceruloplasmin, and transferrin. Acidic drugs commonly bind to albumin, whereas basic drugs more commonly bind to α-1-acid glycoprotein. Only unbound drug is available for distribution into tissues and capable of evoking a pharmacologic response (72, 94, 96, 142, 176). The extent of protein binding is therefore important in determining both pharmacologic response and drug disposition.

Cirrhosis causes a number of alterations that can also influence the binding of drugs within the blood, including *(a)* a decrease in serum albumin levels, *(b)* the appearance of altered or defective plasma proteins, and *(c)* the accumulation of endogenous and exogenous compounds that can displace drugs from protein binding sites. For example, acute viral hepatitis or primary biliary cirrhosis can lead to elevated serum bilirubin levels. The strong affinity of bilirubin for protein binding sites on albumin and the elevated levels are in part responsible for the displacement of some acidic drugs from the protein (15, 211). Taken together, these factors can produce alterations in drug binding to proteins and in the unbound serum drug concentrations. As a result, changes may occur in drug distribution and elimination and pharmacologic response.

With a decrease in drug binding to plasma or blood proteins, more drug may become available for distribution into tissues, increasing the drug's apparent volume of distribution. This change can alter the drug's elimination half-life independently of any change in drug metabolism. The reason for this change is apparent from the dependence of the half-life $(t_{1/2})$ on both its total clearance from the blood (Cl) and its apparent volume of distribution (V_d), according to the equation:

$$t_{1/2} = \frac{0.693 \ V_d}{Cl} \tag{2}$$

As a result of this dependence, the half-life of a drug can be a misleading parameter when attempting to determine the effect(s) of liver disease on drug elimination. For example, an increase in the apparent volume of distribution of a drug may lead to a prolongation in its elimination half-life in the absence of any real change in metabolic drug elimination. The increase in the half-lives of valproic acid (88) and lorazepam (89) in patients with liver disease, in fact, has been explained entirely by an increase in drug distribution secondary to decreased plasma binding rather than by a reduction in clearance.

In addition to influencing drug distribution, changes in protein binding can influence drug elimination. A change in the free fraction of a drug in the blood can lead to an increase in the amount of drug available to the drug-metabolizing enzymes and therefore to an increase in the total clearance of some drugs. This increase can shorten the half-life of a drug in the absence of any change in the activity of drug-metabolizing enzymes. Indeed, the decrease in the half-life of tolbutamide (211) in acute viral hepatitis has been attributed solely to a decrease in its binding to plasma proteins, since it has been shown that even though total (free + bound) clearance of tolbutamide increases, protein binding decreases and free clearance remains unchanged.

These examples indicate that the effect of protein binding on drug disposition is difficult to predict. As shown in Table 4.1, these changes in binding are a function of both type and severity of disease, as well as of the drug itself. Presently, there are no guidelines for predicting the effect of liver disease on drug binding. However, two general rules may provide some

Table 4.1
Changes in the Plasma Protein Binding of Drugs Caused by Liver Disease

Drug	Free Fraction (f_p) in Plasma (%)	Change in f_p with Liver Disease (%)	Significance	Type of Disease	Reference
Amylobarbital	39.3	76	$P < 0.005$	Cirrhosis	106
Azapropazone	0.44	377	$P < 0.05$	Cirrhosis	70
Caffeine	68.7	8.4	$P < 0.01$	Cirrhosis	31
Chlordiazepoxide	3.5	54	$P < 0.05$	Cirrhosis	163
Chlordiazepoxide	3.5	131	$P < 0.01$	Acute hepatitis	163
Chlormethiazole	35.6	24	$P < 0.01$	Cirrhosis	143
Clindamycin	20.8	1	NS	Cirrhosis	11
Clofibrate (CPIB)	2.8	0	NS	Acute hepatitis	50
Clofibrate (CPIB)	2.8	157	$P < 0.05$	Cirrhosis	50
Dapsone	18.5	125	—	Cirrhosis	155
Diazepam	2.2	113	$P < 0.001$	Cirrhosis	85
Diphenylhydantoin	8.3	41	NS	Cirrhosis	4
Diphenylhydantoin	10.8	44	$P < 0.05$	Cirrhosis	62
Diphenylhydantoin	9.9	27	$P < 0.05$	Acute hepatitis	15
Diphenylhydantoin	5.8	309	$P < 0.005$	Hepatic failure	135
Furosemide	4.0	155	$P < 0.001$	Cirrhosis	200
Furosemide	1.9	63	$P < 0.01$	Cirrhosis	5
Hexobarbital	53	1.9	NS	Cirrhosis	218
Lorazepam	6.8	68	$P < 0.01$	Cirrhosis	89
Meperidine	36	−1.6	NS	Cirrhosis	87
Meperidine	42	5.5	NS	Acute hepatitis	108
Morphine	80.1	3.4	NS	Cirrhosis	140
Morphine	64.9	16	$P < 0.05$	Hepatic failure	135
Oxazepam	13.3	6.9	NS	Cirrhosis	178
Oxazepam	13.3	4.9	NS	Acute hepatitis	178
Phenylbutazone	6	67	$P < 0.01$	Cirrhosis	205
Prednisolone	46.5	15	$P < 0.05$	Chronic liver disease	152
Prednisolone	46.5	6.7	NS	Acute hepatitis	152
Propoxyphene	25	8	NS	Cirrhosis	44
Propranolol	6.6	55	$P < 0.05$	Cirrhosis	214
Propranolol	12.2	45	$P < 0.05$	Cirrhosis	20
Quinidine	11	18	$P < 0.05$	Chronic liver disease	144
Quinidine	14.1	194	$P < 0.001$	Cirrhosis	4
Salicylate	27	52	$P < 0.005$	Cirrhosis	22
Salicylate	19.9	30	NS	Chronic liver disease	144
Salicylate	27	18.5	NS	Mixture	205
Sulfadiazine	46	46	$P < 0.01$	Mixture	205
Theophylline	47	33	—	Cirrhosis	147
Theophylline	35	103	$P < 0.001$	Cirrhosis	101
Thiopental	28.0	89	$P < 0.01$	Cirrhosis	43
Tolbutamide	2.2	100	$P < 0.02$	Alcoholic	195
Tolbutamide	6.8	28	$P < 0.01$	Acute hepatitis	211
Triamterene	19.3	71	$P < 0.01$	Cirrhosis	4
Valproic acid	11.3	159	$P < 0.002$	Cirrhosis	88
Valproic acid	11.3	36	—	Acute hepatitis	88
Warfarin	1.2	0	NS	Acute hepatitis	212

insight into the more important factors influencing the extent of change. (a) If protein binding is altered by a particular liver disease, the degree of liver damage will influence the extent of change in drug binding to plasma proteins. (b) Changes in the extent of binding to plasma proteins will tend to be greater for extensively bound drugs (i.e., >60% bound) than for poorly bound drugs (i.e., <60% bound). Although these are general rules that have

their exceptions, they should provide some appreciation for the effects of liver disease on plasma protein binding.

Elimination

Elimination of drug is defined as the irreversible loss of drug from the site of measurement and includes both metabolism and excretion. Clearance is an important parameter that relates drug concentration to the rate of elimination, thereby providing a measure of efficiency of the elimination process. By definition, total or systemic clearance is a measure of the amount of plasma cleared of drug per unit time. This measure can be obtained from measurements of drug concentration in plasma after single doses (Equation 2) or at steady state:

$$Cl = \frac{\text{rate of drug administration}}{Cp_{ss}} \quad (3)$$

where Cp_{ss} is the steady state plasma concentration. Clearance is independent of the mechanism of elimination involved, and if multiple routes of elimination occur concurrently, it provides an estimate of the sum of these processes.

When the rate of elimination is proportional to the amount of drug present, this is known as a first order process. Clearance of drug is constant (linear) over a range of concentrations. Not all drugs undergo first order kinetics; however, in some instances dose-dependent elimination occurs. Clearance in these cases is nonlinear and will vary depending on the achieved concentration of drug.

Clearance can also be described as the efficiency of removal of drug across an organ of elimination, the two major organs being liver and kidney. Hepatic clearance, (Cl_H) reflects the efficiency with which the liver irreversibly removes drug from the blood. It is determined by both the fraction of drug removed or extracted (E) from the blood during passage through the liver and the liver blood flow (Q_H). The relationship between these parameters is given by:

$$Cl_H = Q_H E \quad (4)$$

Drugs that are given orally must first pass through the liver before reaching the systemic circulation. If hepatic enzymes extract drug from the blood as it passes through, then the fraction (F) of the total dose entering the general circulation is reduced. For drugs that are completely absorbed from the gastrointestinal tract, this fraction F (or bioavailability) is determined from the drug's extraction (E) by the liver according to the equation:

$$F = 1 - E \quad (5)$$

The ability of the liver to extract a drug is in turn dependent on three separate factors: (a) the intrinsic activity of metabolic enzymes and transport processes within the liver that irreversibly remove drug from the blood, (b) the fraction of total drug in blood that is free to interact with enzymes responsible for its elimination, and (c) the rate at which drug passes or flows through the liver (146, 165, 209).

The irreversible removal of drug from the blood may be carried out by a number of separate enzymes in the liver. For simplicity, however, the elimination process is often considered as if it is due to only a single enzyme system. Thus, metabolic and transport processes responsible for drug removal by the liver, defined as the free intrinsic drug clearance (Cl^u_{int}), can be described by a simple Michaelis-Menten equation as:

$$Cl^u_{int} = \frac{V_{max}}{(K_m + C^u_L)} \quad (6)$$

where V_{max} represents the maximal rate of irreversible drug elimination by all liver enzymes, K_m is the Michaelis-Menten constant for the overall enzymatic removal process, and C^u_L is the concentration of unbound or free drug in liver.

The second factor that can contribute to the extraction of a drug by the liver is the free fraction of drug in blood (f_B). If the unbound fraction of total drug in blood changes, then the free drug concentration at the site of elimination will also change. For some drugs, changes in binding can alter hepatic extraction by metabolic and transport enzymes in the liver.

Finally, the total amount of drug extracted by the liver is dependent on the rate at which drug is delivered to the enzymes responsible for its elimination. This rate of delivery is determined by the liver blood flow (Q_H) perfusing functional hepatocytes. If intrinsic clearance is high, flow becomes the rate-limiting factor and reductions in flow will not change hepatic extraction, but rather will reduce hepatic clearance. If, on the other hand, intrinsic clearance is low, then as flow is decreased, hepatic extraction will increase and hepatic clearance will not be influenced by blood flow.

The relationship of the extraction (E) of a drug by the liver with its free intrinsic clearance (Cl^u_{int}), free fraction in the blood (f_B), and the total effective liver blood flow (Q_H) is given by:

$$E = \frac{f_B Cl^u_{int}}{(Q_H + f_B Cl^u_{int})} \quad (7)$$

If Equation 7 is now substituted into Equation 4, which defines hepatic clearance, the expression obtained relates hepatic clearance with three variables—f_B, Q_H and Cl^u_{int}. Thus, hepatic clearance may be written as:

$$Cl_H = Q_H E = Q_H \frac{f_B Cl^u_{int}}{(Q_H + f_B Cl^u_{int})} \qquad (8)$$

Although these relationships may appear complex, it is important to recognize that hepatic clearance is determined by only these three physiologic variables, each of which can be changed independently by liver disease. The effect on drug disposition of any one of these variables can be anticipated by knowing the relative importance of each of these variables to that drug's disposition. This concept has been used to provide a framework for the classification of drugs into a system in which those drugs sharing a rate-limiting characteristic are grouped together.

Drugs Classified by Dispositional Characteristics

FLOW-LIMITED DRUGS

When the total intrinsic clearance ($f_B Cl^u_{int}$) of a drug is large relative to liver blood flow (Q_H), such that $E > 0.6$, hepatic clearance of the drug becomes dependent on liver blood flow (Equation 8). The rate at which the liver is able to remove these drugs from the blood is limited by their rate of presentation to the liver. Metabolism and protein binding, theoretically, should not affect hepatic clearance of these drugs. Accordingly, this class of drugs is referred to as blood flow–limited and is sensitive to factors that can alter only the effective liver blood flow (Table 4.2).

ENZYME-LIMITED DRUGS

When the total intrinsic clearance of a drug is small relative to liver blood flow, such that $E < 0.2$, hepatic clearance becomes essentially dependent on the intrinsic activity of liver enzymes (Equation 8). Factors that influence the ability of the liver enzymes to remove drug become more important in altering drug elimination than changes in liver blood flow. Drugs with this characteristic belong to the class referred to as enzyme-limited. This class is further subdivided according to the extent of protein binding.

Enzyme-limited, Binding-insensitive Drugs

For enzyme-limited drugs with low binding to plasma or blood proteins (i.e., < 50% bound), a change in plasma protein binding is not an important factor in altering hepatic drug elimination (Equation 8). This drug class is most affected by factors that change the level or activity of liver enzymes (Cl^u_{int}) responsible for their elimination. Drugs with these characteristics are referred to as enzyme-limited and binding-insensitive (Table 4.2).

Enzyme-limited, Binding-sensitive Drugs

For enzyme-limited drugs that are extensively bound to plasma or blood proteins (i.e., > 85% bound), hepatic clearance is sensitive to changes in protein binding in the blood (f_B) and/or liver enzyme activity (Cl^u_{int}). Drugs with these characteristics are referred to as enzyme-limited, binding-sensitive drugs. Factors that may alter binding to proteins in the blood or the activity of liver enzymes responsible for drug elimination influence the hepatic clearance of these drugs (Table 4.2).

FLOW/ENZYME-SENSITIVE DRUGS

A drug may not be extensively bound or poorly extracted by the liver, but fall somewhere between the flow-limited and enzyme-limited classes. The clearance of these drugs from the blood may be sensitive to changes in liver blood flow, intrinsic clearance by the liver, and in some cases, binding to plasma proteins (Equation 8). Drugs with these characteristics are referred to as flow and enzyme sensitive (Table 4.2).

Table 4.2 lists a number of drugs eliminated by the liver according to this classification. The extraction ratios and plasma protein binding reported are approximate values from subjects with normal liver and kidney function. Drugs are classified according to this scheme to help provide a better appreciation for the importance of pathophysiologic changes produced by liver disease in altering drug disposition.

It is important to emphasize, however, that Table 4.2 is based on information about the handling of drugs by normal, healthy subjects and that certain biological determinants of metabolism (i.e., disease or genetic predisposition) may change the classification of a given drug for an individual patient.

Table 4.2
Characterization of Drugs Eliminated Primarily by the Liver

	Approximate Extraction (E)	Protein Binding (%)	Comments on Effects of Liver Disease
Flow-limited drugs			
Chlormethiazole	0.70	99	Changes in liver blood flow and intrinsic
Labetalol	0.85	40	clearance associated with liver disease
Lidocaine	0.60	65	affect these drugs. The shunting of
Lorcainide	0.65	70	blood around the liver has important
Morphine	0.75	35	effects on the bioavailability of these
Pentazocine	0.60	65	drugs.
Propoxyphene	>0.90	75	
Propranolol	0.65	95	
Verapamil	0.80	92	
Flow/enzyme-sensitive drugs			
Acetaminophen	0.30	20	Changes in liver blood flow, free
Chloramphenicol	0.28	70	intrinsic clearance, and free fraction of
Chlorpromazine	0.30	95	drug in blood may be important for this
Erythromycin	0.30	80	class of drugs.
Isoniazid	0.27	10	
Meperidine	0.50	70	
Methohexital	0.53	—	
Metoprolol	0.56	10	
Nafcillin	0.27	90	
Nortriptyline	0.50	95	
Quinidine	0.27	85	
Ranitidine	0.28	15	
Enzyme-limited, binding-insensitive			
Antipyrine	0.05	10	This class of drugs is most sensitive to
Amylobarbital	0.03	60	changes occurring in the free intrinsic
Caffeine	0.04	31	drug clearance with liver disease.
Cyclophosphamide	0.08	14	
Hexobarbital	0.15	47	
Theophylline	0.05	62	
Enzyme-limited, binding-sensitive			
Cefoperazone	0.04	90	This class of drugs will be influenced by
Chlordiazepoxide	0.02	96	changes in free fraction of drug in blood
Diazepam	0.02	97	and free intrinsic drug clearance. The
Diphenylhydantoin	0.03	92	overall change in drug clearance will be
Fenprofen	0.13	>99	governed by which one of these factors
Indomethacin	0.08	90	changes the most as a result of the
Naproxen	0.005	>99	disease process.
Phenylbutazone	0.01	99	
Rifampin	0.11	85	
Tolbutamide	0.02	98	
Valproic acid	0.02	89	
Warfarin	0.005	99	

It is now known that some people have genetic defects in the metabolism of certain drugs. Fast and slow acetylators of isoniazid have been recognized since the 1950s. More recently, independent genetic polymorphisms have been found for a number of other drugs metabolized by different oxidative enzymes. Poor and extensive metabolizers of debrisoquine, an antihypertensive agent, and mephenytoin, an anticonvulsant, are representative examples of two independent routes of oxidative metabolism. Debrisoquine acts as a flow-limited drug in subjects who are extensive metabolizers, but as an enzyme-limited drug in those who are poor metabolizers (182). Not only will the effect of liver disease have a greater effect on the clearance of this drug in extensive metabolizers than in poor metabolizers, but the effect of factors such as development of portal-systemic shunts will have a marked influence in systemic availability in extensive but not poor metabolizer subjects.

INFLUENCE OF LIVER DISEASE ON DRUG DISPOSITION

As previously mentioned, both dispositional characteristics of a drug and biological determinants of the system involved are important in determining the effects of liver disease on ultimate drug disposition. In the following sections, the effects of liver disease on each of these factors are discussed.

Route of Elimination

Since there are multiple routes of elimination, only some of which involve the liver, it is important to determine which route is utilized for a given drug. For a drug that is excreted unchanged by the kidney, liver disease should have no effect on disposition, provided that there is no secondary or concomitant renal disease.

Figure 4.1 shows the relationship between

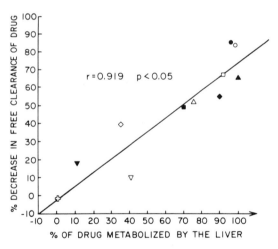

Figure 4.1 Relationship between the percentage of drug eliminated by the liver and the observed percentage decrease in the free clearance of drug in cirrhotic patients. Only drugs that are known or appear to be metabolized via oxidative pathways within the liver have been used for this plot. Each symbol represents the mean percentage change in the free clearance of one, or the average percentage change in free clearance of more than one drug. ⊹ = cefuroxime; ▼ = ampicillin; ◇ = furosemide; ▽ = cimetidine; ■ = nafcillin; △ = cefoperazone; ◆ = caffeine and theophylline; □ = antipyrine; ● = meperidine and propranolol; ○ = diazepam, verapamil, amylobarbital, lorcainide, and valproic acid; ▲ = chlordiazepoxide, chlormethiazole, and hexobarbital.

free clearance and extent of metabolism in cirrhotic patients for several drugs known, or assumed, to undergo oxidative metabolism. This plot was constructed from many different studies and, although all were conducted in cirrhotic patients, the severity of liver disease was not controlled for. The significant correlation found in Figure 4.1 implies a strong relationship between the extent of oxidative metabolism of a drug by the liver and the percentage decrease in its free clearance caused by liver cirrhosis. Liver disease has the greatest effect on those drugs that undergo extensive oxidative metabolism.

Route of Metabolism

For drugs that are metabolized by the liver, the route of metabolism is also important in determining the effects of liver disease on drug disposition. All metabolic pathways are not affected equally by liver disease. For example, the elimination of lorazepam, morphine, and oxazepam, which are primarily metabolized by conjugation with glucuronic acid, is unaltered by liver disease (89, 140, 178). The reason for this fact is unknown. It may reflect the sparing of conjugative pathways of drug metabolism in the liver during liver disease, and/or the importance of other organs to the elimination of drugs by this route. This preservation contrasts with reductions in clearance of drugs that are eliminated by oxidative metabolism.

Routes and Duration of Drug Administration

The effect of liver disease on drug disposition is determined by *(a)* the route of drug administration, *(b)* the class to which the drug belongs (i.e., flow-limited, flow/enzyme-sensitive, or enzyme-limited), and *(c)* duration of drug administration.

As noted previously, drugs that are taken orally, unlike those administered intravenously or intramuscularly, must pass through the liver before reaching the systemic circulation and target tissues. This provides an opportunity for presystemic elimination, particularly for flow-limited drugs, with their high hepatic extractions, which normally have a low bioavailability. For flow-limited drugs, liver disease may reduce the efficiency of drug me-

Table 4.3
Influence of Liver Cirrhosis on the Bioavailability of Flow-limited Drugs

Drug	Bioavailability in Controls	Bioavailability in Cirrhotics	Change in Bioavailability (%)	Reference
Labetalol	0.33	0.63	91	60
Lidocaine	0.33	0.65	97	198
Meperidine	0.48	0.87	81	121
Metoprolol	0.50	0.84	68	154
Pentazocine	0.20	0.70	250	150
Pentazocine	0.18	0.68	278	122
Propranolol	0.38	0.54	42	214
Verapamil	0.22	0.52	136	184
Verapamil	0.14	0.30	114	215

tabolism and considerably increase their bio-availability (Table 4.3). This increased bio-availability, however, is only partially explained by a decrease in the efficiency of drug extraction by liver enzymes. Another important factor contributing to this increase is the rerouting of blood from the portal vein through intrahepatic and extrahepatic portal-systemic shunts in response to portal hypertension caused by liver disease. In severely cirrhotic patients, this shunting may involve 60% or more of portal venous blood flow (49, 192, 193). This shunting allows a large amount of an orally administered drug to bypass the liver altogether and enter the systemic circulation directly. As a result of the changes in bioavailability of flow-limited drugs, peak blood concentrations following single oral dose administration are substantially higher in patients with cirrhosis than in normal subjects. (Fig. 4.2). In contrast, the bioavailability of enzyme-limited drugs is high in normal subjects and remains unaffected in liver disease. Thus, peak concentrations following single oral dose administration are the same in cirrhotic and normal subjects (Fig. 4.2).

The case is somewhat different for chronic oral therapy: drug blood levels accumulate to an approximate steady state situation that is dependent on drug clearance, the fraction of the dose that reaches the systemic circulation, and the dosage interval (Equation 3). Reductions in clearance due to liver disease result in the potential for excessive drug accumulation during chronic therapy for both flow-limited and enzyme-limited drugs (Fig. 4.2). This may require dosage reduction in order to obtain the desired therapeutic objective.

In summary, the influence of liver disease on drug disposition is a function of how a drug is handled in healthy subjects. For flow-limited drugs, initial blood concentrations follow-

ing intravenous or intramuscular administration can be expected to be similar in cirrhotic and normal subjects, whereas peak blood concentrations are higher in cirrhotic patients after single oral dose administration or at steady state during chronic therapy. In contrast, enzyme-limited drugs can be expected to have similar initial blood concentrations after both intravenous and single oral dose administration in cirrhotic and normal subjects, but increased blood concentrations at steady state during chronic therapy in cirrhotic subjects.

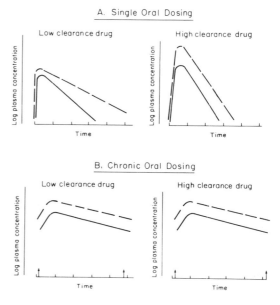

Figure 4.2 The effects of single **(A)** and chronic **(B)** oral dosing on low clearance (enzyme-limited) and high clearance (flow-limited) drugs in patients with cirrhosis *(dashed lines)* and in normal subjects *(solid lines)*. *Arrows* indicate dosage interval for chronic dosing graphs.

Severity of Liver Disease

The type and severity of liver disease are one example of the effect of biological determinants on drug disposition. All drugs that undergo extensive oxidative metabolism are not affected to an equal extent by all liver diseases. Acute viral hepatitis, for example, does not have any effect on the metabolic elimination (Cl_{int}^u) of tolbutamide, warfarin, diphenylhydantoin, or antipyrine (15, 37, 90, 211, 212), whereas it does produce changes in metabolic elimination of hexobarbital, meperidine, and chlordiazepoxide (21, 108, 208). These observations might reflect differences in the degree to which different oxidative pathways of drug elimination are affected by liver disease, but more likely reflect the differences in the severity of the disease process in patients used for the separate studies. Thus, it may not be possible to find any change in the metabolic elimination of drugs in patients with mild or moderate forms of hepatitis. Certainly the levels of cytochrome P-450 drug-metabolizing enzymes are not altered in liver biopsies from such patients (38). With more extensive liver damage due to viral hepatitis or other causes, the level of these enzymes declines (38, 171). This decline should cause a decrease in the free intrinsic clearance of those drugs that are oxidatively metabolized in the liver by this enzyme system.

Drug Interactions in Liver Disease

As stated earlier, patients with liver disease are often on a multidrug regimen. Certain drugs are well known to affect drug metabolism either by induction or inhibition of metabolic enzymes.

Phenobarbital, pentobarbital, tolbutamide, and phenytoin act as metabolic inducers, increasing the synthesis of metabolic enzymes. The administration of enzyme-inducing drugs to patients with moderate liver disease may offset the disease-induced decrease in cytochrome P-450 enzymes. This effect, however, is limited. With an increase in the severity of liver damage, liver reserves may become too depressed for drug administration to exert much of an effect on either the level or activity of these enzymes (38, 188).

Cimetidine, on the other hand, a drug commonly used in the treatment of patients with alcoholic liver disease, has been shown to decrease total plasma clearance of theophylline

(52) and chlordiazepoxide (123) in both control and cirrhotic subjects. It is believed that cimetidine interferes with oxidative metabolism but does not alter hepatic blood flow (123). Consequently, patients with liver disease may have an additional risk of impaired drug metabolism. The study by Nelson and colleagues (123) showed the decrease in plasma clearance of chlordiazepoxide to be greater in the control group than in the cirrhotic group, suggesting that the greater the initial microsomal function, the greater the effect of an inhibitor. However, it should be emphasized that this further decrease in drug metabolism may still be of importance in a patient with liver disease who may already have decreased metabolic function.

Endogenous substances may also affect drug metabolism. Both interferon and interferon inducers have been shown to decrease drug biotransformation (102, 113, 114, 156, 157, 180, 181). The mechanism for this is not completely understood, although it is thought to involve variable depression of the cytochrome P-450 enzymes. This factor has important implications for patients with viral hepatitis, for not only do interferon levels increase with acute infection, but recently exogenous interferon has been used as a treatment for patients with hepatitis B or non-A, non-B viral hepatitis.

RECOMMENDATIONS FOR DOSAGE ADJUSTMENTS

As seen from the discussion of pharmacokinetic considerations in liver disease, it is not easy to predict the effect of disease on drug disposition in individual patients. Although severity of disease seems to play a major role in distribution and elimination of a drug, there is no good predictor of hepatic function. Despite a considerable effort by a number of investigators (8, 14, 31, 148, 177), there is no useful noninvasive test of liver function to guide dosage adjustments. The best that can be said for most of the so-called liver function tests (i.e., serum albumin, prothrombin time, bilirubin, serum glutamic-oxaloacetic and glutamic-pyruvic transaminases (SGOT and SGPT), alkaline phosphatase, etc.) is that they reflect but do not predict the extent of liver damage.

Measuring cytochrome P-450 enzyme levels from liver biopsies might be expected to provide a better measure of the degree to which oxidative drug metabolism in the liver has been damaged. The level of these enzymes, however, has not been found to be a useful predictor of the metabolic elimination of drugs by this organ (188). One explanation for the poor predictive value is that this measure fails to account for total hepatic size (148).

Some measures do exist that correlate with drug clearance, such as tests of antipyrine, aminopyrine, and indocyanine green clearance; however, these studies are not usually conducted as part of a patient's routine clinical evaluation. Moreover, the correlation coefficients usually only approximate 0.6 in most studies, accounting for only 40% or less of variance. Therefore, a good predictor of hepatic function or drug clearance has not been found; and at the present time, there is not a good hepatic counterpart for glomerular filtration rate, which is a reliable indicator of renal function.

Before considering the influence of liver disease on drug dosage requirements, some mention must be made of the use of drugs in general. There are always risks associated with the use of any drugs, and these risks may become particularly pronounced in patients with liver disease. In a prospective, drug-monitoring study of over 2000 patients, Naranjo and colleagues (120) found the frequency of adverse drug reactions (ADRs) to be higher in patients with cirrhosis than in those with renal disease, other liver diseases, or neither liver nor renal disease. In the group of cirrhotic patients, the frequency of ADRs was significantly correlated with the severity of liver dysfunction as measured by a composite clinical and laboratory index. Thus, consideration should be given as to whether the drug is really needed and whether its benefits outweigh the risks. For example, the use of some drugs in patients with liver disease is associated with a particularly high risk and they should be used with great caution or not at all in these patients (Table 4.4). In general, the drugs listed in Table 4.4 fall into three categories: (a) drugs capable of causing liver damage even in normal patients, (b) drugs that can further compromise depressed liver functions often found in liver disease patients, and (c) drugs that can make the complications of liver disease worse. In the above-cited study, diuretics were found to be the most common cause of ADRs and to cause the most severe reactions.

If drug treatment is required and alternatives are available, it is preferable to use a drug whose disposition is least affected by the liver disease (e.g., a drug that is renally excreted or metabolized by glucuronidation). If a drug must

Table 4.4
Drugs That Should Be Used with Caution or Not at All in Liver Disease Patients

Group I: Drugs capable of causing hepatic damage
  Acetaminophen
  Acetylsalicylic acid
  Chlorpromazine
  Erythromycin estolate
  Methotrexate
  Methyldopa
Group II: Drugs that can compromise liver functions
  Anabolic and contraceptive steroids
  Prednisone (in acute viral hepatitis)
  Tetracycline
Group III: Drugs that may make complications of liver disease worse
  Cyclooxygenase inhibitors (indomethacin)
  Diuretics
  Meperidine and other CNS depressants
  Morphine
  Pentazocine
  Phenylbutazone

be prescribed that may be affected by the disease process, then a number of factors need to be considered, including (a) the extent of liver damage, (b) the degree of hepatic elimination of the drug, (c) the degree of protein binding, (d) the class to which the drug belongs (i.e., enzyme-limited, flow/enzyme sensitive, or flow-limited, (e) the route of administration; and (f) the duration of administration.

A considerable amount of information has been gathered over the years regarding disposition of specific drugs in liver disease. Most of this work has been done in cirrhosis, a lesser amount in acute viral hepatitis, and very little in other types of liver disease. To help the clinician, a compilation has been made of the dispositional characteristics of a number of drugs in normal subjects, the route of elimination of these drugs, the effect of liver disease on their disposition, and the recommendations for adjustment of dose (Table 4.5).

For drugs not listed in Table 4.5, general guidelines for dosage adjustment are given in Table 4.6. While these considerations may not be all inclusive, they should provide some guidance as to the extent of dosage change required with liver disease. It should be kept in mind, however, that these may not be the only variables to consider in patients with this condition. For example, as noted earlier, in moderate liver disease the administration of drugs capable of increasing drug metabolism may offset the decline in the metabolic elimination of drugs due to the disease, and the adminis-

Table 4.5
The Dispositional Characteristics in Normal Subjects and in Patients with Liver Disease, Routes of Elimination, and Recommendations for Dose Adjustment for a Variety of Drugs[a]

Drug	Protein Binding (%)	Volume of Distribution (V_d) (liter/kg)	Half-life ($t_{1/2}$) (hr)	Clearance (Cl) (ml/min)	Class	Hepatic/Renal Elimination	Effect of Liver Disease on Drug Disposition	Adjustment of Dose	References
Antibiotic									
Amantadine	—	4.75	20.0	190	—	<10% Hepatic >90% Renal	Negligible unless renal function decreased	None	
Amikacin	5	0.26	2.5	85	—	<5% Hepatic >95% Renal	Negligible unless renal function decreased	None	
Ampicillin	30	0.28	1.0	340	—	<10% Hepatic >90% Renal	$t_{1/2}\uparrow$; $V_d\uparrow$; $Cl\rightarrow$; $f_p?\rightarrow$	None	95
Aztreonam	56	0.15	1.9	70	—	33% Hepatobiliary 66% Renal	$t_{1/2}\uparrow$; $V_d\rightarrow$; $Cl\rightarrow$	Decrease if chronic, high-dosing	98
Carbenicillin	48	0.16	1.0	130	—	<10% Hepatic >90% Renal	Negligible unless renal function decreased	None	59
Cefaclor	24	0.35	1.0	280	—	<10% Hepatic >90% Renal	Negligible unless renal function decreased	None	
Cefamandole	74	0.16	1.0	130	—	<5% Hepatic >95% Renal	Negligible unless renal function decreased	None	
Cefazolin	84	0.15	1.8	68	—	<5% Hepatic >95% Renal	$t_{1/2}\downarrow$; $f_p\uparrow$	None	130
Cefoperazone	90 non-linear	0.20	1.7	80	Enzyme-limited, binding-sensitive	75% Hepatic 25% Renal	$t_{1/2}\uparrow$; $V_d\rightarrow$; $Cl\downarrow$ 60%; $f_p?$	Decrease dose	16, 17, 28, 29, 48
Cefotaxime	36	0.24	1.2	94	—	40% Hepatic 60% Renal	$t_{1/2}\uparrow$; $V_d?$; $Cl?$	Unknown	115
Cefoxitin	73	0.12	1.0	98	—	15% Hepatic 85% Renal	Negligible unless renal function decreased	None	
Ceftazidime	17	0.2	1.7	75	—	10% Hepatic 90% Renal	$t_{1/2}\uparrow$; $V_d?$; Cl slight $\downarrow$	Negligible, unless renal function decreased	139
Ceftriaxone	90	0.14	8.4	16	Enzyme-limited, binding-sensitive	60% Hepatobiliary 40% Renal	$t_{1/2}\rightarrow$; $V_d\uparrow$ if ascites present; $Cl\rightarrow$; $fp\uparrow$	None	190, 191
Cefuroxime	30	0.33	1.2	210	—	<1% Hepatic >99% Renal	Negligible unless renal function decreased	None	133

Table 4.5 (continued)

Drug	Protein Binding (%)	Volume of Distribution (V_d) (liter/kg)	Half-life ($t_{1/2}$) (hr)	Clearance (Cl) (ml/min)	Class	Hepatic/Renal Elimination	Effect of Liver Disease on Drug Disposition	Adjustment of Dose	References
Cephalothin	75	0.30	0.60	470	—	30–50% Hepatic 50–70% Renal	$t_{1/2}$ slight ↑; V_d →; Cl ↓	None	130
Chloramphenicol	70	1.0	3.0	170	Enzyme-limited, binding-sensitive	>90% Hepatic <10% Renal glucuronidation of drug	$t_{1/2}$ ↑; V_d slight ↓; Cl ↓ 65%; f_p →?; unknown if f_p changes	Decrease dose	12, 92, 119
Clindamycin	79	0.58	2.0	160	Enzyme-limited, binding-sensitive	90% Hepatic 10% Renal	$t_{1/2}$ slight ↑; V_d →; Cl ↓ 23%; f_p →	Decrease dose in severe cases	11, 58
Doxycycline	82	—	12.0	195	—	<10% Hepatic >90% Renal	Negligible unless renal function decreased	None	
Erythromycin	80	0.77	1.6	600	Enzyme-limited, binding-sensitive	>90% Hepatic <10% Renal	$t_{1/2}$ ↑; no other information	Decrease dose in moderate or severe disease	54, 91
Gentamicin	< 5	0.25	2.0	100	—	<5% Hepatic >95% Renal	Negligible unless renal function decreased	None	
Isoniazid	<10	0.6	2.0 fast 6.0 slow	480 fast 170 slow	Enzyme-limited, binding-insensitive	85% Hepatic 15% Renal Drug acetylated	$t_{1/2}$ ↑; some assume Cl ↓; genetic differences more important than disease	Decrease dose in severe cases	2, 93
Kanamycin	<10	0.20	3.0	55	—	<5% Hepatic >95% Renal	Negligible unless renal function decreased	None	
Metronidazole	10	0.75	8.0	85	—	>90% Hepatic <10% Renal	$t_{1/2}$ ↑; V_d →; Cl ↓	Decrease dose	30, 36
Nafcillin	90	0.4	1.0	580	Enzyme-limited, binding-sensitive	70% Hepatic 30% Renal	$t_{1/2}$ ↑ but little change; V_d ↓; Cl ↓ 50–60%; fp →?	Decrease dose in moderate or severe disease	105
Neomycin	40	—	2.0	—	—	<5% Hepatic >95% Renal	Negligible unless renal function decreased	None	
Rifampin	85	0.4	2.5	180	Enzyme-limited, binding-sensitive	90% Hepatic 10% Renal	$t_{1/2}$ ↑; V_d?; Cl ↓; f_p?	Decrease in severe disease	78, 153
Streptomycin	35	0.26	2.5	85	—	<5% Hepatic >95% Renal	Negligible unless renal function decreased	None	
Sulphamethoxazole	66	0.17	9.0	15	Enzyme-limited, binding-sensitive	70% Hepatic 30% Renal Drug acetylated	Unknown, but probably little change unless there is severe liver disease	Slight decrease	

Drug				Classification	Elimination	Changes	Dose Recommendation	References
Tobramycin	<5	0.24	2.5	80	—	<5% Hepatic >95% Renal	Negligible unless renal function decreased	None	
Trimethoprim	45	1.5	12.0	96	—	30% Hepatic 70% Renal	Slight unless renal function decreased	None	
Vancomycin	55	0.4	5.0	80	—	<10% Hepatic >90% Renal	$t_{1/2} \uparrow$; $V_d \rightarrow$; $Cl \downarrow$	Decrease dose	23
Analgesic									
Acetaminophen	20	0.9	2.2	350	Flow/enzyme-sensitive	>95% Hepatic <5% Renal Mostly conjugated	$t_{1/2} \uparrow$; V_d?; $Cl \downarrow$ 54%; assume $f_p \rightarrow$; little change in Cl if albumin > 3.5 g/100 ml	Avoid chronic use; single dose—no change	10, 40, 41, 174, 179
Meperidine	65	4.5	4.5	900	Flow/enzyme-sensitive	>95% Hepatic <5% Renal	$t_{1/2} \uparrow$; $V_d \rightarrow$; $Cl \downarrow$ 50%; $f_p \rightarrow$	Decrease oral dose by 50% in cirrhosis or acute viral hepatitis	87, 108, 122, 151
Methadone	80	4.0	28	150	Enzyme-limited, binding-sensitive	80% Hepatic 20% Renal	$t_{1/2} \uparrow$ with severe liver disease; $Cl \rightarrow$; $V_d \uparrow$ slightly	None or decrease	125, 126
Morphine	35	3.7	2.0	1200	Flow-limited	90% GI tract and liver, 10% renal Extensive glucuronidation	$t_{1/2} \rightarrow$; $V_d \rightarrow$; $Cl \rightarrow$; $f_p \rightarrow$, by some reports $f_p \uparrow$	None, but avoid in severe liver disease	135, 140, 141
Pentazocine	65	5.4	4.5	1000	Flow-limited	>95% Hepatic <5% Renal	$t_{1/2} \uparrow$; $V_d \rightarrow$; $Cl \downarrow$ 50%	Decrease oral dose by ⅔	122, 150
Propoxyphene	75	16	12	1200	Flow-limited	>95% GI tract and liver; <2% renal	$t_{1/2} \uparrow$ slightly; V_d?; $Cl \downarrow$ 25%; $f_p \rightarrow$	Decrease oral dose by 50%	44
Anticancer									
Adriamycin	50	2.5	20	100	Enzyme-limited, binding-insensitive	>95% Hepatic <5% Renal Most biliary Active metabolite	$t_{1/2} \uparrow$; V_d?; Cl?; f_p?, assume $f_p \rightarrow$	Unknown	13
Bleomycin	0	0.3	2.0	120	—	40% Hepatic 60% Renal	Unknown; probably not altered greatly	None? Perhaps decrease	
Cyclophosphamide	14	0.6	5.0	120	Enzyme-limited, binding-insensitive	90% Hepatic 10% Renal Active metabolite	$t_{1/2} \uparrow$; $V_d \rightarrow$?; $Cl \downarrow$ 43%; $f_p \rightarrow$?	Unknown	74, 204

Table 4.5 (continued)

Drug	Protein Binding (%)	Volume of Distribution (V_d) (liter/kg)	Half-life ($t_{1/2}$) (hr)	Clearance (Cl) (ml/min)	Class	Hepatic/Renal Elimination	Effect of Liver Disease on Drug Disposition	Adjustment of Dose	References
Cytosine arabinoside	13	2.5	2.5	800	—	Extensive extrahepatic elimination; 40% renal	No data; probably little effect	None	
Etoposide	—	.28	5.6	39	—	65% Hepatic 35% Renal	$t_{1/2} \rightarrow$; $V_d \rightarrow$; $Cl \rightarrow$	None	32, 55
5-Fluorouracil	—	0.5	0.1	—	Flow-limited	Hepatic and extrahepatic; <5% Renal	Some decrease in clearance expected	Probable slight decrease	
Methotrexate	50	0.5	9.0	80	—	15% Hepatic; mostly biliary; 85% Renal	No data; probably little effect. Drug is hepatoxic and should be avoided if possible.	None	
Antiepileptic									
Carbamazepine	75	1.1	18.0 induced	—	Enzyme-limited, binding-sensitive	>98% Hepatic <2% Renal	No data; expect a decrease in clearance and increase in $t_{1/2}$	Probably decrease dose	
Diphenylhydantoin	92	0.65	15.0 non-linear	40	Enzyme-limited, binding-sensitive	>95% Hepatic <5% Renal	AVH $t_{1/2} \rightarrow$; $Cl \rightarrow$; $f_p \uparrow$. Cirrhosis $f_p \uparrow$	Decrease dose in moderate to severe liver disease	15, 62, 135
Phenobarbital	50	0.8	100	8	Enzyme-limited, binding-insensitive	75% Hepatic 25% Renal	$t_{1/2} \uparrow$; presumed $Cl \downarrow$	Decrease with severe liver disease	7
Valproic Acid	89 non-linear	12	0.14	30	Enzyme-limited, binding-sensitive	>98% Hepatic <25% Renal	$t_{1/2} \uparrow$; V_d slightly $\uparrow$; $Cl \downarrow$ 40%; $f_p \uparrow$	Decrease dose	88
Antipyretic/ Antinflammatory									
Antipyrine	<10	0.58	12	50	Enzyme-limited, binding-insensitive	92% Hepatic 8% Renal	$t_{1/2} \uparrow$; $V_d \uparrow$ or $\rightarrow$; $Cl \downarrow$ 60% or more, but actual decrease in Cl depends on disease	Not used clinically	24, 35, 61, 69, 90, 109, 112, 118, 148, 186, 188, 194
Dexamethasone	68	0.75	3.25	260	Flow/enzyme-sensitive	>97% Hepatic <3% Renal	$f_p \rightarrow$; $V_d \rightarrow$; $t_{1/2} \uparrow$; Cl	Decrease dose	76
Fenprofen	>99	0.10	1.5	200	Enzyme-limited, binding-sensitive	>98% Hepatic <2% Renal	No data; would expect $f_p \uparrow$; $t_{1/2} \uparrow$; $Cl \uparrow$ or $\rightarrow$	Decrease dose	

Ibuprofen	>99	0.15 V area/F	2.0	52	Enzyme-limited, binding-sensitive	>99% Hepatic <1% Renal	$t_{1/2}$ slightly ↑ in severe LD; V_d?; Cl?	Decrease in severe liver disease if high doses	73
Indomethacin	90	0.17	8.0	125	Enzyme-limited, binding-sensitive	>98% Hepatic <2% Renal	$t_{1/2}$ ↑; no other information. Assume Cl ↓, f_p ↑	Decrease dose as required	56
Naproxen	99.6	0.10	14.0	5	Enzyme-limited, binding-sensitive	>90% Hepatic <10% Renal	$t_{1/2}$ ↑; V_d →; Cl ↓ 28%; f_p?	Decrease dose in moderate to severe disease	25, 213
Phenylbutazone	98.5	0.17	70	2	Enzyme-limited, binding-sensitive	>99% Hepatic <1% Renal	$t_{1/2}$ ↑ or →; f_p ↑; V_d?; Cl? Assume Cl ↓ with liver disease	Decrease dose	22, 68, 93, 207
Prednisolone	80	0.6	3.0	180	Enzyme-limited, binding-sensitive	>85% Hepatic <15% Renal	$t_{1/2}$ →; V_d →; Cl →; f_p → or ↑. Drug little affected by liver disease.	None	76, 152, 168, 199
Salicylic acid	80–95 dose dependent	0.17 dose dependent	2.4–19	13 in therapeutic range	—	2–30% Renal; dose dependent	$t_{1/2}$ →; V_d →; Cl?; f_p ↑	None	162
Sulfinpyrazone	99	0.06	6.0	23	Enzyme-limited, binding-sensitive	65% Hepatic 35% Renal	No data; would expect some decrease in Cl with liver disease	Slight decrease in dose	
Cardiovascular									
Atenolol	<5	0.55	6.5	55–130	—	10% Hepatic 90% Renal	$t_{1/2}$ →; V_d →; Cl →	None	81
Digitoxin	95	0.60	180	2.5	Enzyme-limited, binding-sensitive	70% Hepatic 30% Renal	$t_{1/2}$ → or ↓; Cl ↑ or →; f_p ↑	None	80, 127, 145
Digoxin	30	6.0	35	150	—	30% Hepatic 70% Renal	Appears negligible	None	100, 104, 219
Disopyramide	80 non-linear	1.0	8	100	—	45% Hepatic 55% Renal	No data; would not expect a tremendous change in liver disease	Probably slight decrease	
Labetalol	50	11.5	3.0	1600	Flow-limited	>95% Hepatic <5% Renal	$t_{1/2}$ →; V_d ↓; Cl → or ↓; f_p?, assume ↑	Decrease oral dose; decrease i.v. dose to much smaller extent	60

Table 4.5 (continued)

Drug	Protein Binding (%)	Volume of Distribution (V_d) (liter/kg)	Half-life ($t_{1/2}$) (hr)	Clearance (Cl) (ml/min)	Class	Hepatic/Renal Elimination	Effect of Liver Disease on Drug Disposition	Adjustment of Dose	References
Lidocaine	65 non-linear	1.1	2.0	1000	Flow-limited	97% Hepatic 3% Renal	$t_{1/2}$ ↑; V_d ↑ or →; Cl ↓ ~ 50%; f_p? Low therapeutic ratio. Decrease in Cl depends on severity of disease	Decrease dose by 50% in severe liver disease	3, 41, 64, 196–198, 210
Lorcainide	70	12.9	8.0	1700	Flow-limited	98% Hepatic 2% Renal	$t_{1/2}$ ↑; V_d →; Cl ↓ 29%; f_p ↑ slightly. Cl_{int} exhibits a very large decrease	Decrease dose	86
Metoprolol	10	3.2	4.0	800	Flow-limited	95% Hepatic 5% Renal	$t_{1/2}$ ↑; V_d ↑ slightly; Cl ↓ 23%; f_p? assumed unaffected	Decrease dose slightly	154
N-Acetyl procainamide	10	1.4	8.0	210	—	20% Hepatic 80% Renal	No data: expect little change unless renal function altered	None	
Nifedipine	98	1.0	3.0	600	Flow-limited, binding-sensitive	100% Hepatic	$t_{1/2}$ ↑; V_d →; Cl ↓; f_p ↑	Decrease dose	82
Pindolol	57	6.2	3.5	300	Enzyme-limited, binding-insensitive	70% Hepatic 30% Renal	Not affected by AVH. Cirrhosis Cl ↓ slightly and renal excretion of drug is increased	Some decrease in severe liver disease	131
Prazosin	97	1.3	3.0	450	Flow-limited	95% Hepatic 5% Renal	No data—would expect $t_{1/2}$ ↑; Cl ↓; f_p ↑	Decrease dose	
Procainamide	15	2.2	3.0	600	—	45% Hepatic 55% Renal Drug acetylated	$t_{1/2}$ ↑; V_d?; Cl? probably decreased slightly	Some minor decrease in dose	34
Propranolol	95	4.0	4.0	850	Flow-limited	>95% Hepatic <5% Renal	$t_{1/2}$ ↑; V_d ↑; Cl ↓ ~ 60%; f_p ↑. Tremendous decrease in Cl_{int}. Flow/enzyme-limited in cirrhosis	Decrease dose depending on extent of damage	20, 146, 214
Quinidine	85	3.0	6.0	330	Flow/enzyme-sensitive	80% Hepatic 20% Renal	$t_{1/2}$ ↑; V_d ↑; Cl →; f_p ↑; Cl_{int} decreased significantly	Decrease dose	4, 79, 144

Drug					Classification	Elimination	Effect in liver disease	Dosage recommendation	References
Tocainide	10	3.0	13	150	Enzyme-limited	60% Hepatic 40% Renal	$t_{1/2} \uparrow$; V_d?; $Cl \downarrow$	Decrease dose	136
Verapamil	92	6.7	3.5	1570	Flow-limited	95% Hepatic 5% Renal	$t_{1/2} \uparrow$; $V_d \uparrow$; $Cl \downarrow$ 60%; $f_p \rightarrow$; Cl_{int} decreases even more than 60%	Decrease dose by 50% in severe liver disease	184, 215
Diuretic									
Bumetanide	?	9.45	1.0	129	—	36% Hepatic 64% Renal	$t_{1/2} \uparrow$; $V_d \downarrow$; $Cl \downarrow$	Minor decrease in dose	103
Furosemide	95	0.15	1.0	170	—	35% Hepatic 65% Renal	$t_{1/2} \uparrow$ or $\rightarrow$; $V_d \uparrow$ or $\rightarrow$; $Cl \rightarrow$; $f_p \uparrow$; the change in f_p compensates for decrease in Cl_{int} of liver	None or slight decrease in severe cases	5, 42, 46, 77, 167, 200, 203
Hydrochlorothiazide	95	1.5	2.5	480	—	<10% Hepatic >90% Renal	No data; probably little affected unless renal function altered	None	
Spironolactone	98	—	20	—	Enzyme-limited, binding-sensitive, and extrahepatic metabolism	>85% Hepatic <15% Renal	No apparent change in drug disposition with liver disease; $t_{1/2} \rightarrow$	None	1, 166
Triamterene	50	2.5	2.0	1000	Flow-limited	95% Hepatic 5% Renal	$Cl \downarrow$; $f_p \uparrow$; expect $t_{1/2} \uparrow$	Decrease dose	202
Sedative/hypnotic									
Amylobarbital	60	1.2	21	35	Enzyme-limited, binding-insensitive	>95% Hepatic <5% Renal	$t_{1/2} \uparrow$; $V_d \rightarrow$; $Cl \downarrow$ 55%; $f_p \uparrow$. Little change if albumin > 3.5 g/100 ml	Decrease dose	106
Chlordiazepoxide	96	0.3	12 age-dependent	20	Enzyme-limited, binding-sensitive	>99% Hepatic <1% Renal	$t_{1/2} \uparrow$; $V_d \uparrow$; $Cl \downarrow$ 60%; $f_p \uparrow$. Both AVH and cirrhosis affect drug	Decrease dose	110, 116, 163, 164, 172
Diazepam	99	1.2	45	28	Enzyme-limited, binding-sensitive	>97% Hepatic <3% Renal	$t_{1/2} \uparrow$; $V_d \uparrow$; $Cl \downarrow$ 50%; $f_p \uparrow$. AVH and cirrhosis increase $T_{1/2}$. Large therapeutic index—safe	Single dose, no change; chronic, decrease dose	9, 19, 57, 84, 85, 107, 128
Hexobarbital	47	1.2	6.0	232	Enzyme-limited, binding-insensitive	>99% Hepatic <1% Renal	$t_{1/2} \uparrow$; $V_d \rightarrow$; $Cl \downarrow$ 62% (Cl decreased in AVH and cirrhosis, $Cl \rightarrow$ in cholestasis); $f_p \rightarrow$	Decrease during chronic dosing	21, 158, 218

Table 4.5 (continued)

Drug	Protein Binding (%)	Volume of Distribution (V_d) (liter/kg)	Half-life ($t_{1/2}$) (hr)	Clearance (Cl) (ml/min)	Class	Hepatic/Renal Elimination	Effect of Liver Disease on Drug Disposition	Adjustment of Dose	References
Lorazepam	90	1.3	12.0	53	Enzyme-limited, binding-sensitive	>98% Hepatic <2% Renal Extensive glucuronidation	$t_{1/2}$ ↑; V_d ↑; Cl →; f_p ↑. Neither AVH nor cirrhosis affects drug dosing	None	89
Methohexital	—	61	2.0	829	Flow/enzyme-sensitive	>90% Hepatic <10% Renal	No data; assume Cl ↓, $t_{1/2}$ ↑	Probably decrease dose	
Midazolam	—	1.3	1.6	624	Flow-limited	>95% Hepatic <5% Renal	$t_{1/2}$ ↑; V_d slightly ↑; Cl ↓	Decrease dose	6, 97
Nitrazepam	87	1.9	26	63	Enzyme-limited	>99% Hepatic <1% Renal Mainly nitroreduction	$t_{1/2}$ →; V_d →; Cl →; f_p ↑	None	71
Oxazepam	90	1.6	6.0	140	Enzyme-limited, binding-sensitive	>99% Hepatic <1% Renal Extensive glucuronidation	$t_{1/2}$ →; V_d →; Cl →; f_p →. Neither AVH nor cirrhosis alters disposition significantly	None	172, 178
Pentobarbital	65	1.0	30	30	Enzyme-limited, binding-sensitive	99% Hepatic <1% Renal	No data; expect Cl ↓, $t_{1/2}$ ↑	Single dose, no change; chronic, lower dose	173
Primidone	19	0.86	17	41	—	60% Hepatic 40% Renal (in children)	$t_{1/2}$ →; V_d slight ↑; Cl slight ↑ in hepatitis	None	149
Temazepam	98	1.2	14	80	—	>98% Hepatic <2% Renal Mainly glucuronidation	$t_{1/2}$ →; V_d →; Cl →; f_p →	None	129
Others									
Alfentanil	90	0.28	1.5	200	Flow/enzyme-sensitive	99% Hepatic 1% Renal	$t_{1/2}$ ↑; V_d →; Cl ↓; f_p ↑ (dose-dependent)	Decrease dose	39
Atracurium	—	0.16	0.33	385		Hofmann elimination; autometabolism	$t_{1/2}$ →; V_d ↑; Cl →; long $t_{1/2}$ of metabolite	Decrease dose if long-term use	206
Caffeine	31	0.54	6.0	63	Enzyme-limited, binding-insensitive	95% Hepatic 5% Renal	$t_{1/2}$ ↑ slightly; V_d →; Cl ↓ 40%; f_p ↑; large therapeutic ratio	None	31

Drug				Classification	Elimination	Effect of liver disease	Dose adjustment	Ref.
Chlormethiazole	64	0.12	7.0	1100	Flow-limited; vitamin B substitute	>99% Hepatic <1% Renal	$t_{1/2}$ ↑; V_d →; Cl ↓ 28%; f_p ↑	Probably not necessary	143
Cimetidine	20	1.1	2.3	550	—	40% Hepatic 60% Renal	$t_{1/2}$ →; V_d ↑ or ↓ or →; Cl → or ↓; f_p changes assumed unimportant. Drug associated with increased incidence of mental confusion in cirrhotics	Decrease dose in severe liver disease	27, 47, 51, 52, 123, 124, 132, 170, 185, 201, 217
Clofibrate (CPIB)	95	0.15	18.0	8	Enzyme-limited, binding-sensitive	90% Hepatic <10% Renal Glucuronidation of metabolite	$t_{1/2}$ →; V_d ↑ slightly; Cl →; f_p ↑. AVH does not alter Cl; cirrhosis does have an effect on Cl_{int} ↓ 50%	Decrease dose in cirrhosis by 50%	49
Diphenhydramine	78	6.5	9.5	696	Flow-limited	>98% Hepatic <2% Renal	$t_{1/2}$ ↑; V_d →; free Cl ↓; total Cl →; f_p ↑	Decrease dose	111
Fentanyl	80	3.5	4.0	750	—	92% Hepatic 8% Renal	$t_{1/2}$ →; V_d →; Cl →	None	53
Ranitidine	15	1.5	2.3	600	—	30% Hepatic 70% Renal	$t_{1/2}$ →; V_d →; Cl → or ↓	None	117, 134, 183, 216
Sulfisoxazole	92	0.15	6.6	20	Enzyme-limited, binding-sensitive	50% Hepatic 50% Renal Acetylation	$t_{1/2}$ →; V_d ↑; Cl ↑; f_p ↑	None	26
Theophylline	52	0.5	8.0	45	Enzyme-limited, binding-insensitive	91% Hepatic 9% Renal	$t_{1/2}$ ↑; V_d → cirrhosis, ↑ hepatitis and cholestasis; Cl ↓ 55%; f_p ↑. Low therapeutic index caution	Decrease dose by 50%	75, 101, 147, 189
Thiopental	85	2.3	9.0	275	Enzyme-limited	>99% Hepatic <1% Renal	$t_{1/2}$ →; V_d →; Cl →; f_p ↑	Uncertain; may need to decrease dose	138
Tolbutamide	98	0.15	5.0	20.0	Enzyme-limited, binding-sensitive	95% Hepatic 5% Renal	$t_{1/2}$ slightly ↑ or →; Cl ↑; f_p ↑. AVH has been reported to increase rate of elimination	None; probably not used in liver disease	211
Warfarin	99	0.20	23	8.0	Enzyme-limited, binding-sensitive	99% Hepatic 1% Renal	$t_{1/2}$ →; V_d →; Cl →; f_p →. AVH no effect, but may be related to extent of liver damage	None; probably not used in liver disease	212

[a] GI, gastrointestinal; AVH, acute viral hepatitis; LD, liver disease.

Table 4.6
Considerations for Drug Dosage Adjustments in Liver Disease Patients

Extent of Change in Drug Dose	Conditions or Requirements to Be Satisfied
No change or minor change in dose	1. Mild liver disease 2. Extensive elimination of drug by kidneys and no renal dysfunction 3. Elimination by pathways of metabolism spared by liver disease 4. Drug is enzyme-limited and given acutely 5. Drug is flow/enzyme-sensitive and only given acutely by i.v. route 6. No alteration in drug sensitivity
Decrease in dose up to 25%	1. Elimination by the liver does not exceed 40% of the dose; no renal dysfunction 2. Drug is flow-limited and given by i.v. route, with no large change in protein binding 3. Drug is flow/enzyme-limited and given acutely by oral route 4. Drug has a large therapeutic ratio
Decrease in dose of greater than 25%	1. Drug metabolism is affected by liver disease; drug administered chronically 2. Drug has a narrow therapeutic range; protein binding altered significantly 3. Drug is flow-limited and given orally 4. Drug is eliminated by kidneys and renal function severely affected 5. Altered sensitivity to drug due to liver disease

tration of drugs that inhibit drug metabolism may further decrease an already depressed level of metabolic function. Age, genetic factors, or smoking can also influence drug disposition and make it difficult to accurately predict dosage requirements. Faced with such a wide array of variables influencing drug disposition, the best advice is still the following: *(a)* use caution when dosing, *(b)* follow blood levels if possible, and *(c)* be alert for signs of drug toxicity.

Acknowledgment

This work was supported in part by United States Public Health Service Grant GM 31304.

References

1. Abshagen U, Rennekamp H, Luszpinski G: Disposition kinetics of spironolactone in hepatic failure after single doses and prolonged treatment. *Eur J Clin Pharmacol* 11:169–176, 1977.
2. Acocella G, Bonollo L, Garimoldi M, Mainardi M, Tenconi LT, Hicolis FB: Kinetics of rifampin and isoniazid administered alone and in combination to normal subjects and patients with liver disease. *Gut* 13:47–53, 1972.
3. Adjepon-Yamoah KK, Himmo J, Prescott LF: Gross impairment of hepatic drug metabolism in a patient with chronic liver disease. *Br Med J* 4:387–388, 1974.
4. Affrime A, Reidenberg MM: The protein binding of some drugs in plasma from patients with alcoholic liver disease. *Eur J Clin Pharmacol* 8:267–269, 1975.
5. Allgulander C, Beerman B, Sjogren, A: Furosemide

pharmacokinetics in patients with liver disease. *Clin Pharmacokinet* 5:570–575, 1980.
6. Allonen H, Zieglar G, Koltz U: Midazolam kinetics. *Clin Pharmacol Ther* 30:653–660, 1981.
7. Alvin J, Meltorse T, Hoyumpa A, Bush MT, Schenker S: The effect of liver disease in man on the disposition of phenobarbital. *J Pharmacol Exp Ther* 192:224–235, 1975.
8. Andreasen PB, Greisen G: Phenazone metabolism in patients with liver disease. *Eur J Clin Invest* 6:21–26, 1976.
9. Andreasen PB, Hendel J, Greisen G, Hvidberg EF: Pharmacokinetics of diazepam in disordered liver function. *Eur J Clin Pharmacol* 10:115–120, 1976.
10. Andreasen PB, Hutters L: Paracetamol (acetaminophen) clearance in patients with cirrhosis of the liver. *Acta Med Scand* [Suppl] 624:99–105, 1979.
11. Avant GR, Schenker S, Alford RH: The effect of cirrhosis on the disposition and elimination of clindamycin. *Am J Dig Dis* 20:223–230, 1975.
12. Azzollini F, Gazzaniga A, Lodola E, Natangelo R: Elimination of chloramphenicol and thiamphenicol in subjects with cirrhosis of the liver. *Int J Clin Pharmacol Ther Toxicol* 6:13–134, 1972.
13. Benjamin RS: Clinical pharmacology of adriamycin (NSC-123127). *Cancer Chemother Rep* 6:183–185, 1975.
14. Bircher J, Blankart R, Halpern A, Hacki W, Laissue J, Preisig R: Criteria for assessment of functional impairment in patients with cirrhosis of the liver. *Eur J Clin Invest* 3:72–85, 1973.
15. Blaschke TF, Meffin, PJ, Melmon KL, Rowland M: Influence of acute viral hepatitis on phenytoin kinetics and protein binding. *Clin Pharmacol Ther* 17:685–691, 1975.
16. Boscia JA, Korzeniowski OM, Kobasa WD, Rocha H, Levison ME, Kaye D: Pharmacokinetics of cefoperazone in normal subjects and patients with hepatosplenic schistosomiasis. *J Antimicrob Chemother* 12:407–410, 1983.
17. Boscia JA, Korzeniowski OM, Snepar R, Kobasa WD,

Levison ME, Kaye D: Cefoperazone pharmacokinetics in normal subjects and patients with cirrhosis. *Antimicrob Agents Chemother* 23:385–389, 1983.

18. Branch RA, James J, Read AE: A study of factors influencing drug disposition in chronic liver disease, using the model drug (+)-propranolol. *Br J Clin Pharmacol* 3:243–249, 1976.

19. Branch RA, Morgan MH, James J, Read AE: Intravenous administration of diazepam in patients with chronic liver disease. *Gut* 17:975–983, 1976.

20. Branch RA, Shand DG: Propranolol disposition in chronic liver disease: a physiological approach. *Clin Pharmacokinet* 1:264–279, 1976.

21. Breimer DD, Zilly W, Richter E: Pharmacokinetics of hexobarbital in acute hepatitis and after apparent recovery. *Clin Pharmacol Ther* 18:433–440, 1975.

22. Brodie MJ, Boobis S: The effect of chronic alcoholic ingestion and alcoholic liver disease on binding of drugs to serum proteins: *Eur J Clin Pharmacol* 13:435–438, 1978.

23. Brown N, Ho DHW, Fong KL, Bogerd L, Maksymiuk A, Bolivar R, Fainstein V, Bodey GP: Effects of hepatic function on vancomycin clinical pharmacology. *Antimicrob Agents Chemother* 23:603–609, 1983.

24. Burnett DA, Barak AJ, Tuma DJ, Sorrell MF: Altered elimination of antipyrine in patients with acute viral hepatitis. *Gut* 17;341–344, 1976.

25. Calvo MV, Dominguez-Gil A, Macias JG, Dietz JL: Naproxen disposition in hepatic and biliary disorders. *Int J Clin Pharmacol Ther Toxicol* 18:242–246, 1980.

26. Cello JP, Oie S: Binding and disposition of sulfisoxazole in alcoholic cirrhosis. *J Pharmacokinet Biopharm* 13:1–12, 1985.

27. Cello JP, Oie J: Cimetidine disposition in patients with Laennec's cirrhosis during multiple dosing therapy. *Eur J Clin Pharmacol* 25:223–229, 1983.

28. Cochet B, Belaieff J, Allaz AF, Rudhardt M, Balant L, Fabre J: Decreased extrarenal clearance of cefoperazone in hepatocellular diseases. *Br J Clin Pharmacol* 11:389–390, 1981.

29. Cochet B, Belaieff J, Allaz AJ, Rudhardt M, Balant L, and Fabre J: Serum levels and urinary excretion of cefoperazone in patients with hepatic insufficiency. *Infection* 9(suppl 1):537–539, 1981.

30. Daneshmend TK, Homeida M, Kaye CM, Elamin AA, Roberts CJC: Disposition of oral metronidazole in hepatic cirrhosis and in hepatosplenic schistosomiasis. *Gut* 23:807–813, 1982.

31. Desmond PV, Patwardhan RV, Johnson RF, Schenker S: Impaired elimination of caffeine in cirrhosis. *Dig Dis Sci* 25:193–197, 1980.

32. D'Incalci M, Rossi C, Zucchetti M, Urso R, Cavalli F, Mangioni C, Williams Y, Sessa C: Pharmacokinetics of etoposide in patients with abnormal renal and hepatic function. *Cancer Res* 46:2566–2571, 1986.

33. Doshi J, Luisada-Oppe A, Leevy CM: Microsomal pentobarbital hydroxylase activity in acute viral hepatitis. *Proc Soc Exp Biol Med* 140:492–495, 1975.

34. duSouich P, Erill S: Metabolism of procainamide and p-aminobenzoic acid in patients with chronic liver disease. *Clin Pharmacol Ther* 22:588–595, 1977.

35. El-Raghy I, Back DJ, Osman F, Nafeh MA, Orme M L'E: The pharmacokinetics of antipyrine in patients with graded severity of schistosomiasis. *Br J Clin Pharmacol* 20:313–316, 1985.

36. Farrell G, Baird-Lambert J, Cvejic J, Buchanan N: Disposition and metabolism of metronidazole in patients with liver failure. *Hepatology* 4:722–726, 1984.

37. Farrell GC, Cooksley WGE, Hart P, Powell LW: Drug metabolism in liver disease. Identification of patients with impaired hepatic drug metabolism. *Gastroenterology* 75:580–588, 1978.

38. Farrell GC, Cooksley WGE, Powell LW: Drug metabolism in liver disease: Activity of hepatic microsomal metabolizing enzymes. *Clin Pharmacol Ther* 26:483–492, 1979.

39. Ferrier C, Marty J, Bouffard Y, Haberer JP, Levron JC, Duvaldestin P: Alfentanil pharmacokinetics in patients with cirrhosis. *Anesthesiology* 62:480–484, 1985.

40. Forrest JA, Adriaenssens P, Finlayson NDC, Prescott LF: Paracetamol metabolism in chronic liver disease. *Eur J Clin Pharmacol* 15:427–431, 1979.

41. Forrest JAH, Finlayson NDC, Adjepon-Yamoah KK, Prescott LF: Antipyrine, paracetamol, and lidocaine elimination in chronic liver disease. *Br Med J* 1:1384–1387, 1977.

42. Fuller R, Hoppel C, Ingalls ST: Furosemide kinetics in patients with hepatic cirrhosis with ascites. *Clin Pharmacol Ther* 30:461–467, 1981.

43. Ghoneim MM, Pandya H: Plasma protein binding of thiopental in patients with impaired renal or hepatic function. *Anesthesiology* 42:545–549, 1975.

44. Giacomini KM, Giacomini JC, Gibson TP, Levy G: Propoxyphene and norpropoxyphene plasma concentrations after oral propoxyphene in cirrhotic patients with and without surgically constructed portacaval shunt. *Clin Pharmacol Ther* 28:417–424, 1980.

45. Giargcau AJ, Chalmers TC: The natural history of cirrhosis. I. Survival with esophageal varices. *N Engl J Med* 268:469–473, 1963.

46. Gonzalez G, Arancibia A, Rivas MI, Caro P and Antezana C: Pharmacokinetics of furosemide in patients with hepatic cirrhosis. *Eur J Clin Pharmacol* 22:315–320, 1980.

47. Grahnen A, Jameson S, Lööf L, Tyllström J, Lindström B: Pharmacokinetics of cimetidine in advanced cirrhosis. *Eur J Clin Pharmacol* 26:347–355, 1984.

48. Greenfield RA, Gerber AU, Craig WA: Pharmacokinetics of cefoperazone in patients with normal and impaired hepatic and renal function. *Rev Infect Dis* 5(suppl 1):S127–S136, 1983.

49. Groszman R, Kotelanski B, Khatri IM, Cohn JN: Quantitation of portasystemic shunting from the splenic and mesenteric beds in alcoholic liver disease. *Am J Med* 53:715–722, 1972.

50. Gugler R, Kurten JW, Jensen CJ, Klehr U, Hartlapp J: Clofibrate disposition in renal failure and acute and chronic liver disease. *Eur J Clin Pharmacol* 15:341–347, 1979.

51. Gugler R, Muller Liebenau B, Somogyi A: Altered disposition and availability of cimetidine in liver cirrhotic patients. *Br J Clin Pharmacol* 14:421–429, 1982.

52. Gugler R, Wolf M, Hansen HH, Jensen JC: The inhibition of drug metabolism by cimetidine in patients with liver cirrhosis. *Klin Wochenschr* 62:1126–1131, 1984.

53. Haberer JP, Schoeffler P, Couderc E, Duvaldestin P: Fentanyl pharmacokinetics in anaesthetized patients with cirrhosis. *Br J Anaesth* 54:1267–1270, 1982.

54. Hall KW, Nightingale CH, Gibaldi M, Nelson E, Bates TR, Disanto AR: Pharmacokinetics of erythromycin in normal and alcoholic liver disease subjects. *J Clin Pharmacol* 22:321–325, 1982.

55. Hande KR, Wedlund PJ, Noone RM, Wilkinson GR, Greco FA, Wolff SN: Pharmacokinetics of high-dose etoposide (VP-16-213) administered to cancer patients. *Cancer Res* 44:379–382, 1984.

56. Helleberg L: Clinical pharmacokinetics of indomethacin. *Clin Pharmacokinet* 6:245–258, 1981.

57. Hepner GW, Vesell ES, Lipton A, Harvey HA, Wilkinson GR, Schenker S: Disposition of aminopyrine, antipyrine, diazepam and indocyanine green in patients with liver disease or on anticonvulsant drug therapy: diazepam breath test and correlations in drug elimination. *J Lab Clin Med* 90:440–456, 1977.

58. Hinthorn DR, Baker LH, Romig DR, Hassanien K, Liu C: Use of clindamycin in patients with liver disease. *Antimicrob Agents Chemother* 9:498–501, 1976.

59. Hoffman TA, Cestero R, Bullock WE: Pharmacodyn-

amics of carbenicillin in hepatic and renal failure. *Ann Intern Med* 73:173–178, 1970.

60. Homeida M, Jackson L, Roberts CJC: Decreased first-pass metabolism of labetalol in chronic liver disease. *Br Med J* 2:1048–1050, 1978.

61. Homeida M, Roberts CJC, Halliwell M, Read AE, Branch RA: Antipyrine clearance per unit volume liver: an assessment of hepatic function in chronic liver disease. *Gut* 20:596–601, 1979.

62. Hooper WD, Bochner F, Eadie MJ, Tyrer JH: Plasma protein binding of diphenylhydantoin. Effects of sex hormones, renal and hepatic disease. *Clin Pharmacol Ther* 15:276–282, 1974.

63. Horn T, Christofferson P, Henriksen JH: Alcoholic liver injury: defenestration in noncirrhotic livers—a scanning electron microscopic study. *Hepatology* 7:77–82, 1987.

64. Huet P, Lelorier J: Effects of smoking and chronic hepatitis B on lidocaine and indocyanine green kinetics. *Clin Pharmacol Ther* 28:208–215, 1980.

65. Huet P-M, Goresky CA, Villeneuve J-P, Marleau D, Lough JO: Assessment of liver microcirculation in human cirrhosis. *J Clin Invest* 70:1234–1244, 1982.

66. Huet P-M, Pomier-Layrargues G, Villeneuve J-P, Varin F, Viallet A: Intrahepatic circulation in liver disease. *Semin Liver Dis* 6:277–286, 1986.

67. Huet P-M, Villeneuve J-P, Pomier-Layrargues G, Marleau D: Hepatic circulation in cirrhosis. *Clin Gastroenterol* 14:155–168, 1985.

68. Hvidberg EF, Andreasen PB, Ranek L: Plasma half-life of phenylbutazone in patients with impaired liver function. *Clin Pharmacol Ther* 15:171–177, 1974.

69. Ishizaki T, Chiba K, Sasaki T: Antipyrine clearance in patients with Gilbert's syndrome. *Eur J Clin Pharmacol* 27:297–302, 1984.

70. Jahnchen E, Blanck KJ, Breuing KH, Gilfrich HJ, Meinertz T, Trenk D: Plasma protein binding of azapropazone in patients with kidney and liver disease. *Br J Clin Pharmacol* 11:361–367, 1981.

71. Jochemsen R, Van Beusekom BR, Spoelstra P, Janssens AR, Breimer DD: Effect of age and liver cirrhosis on the pharmacokinetics of nitrazepam. *Br J Clin Pharmacol* 15:295–302, 1983.

72. Johannessen SI, Gerna M, Bakke J, Strandjord RE, Morselli PL: CSF concentrations and serum protein binding of carbamazepine and carbamazepine-10gll-epoxide in epileptic patients. *Br J Clin Pharmacol* 3:575–582, 1976.

73. Juhl RP, VanThiel DH, Dittert LW, Albert KS, Smith RB: Ibuprofen and sulindac kinetics in alcoholic liver disease. *Clin Pharmacol Ther* 34:104–109, 1983.

74. Juma FD: Effect of liver failure on the pharmacokinetics of cyclophosphamide. *Eur J Clin Pharmacol* 26:591–593, 1984.

75. Jusko WJ, Gardner MJ, Mangione A, Shentag JJ, Koup JR, Vance JW: Factors affecting theophylline clearances: age, tobacco, marijuana, cirrhosis, congestive heart failure, obesity, oral contraceptives, benzodiazepines, barbiturates and ethanol. *J Pharm Sci* 68:1358–1366, 1979.

76. Kawai S, Ichikawa Y, Homma M: Differences in metabolic properties among cortisol, prednisolone, and dexamethasone in liver and renal diseases. Accelerated metabolism of dexamethasone in renal failure. *J Clin Endocrinol Metab* 60:848–854, 1985.

77. Keller E, Hoppe-Seyler G, Mumm R, Schollmeyer P: Influence of hepatic cirrhosis and end-stage renal disease on pharmacokinetics and pharmacodynamics of furosemide. *Eur J Clin Pharmacol* 20:27–33, 1981.

78. Kenny MT, Strates B: Metabolism and pharmacokinetics of the antibiotic rifampin. *Drug Metab Rev* 12:159–218, 1981.

79. Kessler KM, Humphries WC, Black M, Spann JF: Quinidine pharmacokinetics in patients with cirrhosis or receiving propranolol. *Am Heart J* 96:627–635, 1978.

80. Kirch W, Ohnhaus EE, Dylewicz P, Pabst J, Storstein L: Bioavailability and elimination of digitoxin in patients with hepatorenal insufficiency. *Am Heart J* 111:325–329, 1986.

81. Kirch W, Schäfer-Korting M, Mutschler E, Ohnhaus EE, Braun W: Clinical experience with atenolol in patients with chronic liver disease. *J Clin Pharmacol* 23:171–177, 1983.

82. Kleinbloesem CH, van Harten J, Wilson JPH, Danhof M, van Brummelen P, Breimer DD: Nifedipine: kinetics and hemodynamic effects' in patients with liver cirrhosis after intravenous and oral administration. *Clin Pharmacol Ther* 40;21–28, 1986.

83. Klinger EL, Vaamonde CA, Vaamonde LS, Lancestremere RG, Morosi HJ, Frisch E, Papper S: Renal function changes in cirrhosis of the liver. *Arch Intern Med* 125:1010–1015, 1970.

84. Klotz U, Antonin KH, Brugel H, Bieck PR: Disposition of diazepam and its major metabolite desmethyldiazepam in patients with liver disease. *Clin Pharmacol Ther* 21:430–436, 1977.

85. Klotz U, Avant GR, Hoyumpa A, Schenker S, Wilkinson GR: The effects of age and liver disease on the disposition and elimination of diazepam in adult man. *J Clin Invest* 55:347–359, 1975.

86. Klotz U, Fischer C, Muller-Seydlitz P, Schulz J, Mueller WA: Alterations in the disposition of differently cleared drugs in patients with cirrhosis. *Clin Pharmacol Ther* 26:221–227, 1979.

87. Klotz U, McHorse TS, Wilkinson GR, Schenker S: The effect of cirrhosis on the disposition and elimination of meperidine in man. *Clin Pharmacol Ther* 16:667–675, 1974.

88. Klotz U, Rapp T, Müller WA: Disposition of valproic acid in patients with liver disease. *Eur J Clin Pharmacol* 13:55–60, 1978.

89. Kraus JW, Desmond PV, Marshall JP, Johnson RF, Schenker S, Wilkinson GR: Effects of aging and liver disease on disposition of lorazepam. *Clin Pharmacol Ther* 24:411–419, 1978.

90. Krausz Y, Zylber-Katz E, Levy M: Antipyrine clearance and its correlation to routine liver function tests in patients with liver disease. *Int J Clin Pharmacol Ther Toxicol* 18:253–257, 1980.

91. Kroboth PD, Brown A, Lyon JA, Kroboth FJ, Juhl RP: Pharmacokinetics of single-dose erythromycin in normal and alcohol liver disease subjects. *Antimicrob Agents Chemother* 21:135–140, 1982.

92. Kunin CM, Glazko AJ, Finland M: Persistence of antibiotics in blood of patients with acute renal failure. Chloramphenicol and its metabolic products in the blood of patients with severe renal disease or hepatic cirrhosis. *J Clin Invest* 38:1498–1508, 1959.

93. Levi AJ, Sherlock S, Walker D: Phenylbutazone and isoniazid metabolism in patients with liver disease in relation to previous drug therapy. *Lancet* 1:1275–1279, 1968.

94. Levy G: Effect of plasma protein binding of drugs on duration and intensity of pharmacological activity. *J Pharm Sci* 65:1264–1265, 1976.

95. Lewis GP, Jusko WJ: Pharmacokinetics of ampicillin in cirrhosis. *Clin Pharmacol Ther* 18:475–484, 1975.

96. Lima JJ, Boudoulas H, Blanford M: Concentration-dependence of disopyramide binding to plasma protein and its influence on kinetics and dynamics. *J Pharmacol Exp Ther* 219:741–747, 1981.

97. MacGilchrist AJ, Birnie GG, Cook A, Scobie G, Murray T, Watkinson G, Brodie MJ: Pharmacokinetics and pharmacodynamics of intravenous midazolam in patients with severe alcoholic cirrhosis. *Gut* 27:190–195, 1986.

98. MacLeod CM, Bartley EA, Payne JA, Hudes E, Vernam K, Devlin RG: Effects of cirrhosis on kinetics of aztreonam. *Antimicrob Agents Chemother* 26:493–497, 1984.

99. Mak KM, Lieber CS: Alterations in endothelial fenestrations in liver sinusoids of baboons fed alcohol: a scanning electron microscopic study. *Hepatology* 4:386–391, 1984.

100. Malini PL, Sarti F, Dal Monte PR, Grepioni A, Boschi S, Ambrosioni E: Effect of chronic liver disease on plasma levels and metabolism of digoxin and beta-methyl digoxin. *Int J Clin Pharmacol Res* 1:21–27, 1982.

101. Mangione A, Inhoff TE, Lee RV, Shum LY, Jusko WJ: Pharmacokinetics of theophylline in hepatic disease. *Chest* 73:616–622, 1978.

102. Mannering GJ, Renton KW, el Azhary R, Deloria LB: Effects of interferon-inducing agents on hepatic cytochrome P-450 drug metabolizing systems. *Ann NY Acad Sci* 350:314–331, 1980.

103. Marcantonio LA, Auld WHR, Murdock WR, Purohit R, Skellern GG, Howes CA: The pharmacokinetics and pharmacodynamics of the diuretic bumetanide in hepatic and renal disease. *Br J Clin Pharmacol* 15:245–252, 1983.

104. Marcus FI, Kapadia GG: The metabolism of tritiated digoxin in cirrhotic patients. *Gastroenterology* 47:517–524, 1964.

105. Marshall JP, Salt WB, Elam RO, Wilkinson GR, Schenker S: Disposition of nafcillin in patients with cirrhosis and extrahepatic biliary obstruction. *Gastroenterology* 73:1388–1392, 1977.

106. Mawer GE, Miller NE, Turnberg LA: Metabolism of amylobarbitone in patients with chronic liver disease. *Br J Pharmacol* 44:549–560, 1972.

107. McConnell JB, Curry SH, Davis M, Williams R: Clinical effects and metabolism of diazepam in patients with chronic liver disease. *Clin Sci* 63:75–80, 1982.

108. McHorse TS, Wilkinson GR, Johnson RF, Schenker S: Effect of acute viral hepatitis in man on the disposition and elimination of meperidine. *Gastroenterology* 68:775–780, 1975.

109. Mehta MU, Venkataramanan R, Burckart GJ, Ptachcinski RJ, Yang SL, Gray JA, Van Thiel DH, Starzl TE: Antipyrine kinetics in liver disease and liver transplantation. *Clin Pharmacol Ther* 39:372–377, 1986.

110. Mendenhall CL, Robinson JD, Morgan DD: Chlordiazepoxide, librium (L), therapy in hepatic insufficiency. *Gastroenterology* 69:845, 1975.

111. Meredith CG, Christian CD Jr, Johnson RF, Madhavan SV, Schenker S: Diphenhydramine disposition in chronic liver disease. *Clin Pharmacol Ther* 35:474–479, 1984.

112. Miguet J-P, Vuitton D, Deschamps J-P, Allemand H, Joanne C, Bechtel P, Carayon P: Cholestasis and hepatic drug metabolism: comparison of metabolic clearance rate of antipyrine in patients with intrahepatic or extrahepatic cholestasis. *Dig Dis Sci* 26:718–722, 1981.

113. Morahan PS, Munson AE, Regelson W, Commerford SL, Hamilton LD: Antiviral activity and side effects of polyriboinosinic-cytidylic acid complexes as affected by molecular size. *Proc Natl Acad Sci USA* 69:842–846, 1972.

114. Morahan PS, Regelson W, Munson AE: Pyran and polyribonucleotides: differences in biological activities. *Antimicrob Agents Chemother* 2:16–22, 1972.

115. Moreau L, Durand H, Biclet P: Cefotaxime concentrations in ascites. *J Antimicrob Chemother* 6(suppl A):121–122, 1980.

116. Morgan DD, Robinson JD, Mendenhall CL: Clinical pharmacokinetics of chlordiazepoxide in patients with alcoholic hepatitis. *Eur J Clin Pharmacol* 19:279–285, 1981.

117. Morichau-Beauchant M, Houin G, Mavier P, Alexandre C, Dhumeaux D: Pharmacokinetics and bioavailability of ranitidine in normal subjects and cirrhotic patients. *Dig Dis Sci* 31:113–118, 1986.

118. Narang APS, Datta DV, Nath N, Mathur VS: Impairment of hepatic drug metabolism in patients with acute viral hepatitis. *Eur J Drug Metab Pharmacokinet* 7:255–258, 1982.

119. Narang APS, Datta DV, Nath N, Mathur VS: Pharmacokinetic study of chloramphenicol in patients with liver disease. *Eur J Clin Pharmacol* 20:479–483, 1981.

120. Naranjo CA, Busto U, Janecek E, Ruiz I, Roach CA, Kaplan K: An intensive drug monitoring study suggesting possible clinical irrelevance of impaired drug disposition in liver disease. *Br J Clin Pharmacol* 15:451–458, 1983.

121. Naranjo CA, Busto U, Mardones R: Adverse drug reactions in liver cirrhosis. *Eur J Clin Pharmacol* 13:429–434, 1978.

122. Neal EA, Meffin PJ, Gregory PB, Blaschke TF: Enhanced bioavailability and decreased clearance of analgesics in patients with cirrhosis. *Gastroenterology* 77:96–102, 1979.

123. Nelson DC, Avant GR, Speeg KV Jr, Hoyumpa AM Jr, Schenker S: The effect of cimetidine on hepatic drug elimination in cirrhosis. *Hepatology* 5:305–309, 1985.

124. Nouel O, Bernuau J, Lebar M, Rueff B, Benhamou JP: Cimetidine-induced mental confusion in patients with cirrhosis. *Gastroenterology* 79:780–781, 1980.

125. Novick DM, Kreek MJ, Arns PA, Lau LL, Yancovitz SR, Gelb AM: Effect of severe alcoholic liver disease on the disposition of methadone in maintenance patients. *Alcoholism* 9;349–354, 1985.

126. Novick DM, Kreek MJ, Fanizza AM, Yancovitz SR, Gelb AM, Stenger RJ: Methadone disposition in patients with chronic liver disease. *Clin Pharmacol Ther* 30:353–362, 1981.

127. Ochs HR, Greenblatt DJ, Bodem G, Dengler HJ: Disease-related alterations in cardiac glycoside disposition. *Clin Pharmacokinet* 7:434–451, 1982.

128. Ochs HR, Greenblatt DJ, Eckardt B, Harmatz JS, Shader RI: Repeated diazepam dosing in cirrhotic patients: accumulation and sedation. *Clin Pharmacol Ther* 33:471–476, 1983.

129. Ochs HR, Greenblatt DJ, Verburg-Ochs B, Matlis R: Temazepam clearance is unaltered in cirrhosis. *Am J Gastroenterol* 81:80–84, 1986.

130. Ohashi K, Tsunoo M, Tsuneoka K: Pharmacokinetics and protein binding of cefazolin and cephalothin in patients with cirrhosis. *J Antimicrob Chemother* 17:347–351, 1986.

131. Ohnhaus EE, Münch U, Meier J: Elimination of pindolol in liver disease. *Eur J Clin Pharmacol* 22:247–251, 1982.

132. Okolicsanyi L, Venuti M, Orlando R, Lirussi R, Nassuato G, Benvenuti C: Oral and intravenous pharmacokinetics of cimetidine in liver cirrhosis. *Int J Clin Pharmacol Toxicol* 20:482–487, 1982.

133. Okolicsanyi L, Venuti M, Orlando R, Xerri L, Pugina M: Pharmacokinetic studies of cefuroxime in patients with liver cirrhosis. *Arzneimittelforschung* 7:777–782, 1982.

134. Okolicsanyi L, Venuti M, Strazzabosco M, Orlando R, Nassuato G, Iemmolo RM, Lirussi R, Muraca M, Pastorino AM, Castelli G: Oral and intravenous pharmacokinetics of ranitidine in patients with liver cirrhosis. *Int J Clin Pharmacol Ther Toxicol* 22:329–332, 1984.

135. Olsen GD, Bennett WM, Potter GA: Morphine and phenytoin binding to plasma proteins in renal and hepatic failure. *Clin Pharmacol Ther* 17:677–684, 1976.

136. Oltmanns D, Pottage A, Endell W: Pharmacokinetics of tocainide in patients with combined hepatic and renal dysfunction. *Eur J Clin Pharmacol* 25:787–790, 1983.

137. Orrego H, Medline A, Blendis LM, Rankin JG, Kreaden DA: Collagenisation of the Disse space in alcoholic liver disease. *Gut* 20:673–679, 1979.

138. Pandele G, Chaux F, Salvadori C, Farinotti M, Duvaldestin P: Thiopental pharmacokinetics in patients with cirrhosis. *Anesthesiology* 59:123–126, 1983.

139. Pasko MT, Beam TR, Spooner JA, Camara DS: Safety and pharmacokinetics of ceftazidime in patients with chronic hepatic dysfunction. *J Antimicrob Chemother* 15:365–374, 1985.

140. Patwardhan R, Johnson R, Sheehan J, Desmond P, Wilkinson G, Hoyumpa A, Branch R, Schenker S: Morphine metabolism in cirrhosis. *Gastroenterology* 80:1344, 1981.

141. Patwardhan RV, Johnson RF, Hoyumpa A, Sheehan JJ, Desmond PV, Wilkinson GR, Branch RA, Schenker S: Normal metabolism of morphine in cirrhosis. *Gastroenterology* 81:1006–1011, 1981.

142. Pearson RM, Breckenridge AM: Renal function, protein binding and pharmacological response to diazoxide. *Br J Clin Pharmacol* 3:169–175, 1976.

143. Pentikainen PJ, Neuvonen PJ, Jostell K-G: Pharmacokinetics of chlormethiazole in healthy volunteers and patients with cirrhosis of the liver. *Eur J Clin Pharmacol* 17:275–284, 1980.

144. Perez-Mateo M, Erill S: Protein binding of salicylates and quinidine in plasma from patients with renal failure, chronic liver disease and chronic respiratory insufficiency. *Eur J Clin Pharmacol* 11:225–231, 1977.

145. Perrier D, Mayersohn M, Marcus FI: Clinical pharmacokinetics of digitoxin. *Clin Pharmacokinet* 2:292–311, 1977.

146. Pessayre D, Lebrec D, Descatorie V, Peignoux M, Benhamou J-P: Mechanism for reduced drug clearance in patients with cirrhosis. *Gastroenterology* 74:566–571, 1978.

147. Piafsky KM, Sitar DS, Rangno Re, Oglivie RI: Theophylline disposition in patients with hepatic cirrhosis. *N Engl J Med* 296:1495–1497, 1977.

148. Pirttiaho HI, Sotaniemi EA, Ahlqvist J, Pitkanen U, Pelkonen RO: Liver size and indices of drug metabolism in alcoholics. *Eur J Clin Pharmacol* 13:61–67, 1978.

149. Pisani F, Perruca E, Primerano G, D'Agostino AA, Petrelli RM, Fazio A, Oteri G, Di Perri R: Single-dose kinetics of primidone in acute viral hepatitis. *Eur J Clin Pharmacol* 27:465–469, 1984.

150. Pond SM, Tong T, Benowitz NL, Jacob P: Enhanced bioavailability of pethidine and pentazocine in patients with cirrhosis of the liver. *Aust NZ J Med* 10:515–519, 1980.

151. Pond SM, Tong T, Benowitz NL, Jacob P, Rigod J: Presystemic metabolism of meperidine to normeperidine in normal and cirrhotic subjects. *Clin Pharmacol Ther* 30:183–188, 1981.

152. Powell LW, Axelsen E: Corticosteroids in liver disease: studies on the biological conversion of prednisone to prednisolone and plasma protein binding. *Gut* 13:690–696, 1972.

153. Pozzi E, Menghini P: Blood levels of rifampicin in liver diseases. *Int J Clin Pharmacol* 10:44–49, 1974.

154. Regardh, G-G, Jordo L, Ervik M, Lundborg P, Olsson R, Ronn O: Pharmacokinetics of metoprolol in patients with hepatic cirrhosis. *Clin Pharmacokinet* 6:375–388, 1981.

155. Reidenberg MM, Affrime M: Influence of disease on binding of drugs to plasma proteins. *Ann NY Acad Sci* 226:115–126, 1973.

156. Renton KW, Mannering GJ: Depression of hepatic cytochrome P-450–dependent monooxygenase systems with administered interferon inducing agents. *Biochem Biophys Res Commun* 73:343–348, 1976.

157. Renton KW, Mannering GJ: Depression of the hepatic cytochrome P-450 mono-oxygenase system by administered tilorone (2,7-bis (2-(diethylamino) ethoxy) fluoren-9-one dihydrochloride). *Drug Metab Dispos* 4:223–231, 1976.

158. Richter E, Breimer DD, Zilly W: Disposition of hexobarbital in intra- and extrahepatic cholestasis in man and the influence of drug metabolism–inducing agents. *Eur J Clin Pharmacol* 17:197–202, 1980.

159. Ring-Larsen H: Renal blood flow in cirrhosis: relation to systemic and portal haemodynamics and liver function. *Scand J Clin Lab Invest* 37:635–642, 1977.

160. Ring-Larsen H, Birger H, Henriksen JH, Christensen NJ: Sympathetic nervous activity and renal and systemic hemodynamics in cirrhosis: plasma norepinephrine concentration, hepatic extraction, and renal release. *Hepatology* 2:304–310, 1982.

161. Ring-Larsen H, Henriksen JH: Pathogenesis of ascites formation and hepatorenal syndrome: humoral and hemodynamic factors. *Semin Liver Dis* 6:341–352, 1986.

162. Roberts MS, Rumble RH, Wanwimolruk S, Thomas D, Brooks PM: Pharmacokinetics of aspirin and salicylate in elderly subjects and in patients with alcoholic liver disease. *Eur J Clin Pharmacol* 25:253–261, 1983.

163. Roberts RK, Wilkinson GR, Branch RA, Schenker S: Effect of age and parenchymal liver disease on the disposition and elimination of chlordiazepoxide (Librium). *Gastroenterology* 75:479–485, 1978.

164. Robinson JD, Whitney HAK Jr, Guisti DL, Morgan DD, Mendenhall CL: The absorption of intramuscular chlordiazepoxide (Librium) in patients with severe alcoholic liver disease. *Int J Clin Pharmacol Ther Toxicol* 21: 433–438, 1983.

165. Rowland M, Benet LZ, Graham GG: Clearance concepts in pharmacokinetics. *J Pharmacol Biopharm* 1:123–136, 1973.

166. Sadee W, Schroder R, V Leitner E, Dagcioglu M: Multiple dose kinetics of spironolactone and canrenoate-potassium in cardiac and hepatic failure. *Eur J Clin Pharmacol* 7:195–200, 1974.

167. Sawhney VK, Gregory PB, Swezey SE, Blaschke TF: Furosemide disposition in cirrhotic patients. *Gastroenterology* 81:1012–1016, 1981.

168. Schalm SW, Summerskill Wolt J, Go VLW: Prednisone for chronic active liver disease: pharmacokinetics, including conversion to prednisolone. *Gastroenterology* 72:910–913, 1977.

169. Schenker S, Breen KJ, Hoyumpa AM: Hepatic encephalopathy: current status. *Gastroenterology* 66:121–151, 1974.

170. Schentag JJ, Cerra FB, Calleri GM, Leising ME, French MA, Bernhard H: Age, disease, and cimetidine disposition in healthy subjects and chronically ill patients. *Clin Pharmacol Ther* 29:737–743, 1981.

171. Schoene B, Fleischmann RA, Remmer H: Determination of drug metabolizing enzymes in needle biopsies of human liver. *Eur J Clin Pharmacol* 4:65–73, 1972.

172. Sellers EM, Greenblatt DJ, Giles HG, Naranjo CA, Kaplan H, MacLeod SM: Chlordiazepoxide and oxazepam disposition in cirrhosis. *Clin Pharmacol Ther* 26:240–246, 1979.

173. Sessions JT, Minkel HP, Bullard JC, Ingelfinger FJ: The effect of barbiturates in patients with liver disease. *J Clin Invest* 33:1116–1127, 1954.

174. Shamszad M, Soloman H, Mobarhan S, Iber FL: Abnormal metabolism of acetaminophen in patients with alcohol liver disease. *Gastroenterology* 69:865, 1975.

175. Shear L, Kleinerman J, Gabuzda GJ: Renal failure in patients with cirrhosis of the liver. *Am J Med* 39:184–198. 1965.

176. Shoeman DW, Azarnoff DL: Diphenylhydantoin potency and plasma protein binding. *J Pharmacol Exp Ther* 195:84–86, 1975.

177. Shreeve WW, Shoop JD, Ott DG, McInteer BB: Test for alcoholic cirrhosis by conversion of ^{14}C- or ^{13}C-galactose to expired CO_2. *Gastroenterology* 71:98–101, 1976.

178. Shull HJ, Wilkinson GR, Johnson R and Schenker S: Normal disposition of oxazepam in acute viral hepatitis and cirrhosis. *Ann Intern Med* 84:420–425, 1976.

179. Siegers C-P, Oltmanns D, Younes M: Effect of alcohol and chronic liver disease on the metabolic disposal of paracetamol in man. *Hepatogastroenterology* 28:304, 1981.

180. Singh G, Renton KW: Homogeneous interferon from

E. coli depresses hepatic cytochrome P-450 and drug biotransformation. *Biochem Biophys Res Commun* 106:1256–1261, 1982.

181. Singh G, Renton KW: Interferon-mediated depression of cytochrome P-450–dependent drug biotransformation. *Mol Pharmacol* 20:681–684, 1981.

182. Sloan TP, Lancaster R, Shah RR, Idle JR, Smith RL: Genetically determined oxidation capacity and the disposition of debrisoquine. *Br J Clin Pharmacol* 15:443–450, 1983.

183. Smith IL, Ziemniak JA, Bernhard H, Eshelman FN, Martin LE, Schentag JJ: Ranitidine disposition and systemic availability in hepatic cirrhosis. *Clin Pharmacol Ther* 35:487–494, 1984.

184. Somogyi A, Albrecht M, Kliens G, Schafer K, Eichelbaum M: Pharmacokinetics, bioavailability and ECG response of verapamil in patients with liver disease. *Br J Clin Pharmacol* 12:51–60, 1981.

185. Sonne J, Poulsen HE, Dossing M, Larsen NE, Andreasen PB: Cimetidine clearance and bioavailability in hepatic cirrhosis. *Clin Pharmacol Ther* 29:191–197, 1981.

186. Sotaniemi EA, Luoma PV, Jarvensiva PM, Sotaniemi KA: Impairment of drug metabolism in polycystic nonparasitic liver disease. *Br J Clin Pharmacol* 8:331–335, 1979.

187. Sotaniemi EA, Niemalä O, Risteli L, Stenbäck F, Pelkonen RO, Lahtela JT, Risteli J: Fibrotic process and drug metabolism in alcoholic liver disease. *Clin Pharmacol Ther* 40:46–55, 1986.

188. Sotaniemi EA, Pelkonen RO, Puukka M: Measurement of hepatic drug-metabolizing enzyme activity in man. *Eur J Clin Pharmacol* 17:267–274, 1980.

189. Staib AH, Schuppan D, Lissner R, Zilly W, Bomhard GV, Richter E: Pharmacokinetics and metabolism of theophylline in patients with liver diseases. *Int J Clin Pharmacol Ther Toxicol* 18:500–502, 1980.

190. Stoeckel K, Koup JR: Pharmacokinetics of ceftriaxone in patients with renal and liver insufficiency and correlations with a physiologic nonlinear protein. *Am J Med* 19:26–32, 1984.

191. Stoeckel K, Tuerk H, Trueb V, McNamara PJ: Single-dose ceftriaxone kinetics in liver insufficiency. *Clin Pharmacol Ther* 36:500–509, 1984.

192. Syrota A, Paraf A, Gaudebout C, Desgrez A: Significance of intra- and extrahepatic portasystemic shunting in survival of cirrhotic patients. *Dig Dis Sci* 26:878–885, 1981.

193. Syrota A, Vinot J-M, Paraf A, Roucayrol JC: Scintillation splenoportography: hemodynamic and morphological study of the portal circulation. *Gastroenterology* 71:652–659, 1976.

194. Teunissen MWE, Spoelstra P, Koch CW, Weeds B, Van Duyn W, Janssens AR, Breimer DD: Antipyrine clearance and metabolite formation in patients with alcoholic cirrhosis. *Br J Clin Pharmacol* 18:707–715, 1984.

195. Thiessen JJ, Sellers EM, Denbeigh P, Dolman L: Plasma protein binding of diazepam and tolbutamide in chronic alcoholics. *J Clin Pharmacol* 16:345–351, 1976.

196. Thomson PD, Melmon KL, Richardson JA, Cohn K, Steinbrunn W, Cudihee R, Rowland M: Lidocaine pharmacokinetics in advanced heart failure, liver disease, and renal failure in humans. *Ann Intern Med* 78:499–508, 1973.

197. Thomson PD, Rowland M, Melmon KL: The influence of heart failure, liver disease, and renal failure on the disposition of lidocaine in man. *Am Heart J* 82:417–421, 1971.

198. Tschang C, Steiner JA, Hignite CE, Huffman DH, Azarnoff DL: Systemic availability of lidocaine in patients with liver disease (abstract). *Clin Res* 25:609A, 1977.

199. Uribe M, Summerskill WHJ, Go VLW: Comparative serum prednisone and prednisolone concentrations following administration to patients with chronic active liver disease. *Clin Pharmacokinet* 7:452–459, 1982.

200. Verbeeck RK, Patwardhan RV, Villeneuve J-P, Wilkinson GR, Branch RA: Furosemide disposition in cirrhosis. *Clin Pharmacol Ther* 31:719–725, 1982.

201. Villeneuve J-P, Fortunet-Fouin H, Arsene D: Cimetidine kinetics and dynamics in patients with severe liver disease. *Hepatology* 3:923–927, 1983.

202. Villeneuve J-P, Rocheleau F, Raymond G: Triamterene kinetics and dynamics in cirrhosis. *Clin Pharmacol Ther* 35:831–837, 1984.

203. Villeneuve J-P, Verbeeck RK, Wilkinson GR, Branch RA: Furosemide kinetics and dynamics in patients with cirrhosis. *Clin Pharmacol Ther* 40:14–20, 1986.

204. Wagner VT, Heydrich D, Bartels H, Hohorst HJ: The influence of damaged liver parenchyma, renal insufficiency and hemodialysis on the pharmacokinetics of cyclophosphamide and its activated metabolites. *Arzneimittelforschung* 30:1588–1592, 1980.

205. Wallace S, Brodie MJ: Decreased drug binding in serum from patients with chronic hepatic disease. *Eur J Clin Pharmacol* 9:429–432, 1976.

206. Ward S, Weatherley BC: Pharmacokinetics of atracurium and its metabolites. *Br J Anaesth* 58:6S–10S, 1986.

207. Weiner M, Chenkin T, Burns JJ: Observations on the metabolic transformation and effects of phenylbutazone in subjects with hepatic disease. *Am J Med Sci* 228:36–39, 1954.

208. Wilkinson GR: The effects of liver disease and aging on the disposition of diazepam, chlordiazepoxide, oxazepam and lorazepam in man. *Acta Psychiatr Scand* 274:561–573, 1978.

209. Wilkinson GR, Shand DG: A physiological approach to hepatic drug clearance. *Clin Pharmacol Ther* 18:377–390, 1975.

210. Williams RL, Blaschke TF, Meffin PJ, Melman KL, Rowland M: Influence of viral hepatitis on the disposition of two compounds with high clearance: lidocaine and indocyanine green. *Clin Pharmacol Ther* 20:290–299, 1976.

211. Williams RL, Blaschke TF, Meffin PJ, Melmon KL, Rowland M: Influence of acute viral hepatitis on disposition and plasma binding of tolbutamide. *Clin Pharmacol Ther* 21:301–309, 1977.

212. Williams RL, Schary WL, Blaschke TF, Meffin PJ, Melmon KL, Rowland M: Influence of acute viral hepatitis on disposition and pharmacological effect of warfarin. *Clin Pharmacol Ther* 20:90–97, 1976.

213. Williams RL, Upton RA, Cello JP, Jones RM, Blitstein M, Kelly J, Nierenburg D: Naproxen disposition in patients with alcoholic cirrhosis. *Eur J Clin Pharmacol* 27:291–296, 1984.

214. Wood AJJ, Kornhauser DM, Wilkinson GR, Shand DG, Branch RA: The influence of cirrhosis on steady-state blood concentrations of unbound propranolol after oral administration. *Clin Pharmacokinet* 3:478–487, 1978.

215. Woodcock BG, Rietbrock I, Vohringer HF, Rietbrock N: Verapamil disposition in liver disease and intensive care patients: kinetics, clearance and apparent blood flow relationships. *Clin Pharmacol Ther* 29:27–34, 1981.

216. Young CJ, Daneshmend TK, Roberts CJC: Effects of cirrhosis and aging on the elimination and bioavailability of ranitidine. *Gut* 23:819–823, 1982.

217. Ziemniak JA, Bernhard H, Schentag JJ: Hepatic encephalopathy and altered cimetidine kinetics. *Clin Pharmacol Ther* 34:375–382, 1983.

218. Zilly W, Breimer DD, Richter E: Hexobarbital disposition in compensated and decompensated cirrhosis of the liver. *Clin Pharmacol Ther* 23:525–533, 1978.

219. Zilly W, Richter E, Rietbrock E: Pharmacokinetics and metabolism of digoxin- and β-methyl-digoxin-12α-^{3}H in patients with acute viral hepatitis. *Clin Pharmacol Ther* 17:302–309, 1975.

5

Pediatric Pharmacotherapy

Daniel A. Notterman, M.D., F.A.A.P.

Children develop and grow, and their response to drug therapy is conditioned by age, size, and stage of development. It is axiomatic that the change in body size associated with growth is a factor in determining dosage and response. However, even when the effect of size is accommodated, age and maturity exert a profound effect on response to pharmacotherapy. The influence of developmental factors is modulated, and usually amplified, by the imposition of critical illness, multiple organ system failure, heredity, and coadministration of other drugs. In infants and small children, vagaries of drug delivery systems and administration techniques assume significance (51, 64, 87, 110, 144, 145). This chapter provides a review of selected aspects of pediatric clinical pharmacology. It is not intended as, and does not include, a compendium of pediatric drug dosages. The pharmacology of individual agents is reviewed in greater detail in other chapters. The purpose here is to describe specific features that distinguish pharmacologic responses of children from those of adults, and to indicate, when possible, which observed pharmacologic differences are likely to result in important clinical differences.

Age-related differences in response are both pharmacokinetic and pharmacodynamic in origin (7, 18, 149, 151). The pharmacokinetic description concerns the relationship, over time, between drug *dosage* and drug *concentration*. The pharmacodynamic description concerns the relationship between this concentration and the resulting *response*. Narrowly construed, "pharmacodynamics" means "sensitivity," and applies to the relationship between unbound drug concentration (theoretically at the site of action; in practice, in the plasma) and magnitude of effect. Broadly conceived, pharmacodynamics comprises all of the biochemical and physiologic effects of a substance (149). Sensitivity is graphically represented in several ways (149); most often

as a plot of the log of drug concentration versus intensity of pharmacologic response. Figure 7.1, described in more detail in a subsequent section, is from a study by Driscoll and associates (38), and displays the pharmacodynamic relationship between dopamine concentration and the resulting inotropic effect in puppy ventricles from animals of different ages. Figure 7.2 illustrates an age-related pharmacodynamic effect from a study involving the elderly (139). It indicates that increasing age is associated with a reduction in the concentration of diazepam needed to induce a specified degree of hypnosis. By measuring diazepam concentration (rather than simply dosage), the

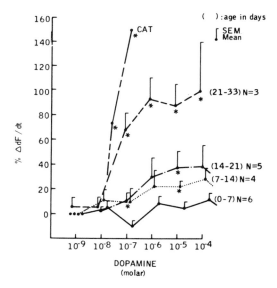

Figure 5.1 Inotropic ($\%\Delta dF/dt$) dose-response curves of puppy ventricles and adult cat ventricle treated with dopamine. There is an increasing inotropic responsiveness with age of isolated puppy ventricle to dopamine.* $P < 0.05$ using puppies 0–7 days old as control. (From Driscoll DJ, Gillette PC, Ezrailson EG, et al: Inotropic response of the neonatal canine myocardium to dopamine. *Pediatr Res* 12:42, 1978.)

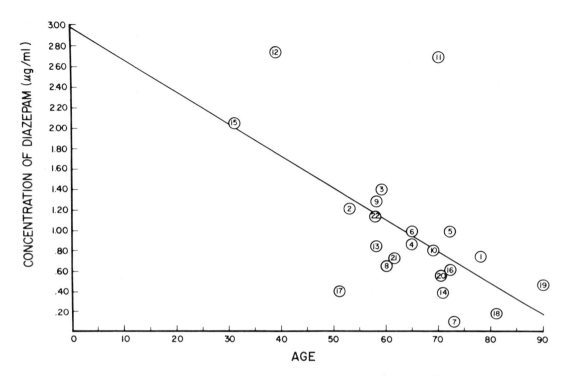

Figure 5.2. Relationship between age (31–90 years) of patient and plasma concentration of diazepam causing failure to respond to vocal but not painful stimuli. $P < 0.01$. (From Reidenberg MM, Levy M, Warner H, et al: Relationship between diazepam dose, plasma level, age and central nervous system depression. *Clin Pharmacol Ther* 23:371, 1978.)

investigators have excluded the hypothesis that a pharmacokinetic difference accounts for lower diazepam dosage requirements. Unfortunately, similar work is quite uncommon in the pediatric age group (7, 18), and experimentally proven differences in sensitivity between adults and children are not well documented.

A fundamental requirement for pharmacodynamic analysis is that there be precise pharmacokinetic information regarding the drug of interest *in the population in question.* Such is gradually becoming available in the pediatric age group.

PHARMACODYNAMIC VARIATION

Pharmacodynamic differences between the responses of pediatric patients and adult patients will be considered in the context of (a) unique effects in children, (b) adverse effects, and (c) therapeutically desired effects. This last category will focus on the catecholamines.

Unique Effects

Drugs may have unique effects in children. Many substances disturb patterns of growth and differentiation that occur only during particular phases of life (94). Notable in this regard are teratogens, which have unique, adverse effects on the fetus (18, 94, 97, 144, 163). To a certain extent, children share this special vulnerability with the fetus until growth and development cease at maturity. Thus, the tetracyclines affect bone growth in the fetus and newborn infant (28), as well as development of the teeth in children less than 6 years of age (66, 194). Corticosteroids, among their other adverse effects, suppress the linear growth of children (93), an effect that cannot occur in adults.

Cartilage toxicity is also a concern with nalidixic acid (170) and related fluoroquinoline antibiotics such as ciprofloxacin and norfloxacin (74, 113). It has been suggested that these newly developed quinoline derivatives, which are likely to have important critical care applications, be avoided in children until skeletal growth is complete (74, 113).

Adverse Effects

INCREASED OCCURRENCE OR SENSITIVITY

Metoclopramide and other dopamine antagonists such as prochlorperazine (Compazine), haloperidol, and chlorpromazine, have a variety of potential critical care indications (82, 100, 141, 183). These drugs produce acute dystonic reactions much more frequently in children and adolescents than in adults (9, 10, 172). A pharmacokinetic basis for this increase in dystonic reactions has been examined and rejected (9). The increase in CNS sensitivity to a variety of dopamine antagonists might be caused by the greater concentration of dopamine-2 receptors in the brains of young subjects (190).

Verapamil, a calcium entry blocking agent, is used to treat supraventricular tachycardia and other atrial dysrhythmias in children (65, 133, 166). There are clinical reports of infants developing acute, severe cardiorespiratory failure following administration of the drug (43, 56, 135). For this reason, verapamil should not be administered to individuals less than 1 year of age (43, 56, 135).

In infants, elastic and resistive properties of the lung entail optimal efficiency at high respiratory rates with low tidal volumes (131). Thus, the resting respiratory rate is higher, and the infant responds to the need for hyperventilation by increasing rate in preference to tidal volume (131). The need to maintain rapid respiratory rates implies greater sensitivity to respiratory depressants. Indeed, some years ago, Way and associates (181) demonstrated that compared with adults, infants required one-third the dose of morphine (on a weight normalized basis) for comparable depression in CO_2 sensitivity. Pharmacokinetic factors were not excluded, and further work on the effect of depressant drugs on the immature respiratory system would be useful.

DECREASED OCCURRENCE OR SENSITIVITY

Children enjoy relative protection from the adverse effects of several drugs. In most cases, the mechanism responsible for the relative immunity of youth has not been determined.

Several drugs cause hepatic injury less frequently in children than in adults. These include isoniazid (6, 41, 49, 116, 167), halothane (20, 24, 45, 96, 99, 180), and acetaminophen (4, 48, 111, 152, 153, 171).

Therapy with isoniazid (INH) is associated with asymptomatic increases in hepatic enzymes in 10–20% of adults (6, 41). In children 9–14, 17% had elevations of serum glutamic-oxaloacetic transaminase (SGOT) or glutamic-pyruvic transaminase (SGPT), similar to the proportion in adults (167). INH hepatitis, a potentially fatal disorder, develops in some individuals receiving the drug. The risk of developing INH hepatitis increases with age: 0 per 1000 in patients less than 20 years of age, 3 per 1000 for those 20–34 years of age, 12 per 1000 for those 35–49 years old, 23 per 1000 for those 50–65 years of age, and 8 per 1000 for those older than 65 years (49). Despite occasional reports of INH hepatitis in children (167), usually when INH and rifampin are coadministered (116), the incidence is still extremely low, and measurement of SGOT is not routinely performed in children receiving INH alone. Neither the mechanism of INH hepatitis, nor the reason for the relative protection of youth, has been elucidated.

Although there are isolated case reports to the contrary (24, 180), halothane hepatotoxicity appears to be extremely rare in children, even following multiple exposures to the drug, which increases risk in adults (180). Again, the mechanism of protection is unknown.

Acetaminophen produces marked elevation (>1000 IU/liter) of SGOT following ingestion of a substantial overdose (>150 mg/kg) (152). Without administration of an antidote, such as N-acetylcysteine (153), severe hepatitis occurs in 10%, with an associated mortality of 10–20% (48). Of individuals with potentially toxic acetaminophen levels, 5.5% of those less than 12 years of age had SGOT levels above 1000 IU/liter, while 29% of those older than 12 years had an increase of this magnitude (152). The protection conferred by young age has been related to ingestion of relatively small quantities of drug and to early emesis (152, 153). This fact is not the only explanation, since severe hepatotoxicity in children is rare even in the presence of levels associated with severe injury to adults (152). Children younger than about 9 years of age conjugate acetaminophen with sulfate as well as glucuronate (171). It is suggested that this additional pathway of detoxification reduces flux through the mixed function oxidase pathway implicated in acetaminophen hepatotoxicity (152, 171); or, that children have increased availability of glutathione, used to detoxify acetaminophen metabolites (152). These explanations remain speculative. Cases of severe acetaminophen toxicity, and death, have occurred in children (4, 111). Thus, children who ingest a potentially toxic quantity should be fully evaluated and treated with N-acetylcysteine if the concentration of acetaminophen exceeds the "probable risk" line of the Rumack nomogram (153), or if more than 150 mg/kg has been ingested and a serum level cannot be determined within 16 hours of ingestion (152).

Aminoglycoside ototoxicity and nephrotoxicity are probably less common in infants and children than in adults (31, 72, 98, 136). This subject has been recently reviewed (98). There is experimental and clinical evidence that the kidney of the infant or child is more tolerant of aminoglycoside exposure (31, 72). Enzymuria, a marker of renal tubular injury, is less in infants and children following treatment with an aminoglycoside, and there is less renal accumulation of these drugs in infants (72). In an analysis of controlled studies to date, the incidence of cochlear and vestibular toxicity was not found to be greater in infants receiving aminoglycosides than in control subjects (98). The relatively low incidence of aminoglycoside toxicity in infants and children should not be taken as evidence that these drugs are innocuous (98). The usual precautions for minimizing aminoglycoside toxicity, including therapeutic drug monitoring when appropriate, are indicated.

Infants tolerate higher serum concentrations of digoxin than do older children or adults (71, 118, 122), although some investigators dispute this observation (70). Lessened susceptibility to glycoside-induced arrhythmias may be a result of decreased norepinephrine content and sympathetic innervation of ventricular myocardium (54, 70, 80, 122); increased vagal tone (127); and/or a healthier myocardium without superimposed coronary artery disease (122).

Three other points should be mentioned. *First*, the observation that infants tolerate higher concentrations of digoxin without manifesting toxicity does not mean that they require higher concentrations in order to achieve therapeutic benefit. In fact, no therapeutic advantage accrues to maintaining serum digoxin levels greater than those associated with therapeutic efficacy (1–2 ng/ml) in adults (106, 122, 124, 130). Infants with relatively high, and rela-

tively low, digoxin levels have comparable shortening of systolic time intervals (130, 154). An average level of 1.3 ng/ml provides adequate cardiac functional improvement in infants with congestive heart failure (122, 124). *Second*, when normalized by weight, the dose of digoxin needed to achieve a particular digoxin concentration is larger in infants than adults (106, 122, 124). This fact represents a true pharmacokinetic difference between the two populations, and is reflected in different dosage requirements (106, 122). As discussed, this pharmacokinetic observation does not mean that infants are less sensitive to the drug. *Third*, the recent discovery of an endogenous digoxin-like substance that interacts with digoxin assays employing antibody systems (173, 174) means that much of the recent information concerning digoxin pharmacokinetics and dosage in infants and patients with hepatic or renal failure may need revision.

Serious theophylline toxicity is life-threatening and is manifest by seizures and cardiac rhythm disturbances. In adults, these events have been noted at concentrations of less than 50 mg/liter (23, 197). Children seem less sensitive to acute intoxications. In one prospective study, seizures or life-threatening rhythm disturbances did not occur when the concentration was less than 100 mg/liter (57). This observation has been incorporated into guidelines for managing theophylline overdosage in children: aggressive methods for reducing theophylline concentration, such as charcoal hemoperfusion (121) or hemodialysis (84, 132) are avoided in acute intoxications unless the concentration of theophylline exceeds 80–100 mg/liter or a life-threatening event has occurred (1). Peritoneal dialysis is ineffective in removing theophylline (101), and its use is contraindicated.

Therapeutically Desired Effects

CARDIAC GLYCOSIDES

An earlier incorrect belief that infants require higher serum concentrations of digoxin to achieve comparable pharmacologic effect is discussed above.

NEUROMUSCULAR BLOCKING AGENTS

Newborns and infants respond differently from older children and adults to neuromuscular blocking agents. They require smaller dosages of competitive (nondepolarizing) agents such as pancuronium and d-tubocurarine (11, 12, 29, 188, 192). This probably represents a pharmacodynamic increase in sensitivity. Electrophysiologic examination of the young infants' (<12 weeks) neuromuscular junctions indicates similarities to those of adult myasthenics (11). The dose of d-tubocurarine or pancuronium needed to induce paralysis is much lower in young infants: Bennett and associates (12) found that 40 μg/kg of pancuronium produced apnea in the 1-day-old infant, whereas 92 μg/kg was required at one month. Similar results have been reported with d-tubocurarine (11, 188). This difference persists even when d-tubocurarine is prescribed on the basis of surface area (neonate: 4.1 mg/m²; adult: 7.0 mg/m²) (29). The reduced dosage requirement of infants cannot be explained on a pharmacokinetic basis, since clearance is greater in infants than in adults (117). In contrast, equal doses of succinylcholine, per unit weight, yield a shorter duration of apnea in infants than in adults (29, 30, 188). On the basis of body weight, infants require twice the adult dose to produce equivalent degrees of blockade (115). The discrepancy is attenuated when dose is normalized to body surface area rather than mass, and a uniform dose of 40 mg/m² produces equivalent duration of effect

Table 5.1
Dosage of Neuromuscular Blocking Drugs in Children[a,b]

Drug	Dose (mg/kg)
Succinylcholine	
Newborns, infants	2
Children, adolescents, adults	1
Pancuronium	
Newborn–1 week	0.03
1–2 weeks	0.06
2–4 weeks	0.09
>4 weeks (continuous infusion 0.1 mg/kg/hr; slightly lower dose may be adequate)	0.1
d-Tubocurarine	
Newborn–1 week	0.2
1–2 weeks	0.3
2–4 weeks	0.4
4–6 weeks	0.5
>6 weeks	0.6

[a] Adapted from Nugent SK, Laravuso R, Rogers MC: Pharmacology and use of muscle relaxants in infants and children. J Pediatr 94:481, 1979.
[b] Note that dose of succinylcholine is greater in infants, but doses of pancuronium and d-tubocurarine are smaller.

in infants and adults (29, 188). As discussed in a later section ("Adjustment for Size"), this finding suggests a pharmacokinetic rather than true pharmacodynamic basis for the apparent decrease in sensitivity of infants to succinylcholine. In line with this conclusion, the elimination half-life of succinylcholine is shorter in infants than in older children and adults (188).

Dosage guidelines incorporate these observations, and are summarized in Table 5.1.

SYMPATHOMIMETIC AGENTS

It has been suggested that the immature cardiovascular system responds differently to inotropic agents, including exogenously administered catecholamines. Structural and physiologic cardiovascular differences between the fetus, infant, child, and adult have been summarized (5, 25, 52, 53, 127, 195) and will not be explored in detail. The clinical pharmacology of sympathomimetic agents, particularly the catecholamines, is reviewed in Chapter 12. The following discussion highlights differences between adults, children, and infants that are of particular relevance to the clinical use of catecholamine infusions.

Driscoll and coworkers (38) examined the inotropic response of isolated, perfused ventricles from puppies of different ages as the preparations were exposed to perfusate containing varying concentrations of dopamine and isoproterenol. Figure 5.1 displays the data obtained when dopamine was in the perfusate. Sensitivity increased with increasing puppy age from 0–7 days to 21–33 days. This relationship was ablated by pretreatment with reserpine, and was not noted when isoproterenol was tested. These observations suggested that the blunted inotropic response to dopamine of preparations from younger animals resulted from incomplete sympathetic innervation and reduced norepinephrine stores. Relative deficiencies of sympathetic innervation have been repeatedly demonstrated in newborn animals (52, 54, 58, 127). This fact has not been evaluated in human infants, and the timing of complete myocardial innervation has not been elucidated (54). Others have also observed cardiac subsensitivity to exogenous catecholamines (39, 146). However, results have varied between laboratories, even when the same species was examined. For example, Rockson and associates (146), administered bolus injections of isoproterenol to intact puppies, and unlike

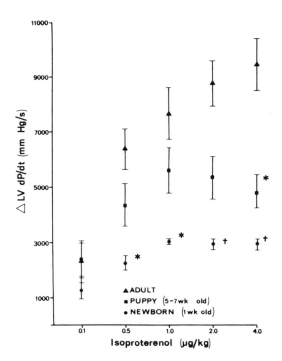

Figure 5.3 Inotropic dose-response curves to iso-proterenol for adult, 1-week-old, and 5- to 7-week-old puppies. The mean inotropic response of newborn animals was blunted throughout the dose-response range, and the maximal stimulation was achieved at a much lower dose of isoproterenol at this stage of development. Responses significantly different from adults are noted by *(P < 0.05) and +(P < 0.01). (From Rockson SG, Homcy CJ, Quinn P, et al: Cellular mechanisms of impaired adrenergic responsiveness in neonatal dogs. *J Clin Invest* 67:319, 1981.)

Driscoll and associates (38) found that there was a close relationship between age and inotropic response to isoproterenol (Fig. 5.3). Geis and coworkers (58) reported that compared with adult dogs, puppies responded equally well to isoproterenol and exhibited a greater chronotropic response to norepinephrine. Methodologic rather than physiologic differences may play a role in the diversity of these observations. The subtlety of potential experimental artifact was reemphasized by Park and colleagues (123) who showed that the age-dependent difference in inotropic response of right atrial rabbit tissue to isoproterenol disappeared when the preparations were tested at 38°C rather than 26° or 32°C. Thus, the presumed age-dependent difference in inotropic response to β-agonists may be an age-dependent difference in temperature sensitivity.

The immature heart has a greater proportion of noncontractile relative to contractile tissue (52, 53) and has a lower compliance (53, 127, 147, 148). Stroke volume is smaller when normalized to weight (127). Decreased compliance and stroke volume imply that the immature heart has a limited "preload reserve" (53, 127). The increase in stroke volume that follows volume loading is smaller than expected (147, 148). Newborn ventricles exhibit greater interdependence than those from adult animals (147), which is also expected to limit the efficacy of volume loading. A high baseline heart rate (127), coupled with limited ability to augment stroke volume, impairs the ability of the heart to increase cardiac output. Stroke volume may not be augmented by the usual inotropic agents; increases in cardiac output may depend on drug-induced acceleration of heart rate (53, 127). It is in this context that Friedman and George (53) have referred to the limited "total functional reserve" of the infant heart.

The cardiovascular response to catecholamines may also be limited by differences in the number and function of adrenergic receptors. Binding studies of peripheral white blood cells indicate that β-adrenergic receptor number may be reduced in infants and children (140, 143). It is not certain that the number of β-receptors on peripheral white cells reflects the number in the myocardium. Work in the elderly (178) and in patients with heart failure (63) suggests that this fact may be so. Evidence against a role for the adrenergic receptor in neonatal cardiac subsensitization was provided by Rockson and associates (146), who observed that the density of β-adrenergic binding sites was *increased* in immature animals, and that these receptors generated cyclic AMP appropriately, even though the inotropic response to isoproterenol and norepinephrine was reduced. This finding was thought to represent an adaptive response to decreased myocardial innervation, but suggests that diminished number and function of receptors does not play a major role in the limited response of immature animals to catecholamines.

Studies in nonhuman neonates have shown age-related or maturational-related differences in α- and β-adrenergic receptor content of lung, brain, liver, platelets, and fat cells (184). It would not be surprising if these differences produced qualitative and quantitative alterations in noncardiovascular pharmacologic effects of catecholamine infusions. Postnatal changes in vascular responsiveness to adrenergic agents have been extensively explored. Decreased vascular sensitivity to a variety of catecholamines has been a fairly constant (5, 21, 42) but not invariant (42) finding in immature animals. The newborn pig requires a higher dose of isoproterenol than does the adult to reduce vascular resistance (22), and sheep display greater sensitivity to both norepinephrine and isoproterenol with increasing fetal and postnatal age (5). Interestingly, the authors of this study related increasing sensitivity to closure of vascular shunts rather than to maturation of the neuroeffector system. These in vivo experiments are supported by in vitro work with isolated vascular muscle strips and rings, and experiments in which the microvasculature is directly observed. This work has been recently reviewed (42).

In addition to deficiencies in adrenergic innervation and receptor number, the immature cardiovascular system displays limited reflex integration. Hydralazine does not evoke reflex tachycardia in the rat until 14 days of age (8).

In human infants and children, several published clinical studies have evaluated the use of dopamine or dobutamine. Surprisingly, these studies do not provide unambiguous evidence that pediatric patients display a diminished or different response to catecholamines; in fact, the contrary may be true.

Lang and coworkers (86) treated five children (age, 1–24 months; mean age, 8 months) with dopamine following cardiovascular surgery. For the group as a whole, neither heart rate, blood pressure, nor cardiac output increased significantly at infusion rates less than 15 μg/kg/min. Increases in cardiac output were related to higher heart rate rather than greater stroke volume. Adults display increases in blood pressure and cardiac output at infusion rates below 5–10 μg/kg/minute and increases in heart rate below 10 μg/kg/minute (13, 27, 60, 168, 187). Lang's study has been taken to support the view that the cardiovascular system of infants and children is less sensitive to dopamine (53). However, the study was uncontrolled and included a heterogeneous group of patients. Driscoll and associates (40) evaluated dopamine in 24 children (age, 2 days to 18 years; mean age, 39 months) with shock of disparate medical and surgical causes (20 of 24 had congenital heart disease). The infusion was started at 2–10 μg/kg/min and titrated to desired response. More than half of the subjects responded favorably to the infusion ($\geq$15% increase in systolic blood pressure), at a mean dosage in responders of 8.3 $\pm$ 1.5 μg/kg/min. In

this group, blood pressure increased significantly, but heart rate did not. The study design did not permit evaluation of a dose-response relationship. Perez and colleagues (125) observed that a group of five hypotensive newborn infants studied prospectively required a dopamine infusion rate of greater than 20 μg/kg/min to achieve adequate blood pressure, capillary refill, and urine output. The average infusion rate of dopamine required to increase mean arterial pressure from 27 to 54 mm Hg was 25 $\pm$ 10 μg/kg/min, and the highest dosage was 50 μg/kg/min. At this dosage, urine output increased and there was no clinical evidence of cutaneous vasoconstriction. Since infusion rates of this magnitude in adults are often associated with marked peripheral vasoconstriction, Perez and associates interpreted their findings to support the concept of cardiac and peripheral vascular subsensitivity to catecholamines during infancy. In contrast, in a placebo-controlled study of infants, DiSessa and associates (35) observed that relatively modest (2.5 μg/kg/min) dosages of dopamine were associated with improvement in blood pressure and myocardial performance, evaluated by echocardiogram; Seri and coworkers (161) made similar observations.

These clinical studies do not permit firm conclusions. The subjects had diverse underlying and coexisting conditions, including structural cardiac disease, recent cardiac operation, asphyxia, pulmonary hypertension, and septicemia. Indications for pressor therapy, volume status, and measure of pharmacologic response were not standardized. A large variety of factors other than age and development, reviewed elsewhere in this text, are known to affect adrenergic receptor function and cardiovascular response to catecholamine infusion (27, 195, 196). These factors were not controlled. Plasma dopamine levels were not measured, and pharmacokinetic data in a population of critically ill children are not available.

Padbury and colleagues (120) incorporated measurement of dopamine concentration with assessment of cardiovascular response in newborn infants. Infusion rates as low as 0.5–1.0 μg/kg/min were associated with important effects on blood pressure and cardiac output. Heart rate increased at infusion rates of 2–3 μg/kg/min. The calculated thresholds for changes in selected hemodynamic functions are listed in Table 5.2. As indicated in Figure 5.4, there was a conventional log-linear relationship between dopamine concentration and several hemodynamic variables. The dopa-

Table 5.2
Concentration of Dopamine and Associated Dopamine Infusion Rate That Produce Threshold Response of Mean Blood Pressure (MBP), Systolic Blood Pressure (SBP), and Heart Rate (HR) in 14 Newborn Infants[a]

Effect	Dopamine Concentration (pg/ml ± SEM)	Infusion Rate (μg/kg/min)
MBP increase	14,000 ± 3500	0.5–1.0
SBP increase	18,000 ± 4500	1–2
HR increase	35,000 ± 5000	2–3

[a] Data from Padbury JF, Agata Y, Baylen BG, et al: Dopamine pharmacokinetics in critically ill newborn infants. *J Pediatr* 110:293, 1987.

mine clearance reported by Padbury and associates was 48–60 ml/kg/min, and did not correlate with age or birth weight. Clearance values of this magnitude have been observed in the pediatric age group by other workers (Notterman, unpublished data; Zaritsky, personal communication, 1987), and are not ap-

preciably different from those recorded in studies of adults (68, 77). This excludes a pharmacokinetic basis for Padbury's observation that newborn infants are as sensitive to dopamine as older children or adults. Table 5.3 summarizes several studies of dopamine pharmacodynamics and pharmacokinetics.

The hemodynamic effects of dobutamine in children have been examined in several studies (15, 37, 126, 156, 169). None contains pharmacokinetic measurements, and such information has not been developed in the pediatric age group. Detailed pharmacodynamic and kinetic information is available for healthy and acutely ill adults (79, 89, 90).

Age-related differences in response to dobutamine have not been consistently observed. In addition to the anticipated increase in cardiac output and stroke volume, Driscoll and Gillette (37) found a fairly consistent increase in systemic vascular resistance, contrary to the behavior of adults with congestive heart failure (81, 89). Driscoll's subjects had structural con-

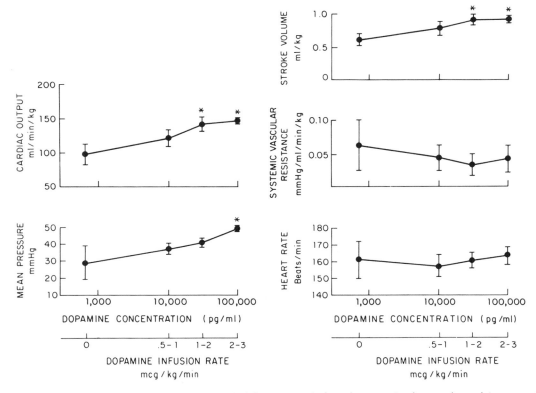

Figure 5.4. Sequential cardiac output, mean arterial pressure, stroke volume, systemic vascular resistance, and heart rate in four infants during dopamine infusions. Dopamine infusion rates are ranges calculated from dopamine clearance values. (Adapted and redrawn from Padbury JF, Agata Y, Baylen BG, et al: Dopamine pharmacokinetics in critically ill newborn infants. *J Pediatr* 294:293, 1987.)

Table 5.3
Dopamine Response Threshold for Heart Rate (HR), Systolic Blood Pressure (SBP), Systemic Vascular Resistance (SVR), and Stroke Volume (SV) in Selected Studies[a,b]

Investigators	No. of Subjects	Age (Condition)	Response Threshold								Clearance (ml/kg/min)
			Infusion Rate (μg/kg/min)				Dopamine Concentration (ng/ml)				
			HR	SBP	SVR	SV	HR	SBP	SVR	SV	
Lang et al (86)	5	1–24 months (post CVS)	15	15	NS	NS (CO-15)	Not measured				NM
Driscoll et al (40)	24	2 days—18 years (18–24 post CVS)	NS	8.3°	NM	NM	Not measured				NM
Seri et al (161)	18	Premature infant (hyaline membrane disease)	8	2	NM	NM	Not measured				NM
Padbury et al (120)	14	Premature/term infants (medical shock)	2–3	0.5–1.0	NM	NM	35	18	NM	NM	48–60
Jarnberg et al (77)	10	32–61 years (post elective surgery)	5†	5†	NM	NM	79	79	NM	NM	70–75
Gundert-Remy et al (68)	5	24–34 years (healthy adults)	6*	6*	NM	NM	74	74	NM	NM	61–85

[a] Data from references 40, 68, 77, 86, 120, 161.
[b] For studies involving adults, only those in which dopamine concentration was measured are included. Response threshold in terms of plasma dopamine concentration and infusion rate is included when available. NS, no significant change at dosage range tested; NM, variable not measured; °, group mean; †, 2 or 5 μg/kg/min tested, no intermediate infusion rate; *, approximate infusion rates calculated from data provided by author; CVS, cardiovascular surgery.

genital heart disease, and most were not in heart failure—these differences, rather than age, probably account for the disparity. Perkin and Levin (126) found dobutamine to be effective in augmenting cardiac output and stroke volume in a variety of conditions associated with shock. Subjects younger than 12 months displayed a trend (not statistically significant) toward an attenuated response to the inotropic effect of the drug. These younger subjects also responded to infusion of dobutamine with an increase in pulmonary capillary wedge pressure. An adverse effect on pulmonary capillary wedge pressure has not been observed in other studies involving children or adults, and would stand as one of the few documented differences between the responses of infants and adults to catecholamine infusion. In newborn infants with "heart failure" of diverse etiology, Stopfkuchen and associates (169) found that abnormal left ventricular systolic time intervals changed significantly during infusion of dobutamine. This change was associated with a significant chronotropic effect. Schranz and coworkers (156) documented a substantial positive inotropic effect with little acceleration of heart rate in 12 children with shock of various etiologies.

In children emerging from cardiopulmonary bypass, dobutamine may not be a desirable agent because of undesirable chronotropy and slight improvement in stroke volume (17). A small left ventricle is thought to limit the inotropic effect of dobutamine in children who are recovering from repair of tetralogy of Fallot (15). In these children, increases in cardiac output depend on dobutamine-associated increases in heart rate. More work will be needed to clarify the relative importance of development, type of structural lesion, and cardiopulmonary bypass in producing these differences.

Work in infants and adults has not as yet documented systematic age-related differences in catecholamine pharmacokinetics or pharmacodynamics. This fact is surprising because of the extensive work in animals that supports reduced responsiveness to catecholamines in the young. The extent of our knowledge in humans, however, is limited by methodologic problems and by the virtual absence of pharmacokinetic data in infants and children. There is detailed pharmacokinetic and pharmacodynamic information concerning each of the clinically employed catecholamines in healthy and, to a limited extent, critically ill adults (32, 33, 47, 62, 88, 89, 165). Recent developments in analytic chemistry presage an exten-

sion of this knowledge to the pediatric age group and to critically ill patients of any age.

PHARMACOKINETIC VARIATION

The weight of the average 18-year-old male, 63 kg, exceeds that of the average term newborn infant, 3.4 kg (94), by a factor of 19. Expressed in terms of surface area, this factor becomes 8.5. Thus, it is not surprising that infants and children require smaller dosages than adults. In this section, the effect of changing size and function on pharmacokinetics will be examined. Such alterations affect each of the major aspects of drug disposition: absorption, distribution (including protein binding), biotransformation, and excretion of changed and unchanged drug (18, 106, 142, 151). Lack of awareness of the need to account for altered function as well as altered size has been responsible for serious therapeutic misadventures such as the "gray syndrome" (182) of the 1960s (neonatal chloramphenicol toxicity) and the "gasping syndrome" (50, 59) of the 1980s (neonatal benzyl alcohol toxicity).

Special Problems in Drug Delivery to Children

Children require and tolerate smaller volumes of intravenous fluid than do adults. This fact limits the volume of intravenously administered fluid in which a drug can be diluted and the maximum rate at which the drug can be infused. These problems are magnified by the imposition of fluid limits associated with critical cardiac, respiratory, or renal disease.

Dilution volumes of intravenous medications can be adjusted, but physical properties of many drugs, as well as concern for safety, place a limit on maximum drug concentration. Current recommendations for dilution of several drugs employed in pediatric critical care are listed in Table 5.4. These recommendations (51, 110) are based on both clinical observation and pharmaceutical information concerning solubility and stability, but may not have been subjected to experimental testing.

Low intravenous flow rates result in a substantial delay before delivery of drug actually starts or is completed. The magnitude of this delay depends on the rate of infusion, the drug dosage volume, and the site of introduction of

Table 5.4
Maximum Drug Concentrations for Intravenous Infusion in Infants and Children[a,b]

Drug	Concentration
Antibiotics	
Acyclovir	7 mg/ml
Amikacin	6 mg/ml
Amphotericin	0.1 mg/ml
Beta-lactam	50–100 mg/ml
Chloramphenicol	50–100 mg/ml
Clindamycin	6 mg/ml
Erythromycin	
lactobionate	5 mg/ml
Gentamicin	2 mg/ml
Imipenem	5 mg/ml
Kanamycin	6 mg/ml
Metronidazole	8 mg/ml
Penicillin G	50–100,000 units/ml
Sulfamethoxazole/	
trimethoprim	1 ml/15 ml
Tobramycin	2 mg/ml
Vancomycin	5 mg/ml
Vidarabine	0.45 mg/ml
Miscellaneous	
Aminophylline	1 mg/ml
Bretylium tosylate	10 mg/ml
Catecholamine	Varies
Ethacrynate	1 mg/ml
Lidocaine	Varies
Magnesium sulfate	10 mg/ml
Methyldopa	10 mg/ml

[a] Adapted from Nelson JD: *Pocketbook of Pediatric Antimicrobial Therapy,* ed 7. Baltimore, Williams & Wilkins, 1987; Ford DC, Leist ER, Algren JT: *Guidelines for Administration of Intravenous Medications to Pediatric Patients,* ed 2. Bethesda, American Society of Hospital Pharmacists, 1984; and information provided by manufacturers.
[b] Intravenous push injection, when appropriate, may require different dilution. Information represents literature consensus and may not have been evaluated by appropriate pharmaceutical tests.

the drug into the intravenous tubing. The length of delay can be surprising. For example, when drug is added to the fluid reservoir of a system in which the rate of flow is 25 ml/hr, delivery of drug does not begin for nearly 2 hours and is not complete for 4 hours (145). Delayed drug delivery has several untoward consequences, which were recently summarized by Roberts (125). (*a*) In one study, 36% of the total daily dose of certain intravenous medications was inadvertently discarded when intravenous sets were routinely changed. (*b*) Therapeutic drug monitoring becomes inaccurate when the precise time of delivery of drug cannot be determined. (*c*) When the rate of infusion is less than or equal to the drug's elimination rate, plasma drug levels will be negligible. Clearly,

precise knowledge of the characteristics of drug delivery systems must be an important consideration in devising treatment plans.

Gould, Roberts, and Leff (64, 87, 145) evaluated several methods of intravenous drug delivery; based on their experiments, they developed a plan for the selection of an appropriate drug delivery system (Figs. 5.5 and 5.6). The reader is referred to the original publications for details (64, 87, 145).

Absorption

Absorption of drug occurs from the gastrointestinal tract (mouth, stomach, small intestine, rectum), from intramuscular or subcutaneous sites of injection, from the skin, and from lung. Agents that are administered by vein or artery bypass the process of absorption.

The effect of age on enteral absorption is not uniform and is difficult to predict. Newborns absorb drugs more slowly, but not necessarily less completely than older children and adults (18, 105, 106, 144). Drugs known to be well absorbed when given orally may not be available in a form suitable for administration to young children. For example, when isoniazid tablets are crushed and administered with applesauce, as some recommend, the INH is poorly absorbed. This practice has led to failed treatment of tuberculous meningitis (114). Untested, extemporaneous forms of medication should not be administered to children.

Absorption from intramuscular sites has not been broadly examined in children, although some antibiotics display excellent bioavailability (78, 109). This route is not recommended for use with critically ill children.

In the past, rectal suppository administration was frequently prescribed for drugs such as phenobarbital, aspirin, acetaminophen, aminophylline, belladonna, opium, and others. Rectal suppository administration is generally not desirable in the critical care setting, and many substances are slowly and unpredictably absorbed by this route (18). Therapeutic failure and severe intoxication have occurred with rectal administration of aminophylline (18, 112). Recently, however, rectal administration of solutions of diazepam or sodium valproate (104, 176) has been suggested for control of status epilepticus.

Transdermal drug delivery has not been exploited in therapy of children. Since percutaneous absorption is facilitated by the relatively thin stratum corneum of the infant and child

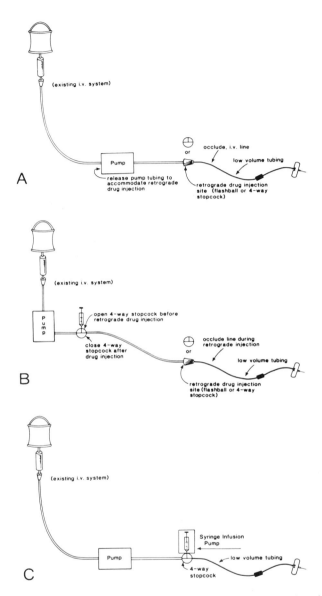

Figure 5.5. **A,** Construction of an intravenous system for manual retrograde injection. An injection site (flashball or stopcock) and low-volume extension tubing are located at the distal end of the existing intravenous set-up. **B,** Construction of intravenous system for retrograde injection modified for a volume infusion pump device unable to accept retrograde injection. System consists of existing intravenous set-up to which is attached an extension set with a proximal four-way stopcock and distal flashball injection site. A large-volume syringe is attached to the four-way stopcock and acts as an overflow reservoir for the intravenous fluid displaced by the dose volume. **C,** Construction of mechanical (syringe) infusion system. A four-way stopcock and low-volume extension tubing are attached distal to the existing intravenous system. The dosing syringe is attached directly to the four-way stopcock before placement on the syringe infusion device. For details see original sources. (Adapted from Leff RD, Roberts RJ: Methods of intravenous drug administration in the pediatric patient. *J Pediatr* 98:681, 1981; and Roberts RJ: Intravenous administration of medications in pediatric patients: problems and solutions. *Pediatr Clin North Am* 28:23, 1986.)

Steps

#1. On admission establish only a "basic" I.V. set-up which includes I.V. fluid container, volume control device (Metriset) and associated I.V. tubing connected directly to venous catheter (butterfly, abocath, etc.).

#2. On the basis of **I.V. FLOW RATE** and **DOSE VOLUME** select the appropriate system (retrograde or syringe infusion).

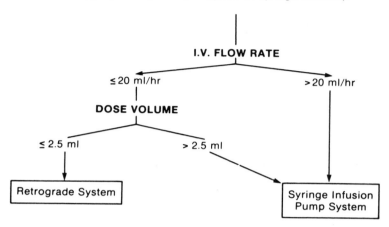

Figure 5.6. Selection of an appropriate method (retrograde versus syringe infusion pump system) for intravenous drug administration based on intravenous flow rate and dose volume. (From Roberts RJ: Intravenous administration of medications in pediatric patients: problems and solutions. *Pediatr Clin North Am* 28:23, 1986.)

(106), both therapeutic and toxic effects of topically applied substances will be greater than in adults. Numerous examples of inadvertent systemic absorption and toxicity in infants have been recorded (26, 46, 61, 76, 107, 150, 155, 162, 189). The pediatric intensive care physician should be cautious about application of presumably innocuous substances to the integument of these patients. Viscous lidocaine has produced seizures following topical application to the oral mucosa (150), and delirium has been reported after administration of aerosolized tripelennamine, an antihistamine (155).

Intraosseous administration of emergency medications has been reintroduced (14, 75, 119, 164). The technique is simple, rapid, and is not associated with major complications. Following intraosseous administration, brisk appearance in the bloodstream has been documented for several emergency drugs: catecholamines, calcium, bicarbonate, blood, colloid, and saline (119, 164). Intraosseous administration permits continuous infusion of catecholamines and resuscitation fluid, and permits bolus injection of most standard emergency medications. This is an important advantage over the intratracheal route (179). Con-

sidering the difficulty in securing vascular access during a cardiorespiratory or hemodynamic emergency, intraosseous administration is the method of choice for administration of emergency drugs and fluids when intravenous access cannot be secured within a few minutes. This method is preferred over intracardiac administration (119).

Distribution

Distribution refers to the movement of drug from the central compartment to peripheral compartments and ultimately, to the site of action and elimination. Changes in volume of distribution (V_d) result in reciprocal changes in the drug concentration (C) following a single drug dose or during repetitive drug dosing.

Distribution is affected by several parameters, including the cardiac output, individual organ blood flow, composition and relative size of body compartments, pH of body fluids, and extent of drug binding to plasma proteins and peripheral tissues (79, 83, 106, 151). Important age-related changes include differ-

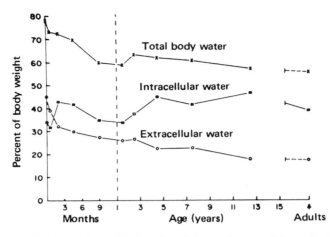

Figure 5.7. Developmental changes in total body, intracellular, and extracellular water in infants and children. The changes are expressed as percentages of body weight. (From Rane A, Wilson JT: Clinical pharmacokinetics in infants and children. In Gibaldi M, Prescott L (eds): *Handbook of Clinical Pharmacokinetics.* New York, ADIS Health Science Press, 1983. Data from Friis-Hansens B: *Pediatrics* 28:169, 1961.)

ences in body composition and protein binding.

BODY COMPOSITION

In the neonate, infant, and child, the various body compartments have a different absolute and relative size than in adults. The size and composition of these compartments vary continuously. As indicated in Figure 5.7, total body water (expressed as percentage of body weight) decreases from about 80% in the newborn infant to 60% in the adult, whereas extracellular water (ECW) decreases from 45% to 20% during the same interval (138). Conversely, expressed as a function of body surface area, ECW is relatively constant (7, 18). As a percentage of body mass, adipose tissue doubles during the first year of life. In the infant, skeletal muscle mass is reduced, and the brain and liver are much larger in relation to body weight than they are in the adult (106).

PROTEIN BINDING

Many drugs are less avidly bound to plasma proteins in the neonate and infant than they are in the older patient (18, 106, 144, 191). Decreased binding affects acidic drugs (e.g., phenytoin), which are bound to albumin (175), as well as basic drugs (e.g., lidocaine), which are bound to α_1-glycoprotein (16, 128, 191). Reduced binding to plasma proteins is associated with at least three potentially important effects: (*a*) increase in apparent volume of distribution (V_d) (144); (*b*) decrease in the total

plasma drug concentration following a standard dosage (151, 185); and (*c*) decrease in the range of total plasma drug concentrations associated with both therapeutic efficacy and toxicity. These effects are important for extensively protein-bound drugs that have a low hepatic extraction ratio (151, 185).

Although the protein binding of many drugs is reduced in the newborn, these observations have not been extended into later infancy (105, 106, 144). Reduced binding is of definite clinical importance for drugs that are both extensively bound and subject to therapeutic drug monitoring. Phenytoin (91, 175) is the usual example. When an infant or young child is treated with this anticonvulsant, the free rather than the total phenytoin concentration should be monitored. Other extensively bound drugs with reduced binding in early infancy include quinidine (129), diazepam (108), furosemide (108), some antibiotics (18, 106), propranolol, and thiopental (18). However, the effect on therapy has not been delineated, and it would be incorrect to assume that these alterations in protein binding must be clinically important. Further investigation is warranted. Protein binding of certain neuromuscular blocking agents is reduced in infancy (188, 192), but the substances are so weakly bound in adults (192) that this observation is not likely to have clinical significance.

Changes in protein binding affect other kinetic functions and calculations, including clearance and volume of distribution. These are reviewed in several publications (106, **144,**

151, 175, 177, 185), which include a discussion of the manner in which efficiency of hepatic extraction interacts with the extent of protein binding to affect total and unbound drug clearance. The net effect of greater ECW, diminished protein binding, and the relatively large brain and liver in the infant is to increase, on a weight-normalized basis, the V_d of most drugs (106, 151). This change in V_d does not necessarily entail a larger dosage of these drugs, because of the countervailing influence of reduced elimination.

Binding of unconjugated bilirubin to plasma proteins is affected by drug therapy (18). This subject has been extensively reviewed, and is not considered in this chapter.

Elimination

Elimination of drug from the body occurs by two processes: biotransformation (metabolism) and excretion (91, 151). Age-related differences in both processes are well described and are of clinical importance.

BIOTRANSFORMATION

Drug biotransformation is divided into two phases: phase 1 and phase 2 (186). Phase 1 reactions are catalyzed by oxidoreductases and hydroxylases, which produce carboxyl, epoxide, hydroxyl, amino, and sulfur groups (36, 95). These reactive groups promote elimination and permit phase 2 conjugation reactions with moieties such as acetate, amino acids, glucuronic acid, sulfate, and glutathione. Conjugation leads to more polar products that are readily eliminated via the kidney or gastrointestinal tract. The hepatic contribution to biotransformation is the largest and best characterized (177). Hepatic phase 1 and phase 2 reactions are both depressed in the neonate, but increase during later infancy and childhood, often to rates much greater than those seen in the adult (106).

Phase 1 Reactions

Phase 1 biotransformation of many drugs is slow in newborn infants (105, 106, 144). At birth, the cytochrome P-450 content of the liver is only 28% of the adult level. Activity of a variety of monooxygenases is depressed to less than 50% of adult activity (177). Depressed rates of metabolism persist for a variable but substantial period of time. Table 5.5 indicates selected compounds that display im-

Table 7.5
Selected Drugs That Undergo Oxidation: Plasma Half-lives in Full-term Newborns and Adults[a]

Drug	Elimination Half-life (hr)	
	Newborns	Adults
Aminopyrine	30–40	2–4
Bupivacaine	25	1.3
Caffeine	95	4
Carbamazepine	8–28	21–36
Diazepam	25–100	15–25
Indomethacin	14–20	2–11
Lidocaine	2.9–3.3	1.0–2.2
Meperidine	22	3–4
Mepivacaine	8.7	3.2
Nortriptyline	56	18–22
Phenobarbital	28–43	36–38
Phenylbutazone	21–34	12–30
Phenytoin	21	11–29
Theophylline	24–36	3–9
Tolbutamide	10–40	4.4–9

[a] Adapted from Rane A: Basic principle of drug disposition and action. In Yaffe SJ (ed): *Pediatric Pharmacology*. New York, Grune & Stratton, 1980; and Morselli PL, Franco-Morselli R, Bossi L: Clinical pharmacokinetics in newborns and infants. *Clin Pharmacokinet* 5:485, 1980.

paired oxidation reactions. This category of reaction is most consistently impaired in the newborn period (95, 137). In contrast, demethylation reactions, as illustrated by diazepam, are relatively intact (18, 106), indicating that each class of compound must be individually evaluated.

As expected, the newborn and young infant display reduced oxidative activity toward theophylline and caffeine. Instead of undergoing N-demethylation as in adults, theophylline is N-methylated to caffeine (69), a compound with similar biologic activity. By 7–9 months of age, the adult metabolic pattern is attained (69). This fact illustrates that not only is biotransformation slower, as a rule, in early infancy, but the end products may be different.

Deficient phase 1 activity is not limited to the mixed function oxidase system. Other enzymes known to be deficient in the newborn are reviewed elsewhere (95, 106, 107), and include (with their substrates in parentheses) alcohol dehydrogenase (ethyl alcohol, methyl alcohol, chloral hydrate), plasma esterase (local anesthetics), and N-acetyltransferase (INH, hydralazine) (102).

Phase 2 Reactions

Conjugation reactions are also limited at birth. Glucuronic acid conjugation is severely im-

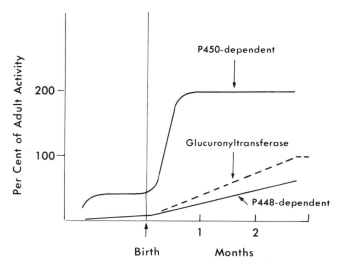

Figure 5.8. Developmental pattern of cytochrome P-450— and P-448—dependent reactions and of UDP-glucuronyltransferase in human liver. (From Vessey DA: Hepatic metabolism of drugs and toxins. In Zakim D, Boyer TD (eds): *Hepatology.* Philadelphia, WB Saunders, 1982.)

paired for some (not all) compounds; this is implicated in intoxication with chloramphenicol (182). Sulfate and glycine conjugation are well preserved in the neonate, and sulfonation of steroids occurs at near adult rates (95). Thus, as with phase 1 reactions, generalization regarding the effect of immaturity on phase 2 reactions can be misleading. Each reaction must be individually evaluated.

Maturation of Biotransformation

Concurrent with the maturation of hepatic biotransformation (Fig. 5.8), there is a dramatic acceleration of the elimination rates of many

compounds (106, 151). Beyond early infancy, children metabolize many substances more rapidly than do adults. As Morselli and associates (106) indicate, disposition rates that are less than 30% of adult values in the newborn become several-fold greater than adult values by the end of the first year of life. The intensive care physician caring for infants and children thus encounters a heterogeneous population of subjects with regard to drug elimination. Figures 5.9 and 5.10 vividly illustrate the effect of age on elimination half-life $(t_{1/2})$ and maintenance dosage requirement. Detailed information about maturation of hepatic biotransformation is available (18, 95, 106, 144, 151, 177).

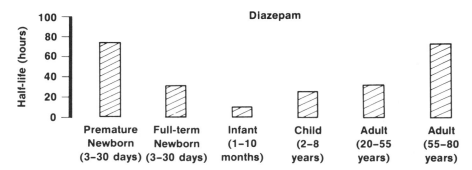

Figure 5.9. The elimination half-life of diazepam is shortest in the infant and longest in the newborn and the elderly. (From Rowland M, Tozer TN; *Clinical Pharmacokinetics.* Philadelphia, Lea & Febiger, 1980. Adapted from the data of Morselli PL: *Drug Disposition During Development.* New York, Spectrum Publications, 1977; and Klotz U, Avant GR, Hoyumpa A, et al: The effect of age and liver disease on the disposition and elimination of diazepam in adult man. *J Clin Invest* 55:347, 1975.)

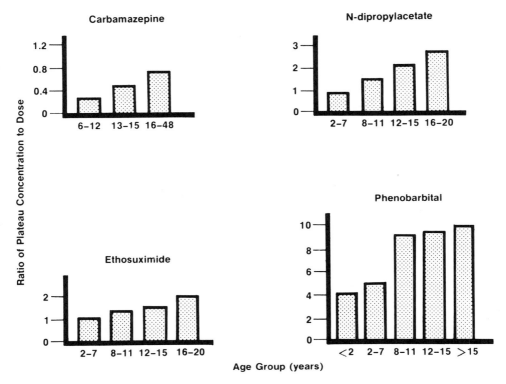

Figure 5.10. Plateau plasma drug concentrations of several antiepileptic drugs after chronic oral medication in children. An increased clearance per kilogram of body weight explains the lower ratio of concentration: dose per kilogram in the youngest children. (From Rowland M, Tozer TN: *Clinical Pharmacokinetics*. Philadelphia, Lea & Febiger, 1980. Adapted from the data of Morselli PL: Antiepileptic drugs. In Morselli PL (ed): *Drug Disposition During Development*. New York, Spectrum Publications, 1977.)

RENAL ELIMINATION

At birth, many aspects of renal function are reduced, even when normalized to body weight or to surface area. In full-term neonates, the glomerular filtration rate (GFR) is 2–4 ml/min (15 ml/min/1.73 m²) (3, 67). It doubles during the first 2 weeks of life. When normalized to surface area, adult rates of filtration (90–130 ml/min/1.73 m²) are achieved by 6 months of age (3). Thereafter, there is a linear relation between GFR and body surface area (Fig. 5.11). Tubular function is also reduced in the newborn, and maturation of tubular function is slower than maturation of glomerular filtration (18). Neonates display decreased transport capacity for a variety of substances, including acids, bases, glucose, protein, and bicarbonate (3, 67, 106).

Many substances are eliminated by the kidney in unchanged form. Whether it be due to immaturity or to disease, reduced renal function decreases clearance and prolongs elimination half-life. This may entail a reduction in

dosage. Rane and Wilson (138) have elegantly shown how reduced glomerular filtration or tubular secretion in the infant can affect drug $t_{1/2}$. They examined two drugs—p-aminohippurate, assumed to be eliminated exclusively by tubular secretion, and inulin, assumed to be eliminated exclusively by glomerular filtration. Based on age-appropriate V_d and measured total body clearances (*Cl*) for these substances, it is simple to calculate resulting elimination half-life, since:

$$t_{1/2} = \frac{0.693 \times V_d}{Cl} \quad (1)$$

The calculations are shown in Table 5.6. Inulin, representing drugs that are cleared by filtration (e.g., aminoglycosides), displays a 50% increase in its $t_{1/2}$ in the infant compared with the adult. p-Aminohippurate, representing drugs cleared by tubular secretion (e.g., penicillin), displays a 3-fold increase in its $t_{1/2}$. These theoretic calculations conform reasonably well to measured values (134). As renal

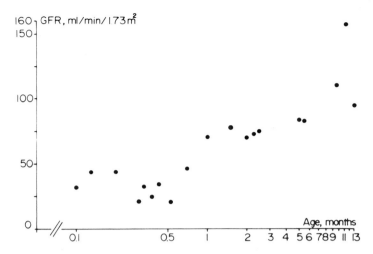

Figure 5.11. Glomerular filtration rate *(GRF)* during the first year of life, related to the logarithm of age. Determined by inulin disappearance curve. (From Aperia A, Broberger O, Thodenius K, et al: Development of renal control of salt and fluid homeostasis during the first year of life. *Acta Paediatr Scand* 64:393, 1975.)

function matures (Fig. 5.11), these values approach those seen in adults.

Generalization is problematic, since renal elimination of some drugs is either unchanged in infancy (e.g., colistin) (134) or actually greater than in adults. The latter is the case for lidocaine (103) and digoxin (122), and may represent maturation of filtration prior to tubular reabsorptive function (124).

Digoxin elimination provides an interesting example of maturation of renal function. In neonates, clearance of this drug is lower than in older infants and children, reflecting immature rates of filtration and elimination (106, 122). Clearance of digoxin increases between the 2nd and 3rd month of life, to the extent that it is greater in children than in adults (92, 106, 122). A portion of this increase in clearance can be attributed to the fact that the V_d of digoxin is 1.5–2 times greater in the child than the adult ($Cl = K_e \times V_d$, where K_e is elimi-

nation rate constant). An additional factor is that in children, but not adults, glomerular filtration of digoxin is augmented by secretion (92). During adolescence, net tubular secretion and total renal clearance of digoxin decrease toward adult values. This decrease is correlated with sexual maturity stage (Tanner stage 4–5) rather than chronologic age (92). A relationship between sexual maturity (rather than size or age) and drug elimination rate may also have significance for drugs other than digoxin.

Impairment of Renal Drug Elimination by Disease

Serum creatinine is lower in the pediatric age group than in healthy adults. By the 5th day of life, the plasma creatinine is 0.40 ± 0.02 mg/dl (67). During the balance of childhood (up to 18 years of age), creatinine values are

Table 5.6
Calculation of Half-life for a Proposed Drug with the Same Clearance as Inulin (Glomerular Filtration) or p-Aminohippuric Acid (PAH) (Tubular Secretion) in an Infant (1.5 months old) and Adult[a,b]

	ECW		Inulin		PAH	
Weight (kg)	% of Weight	Total Volume (ml)	Clearance (ml/min)	$t_{1/2}$ (min)	Clearance (ml/min)	$t_{1/2}$ (min)
4.5	32	1,440	10	100	25	40
70.0	18	12,600	130	67	650	13

[a] Rane A, Wilson JT: Clinical pharmacokinetics in infants and children. In Gibaldi M, Prescott L (eds): *Handbook of Clinical Pharmacokinetics.* New York, ADIS Health Science Press, 1983.
[b] The drug distributes in the extracellular water space (ECW). Calculation is based on $t_{1/2} = 0.693 \times V_d \times Cl^{-1}$.

Table 5.7
Method for Calculating Cl_{cr} in Children Aged 1 Week to 21 Years[a,b]

Cl_{cr} (ml/min/1.73 m^2) = length (cm) $\times$ k/P_{cr} (mg/dl)	
Age	k
Infant (1–52 weeks)	0.45
Child (1–13 years)	0.55
Adolescent (14–21 years)	
Male	0.7
Female	0.55

[a] Based on Schwartz and associates (157–159).
[b] This method is valid for individuals without severe muscle wasting and with stable plasma creatinine (P_{cr}) values.

lower than 0.8 mg/dl in healthy individuals (160), reflecting lesser muscle mass. Creatinine values that would be considered normal in young and middle-aged adults can represent significant degrees of renal dysfunction in the child.

Modifying drug dosage to account for impaired renal function depends on an estimate of the extent of impairment. This usually involves measurement or estimation of creatinine clearance. Timed urine collection is difficult in the child, and may not be complete before therapeutic decisions are necessary. However, unless age is taken into account, an isolated serum creatinine measurement does not provide an accurate estimate of renal function. For example, at 6 months of age, a serum creatinine value of 1.0 mg/dl is associated with a clearance of approximately 30 ml/min/1.73 m^2. At 20 years, the same creatinine level indicates a clearance of approximately 115 ml/min/1.73 m^2. Fortunately, it is possible to accurately estimate creatinine clearance from knowledge of the patient's age, sex, length, and plasma creatinine (157–159). The equation and appropriate constants are indicated in Table 5.7.

Adjustment of dosage in renal failure is discussed in detail in Chapter 2, and is briefly considered here. The creatinine clearance is estimated using the method indicated in Table 5.7. The following equation is used to estimate corrected dosage:

$$D_r = D_n \times [1 - f(1 - R)] \quad (2)$$

where R, the fraction of remaining renal function, is given by

$$R = \frac{\text{estimated } Cl_{cr} \text{ of patient (per 1.73 m}^2)}{\text{normal } Cl_{cr} \text{ for age (per 1.73 m}^2)} \quad (3)$$

During the first year of life, normal Cl_{cr} for age is estimated as shown in Figure 5.11. Subse-

quently, it is assumed to be 100 ml/min/1.73 m^2. Other terms in Equation 2 are as follows: f, fraction of drug excreted unchanged by the kidney in a normal subject (Table 5.8); D_r, daily dose during renal failure; and D_n, daily dose in a normal subject (of the same age). D_r, the total daily dose during renal failure, can be delivered by administering the usual dose at an extended interval, or by offering a reduced dose at the usual interval. It may be most appropriate both to reduce individual dose and to extend dosing interval. Further details are available in a number of publications (2, 34, 44, 142, 151).

EXAMPLE: A 3-year-old child (weight, 15 kg; length, 96 cm) with a serum creatinine of 1.2 mg/dl requires gentamicin ($f = 1.0$). The usual dosage for this age is 5 mg/kg/day (75

Table 5.8
Fraction of Dose Excreted Unchanged in Urine (f) with Normal Renal Function[a,b]

Drug	f
Antibiotics	
*Acyclovir	0.9
*Aminoglycosides	1.0
*Ampicillin	0.9
Amphotericin	0
Erythromycin	0.1
*Cefazolin	0.7
Cefoperazone	0.3
*Cefoxitin	0.9
*Ceftazidime	0.9
*Cefuroxime	0.9
Chloramphenicol	0
*Ganciclovir	1.0
*Imipenem/cilastin	0.7
*Methicillin	0.9
Nafcillin	<0.2
*Oxacillin	0.8
*Penicillin	0.9
Rifampin	0
*Sulfamethoxazole	0.9
*Trimethoprim	0.7
*Vancomycin	1.0
Miscellaneous	
*Cimetidine	0.8
*Digoxin	0.7
*Lithium	1.0
*Ranitidine	0.7

[a] From Rowland M, Tozer TN: *Clinical Pharmacokinetics.* Philadelphia, Lea & Febiger, 1980; Nelson JD: *Pocketbook of Pediatric Antimicrobial Therapy,* ed 7. Baltimore, Williams & Wilkins, 1987; and manufacturers' information.
[b] f may change in the presence of renal or hepatic disease. *Indicates that dosage reduction may be necessary with clinically significant renal dysfunction. Individual product information should be consulted.

mg), divided into three 8-hourly doses. The corrected dosage for this child is calculated as follows:

1. Creatinine clearance of patient:

$$Cl_{cr} = \frac{0.55 \times 96 \text{ cm}}{1.2 \text{ mg/dl}}$$

$$= 44 \text{ ml/min/m}^2$$

2. Calculation of dosage:

$$R = \frac{44 \text{ ml/min/m}^2}{100 \text{ ml/min/m}^2}$$

$$= 0.44$$

$$D_r = 75 \text{ mg/day} \times [1 - 1.0 \, (1 - 0.44)]$$
$$= 33 \text{ mg/day}$$

This dosage can be given at the usual (8-hour interval, 11 mg every 8 hours, or at an extended interval, 33 mg every 24 hours. The 8-hourly schedule prevents prolonged subtherapeutic concentrations, whereas the 24-hourly schedule permits the usual peak, trough, and mean drug concentrations.

This presentation does not take into account excretion of products of hepatic drug metabolism by the kidney or the effect of altered renal function on drug metabolism in the liver and other organs. These subjects are reviewed in Chapters 1–4 and elsewhere (2, 144, 151).

Exchange Transfusion

Exchange transfusion is performed in neonates for control of hyperbilirubinemia. In older infants and children, this procedure is occasionally advocated for therapy of diverse hematologic and metabolic conditions. Usually, a double volume exchange is performed, although "partial" exchange transfusions employing lesser volumes are occasionally employed. Exchange of the blood volume represents an additional mode of elimination and perturbs distribution. Lackner (85) presented the following equation for estimating the fraction of drug removed (f_x) as a result of an exchange transfusion of volume (V).

$$f_x = 1 - e^{-V/V_d} \tag{4}$$

In most instances, the amount of drug loss is trivial (<20%). With the possible exception of theophylline ($f_x = 32.4\%$), specific drug replacement is not necessary unless exchanges are numerous or greater than two blood volumes.

Adjustment for Size

Adjusting dosage to body size can be complex: Ritschel (142) was able to count no less than 23 separate approaches, employing a total of 52 different equations! Most methods involve adjustment for body weight or adjustment for body surface area.

Adjustments for body weight have the advantage of simplicity and familiarity. In most reference sources, pediatric dosages are presented in terms of body weight. The theoretic and practical objection to this method is that the weight-normalized dosage of many drugs increases as weight decreases. If a constant per unit weight dosage is employed, small individuals (children) will receive too small a dose.

Basing dosage on surface area has the apparent advantage of *approximating* constant dosage over a wide range of body size and age. This supposition is illustrated in Figure 5.12 for theophylline (193), and was discussed earlier in connection with succinylcholine. It is true of a variety of drugs used in critical care (18, 55).

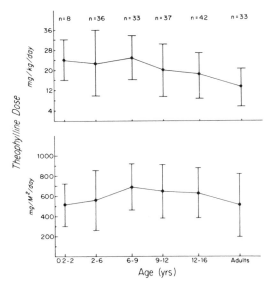

Figure 5.12. Weight-adjusted *(upper)* and body surface area—adjusted *(lower)* theophylline dose requirements (mean ± 2 SD). Dosage was adjusted to maintain peak serum theophylline concentrations between 10 and 20 µg/ml during chronic therapy. (From Wyatt R, Weinberger M, Hendeles L: Oral theophylline dosage for the management of chronic asthma. *J Pediatr* 92:125, 1978.)

The relative linearity between surface area and dosage is predicated on the pharmacokinetic observation that clearance (Cl) is determined by both elimination rate constant (K_e) and volume of distribution (V_d): $Cl = K_e \times V_d$. For many drugs, V_d is related to the volume of the extracellular water. ECW increases relative to mass as size decreases (Fig. 5.11). However, ECW remains nearly constant relative to surface area as size decreases. Thus, relative to mass, clearance increases with decreasing size; relative to surface area, clearance remains constant. Recall that clearance determines dosage (dosage = clearance × concentration). Thus, per kilogram dosage increases with decreasing size, while per meter squared dosage remains *relatively* constant.

Other physiologic processes that affect drug disposition are also directly related to surface area rather than mass. These include cardiac output, GFR, intestinal surface area, and hepatic blood flow (18, 55).

The apparently constant relationship between surface area and dosage leads many to advocate this method of normalization. While there are compelling reasons to employ surface area normalization—(a) during new drug development trials (55); (b) for extrapolation from dosages in adults; and (c) at extremes of weight (obesity, malnutrition) (142)—there appears to be no intrinsic advantage in routine clinical practice. Calculation of surface area is laborious and many nomograms are inaccurate (19). For theophylline, use of surface area–normalized dosages does not reduce interpatient variability (193).

The relative constancy of surface area–normalized dosages should not obscure the real increases in elimination rate that are typical in the preadolescent child (Figs. 5.9 and 5.10). In these individuals, more rapid elimination is signified by a shorter $t_{1/2}$, and will be manifest whether the dosage is calculated on the basis of surface area or weight. For example, the $t_{1/2}$ of theophylline is 3.4 hours at 2.5 years of age and 8.2 hours in healthy, nonsmoking adults (mean, 26 years) (73). The $t_{1/2}$ of phenytoin ranges from 2 to 7 hours in later infancy and from 12 to 40 hours in the adult (138). Drugs such as these also have a narrow therapeutic range, and large fluctuations around the mean steady state concentration should be avoided. This approach requires administration at intervals equal to or less than the $t_{1/2}$. Hence the need, in children, for more frequent division of daily dose, or for formulation of sustained release preparations.

CONCLUSION

The axiom that children are not merely small adults is nowhere more manifest than in consideration of pediatric pharmacotherapy. Pharmacodynamic and pharmacokinetic differences between children and adults are common and important; these differences are derived from the significant changes in human physiology that attend growth and development. Knowledge of basic pharmacological principles guides the clinician in adapting information derived from experience in adults to children; but, these basic (and general) principles must be supplemented by rigorous and detailed knowledge of specific drugs and their application to children.

References

1. Albert S: Aminophylline toxicity. *Pediatr Clin N Am* 34:61, 1987.
2. Anderson RJ: Drug prescribing for patients in renal failure. *Hosp Pract*, February 1983.
3. Aperia A, Broberger O, Thodenius K, et al: Development of renal control of salt and fluid homeostasis during the first year of life. *Acta Paediatr Scand* 64:393, 1975.
4. Arena JM, Rourk MH Jr, Sibrack CD: Acetaminophen: report of an unusual poisoning. *Pediatrics* 61:68, 1978.
5. Assali NS, Brinkman CR, Woods JR, et al: Development of neurohumoral control of fetal, neonatal, and adult cardiovascular functions. *Am J Obstet Gynecol* 129:748, 1977.
6. Bailey WC, Weill H, DeRoven, et al: The effect of isoniazid on transaminase levels. *Ann Intern Med* 81:200, 1974.
7. Barthels H: Drug therapy in childhood: what has been done and what has to be done. *Pediatr Pharmacol* 3:31, 1983.
8. Bartolome J, Mills E, Lau C, et al: Maturation of sympathetic neurotransmission in the rat heart. V. Development of baroceptor control of sympathetic tone. *J Pharmacol Exp Ther* 215:596, 1980.
9. Bateman DN, Croft AW, Nicholson E, et al: Dystonic reactions and the pharmacokinetics of metoclopramide in children. *Br J Clin Pharmacol* 15:557, 1983.
10. Bateman DN, Rawlins MD, Simpson JM: Extrapyramidal reactions to prochlorperazine and haloperidol in the United Kingdom. *Q J Med* 59:549, 1986.
11. Bennett EJ, Ignacio A, Patel K, et al: Tubocurarine and the neonate. *Br J Anaesth* 48:687, 1976.
12. Bennett EJ, Ramamurthy S, Dalal FY, et al: Pancuronium and the neonate. *Br J Anaesth* 47:75, 1975.
13. Beregovich J, Bianchi C, Rubler S: Dose-related hemodynamic and renal effects of dopamine in congestive heart failure. *Am Heart J* 87:550, 1974.
14. Berg RA: Emergency infusion of catecholamines into bone marrow. *Am J Dis Child* 138:810, 1984.
15. Berner M, Rouge JC, Friedli B: The hemodynamic effect of phentolamine and dobutamine after open heart operations in children: influence of the underlying heart defect. *Ann Thorac Surg* 35:643, 1983.
16. Bienvenu J, Sann L, Bienvenu F, et al: Laser nephelometry of orosomucoid in serum of newborns: refer-

ence intervals and relation to bacterial infections. *Clin Chem* 27:721, 1981.

17. Bohn DJ, Poirier CS, Edmonds JF, et al: Hemodynamic effects of dobutamine after cardiopulmonary bypass in children. *Crit Care Med* 8:367, 1980.

18. Boreus LO: *Principles of Pediatric Pharmacology.* New York, Churchill Livingstone, 1982.

19. Brion L, Fleischman AR, Schwartz GJ: Evaluation of four length-weight formulas for estimating body surface area in newborn infants. *J Pediatr* 107:801, 1985.

20. Brown BR Jr: Halothane hepatitis revisted. *N Engl J Med* 313:1347, 1985.

21. Buckley NM, Brazeau P, Gootman P: Maturation of circulatory responses to adrenergic stimuli. *Fed Proc* 42:1643, 1983.

22. Buckley NM, Gootman PM, Yellin EL, et al: Age related cardiovascular effects of catecholamines in anesthetized piglets. *Circ Res* 45:282, 1979.

23. Bukowsky M, Nakatsu K, Munt PW: Theophylline reassessed. *Ann Intern Med* 101:63, 1984.

24. Carney FT, Van Dyke RA: Halothane hepatitis: a critical review. *Anesth Analg* 51:135, 1972.

25. Casella ES, Rogers MC, Zahka KG: Developmental physiology of the cardiovascular system. In Rogers MC (ed): *Textbook of Pediatric Intensive Care.* Baltimore, Williams & Wilkins, 1987.

26. Chabrolle JP, Rossier A: Goitre and hypothyroidism in the newborn after cutaneous absorption of iodine. *Arch Dis Child* 53:495, 1978.

27. Chernow B, Rainey TG, Lake CR: Endogenous and exogenous catecholamines in critical care medicine. *Crit Care Med* 10:409, 1982.

28. Cohlan SQ, Bevelander G, Tiamsic T: Growth inhibition of prematures receiving tetracycline: clinical and laboratory investigation. *Am J Dis Child* 105:453, 1963.

29. Cook DR: Muscle relaxants in infants and children. *Anesth Analg* 60:335, 1981.

30. Cook DR, Fischer CG: Neuromuscular blocking effects of succinylcholine in infants and children. *Anesthesiology* 42:662, 1975.

31. Cowan RH, Jukkola AF, Arant BS: Pathophysiologic evidence of gentamicin nephrotoxicity in neonatal puppies. *Pediatr Res* 14:1204, 1980.

32. Cryer PE: Physiology and pathophysiology of the human sympathoadrenal neuroendocrine system. *N Engl J Med* 303:436, 1980.

33. Cryer PE, Rizza RA, Haymond MW, et al: Epinephrine and norepinephrine are cleared through beta-adrenergic, but not alpha-adrenergic, mechanisms in man. *Metabolism* 29:1114, 1980.

34. Dettli L: Drug dosage in renal disease. In Gibaldi M, Prescott L (eds): *Handbook of Clinical Pharmacokinetics.* New York, ADIS Health Science Press, 1983.

35. DiSessa TG, Leitner M, Ching CT, et al: The cardiovascular effects of dopamine in the severely asphyxiated neonate. *J Pediatr* 99:772, 1981.

36. Drayer DE: Pathways of drug metabolism in man. *Med Clin North Am* 58:927, 1974.

37. Driscoll DJ, Gillette PC: Hemodynamic effects of dobutamine in children. *Am J Cardiol* 43:581, 1979.

38. Driscoll DJ, Gillette PC, Ezrailson EG, et al: Inotropic response of the neonatal canine myocardium to dopamine. *Pediatr Res* 12:42, 1978.

39. Driscoll DJ, Gillette PC, Lewis RM, et al: Comparative hemodynamic effects of isoproterenol, dopamine, and dobutamine in the newborn dog. *Pediatr Res* 13:1006, 1979.

40. Driscoll DJ, Gillette PC, McNamara DG: The use of dopamine in children. *J Pediatr* 92:309, 1978.

41. Drugs for tuberculosis. *Med Lett Drugs Ther* 24:17, 1982.

42. Duckles SP, Banner W Jr: Changes in vascular smooth muscle reactivity during development. *Annu Rev Pharmacol Toxicol* 24:65, 1984.

43. Epstein ML, Kiel EA, Victorica BE: Cardiac decompen-

44. Fabre J, Balant L: Renal failure. In Gibaldi M, Prescott L (eds): *Handbook of Clinical Pharmacokinetics.* New York, ADIS Health Science Press, 1983.

45. Farrell G, Prendergast D, Murray M: Halothane hepatitis. Detection of a constitutional susceptibility factor. *N Engl J Med* 313;1310, 1985.

46. Filloux F: Toxic encephalopathy caused by topically applied diphenhydramine. *J Pediatr* 108:1018, 1986.

47. Fitzgerald GA, Barnes P, Hamilton CA, et al: Circulating adrenaline and blood pressure: the metabolic effects and kinetics of infused adrenaline in man. *Eur J Clin Invest* 10:401, 1980.

48. Flower RJ, Moncada S, Vane JR: Analgesic-antipyretics and anti-inflammatory agents; drugs used in the treatment of gout. In Gilman AG, Goodman LS, Roll TW, Murad F (eds): *The Pharmacological Basis of Therapeutics,* ed 7. New York, Macmillan, 1985.

49. Food and Drug Administration: *FDA Drug Bull* 8:11, 1978.

50. Food and Drug Administration: *FDA Drug Bull* 12:10, 1982.

51. Ford DC, Leist ER, Algren JT: *Guidelines for Administration of Intravenous Medications to Pediatric Patients,* ed 2. Bethesda, American Society of Hospital Pharmacists, 1984.

52. Friedman WF: The intrinsic physiologic properties of the developing heart. *Prog Cardiovasc Dis* 15:87, 1972.

53. Friedman WF, George BL: New concepts and drugs in the treatment of congestive heart failure. *Pediatr Clin North Am* 31:1197, 1984.

54. Friedman WF, Pool PE, Jacobiwitz D, et al: Sympathetic innervation of the developing rabbit heart. Biochemical and histochemical comparisons of fetal, neonatal, and adult myocardium. *Circ Res* 23:25, 1968.

55. Garson A: Dosing the newer antiarrhythmic drugs in children: considerations in pediatric pharmacology. *Am J Cardiol* 57:1405, 1986.

56. Garson A: Medicolegal problems in the management of cardiac arrhythmias in children. *Pediatrics* 79:84, 1987.

57. Gaudreault P, Wason S, Lovejoy FH Jr: Acute pediatric theophylline overdose: a summary of 28 cases. *J Pediatr* 102:474, 1983.

58. Geis WP, Tatooles CJ, Priola DV: Factors influencing neurohumoral control of the heart in the newborn dog. *Am J Physiol* 228:1685, 1975.

59. Gershanik J, Boecler B, Ensley H, et al: The gasping syndrome and benzyl alcohol poisoning. *N Engl J Med* 307:1384, 1982.

60. Goldberg LI: Dopamine—clinical use of an endogenous catecholamine. *N Engl J Med* 291:707, 1974.

61. Goldbloom RB, Goldbloom A: Boric acid poisoning, *J Pediatr* 43:631, 1953.

62. Goldstein DS, Zimlichman R, Stull R, et al: Plasma catecholamine and hemodynamic responses during isoproterenol infusions in humans. *Clin Pharmacol Ther* 40:233, 1986.

63. Gordon EP, Bristow MR, Laser JA, et al: Correlation between beta-adrenergic receptors in human lymphocytes and heart. *Circulation* 68:99, 1983.

64. Gould T, Roberts RJ: Therapeutic problems arising from the intravenous route for drug administration. *J Pediatr* 95:465, 1979.

65. Greco R, Musto B, Arienzo V: Treatment of paroxysmal supraventricular tachycardia in infancy with digitalis, adenosine-5-triphosphate, and verapamil: a comparative study. *Circulation* 66:504, 1982.

66. Grossman ER, Walchek A, Freedman H, et al: Tetracycline and permanent teeth: the relation between dose and tooth color. *Pediatrics* 47:567, 1971.

67. Guignard JP: Renal function in the newborn infant. *Pediatr Clin North Am* 29:777, 1982.

68. Gundert-Remy U, Penzien J, Hildebrandt R, et al: Cor-

sation following verapamil therapy in infants with supraventricular tachycardia. *Pediatrics* 75:737, 1983.

relation between the pharmacokinetics and pharmacodynamics of dopamine in healthy subjects. *Eur J Clin Pharmacol* 26:163, 1984.

69. Haley TJ: Metabolism and pharmacokinetics of theophylline in human neonates, children, and adults. *Drug Metab Rev* 14:295, 1983.

70. Halkin H, Radomsky M, Blieden L, et al: Steady state serum digoxin concentration in relation to digitalis toxicity in neonates and infants. *Pediatrics* 61:184, 1978.

71. Hayes GJ, Butler VP Jr, Gersony WM: Serum digoxin studies in infants and children. *Pediatrics* 52:561, 1973.

72. Heimann G: Renal toxicity of aminoglycosides in the neonatal period. *Pediatr Pharmacol* 3:251, 1983.

73. Hendeles L, Massanari M, Weinberger M: Theophylline. In Evans WE, Schentag JJ, Jusko WJ (eds): *Applied Pharmacokinetics: Principles of Therapeutic Drug Monitoring*, ed 2. Spokane, Applied Therapeutics, 1986.

74. Hooper DC, Wolfson JS: The fluoroquinolones: pharmacology, clinical uses and toxicities in humans. *Antimicrob Agents Chemother* 28:716, 1985.

75. Iserson KV, Criss E: Intraosseous infusions: a usable technique. *Am J Emerg Med* 4:540, 1986.

76. James LS: Hexachlorophene. *Pediatrics* 49:492, 1972.

77. Jarnberg PO, Bengesson L, Erstrand J, et al: Dopamine infusion in man. Plasma catecholamine levels and pharmacokinetics. *Acta Anaesthesiol Scand* 25:334, 1981.

78. Kaplan JM, McCracken GH Jr, Horton CJ, et al: Pharmacologic studies in neonates given large dosages of ampicillin. *J Pediatr* 84:571, 1974.

79. Kates RE, Leier CV: Dobutamine pharmacokinetics in severe heart failure. *Clin Pharmacol Ther* 24:537, 1978.

80. Kelliher GJ, Roberts J: Effect of age on the cardiotoxic action of digitalis. *J Pharmacol Exp Ther* 197:10, 1976.

81. Kho TL, Henquet JW, Punt R, et al: Influence of dobutamine and dopamine on hemodynamics and plasma concentrations of noradrenaline and renin in patients with low cardiac output following acute myocardial infarction. *Eur J Clin Pharmacol* 18:213, 1980.

82. Kittinger JW, Sandler RS, Heizer WD: Efficacy of metoclopramide as an adjunct to duodenal placement of small bore feeding tubes: a randomized, placebo-controlled, double-blind study. *J Parenter Enteral Nutr* 11:33, 1987.

83. Klotz U: Pathophysiology and disease-induced changes in drug distribution volume. In Gibaldi M, Prescott L (eds): *Handbook of Clinical Pharmacokinetics*. New York, ADIS Health Science Press, 1983.

84. Krishna GG, Zahrowski JJ, Nissenson AR, et al: Hemodialysis for theophylline overdose. *Dial Transplant* 12:40, 1983.

85. Lackner TE: Drug replacement following exchange transfusion. *J Pediatr* 100:811, 1982.

86. Lang P, Williams RG, Norwood WI, et al: Hemodynamic effects of dopamine in infants after corrective cardiac surgery. *J Pediatr* 96:630, 1980.

87. Leff RD, Roberts RJ: Methods of intravenous drug administration in the pediatric patient. *J Pediatr* 98:631, 1981.

88. Legan E, Chernow B: Catecholamine response to acute illness. *Semin Respir Med* 7:88, 1985.

89. Leier CV, Unverferth DV, Kates RE: The relationship between plasma dobutamine concentrations and cardiovascular responses in cardiac failure. *Am J Med* 66:238, 1979.

90. Leier CV, Unverferth DV: Dobutamine. *Ann Intern Med* 99:490, 1983.

91. Levy RH, Bauer LA: Basic pharmacokinetics. *Ther Drug Monit* 8:47, 1986.

92. Linday LA, Drayer DE, Kahn MAA, et al: Pubertal changes in net renal tubular secretion of digoxin. *Clin Pharmacol Ther* 35:438, 1984.

93. Leob JN: Corticosteroids and growth. *N Engl J Med* 295:547, 1976.

94. Lowrey GH: *Growth and Development of Children*, ed 7. Chicago, Year Book, 1978.

95. Mannering GJ: Drug metabolism in the newborn. *Fed Proc* 44:2302, 1985.

96. Marshall BE, Wollman H: General anesthetics. In Gilman AG, Goodman LS, Roll TW, Murad F (eds): *The Pharmacological Basis of Therapeutics*, ed 7. New York, Macmillan, 1985.

97. McBride WG: Thalidomide and congenital abnormalities. *Lancet* 2:1358, 1961.

98. McCracken GH Jr: Aminoglycoside toxicity in infants and children. *Am J Med* 80:172, 1986.

99. McLain GE, Sipes IG, Brown BR Jr: An animal model of halothane hepatotoxicity: roles of enzyme induction and hypoxia. *Anesthesiology* 91:321, 1979.

100. Metoclopramide for gastroesophageal reflux. *Med Lett Drugs Ther* 27:21, 1985.

101. Micelli JN, Bidani A, Aronow R: Peritoneal dialysis of theophylline. *Clin Toxicol* 14:539, 1979.

102. Miceli JN, Olson, WA, Cohen SN: Elimination kinetics of isoniazid in the newborn infant. *Dev Pharmacol Ther* 2:225, 1981.

103. Mihaly GW, Moore RG, Thomas JW, et al: The pharmacokinetics and metabolism of the anilide local anesthetics in neonates. *Eur J Clin Pharmacol* 13:143, 1978.

104. Milligan N, Dhillon S, Richens A, et al: Rectal diazepam in the treatment of absence status: a pharmacodynamic study. *J Neurol Neurosurg Psychiatry* 44:914, 1981.

105. Morselli PL: Clinical pharmacokinetics in neonates. *Clin Pharmacokinet* 1:81, 1976.

106. Morselli PL, Franco-Morselli R, Bossi L: Clinical pharmacokinetics in newborns and infants. *Clin Pharmacokinet* 5:485, 1980.

107. Mullick FC: Hexachlorophene toxicity. Human experience at the Armed Forces Institute of Pathology. *Pediatrics* 51:395, 1973.

108. Nau H, Luck W, Kuhnz W, et al: Serum protein binding of diazepam, desmethyldiazepam, furosemide, indomethacin, warfarin, and phenobarbital in human fetus, mother, and newborn infant. *Pediatr Pharmacol* 3:219, 1983.

109. Nelson JD: Antimicrobial drugs. In Yaffe SJ (ed): *Pediatric Pharmacology*. New York, Grune & Stratton, 1980.

110. Nelson JD: *Pocketbook of Pediatric Antimicrobial Therapy*, ed 7. Baltimore, Williams & Wilkins, 1987.

111. Nogen AG, Bremner JE: Acetaminophen overdosage in a young child. *J Pediatr* 92:832, 1978.

112. Nolke AC: Severe toxic effects from aminophylline and theophylline suppositories in children. *JAMA* 161:693, 1956.

113. Norfloxacin. *Med Lett Drugs Ther* 29:25, 1987.

114. Notterman DA, Nardi M, Saslow JG: Effects of dose formulation on isoniazid absorption in two young children. *Pediatrics* 77:850, 1986.

115. Nugent SK, Laravuso R, Rogers MC: Pharmacology and use of muscle relaxants in infants and children. *J Pediatr* 94:481, 1979.

116. O'Brien RJ, Long MW, Cross FS, et al: Hepatotoxicity from isoniazid and rifampin among children treated for tuberculosis. *Pediatrics* 72:491, 1983.

117. O'Keefe, Gregory GA, Stanski DR, et al: d-Tubocurarine: pharmacodynamics and kinetics in children. *Anesthesiology* 51:S270, 1979.

118. O'Mally K, Coleman EN, Doig WB, et al: Plasma digoxin levels in infants. *Arch Dis Child* 48:99, 1973.

119. Orlowski JP: My kingdom for an intravenous line. *Am J Dis Child* 138:803, 1984.

120. Padbury JF, Agata Y, Baylen BG, et al: Dopamine pharmacokinetics in critically ill newborn infants. *J Pediatr* 110:293, 1987.

121. Papadopoulou AL, Novello AC: The use of hemoper-

fusion in children. *Pediatr Clin North Am* 29:1039, 1982.

122. Park MK: Use of digoxin in infants and children with specific emphasis on dosage. *J Pediatr* 108:871, 1986.
123. Park MK, Johnson JM, Hayashi S: Is age dependent difference in inotropic responses to isoproterenol temperature dependent? *Pediatr Res* 20:208A, 1986.
124. Park MK, Ludden T, Arom KV, et al: Myocardial vs serum digoxin concentrations in infants and adults. *Am J Dis Child* 136:418, 1982.
125. Perez CA, Reimer JM, Schreiber MD, et al: Effect of high dose dopamine on urine output in newborn infants. *Crit Care Med* 14:1045, 1986.
126. Perkin RM, Levin DL: Dobutamine: a hemodynamic evaluation in children with shock. *J Pediatr* 100:97, 1982.
127. Perloff WH: Physiology of the heart and circulation. In Swedlow DB, Raphaely RC (eds): *Cardiovascular Problems in Pediatric Critical Care*. New York, Churchill Livingstone, 1986.
128. Piafsky, KM: Disease induced changes in the plasma binding of basic drugs. *Clin Pharmacokinet* 5:246, 1980.
129. Pikoff AS, Kessler KM, Singh S, et al: Age related differences in the protein binding of quinidine. *Dev Pharmacol Ther* 3:108, 1981.
130. Pinsky WW, Jacobsen JR, Gillette PC, et al: Dosage of digoxin in premature infants. *J Pediatr* 96:639, 1976.
131. Polgar G, Weng TR: The functional development of the respiratory system. *Am Rev Respir Dis* 120:625, 1979.
132. Pond AM: Diuresis, dialysis, and hemoperfusion. *Emerg Med Clin North Am* 2:29, 1984.
133. Porter CJ, Garson A, Gillette PC: Verapamil: an effective calcium blocking agent for pediatric patients. *Pediatrics* 71:748, 1983.
134. Prandota J: Clinical pharmacokinetics of changes in drug elimination in children. *Dev Pharmacol Ther* 8:311, 1985.
135. Radford D: Side effects of verapamil in infants. *Arch Dis Child* 58:465, 1983.
136. Rajchgot P, Prosber CG, Soldins S, et al: Aminoglycoside related nephrotoxicity in the premature newborn. *Clin Pharmacol Ther* 35:394, 1984.
137. Rane A: Basic principle of drug disposition and action. In Yaffe SJ (ed): *Pediatric Pharmacology*. New York, Grune & Stratton, 1980.
138. Rane A, Wilson JT: Clinical pharmacokinetics in infants and children. In Gibaldi M, Prescott L (eds): *Handbook of Clinical Pharmacokinetics*. New York, ADIS Health Science Press, 1983.
139. Reidenberg MM, Levy M, Warner H, et al: Relationship between diazepam dose, plasma level, age and central nervous system depression. *Clin Pharmacol Ther* 23:371, 1978.
140. Reinhardt D, Zehmisch T, Becker B, et al: Age dependency of alpha and beta-adrenoreceptor on thrombocytes and lymphocytes of asthmatic and nonasthmatic children. *Eur J Pediatr* 142:111, 1984.
141. Ricci DA, Saltzman MB, Meyer C, et al: Effect of metoclopramide in diabetic gastroparesis. *J Clin Gastroenterol* 7:25, 1985.
142. Ritschel WA: *Handbook of Basic Pharmacokinetics*, ed 2. Hamilton, Drug Intelligence Publications, 1980.
143. Roan Y, Galant SP: Decreased neutrophil beta adrenergic receptors in the neonate. *Pediatr Res* 16:591, 1982.
144. Roberts RJ: *Drug Therapy in Infants*. Philadelphia, WB Saunders, 1984.
145. Roberts RJ: Intravenous administration of medications in pediatric patients: problems and solutions. *Pediatr Clin North Am* 28:23, 1986.
146. Rockson SG, Homcy CJ, Quinn P, et al: Cellular mechanisms of impaired adrenergic responsiveness in neonatal dogs. *J Clin Invest* 67:319, 1981.

147. Romero T, Covell J, Freidman WF: A comparison of pressure volume relations of the fetal, newborn and adult heart. *Am J Physiol* 222:1285, 1972.
148. Romero T, Friedman WF: Limited left ventricular response to volume overload in the neonatal period: a comparative study with the adult animal. *Pediatr Res* 13:910, 1979.
149. Ross EM, Gilman AG: Pharmacodynamics: mechanisms of drug action and the relationship between drug concentration and effect. In Gilman AG, Goodman LS, Roll TW, Murad F (eds): *The Pharmacological Basis of Therapeutics*, ed 7. New York, Macmillan, 1985.
150. Rothstein P, Dornbusch J, Shaywitz BA: Prolonged seizures associated with the use of viscous lidocaine. *J Pediatr* 101:461, 1982.
151. Rowland M, Tozer TN: *Clinical Pharmacokinetics*. Philadelphia, Lea & Febiger, 1980.
152. Rumack BH: Acetaminophen overdose in young children. *Am J Dis Child* 138:428, 1984.
153. Rumack BH, Peterson RC, Koch G, et al: Acetaminophen overdose. *Arch Intern Med* 141:380, 1981.
154. Sandor GGS, Bloom KR, Izukawa T, et al: Noninvasive assessment of left ventricular function related to serum digoxin levels in neonates. *Pediatrics* 65:541, 1980.
155. Schipioe PG: An unusual case of antihistamine poisoning. *J Pediatr* 71:589, 1967.
156. Schranz D, Stopfkuchen H, Jungst BK, et al: Hemodynamic effects of dobutamine in children with cardiovascular failure. *Eur J Pediatr* 139:4, 1982.
157. Schwartz GJ, Feld LG, Langford DJ: A simple estimate of glomerular filtration rate in full term infants during the first year of life. *J Pediatr* 104:849, 1984.
158. Schwartz GJ, Haycock GB, Edelmann CM Jr, et al: A simple estimate of glomerular filtration rate in children derived from body length and plasma creatinine. *Pediatrics* 58:259, 1976.
159. Schwartz GJ, Haycock GB, Gauthier B: A simple estimate of glomerular filtration rate in adolescent boys. *J Pediatr* 106:522, 1985.
160. Schwartz GJ, Haycock GB, Spitzer A: Plasma creatinine and urea concentration in children: normal values for age and sex. *J Pediatr* 88:828, 1976.
161. Seri I, Tulassay T, Kiszel J, et al: Cardiovascular response to dopamine in hypotensive preterm neonates with severe hyaline membrane disease. *Eur J Pediatr* 142:3, 1984.
162. Shawn DH, McGuigan MA: Poisoning from dermal absorption of promethazine. *Can Med Assoc J* 130:1460, 1984.
163. Shaywitz SE, Caparulo BK, Hodgson ES: Developmental language disability as a consequence of prenatal exposure to ethanol. *Pediatrics* 68:850, 1981.
164. Shoor PM, Berryhill RE, Benumof JL: Intraosseous infusion: pressure-flow relationship and pharmacokinetics. *J Trauma* 19:772, 1979.
165. Silverberg AB, Shah SD, Haymond MW, et al: Norepinephrine: hormone and neurotransmitter in man. *Am J Physiol* 234:E252, 1978.
166. Singh BN, Nademanee K, Baky SH: Calcium antagonists. Clinical use in the treatment of arrhythmias. *Drugs* 25:125, 1983.
167. Spyridis P, Sinaniotis C, Papadea I, et al: Isoniazid liver injury during chemoprophylaxis in children. *Arch Dis Child* 94:65, 1979.
168. Stoner JD, Bolen JL, Harrison DC: Comparison of dobutamine and dopamine in treatment of severe heart failure. *Br Heart J* 39:536, 1977.
169. Stopfkuchen H, Schranz R, Huth R, et al: Effects of dobutamine on left ventricular performance in newborns as determined by systolic time intervals. *Eur J Pediatr* 146:135, 1987.
170. Tatsumi H, Senda H, Yatera S, et al: Toxicological studies on pipemidic acid. V. Effect on diarthrodial

joints of experimental animals. *J Toxicol Sci* 3:357, 1978.

171. Tenenbein M: Pediatric toxicology: Current controversies and recent advances. Clinical and recent advances. *Curr Probl Pediatr* 16:185, 1986.

172. Terrin BN, McWilliams NB, Maurer HM: Side effects of metoclopramide as an antiemetic in childhood cancer chemotherapy. *J Pediatr* 104:138, 1984.

173. Valdes R Jr: Endogenous digoxin-like immunoreactive factors: impact on digoxin measurement and potential physiological implications. *Clin Chem* 31:1985, 1985.

174. Valdes R Jr, Graves SW, Brown BA: Endogenous substance in newborn infants causing false-positive digoxin measurements. *J Pediatr* 152:947, 1983.

175. Vallner JJ: Binding of drugs by albumin and plasma protein. *J Pharm Sci* 66:447, 1977.

176. van-der-Kleijn E, Baars AM, Vree TB, et al: Clinical pharmacokinetics of drugs used in the treatment of status epilepticus. *Adv Neurol* 34:421, 1983.

177. Vessey DA: Hepatic metabolism of drugs and toxins. In Zakim D, Boyer TD (eds): *Hepatology*. Philadelphia, WB Saunders, 1982.

178. Vestal RE, Wood AJJ, Shand DG: Reduced beta-adrenoreceptor sensitivity in the elderly. *Clin Pharmacol Ther* 26:181, 1979.

179. Ward JT: Endotracheal drug therapy. *Am J Emerg Med* 1:71, 1983.

180. Warner LO, Beach TP, Garvin JP: Halothane and children. The first quarter century. *Anesth Analg* 63:838, 1984.

181. Way WL, Costley EC, Way EL: Respiratory sensitivity of the newborn infant to meperidine and morphine. *Clin Pharmacol Ther* 6:454, 1962.

182. Weiss CF, Glazko AJ, Weston JK: Chloramphenicol in the newborn infant. *N Engl J Med* 262:787, 1960.

183. Whately K, Turner WW Jr, Dey M, et al: When does metoclopramide facilitate transpyloric intubation? *J Parenter Enteral Nutr* 8:679, 1984.

184. Whitsett JA, Noguchi A, Moore JJ: Developmental aspects of alpha and beta-adrenergic receptors. *Semin Perinatol* 6:125, 1982.

185. Wilkinson GR, Shand DC: A physiologic approach to hepatic drug clearance. *Clin Pharmacol Ther* 7:377, 1975.

186. Williams RT: *Detoxification Mechanisms*. John Wiley & Sons, New York, 1959.

187. Wilson RF, Sibbald WJ, Jaanimagi JL: Hemodynamic effects of dopamine in critically ill septic patients. *J Surg Res* 20:163, 1976.

188. Wingard LB, Cook DR: Clinical pharmacokinetics of muscle relaxants. *Clin Pharmacokinet* 2:330, 1977.

189. Wolff JA: Methemoglobinemia due to benzocaine. *Pediatrics* 20:915, 1957.

190. Wong DF, Wagner HN, Dannals RF, et al: Effects of age on dopamine and serotonin receptors measured by positron tomography of the living human brain. *Science* 226:1393, 1984.

191. Wood M, Wood AJJ: Changes in plasma drug binding and alpha$_1$-acid glycoprotein in mother and newborn infant. *Clin Pharmacol Ther* 4:522, 1981.

192. Wood M, Wood AJJ: Neuromuscular blocking agents. In Wood M, Wood AJJ (eds): *Drugs and Anesthesia*. Baltimore, Williams & Wilkins, 1982.

193. Wyatt R, Weinberger M, Hendeles L: Oral theophylline dosage for the management of chronic asthma. *J Pediatr* 92:125, 1978.

194. Yaffe SJ, Bierman CW, Cann HM, et al: Requiem for tetracyclines. *Pediatrics* 55:142, 1975.

195. Zaritsky A, Chernow B: Use of catecholamines in pediatrics. *J Pediatr* 105:341, 1984.

196. Zaritsky AL, Eisenberg MG: Ontogenetic considerations in the pharmacotherapy of shock. In Chernow B, Shoemaker W (eds): *Critical Care—State of the Art*. Fullerton, Society of Critical Care Medicine, 1986, vol 7.

197. Zwillich CW, Sutton FD, Neff TA, et al: Theophylline-induced seizures in adults. *Ann Intern Med* 82:784, 1975.

6

Resuscitation Pharmacology

Arno L. Zaritsky, M.D.
Allan S. Jaffe, M.D.

The goals of cardiopulmonary resuscitation are *(a)* to restore stable circulatory and ventilatory function, and *(b)* to maintain vital critical organ function until such stabilization can be achieved. Early definitive care (usually defibrillation in adults and ventilatory support in infants) whenever possible is the first priority. Thereafter, the maintenance of circulatory and ventilatory function (with chest compression and assisted ventilation) and pharmacologic interventions aimed at facilitating the reestablishment of more normal cardiopulmonary functioning may improve the success of subsequent efforts. Treatment with pharmacologic agents has the potential to:

1. Suppress ventricular tachycardia and/or fibrillation;
2. Maintain coronary and cerebral perfusion until the restoration of more normal cardiopulmonary function;
3. Evoke a rhythm more apt to be associated with an adequate blood pressure in patients with asystole or electromechanical dissociation;
4. Correct hypoxemia and acidosis;
5. Improve hemodynamics.

These goals are similar in all arrest situations, although there may be some unique circumstances (e.g., trauma) in which additional therapies may also be required. This chapter provides a review of the pharmacology, indications, dosages, and potential complications of each agent used during resuscitation. Indications and dosage recommendations are consistent with recently published guidelines (120).

GENERAL GUIDELINES FOR ADMINISTERING MEDICATIONS

During cardiac arrest, intravenous drug administration is preferred. Central venous drug administration produces higher and more rapid peak drug concentrations than peripheral injections during resuscitations (40). This is a potentially important factor for agents with dose-dependent effects on the arterial circulation, such as epinephrine (100).

However, the placement of a central "line" is time consuming, requires the discontinuation of compressions and ventilations, usually for a potentially deleterious duration, and is associated with substantial morbidity to adjacent structures. In the past, an advocacy for the placement of central lines via the femoral vein obviated some of these considerations. However, unless a long catheter can be advanced into the chest (this is more easily accomplished in pediatric than adult patients), this route should not be used since blood flow below the diaphragm is much lower than blood flow above the diaphragm (31). In adults the brachial vein (120) is the site of choice for the placement of an intravenous line. To enhance delivery to the central circulation, each peripheral venous injection should be followed by a bolus of 50 ml of normal saline.

In pediatric patients, rapid intravenous access can be difficult in general (108), and cannulation of the superior vena caval system is particularly difficult. It has not been established that the difference in blood flow between the upper and lower parts of the body during chest compression in adults also occurs in infants, in whom higher cardiac outputs are induced in part by direct cardiac compression (112). Therefore, in infants any venous access site is acceptable. The administration of intravenous drugs should be followed, as in the adult, with an injection of saline (a smaller amount is required). Intraosseous injection (usually via the tibia) also can be used to provide an access site for the administration of fluids and drugs (109) including catecholamines (89).

If intravenous access is not readily available, endotracheal administration of certain drugs (e.g., epinephrine and atropine) can be utilized (135). Optimal endotracheal doses have not been totally defined. In some animal studies as much as 10 times the intravenous dose of epinephrine is required to produce the same hemodynamic effects (103). However, in general, the upper range of the intravenous dose is chosen for endotracheal use (120). Although it may be possible to administer other agents endotracheally, such as lidocaine, bretylium, isoproterenol, and/or propranolol (81, 102, 113), because they are generally used relatively late during the resuscitation sequence, intravenous access is usually available by that time. When utilizing the endotracheal route, medications should be instilled deeply into the trachea either using a catheter positioned beyond the end of the endotracheal tube or by discontinuing compressions and ventilations during the instillation and thereafter hyperventilating the patient (102).

Pressors are often used to support the circulation once a stable rhythm has been restored. Catecholamines are compatible with many intravenous solutions (normal saline, 0.45N saline, Ringer's lactate and 10% dextrose and water), but 5% dextrose and water usually is preferred. Post arrest, catecholamine infusions should be initiated at a sufficiently rapid rate to clear the intravenous tubing of other solutions; otherwise a substantial delay may occur before a drug effect is observed, particularly in pediatric patients in whom lower infusion rates are typical. Toxicity is avoided by using the lowest possible dose that achieves the desired effect and decreasing the infusion rate as rapidly as possible. Catecholamines should not be mixed in the same intravenous solution bag with alkaline solutions (e.g., bicarbonate, phenytoin, or aminophylline) because catecholamines are autooxidized by basic solutions (89).

ESSENTIAL RESUSCITATION MEDICATIONS

Oxygen

PHARMACOLOGY

Many factors contribute to severely impaired oxygenation during cardiac arrest. Exhaled gas delivered during mouth-to-mouth rescue breathing provides only 16–17% oxygen, which at best produces an alveolar oxygen tension of 80 torr (normal oxygen tension in room air is approximately 104 torr, depending in part on altitude). Cardiopulmonary resuscitation is accompanied by right-to-left intrapulmonary shunting, mismatches between ventilation and perfusion (96) impairing oxygen delivery, and often by aspiration and/or pulmonary edema inhibiting oxygen transport across the alveolus. Because properly performed chest compression only delivers 25–35% of a normal cardiac output (133), oxygen delivery to the tissues is additionally impaired. To compensate, tissue extraction increases, and mixed venous oxygen tension is low. The admixture of this highly desaturated venous blood with poorly oxygenated "arterial" blood further decreases arterial oxygen tension. The net result is that oxygen delivery is markedly compromised during cardiac arrest and resuscitation.

Hypoxemia at the tissue level leads to anaerobic metabolism, lactic acid production, and local acidosis, augmenting intracellular acidosis and cellular dysfunction and eventually leading to cell death. Acidosis also results in vasodilation locally, which may compromise further vital organ perfusion by leading to peripheral pooling and by lowering central aortic pressures and thus diastolic coronary perfusion pressure (see "Epinephrine" below). Acidosis may antagonize the action of catecholamines (87); however, the applicability of this concept to the cardiac arrest setting and the doses of epinephrine utilized is unclear (1, 63, 128). For all of these reasons, aggressive attempts to maximize tissue oxygenation are essential. If the baseline oxygen tension is on the steep portion of the oxyhemoglobin saturation curve, even small increments in oxygen tension may markedly improve the delivery of oxygen to the tissues.

INDICATIONS AND DOSE

Oxygen should be provided in the highest concentration possible (usually 100%) during cardiopulmonary resuscitation. There should be no concern about the development of oxygen toxicity during the short exposure that occurs during resuscitation. Oxygen should not be withheld in any patient with hypoxemia, even if chronic lung disease and carbon dioxide retention is present. By increasing arterial oxygen tension, oxygen content in blood and therefore tissue oxygen delivery may be enhanced.

Although the administration of oxygen improves arterial oxygen tension and content, it does not guarantee adequate oxygen delivery to the tissues. Animal (104) and clinical (137) studies have demonstrated that during cardiopulmonary resuscitation there is a progressive fall in mixed venous oxygen tension, probably the best indicator of the adequacy of tissue oxygen delivery, even when arterial oxygen tension is well maintained. Accordingly, additional therapy is needed to improve tissue oxygen delivery.

Epinephrine

PHARMACOLOGY

The pharmacologic actions of epinephrine are complex and dose related (see Chapter 12). The large doses used during a cardiopulmonary resuscitation produce both α-adrenergic and β-adrenergic effects. During cardiopulmonary resuscitation, epinephrine's α-adrenergic effects on vascular tone are of primary importance because aortic diastolic pressure is a critical determinant of the success or failure of resuscitative efforts in animals (90, 110). During compression, aortic and right atrial pressure are equal and there is little or no coronary blood flow. During diastole, there is a small gradient favoring flow. By increasing arterial vasoconstriction via its effects on α-adrenergic tone, epinephrine elevates aortic diastolic pressure and therefore coronary perfusion pressure, increasing coronary blood flow (143). It is unclear whether the concomitant venoconstriction that increases central volumes diminishes or enhances coronary blood flow (39, 93).

In animals, epinephrine also augments cerebral perfusion. Cerebral blood flow can be maintained at approximately 70% of normal levels with a continuous infusion of epinephrine combined with simultaneous ventilation and compression cardiopulmonary resuscitation in some experimental models (85). The increased cerebral blood flow is related in part to increased blood flow to the upper body due to the thoracic pump mechanism of blood flow during chest compression, and occurs at the expense of blood flow to structures below the diaphragm, including the renal and splanchnic beds (62, 85). This action is augmented by the effects of α-adrenergic stimulation, which improve the rigidity of the arterial system so that pressure and therefore flow are enhanced.

The impact of the β-adrenergic effects of epinephrine is more controversial. The inotropic and chronotropic effects increase myocardial oxygen demand, and many have argued that the increased demand may obviate the benefits of increased coronary flow (38). Furthermore, recent data suggest that it is the α-adrenergic rather than the β-adrenergic effects of epinephrine that enhance the susceptibility of ventricular fibrillation from defibrillation (99). These contentions, along with the possible adverse effects of hypertension and/or arrhythmias that may be induced synergistically by the β- plus α-adrenergic effects of epinephrine following restoration of spontaneous circulation (these effects tend to be worse following intrapulmonary injection of epinephrine when the lungs serve as a depot for epinephrine, which is then released during the postresuscitation period (12, 103)), have led some investigators to advocate the replacement of epinephrine with a more pure α-adrenergic agent such as phenylephrine or methoxamine. Although these agents seem equally effective in supporting coronary perfusion and enhancing the restoration of spontaneous circulation and survival, they do not appear to support cerebral blood flow to the same extent as epinephrine (15–18, 62). Epinephrine therefore remains the drug of choice during cardiopulmonary resuscitation.

INDICATIONS AND DOSE

Epinephrine is indicated in the treatment of cardiac arrest, regardless of mechanism, in infants, children, and adults (120). The optimal dose is undefined. In animals, doses in the range of those recommended during resuscitation in humans (7.5–15 μg/kg) do not increase diastolic blood pressure. Doses of 45, 75, and 150 μg/kg must be used to induce a diastolic pressure of 30 mm Hg or more for up to 5 minutes (76). Nonetheless, concentrations of endogenous catecholamines are quite high during cardiopulmonary resuscitation in humans (well beyond the range usually achieved with infusions in patients with shock (142)) and may be synergistic with exogenous infusions. Thus, although the proper dose in patients is speculative, present recommendations are probably low rather than high, and epinephrine in the recommended dose of 7.5–15 μg/kg should be administered at least every 5 minutes during resuscitation. Estimations of dose should be biased toward greater rather than lesser amounts when exact data are unavailable. The upper range of doses (15 μg/kg) should be utilized with endotracheal administration in which absorption is delayed and therefore peak levels are less (57). Epinephrine should not be injected directly into the heart if it can be avoided, since morbidity has been associated with this procedure, including interruption of compressions and ventilation, coronary artery laceration, cardiac tamponade, pneumothorax, and intractable ventricular fibrillation (57).

Epinephrine, like other catecholamines, should not be mixed with bicarbonate since alkaline solutions autooxidize the drug (89).

Atropine

PHARMACOLOGY

Atropine has predominant parasympatholytic effects at clinically relevant doses. It accelerates sinus or atrial pacemakers, and enhances atrioventricular conduction (37) by competitively antagonizing muscarinic receptors and therefore inhibiting vagal tone. Its use in cardiac arrest is based on its cardiac vagolytic actions. At low doses, atropine has central and peripheral parasympathomimetic actions that may induce paradoxical vagotonic effects (32, 74). Atropine is excreted renally and has a half-life in normal individuals of about 2.5 hours (138). Prolonged elimination should be expected during arrest and the postresuscitation period. Thus, doses of more than 2 mg of atropine, which is a totally vagolytic dose for most individuals (97), should not be used during cardiopulmonary arrest.

INDICATIONS AND DOSE

Atropine is the drug of choice for the treatment of bradycardia, regardless of its mechanism, when it is accompanied by hemodynamic compromise or ventricular ectopy. Its benefit in ventricular asystole is based on the supposition that asystole is the end stage of a spectrum of bradycardias and on the apparent benefit observed in small numbers of patients (19) especially those in a hospital setting where there is a very rapid initiation of resuscitation. There is also some enthusiasm for the use of atropine for asystole in the management of outpatient cardiac arrest, but benefit in the outpatient setting is even more speculative (71, 125). Atropine should be used cautiously in the presence of myocardial ischemia or infarction since excessive increases in heart rate may increase the extent of infarction (97) and can on occasion induce ventricular tachycardia or fibrillation (30). Bradycardia in pediatric cardiac arrest patients and in many adult patients with severe pulmonary disease is due most often to hypoxemia and shock, and is best treated by supporting ventilation and circulation.

The recommended doses of atropine are 1.0 mg for asystole and 0.5 mg for symptomatic bradycardia (120), with a minimal dose of 0.5 mg. A total dose of 2.0 mg generally results in full vagal blockage (97). In pediatric patients, the dose is 0.02 mg/kg intravenously or endotracheally, with a minimum dose of 0.1 mg. The dose may be repeated in 5 minutes, up to 1.0 mg in a child and 2.0 mg in an adolescent. As noted above, smaller doses of atropine, less than 0.5 mg in adults and less than 0.1 mg in pediatric patients, can induce paradoxical vagotonic effects (32, 74).

Lidocaine

PHARMACOLOGY

Lidocaine is a class 1 antiarrhythmic agent. Its primary mode of action is by its membrane-stabilizing effects (131), mediated predominantly by blockade of sodium channels (51). Slowing the slope of phase 4 depolarization, reducing automaticity, is one of lidocaine's important modes of antiarrhythmic action (29). Lidocaine has different effects on the duration of the action potential and the effective refractory period in normal and ischemic tissue, which narrow the differences between these tissues and thus may inhibit the propagation of reentrant arrhythmias (78). In normal tissue lidocaine tends to slightly shorten these intervals, whereas in ischemic tissue it prolongs them. Lidocaine also increases the energy required to induce ventricular fibrillation (the ventricular fibrillation threshold) (78, 119), but high plasma levels appear to be required (2, 25). However, lidocaine does not reduce the energy required to terminate ventricular fibrillation (the ventricular defibrillation threshold). Recent data suggest that it may even increase the energy needed, though only modestly (41, 68). Lidocaine has proven to be as effectives as other agents heralded as having antifibrillatory effects (58, 95). This may be because of the lack of true antifibrillatory effects of the agents with which lidocaine was compared; or because most apparent failures of defibrillation are due to the immediate recurrence of ventricular fibrillation, which is inhibited by the effects of lidocaine on the ventricular fibrillation threshold. At high concentrations, lidocaine can depress myocardial contractility (80) and induce hypotension by peripheral vasodilation (134).

Lidocaine is highly protein bound (14) and is cleared by the liver (29). In normal subjects, its volume of distribution is 0.5 liters/kg. Its elimination has both an α-distributive and a β half-life. In normal subjects, the half-life of lidocaine after a bolus injection (its α-distributive half-life) is 8.3 minutes, and its half-life after achieving a steady state with a constant infusion (the β half-life) is 86–108 minutes. Thus, bolus doses of lidocaine are required to obtain therapeutic blood levels until a steady state concentration (reached after five half-lives) is achieved with a constant infusion. One half of the steady state concentration is reached at one half-life. If the therapeutic range is 2–5 μg/ml, a 4 mg/min infusion will achieve a concentration of approximately 2 μg/ml in 86–108 minutes, assuming normal pharmacokinetics. Clinical circumstances in which hepatic blood flow or cardiac output is reduced and those in which the volume of distribution is altered (older patients) will lead to increased levels of lidocaine for any given dose (7). Accordingly, dose adjustments are required in patients with reduced cardiac output to the liver (e.g., those with shock), in those with congestive heart failure or hepatic dysfunction in which hepatic metabolism is reduced, and in those over the age of 70 in whom the volume of distribution and clearance is decreased (7). In addition, after a 24-hour infusion, the ability of the liver to clear lidocaine appears to decrease, mandating a reduced infusion rate if toxicity is to be avoided (33). Although renal disease does not affect the clearance of lidocaine or its volume of distribution, metabolites of lidocaine will accumulate after prolonged infusions (129). There is little information concerning lidocaine levels or pharmacodynamics during cardiopulmonary resuscitation. However, probably as a consequence of the marked reduction in cardiac output, levels after conventional bolus doses are above or within the therapeutic range for at least 20 minutes (26).

Toxic effects of lidocaine usually occur when levels are above the therapeutic range or when the drug is infused very rapidly (26, 33). These effects include central nervous system manifestations such as drowsiness, confusion, numbness and tingling, muscle twitching, and (predominantly) agitation. Seizures requiring treatment can occur.

INDICATIONS AND DOSE

The prophylactic use of lidocaine to prevent ventricular fibrillation in patients highly suspected of having acute myocardial infarction has been widely recommended (10, 120) because of data suggesting that it reduces the incidence of ventricular fibrillation (36, 77). However, many have questioned the risk-benefit ratio on which this recommendation is based, in part because there have been few data to suggest that primary ventricular fibrillation itself is associated with an adverse prognosis (23, 43). Recent data suggest that ventricular fibrillation is indeed associated with an adverse prognosis (132), which should strengthen the advocacy for the drug's routine prophylactic use. If therapy is not initiated prophylactically, traditional indications for the use of lidocaine in suspected acute myocardial infarction include ventricular premature complexes that are more frequent than 6/min, are multiform, encroach on the T wave of the QRS complex, or occur in bursts of two or more in succession (118). In this circumstance, a loading dose of lidocaine can be administered as multiple, slow boluses of 50 mg, every 5 minutes to a total dose of 200–300 mg or at a rate of 20 mg/min to a total dose of 3–5 mg/kg followed by a continuous infusion of 2–4 mg/min for 24 hours (10). The initial doses and the infusion rate should be decreased (many empirically reduce them by 50%) in the presence of congestive heart failure, hepatic dysfunction, patient age above 70 years, or hypotension (41). If the infusion is continued for more than 24 hours, the rate should be reduced by one-half (58).

A similar regimen can also be used in more emergent situations, e.g., when rapid ventricular tachycardia is present, to achieve and maintain therapeutic levels as quickly as possible. In general, lidocaine is the drug of choice for most malignant ventricular arrhythmias, including those induced by digitalis toxicity. Patients with ventricular tachycardia who fail to respond to lidocaine and those severely compromised usually require cardioversion.

During cardiopulmonary resuscitation when an antiarrhythmic agent is required (when ventricular tachycardia or ventricular fibrillation is present), a bolus of 1 mg/kg of lidocaine will provide levels in or above the therapeutic range for at least 20 minutes (80), during which time defibrillation should be reattempted. Since levels are high for so long, only one dose is generally required, although some may prefer to use repetitive doses of 0.5 mg/kg every 8–10 minutes before changing to bretylium (120).

Similar doses of lidocaine, 1 mg/kg, followed by defibrillation are appropriate for pediatric patients with ventricular tachycardia and ventricular fibrillation, although these rhythm disturbances occur in less than 10% of pediatric cardiac arrests and usually as an end result of a primary respiratory disturbance (44). If ventricular tachycardia/fibrillation is not reversed, a second 1 mg/kg bolus of lidocaine is recommended, followed by an infusion of 20–50 μg/kg/min and repeated attempts at defibrillation or cardioversion. The infusion rate of lidocaine for children who have received loading doses of lidocaine and require maintenance infusions should be reduced by at least 50% if shock, congestive heart failure, or hepatic dysfunction is present (120).

Bretylium Tosylate

PHARMACOLOGY

Bretylium is a quarternary ammonium compound with both adrenergic and direct myocardial effects (72, 101). It is classified as a type 3 antiarrhythmic agent. Class 3 antiarrhythmics generally prolong the duration of the action potential and the refractory period by increasing repolarization time. They have little effect on the rate of rise of phase zero or on the resting membrane potential (117). However, these antiarrhythmic effects are observed with more chronic administration. Acute effects in vivo are probably accounted for by adrenergic stimulation, which will shorten refractory periods. Bretylium's adrenergic effects are biphasic. It initially causes the release of norepinephrine from adrenergic nerve terminals, inducing transient (approximately 20 minutes) hypertension, tachycardia, and in some patients increases in cardiac output. Once norepinephrine is depleted, release is inhibited, and by 45–60 minutes hypotension may be present (59, 83). Since bretylium blocks the uptake of norepinephrine, it may potentiate the effects of exogenously administered catecholamines (72). For some time it was thought that the adrenergic effects of bretylium have little to do with its effects on ventricular fibrillation since neither reserpine nor sympathectomy changes the ventricular fibrillation threshold (24). However, more recent data support the hypothesis that bretylium's effects may be critically dependent on the adrenergic milieu (46). Recently it has been proposed that an increased upstroke velocity of phase zero of the action potential due to catecholamine stimulation, in concert with direct myocardial effects of lengthening of the effective refractory period, are essential to the antiarrhythmic mechanism of the agent (94). Bretylium reduces disparities in refractory periods and conduction velocities between ischemic and normal tissues, and delays the conduction of premature impulses into normal tissue contiguous with ischemic zones ("border zones") (49). In experimental animals and in anecdotal reports in patients, bretylium is capable of terminating ventricular fibrillation (4, 11). Bretylium also has been reported to markedly increase the fibrillation threshold (the amount of energy necessary to induce ventricular fibrillation) even when ischemia or reperfusion is present (3, 61, 70). Recently it has been suggested that the effect on ventricular fibrillation threshold may be unique to certain types of models in which ventricular fibrillation is induced and may be nonapplicable to others (46) and/or of a lesser magnitude than initially described (51). Bretylium either does not change or lowers defibrillation threshold (the energy required to terminate ventricular fibrillation) (68, 75, 127). Despite a pharmacologic profile suggesting that bretylium should be more effective than lidocaine in the treatment of ventricular fibrillation, controlled clinical trials have not been able to discern any differences in efficacy of these drugs in treating ventricular fibrillation (58, 95). Possibly, late administration of antiarrhythmic agents during cardiac arrest sequences is responsible for the lack of difference, or additional factors, as yet undetermined, may modulate the effects of these agents during cardiac arrest.

Bretylium is only utilized intravenously. Its effects generally are delayed for 10–15 minutes when used in conventional doses, which usually are diluted and administered slowly or via an infusion to reduce adverse adrenergic effects. The delay is likely due to the need to concentrate the drug in myocardium (3, 49, 111). Higher doses administered as a bolus without dilution are warranted during emergencies such as cardiac arrest and have more immediate effects. Bretylium is excreted unchanged in the urine. When renal function is normal, 72% is excreted within the first 24 hours and 100% by 72 hours (88). Elimination is similar from myocardium and plasma, with an elimination half-life in humans of 4–17 hours (3, 106). Accordingly, dosage adjustments are required for patients with renal failure.

The principal side effect of bretylium is hypotension, especially orthostatic hypotension, and the nausea and vomiting that are frequently associated. It occurs in 50–75% of patients, depending on dose and rapidity of administration (72). Because bretylium impairs the reuptake of catecholamines, it can potentiate the effects of exogenously administered pressors and/or inotropes (72). Other side effects include negative synergism with other antiarrhythmic agents, but the clinical importance of these interactions in critically ill patients is unclear (5, 34, 72); there is also the possibility that digitalis toxicity could be exacerbated by adrenergic stimulation (59). The treatment for severe hypotension due to bretylium relies on tricyclic antidepressants, which block the access of bretylium to sympathetic neurons but do not affect its antiarrhythmic effects (141).

INDICATIONS AND DOSE

Bretylium is indicated for the treatment of ventricular arrhythmias resistant to other treatments or when other treatments are for some reason contraindicated. For ventricular tachycardia with a pulse, bretylium is usually used after lidocaine, and in most instances procainamide, in a dose of 5–10 mg/kg diluted 1:4. Good results have been obtained even in patients with digitalis toxicity despite concerns about catecholamine stimulation (59). Bretylium is administered slowly, over 8–10 min-

utes, and the dose can be repeated once or twice, followed by intermittent bolus doses every 6–8 hours or a continuous infusion of 1–2 mg/min (72). For ventricular tachycardia without a pulse or ventricular fibrillation, bretylium should be used only if lidocaine has been ineffective or is contraindicated, since in clinical trials lidocaine has proven equally effective (58, 95) and avoids the potentially adverse hemodynamic effects of bretylium (45). In general, a trial of only one dose of lidocaine should precede the use of bretylium in adults. The required dose of bretylium is 5 mg/kg given as a bolus, followed by 10 mg/kg if ventricular fibrillation does not respond to defibrillation. Repeated doses of 10 mg/kg can be given every 15–30 minutes to a maximum dose of 30 mg/kg (72). The indications and doses for pediatric arrests are identical to those for adults.

Intravenous Procainamide

PHARMACOLOGY

Procainamide is a type 1A antiarrhythmic agent. It reduces the rate of phase 4 depolarization in isolated ventricular muscle and Purkinje fibers (60), slows ventricular conduction (115), and increases the refractory period of ventricular tissue (114). How these mechanisms prevent ventricular arrhythmias is not totally clear, but the effects on normal tissue and at the site of impulse formation may be important to procainamide's efficacy (116).

The clearance of procainamide is dependent on both hepatic and renal function. Approximately 60% of any given dose is excreted unchanged in the urine (82) if normal renal function is present, and the remainder undergoes N-acetylation in the liver (42). Thus, elimination is reduced during renal failure or in congestive heart failure if renal and/or hepatic perfusion is impaired (73). In addition, patients may be rapid or slow hepatic acetylators of the agent, which can have clinically important effects on plasma levels (21). The N-acetylated derivative has antiarrhythmic properties that are somewhat different from those of the parent compound (64) and is also excreted renally (42).

Although the metabolism of procainamide is complex, the measurement of both the parent compound and the N-acetyl derivative is routinely available, facilitating more chronic treatment. Difficulties in rapidly obtaining therapeutic blood levels make the agent difficult to use in the emergency setting. Procainamide is a ganglionic blocker with significant vasodilating effects, and at high doses some negative inotropic effects (55). These effects limit the rapidity with which procainamide can be administered (55). Accordingly, the agent must be administered cautiously to patients with hypotension and heart failure or to those whose clearance of procainamide may be impaired (those with hepatic and/or renal dysfunction). Since procainamide slows conduction and increases the refractory period, it can induce heart block, widening of the QRS complex (140), and QT_c prolongation and associated arrhythmias (13).

INDICATIONS AND DOSE

Procainamide is indicated for the treatment of malignant ventricular arrhythmias that do not respond to lidocaine or when treatment with lidocaine is contraindicated. It also may be used intravenously to treat supraventricular arrhythmias (50), but is rarely used to treat ventricular fibrillation because it takes too long to achieve therapeutic levels.

The intravenous loading dose is 50 mg every 5 minutes unless hypotension occurs, the QRS complex has widened by more than 50%, 1 g has been administered, or the arrhythmia has been suppressed. In urgent circumstances, up to 20 mg/min have been given, titrated to the same endpoints (50). An alternative regimen utilizes a loading dose of 17 mg/kg given over 1 hour, followed by a maintenance infusion of 2.8 mg/kg/hr. In patients who might clear the agent slowly, the loading dose is reduced to 12 mg/kg and the infusion rate to 1.4mg/kg/hr. With this regimen, some patients have therapeutic levels by 15 minutes (66). There are no unique considerations concerning the use of procainamide in children other than to appreciate that ventricular arrhythmia is a rare cause of cardiac arrest, which more commonly develops secondary to acute respiratory failure (44).

OTHER MEDICATIONS OF POTENTIAL USE

Sodium Bicarbonate

PHARMACOLOGY

During cardiopulmonary arrest, metabolic and respiratory acidosis are inevitable. Respiratory acidosis results from inadequate ventilation and is effectively antagonized by providing assisted ventilation. Metabolic acidosis is due to inadequate tissue oxygenation, which leads to anaerobic metabolism and the production of lactic acid (136). Acute respiratory and acute metabolic acidosis have very different effects on intracellular pH. Acute increases in $Paco_2$ acutely decrease intracellular pH because carbon dioxide diffuses rapidly into cells, whereas acute increases in the extracellular hydrogen ion concentration depress intracellular pH less rapidly because both H^+ and HCO_3^- diffuse across cell membranes relatively slowly. In addition, the production of carbon dioxide via the reaction $H^+ + HCO_3^- \leftrightharpoons H_2O + CO_2$ favors the formation of bicarbonate over carbonic acid by a ratio of 20:1 (107, 122).

The adverse effects of acidosis appear to be related to changes in the intracellular and extracellular pH and carbon dioxide concentration. Ischemia, which is a likely occurrence during cardiopulmonary resuscitation given the poor coronary perfusion and high myocardial oxygen consumption, induces increases in intracellular Pco_2 to as high as 300 mm Hg or greater, and a decrease in intracellular pH to below 6 (47, 48). Intracellular acidosis and hypercarbia have been related to diminished contractile performance and an elevated end-diastolic pressure (27, 28). This effect is accentuated by increases in Pco_2 even when extracellular pH is held constant (28). In addition, acidosis blunts the myocardial and peripheral response to exogenous catecholamines, increases pulmonary vascular resistance, vasodilates systemic vascular beds, and decreases glycolytic pathway activity, thus impairing ATP synthesis (1, 107, 122). There also is concern that a high Pco_2 will reduce diaphragmatic function and exacerbate respiratory distress, especially in infants (65). An appreciation of the effects of intracellular acidosis and the differences in diffusion between CO_2 and H^+ and HCO_3^- ions has led to a substantial rethinking of the use of buffers during cardiopulmonary resuscitation.

Originally, sodium bicarbonate in combination with epinephrine was reported to improve the success of defibrillation and survival during resuscitation. Sodium bicarbonate alone was no better than placebo (105). More recently, in a careful study in which coronary perfusion pressure was maintained near the critical level between poor and good outcome, sodium bicarbonate (1 mEq/kg) failed to affect the success of defibrillation or improve the chances for spontaneous circulation or survival (54). Other studies have also failed to observe a beneficial effect from sodium bicarbonate administration (86, 128). This is thought in part to be because sodium bicarbonate solutions already have a high carbon dioxide content (260–280 mm Hg for each 50 ml) (92). In addition, sodium bicarbonate buffers metabolic acids through the reaction $HCO_3^- + H^+ \leftrightharpoons H_2O + CO_2$. Thus, in the presence of H^+ ion, more carbon dioxide is formed. The combination of the intrinsic CO_2 concentration plus that formed by the above reaction will diminish both extracellular and intracellular pH (98). Thus, it should not be surprising that rapid administration of bicarbonate transiently increases Pco_2 and diminishes left ventricular performance even in the absence of cardiac arrest (69). Similar adverse effects have been observed in the presence of lactic acidosis with hypoxemia. In this setting, sodium bicarbonate (2.5mEq/kg administered over 1 hour) diminished blood pressure, impaired splanchnic blood flow, and markedly decreased liver intracellular pH compared with animals who received saline alone (53). Blood lactate and lactic acid production were substantially augmented in animals treated with bicarbonate. In a model of cardiac arrest, administration of bicarbonate raises arterial pH, but depresses cerebrospinal fluid pH because CO_2 diffuses into the central nervous system more rapidly than H^+ or HCO_3^- ions (8). The diminished mental status observed after resuscitations may be partly due to this acute rise in cerebrospinal fluid Pco_2 and fall in pH. When metabolic acidosis is produced by administration of acid (HCl), or experimental diabetic ketoacidosis, bicarbonate impairs cerebral oxygen availability, probably by decreasing cerebral blood oxygen content and/or tissue oxygen release (20). This fact appears to result from a shift in the oxyhemoglobin dissociation curve to the left due to arterial alkalosis, which impairs tissue oxygen delivery; and/or a reduction in cardiac output due to hypoxic lactic acidosis exacerbated by bicarbonate (20), with concomitant tissue acidosis secondary to organ ischemia. The effects of excess CO_2 cannot be overcome by hyperventilation alone because of the limited pulmonary blood flow induced during compression and ventilation. Because of the low cardiac output (25–33% of normal) (69) only a modest percentage of the CO_2 generated reaches the lungs for elimination by ventilation. Thus, although oxygenated blood may have a low or normal Pco_2, venous blood will have a high Pco_2 and a much lower pH.

This event has been termed the "venous paradox" and is observed during cardiopulmonary resuscitation in patients and experimental animals (137).

In addition to the adverse effects due to a high venous Pco_2, administration of sodium bicarbonate during cardiac arrest may cause hyperosmolarity and hypernatremia (84) and extracellular alkalosis (126). Alkalosis induced by excessive bicarbonate administration may reduce the concentration of ionized calcium, decrease plasma potassium concentration, shift the oxyhemoglobin dissociation curve to the left (inhibiting the release of oxygen), and induce malignant arrhythmias (79). Precipitation of calcium carbonate occurs when bicarbonate is mixed with calcium.

INDICATIONS AND DOSE

Because of the lack of information documenting benefit of bicarbonate during cardiopulmonary resuscitation and the concerns discussed above about the potential morbidity of its use, the most recent American Heart Association guidelines deemphasize the role of sodium bicarbonate in both pediatric and adult resuscitation (120). Bicarbonate should not be used until the airway is secured, adequate ventilation and chest compressions have been administered, and the patient fails to respond to defibrillation, antiarrhythmic therapy, and epinephrine. Acidosis, if present, should be treated with vigorous hyperventilation. Attention to airway management is particularly important in pediatric patients since respiratory failure is a major cause of cardiopulmonary arrest (44).

Following the restoration of spontaneous circulation, the role of bicarbonate is more controversial. Lactate may be "washed out" of reperfused tissue beds with an acute exacerbation of metabolic acidosis. Bicarbonate should only be administered if an adequate pH cannot be achieved with hyperventilation. It is probably unnecessary to treat mild-to-moderate metabolic acidosis (pH > 7.20), especially when due to correctable hemodynamic causes.

When used, the dose of bicarbonate is 1 mEq/kg by slow intravenous infusion, for both adult and pediatric patients. Subsequent doses of 0.5 mEq/kg may be given every 10 minutes as needed. In infants, it is preferable to dilute the bicarbonate 1:1 with sterile water to decrease the hyperosmolarity of the 8.4% solution (120).

Calcium

PHARMACOLOGY

Calcium is essential to the process of excitation-contraction coupling. It enters the cell through voltage-dependent channels and stimulates the intracellular release of calcium from the sarcoplasmic reticulum. The transient increase in intracellular calcium concentration results in activation of actin-myosin coupling through interaction with regulatory proteins. Contraction terminates when calcium is pumped out of the cell or back into the sarcoplasmic reticulum. Normally there is approximately a 10,000-fold concentration gradiant between extracellular and intracellular calcium concentration maintained by energy-requiring mechanisms. Calcium has variable effects on systemic vascular resistance, which in part determine the extent to which increased inotropy induced by calcium affects systemic arterial pressure. If the intracellular calcium concentration becomes elevated, such as following ischemic insults, cell death results, in part through calcium-mediated mechanisms (67).

Hypercalcemia may precipitate or exacerbate digitalis toxicity, leading to severe arrhythmias including life-threatening bradycardias (52). Calcium forms an insoluble precipitate (calcium carbonate) if mixed with bicarbonate, it is sclerosing to peripheral veins, and if it infiltrates into the subcutaneous tissues, can produce a severe chemical burn.

INDICATIONS AND DOSE

Advocacy of the use of calcium in cardiopulmonary arrest was stimulated by the observation that calcium administration resulted in positive inotropic effects in patients after cardiopulmonary bypass (126). These patients may have been rendered hypocalcemic by transfusion. In recent clinical studies, calcium has been ineffective in the treatment of refractory electromechanical dissociation (56, 123) and/or asystole (124).

In addition to lack of data concerning the efficacy of calcium in cardiac arrest, there is also concern that postischemic cell injury (so-called reperfusion injury) is exacerbated by the excessive plasma calcium concentrations known to occur when calcium is administered during cardiopulmonary resuscitation (22, 35).

Thus, calcium should be used during cardiopulmonary resuscitation only to correct suspected hypocalcemia, to reverse the adverse effects of hyperkalemia and/or hypermagnesemia, or to treat calcium channel blocker toxicity (120). There is little information as to the optimal dose. A dose of 2 ml of 10% calcium chloride (elemental calcium, 2–4 mg/kg) is recommended in adults (120). In pediatric patients, a larger dose (10% calcium chloride, 20 mg/kg; elemental calcium, 5–7 mg/kg) is recommended. The dose should be infused slowly, and may be repeated after 10 minutes if required.

Isoproterenol

PHARMACOLOGY

Isoproterenol is a potent, very short-acting synthetic catecholamine with nearly pure β-adrenergic stimulating properties. As such, isoproterenol induces marked changes in heart rate and contractility centrally and is a potent peripheral and coronary vasodilator. It also markedly increases myocardial work (139).

Isoproterenol may induce or exacerbate ischemia in patients with coronary artery disease (130, 139). Because it lowers perfusion pressure, it increases mortality during experimental resuscitation (91). Isoproterenol can induce ventricular arrhythmias, especially in patients with digitalis toxicity (6).

INDICATIONS AND DOSE

Isoproterenol is not indicated during the management of cardiac arrest since it appears to increase mortality (91), and has been supplanted as a pressor/inotrope by dopamine and dobutamine. Its only role at present is for the temporary treatment of life-threatening bradycardia until a pacemaker can be inserted. With the advent of reliable external pacemakers (144) even this indication may be of less importance in the future. When used to treat bradycardia, the dose of isoproterenol required usually is quite low because it has such potent chronotropic effects. Accordingly, the initial dose should be 2 μg/min. Doses as high as 10 μg/min may be needed to maintain an adequate heart rate (usually approximately 60 beats/min).

In pediatric patients, bradycardia is usually due to hypoxia. Attention to ventilation should precede isoproterenol administration. Epinephrine may be preferable to isoproterenol in pediatric patients since it does not induce vasodilation and thus should better maintain coronary perfusion pressure (120). The infusion dose of isoproterenol is 0.1–1.0 μg/kg/min.

References

1. Andersen MN, Borden JR, Mouritzen CV: Acidosis, catecholamines, and cardiovascular dynamics: when doses of acidosis require correction. Ann Surg 166:344, 1967.
2. Anderson JL: Antifibrillatory versus antiectopic therapy. Am J Cardiol 54:7A, 1984.
3. Anderson JL, Patterson E, Corlon M, et al: Kinetics of antifibrillatory effects of bretylium: correlation with myocardial drug concentrations. Am J Cardiol 46:583, 1980.
4. Bacaner M: Bretylium tosylate for suppression of induced ventricular fibrillation. Am J Cardiol 17:528, 1966.
5. Bacaner MB: Treatment of ventricular fibrillation and other acute arrhythmias with bretylium tosylate. Am J Cardiol 21:530, 1968.
6. Becker DJ, Nonkin PM, Bennett LD, et al: Effect of isoproterenol in digitalis cardiotoxicity. Am J Cardiol 12:242, 1962.
7. Benowitz NL: Clinical applications of the pharmacokinetics of lidocaine. In Melmon K (ed): Cardiovascular Drug Therapy. Philadelphia, FA Davis, 1974, p 77.
8. Berenyi KJ, Wolk M, Killip T: Cerebrospinal fluid acidosis complicating therapy of experimental cardiopulmonary arrest. Circulation 52:319, 1975.
9. Berg RA: Emergency infusion of catecholamines into bone marrow. Am J Dis Child 138:810, 1984.
10. Bethesda Conference Report: Thirteenth Bethesda conference: emergency cardiac care. Am J Cardiol 50:365, 1982.
11. Bigger JT, Jr, Jaffe CC: The effect of bretylium tosylate on the electrophysiologic properties of ventricular muscle and Purkinje fibers. Am J Cardiol 27:82, 1971.
12. Bleyaert AL, Sands PA, Safar P, et al: Augmentation of post-ischemic brain damage by severe intermittent hypertension. Crit Care Med 8:41, 1980.
13. Boccardo D, Pitchon R, Weiner I: Adverse reactions and efficacy of high-dose procainamide therapy in resistant tachyarrhythmias. Am Heart J 102:797, 1981.
14. Boyes RN, et al: Pharmacokinetics of lidocaine in man. Clin Pharmacol Ther 12:105, 1971.
15. Brillman JA, Sanders AB, Otto CW, et al: Outcome of resuscitation from fibrillatory arrest using epinephrine and phenylephrine in dogs. Crit Care Med 13:912, 1985.
16. Brown CG, Werman HA, Davis EA, et al: Comparative effects of epinephrine and phenylephrine on regional cerebral blood flow during cardiopulmonary resuscitation (abstract). Ann Emerg Med 15:635, 1986.
17. Brown CG, Werman HA, Davis EA, et al: Effect of high-dose phenylephrine versus epinephrine on regional cerebral blood flow during cardiopulmonary resuscitation (abstract). Ann Emerg Med 15:14, 1986.
18. Brown CG, Werman HA, Hamlin R, et al: The comparative effects of methoxamine and epinephrine on regional cerebral blood flow in a swine model (abstract). Crit Care Med 14:333, 1986.
19. Brown DC, Lewis AJ, Criley JM: Asystole and its treatment: the possible role of the parasympathetic nervous system in cardiac arrest. J Am Coll Emerg Phys 8:448, 1979.
20. Bureau MA, Begin R, Berthiaume Y, et al: Cerebral hypoxia from bicarbonate infusion in diabetic acidosis. J Pediatr 96:968, 1980.
21. Campbell W, Tilstone WJ, Lawson DH, et al: Acetylator phenotype and the clinical pharmacology of slow release procainamide. Br J Clin Pharmacol 3:1023, 1976.
22. Carlon GC, Howland WS, Kahn RC, et al: Calcium chloride administration in normal calcemic critically ill patients. Crit Care Med 8:209, 1980.
23. Carruth JE, Silverman ME: Ventricular fibrillation complicating acute myocardial infarction: reasons against the routine use of lidocaine. Am Heart J 104:545, 1985.
24. Cervoni P, Ellis CH, Maxwell RA: The antiarrhythmic action of bretylium in normal reserpine-pretreated and chronically denervated dog hearts. Arch Int Pharmacodyn 190:91, 1971.
25. Chow MSS, Kluger J, Dipersio DM, et al: Antifibrillatory effects of lidocaine and bretylium immediately post cardiopulmonary resuscitation. Am Heart J 110:938, 1985.
26. Chow MMS, Ronsfeld RAA, Hamilton RA, et al: Effect of external cardiopulmonary resuscitation on lidocaine pharmacokinetics in dogs. J Pharmacol Exp Ther 224:531, 1983.
27. Cingolani HE, Faulkner SL, Mattiazzi AR, et al: Depression of human myocardial contractility with "respiratory" and "metabolic" acidosis. Surgery 77:427, 1975.
28. Cingolani HE, Mattiazzi AR, Blesa ES, et al: Contractility in isolated mammalian heart muscle after acid base changes. Circulation 26:269, 1970.
29. Collinsworth KA, Kalman SM, Harrison DC: The clinical pharmacology of lidocaine as an anti-arrhythmic drug. Circulation 50:1217, 1974.
30. Cooper MJ, Abinader EG: Atropine-induced ventricular fibrillation: case report and review of the literature. Am Heart J 97:225, 1979.
31. Dalsey WC, Barsan WG, Joyce SM, et al: Comparison of superior vena caval and inferior vena caval access using a radioisotope technique during normal perfusion and cardiopulmonary resuscitation. Ann Emerg Med 13:881, 1984.
32. Dauchot P, Gravenstein JS: Bradycardia after myocardial ischemia and its treatment with atropine. Anesthesiology 44:501, 1976.
33. Davidson R, Parker M, Atkinson AJ Jr: Excessive serum lidocaine levels during maintenance infusion: mechanisms and prevention. Am Heart J 104:203, 1982.
34. De Azevedo IM, Wantanabe Y, Dreifus LS: Electrophysiologic antagonism of quinidine and bretylium tosylate. Am J Cardiol 33:633, 1974.
35. Dembo DH: Calcium in advanced life support. Crit Care Med 9:358, 1981.
36. DeSilva RA, Hennekens CH, Lown B, et al: Lignocaine prophylaxis in acute myocardial infarction. An evaluation of randomized trials. Lancet 2:855, 1981.
37. Dhingia R, Amat-y-Leon F, Wyndham C: Electrophysiologic effects of atropine on human sinus node and atrium. Am J Med 38:492, 1976.
38. Ditchey RV: High dose epinephrine does not improve the balance between myocardial oxygen supply and demand during cardiopulmonary resuscitation in dogs (abstract). J Am Coll Cardiol 3:596, 1984.
39. Ditchey RV, Lindenfeld J: Potential adverse effects of volume loading on perfusion of vital organs during closed-chest resuscitation. Circulation 69:181, 1984.
40. Doan LA: Peripheral versus central delivery of medications during CPR. Ann Emerg Med 13(part 2):784, 1984.
41. Dorian P, Fain ES, Davy JM, et al: Lidocaine causes a reversible concentration-dependent increase in defibrillation energy requirements. J Am Coll Cardiol 8:327, 1986.
42. Dreyfuss J, Bigger JR, Jr., Cohen AI, et al: Metabolism of procainamide in rhesus monkey and man. Clin Pharmacol Ther 13:366, 1972.

43. Dunn HM, McComb JM, Kinney CD, et al: Prophylactic lidocaine in the early phase of suspected acute myocardial infarction. *Am Heart J* 110:353, 1985.

44. Eisenberg M, Bergner L, Hallstrom A: Epidemiology of cardiac arrest and resuscitation in children. *Ann Emerg Med* 12:672, 1983.

45. Euler DE, Leman TW, Wallock ME, et al: Deleterious effects of bretylium on hemodynamic recovery from ventricular fibrillation. *Am Heart J* 112:25, 1986.

46. Euler DE, Scanlon PJ: Mechanism of the effect of bretylium on the ventricular fibrillation threshold in dogs. *Am J Cardiol* 55:1396, 1985.

47. Flaherty JT, Schaff HV, Goldman R, et al: Metabolic and functional effects of progressive degrees of hypothermia during global ischemia. *Am J Physiol* 236:H839, 1979.

48. Flaherty JT, Weisfeldt ML, Bulkley BH, et al: Mechanisms of ischemic myocardial cell damage assessed by phosphorus-31 nuclear magnetic resonance. *Circulation* 65:561, 1982.

49. Fujimoto T, Hamamoto H, Peter T, et al: Electrophysiologic effects of bretylium on canine ventricular muscle during acute ischemia and reperfusion. *Am Heart J* 105:966, 1983.

50. Giardina EGV, Heissenbuttel RH, Bigger JT: Intermittent intravenous procaine amide to treat ventricular arrhythmias. *Ann Intern Med* 78:183, 1973.

51. Gintant GA, Hoffman BF, Naylor RE: The influence of molecular form of local anesthetic-type antiarrhythmic agents on reduction of the maximum upstroke velocity of canine cardiac Purkinje fibers. *Circ Res* 52:735, 1983.

52. Gold H, Edward D: The effects of ouabain on the heart in the presence of hypercalcemia. *Am Heart J* 3:45, 1927.

53. Graf H, Leach W, Arieff AI: Metabolic effects of sodium bicarbonate in hypoxic lactic acidosis in dogs. *Am J Physiol* 2249:F630, 1985.

54. Guerci AD, Chandra N, Johnson E, et al: Sodium bicarbonate does not improve resuscitation from ventricular fibrillation in dogs. *Circulation* 74(suppl 4):75, 1986.

55. Harison DC, Sprouse JH, Morrow AG: The antiarrhythmic properties of lidocaine and procaine amide. Clinical and physiologic studies of their cardiovascular effects in man. *Circulation* 28:486, 1963.

56. Harrison FE, Amey BD: Use of calcium in electromechanical dissociation. *Ann Emerg Med* 13:844, 1984.

57. Hasegawa EA: The endotracheal administration of drugs. *Heart Lung* 15:60, 1986.

58. Haynes RE, Chinn TL, Copan MK, et al: Comparison of bretylium tosylate and lidocaine in management of out-of-hospital ventricular fibrillation. A randomized clinical trial. *Am J Cardiol* 48:353, 1981.

59. Heissenbuttel RH, Bigger JT: Bretylium tosylate: a newly available antiarrhythmic drug for ventricular arrhythmias. *Ann Intern Med* 91:229, 1979.

60. Hoffman BG: The action of quinidine and procainamide on single fibers of dog ventricle and specialized conducting systems. *An Acad Bras Cienc* 29:365, 1958.

61. Holland K, Patterson E, Lucches BR, et al: Prevention of ventricular fibrillation in a conscious canine model of sudden coronary death. *Am Heart J* 105:711, 1983.

62. Holmes HR, Babbs CF, Voorhees WD, et al: Influence of adrenergic drugs upon vital organ perfusion during CPR. *Crit Care Med* 8:137, 1980.

63. Houle DB, Weil MH, Brown EB, et al: Influence of respiratory acidosis on ECG and pressor response to epinephrine, norepinephrine and metaraminol. *Proc Soc Exp Biol Med* 94:561, 1957.

64. Jaillon P, Winkle RA: Electrophysiologic comparative study of procainamide and N-acetyl-procainamide in anesthetized dogs: concentration response relationships. *Circulation* 58:1385, 1979.

65. Juan G, Calverley P, Talamo C, et al: Effect of carbon dioxide on diaphragmatic function in human beings. *N Engl J Med* 310:874, 1984.

66. Kastor JA, Josephson ME, Guss SB, et al: Human ventricular refractoriness. II: Effects of procainamide. *Circulation* 56:462, 1977.

67. Katz A, Tenter M: Cellular calcium and cardiac cell death. *Am J Cardiol* 44:188, 1979.

68. Kerber RE, Pandian NG, Jensen SR, et al: Effect of lidocaine and bretylium on energy requirement for transthoracic defibrillation. Experimental studies. *J Am Coll Cardiol* 7:397, 1986.

69. Kindig NB, Filley GF: Intravenous bicarbonate may cause transient intracellular acidosis. *Chest* 83:712, 1983.

70. Kniffen FJ, Lomas TE, Counsell RE, et al: The antiarrhythmic and antifibrillatory actions of bretylium and its o-iodobenzyltrimethylammonium analog. UM-360. *J Pharmacol Exp Ther* 192:120, 1975.

71. Knoebel SB, McHenry PL, Phillips JF, et al: Atropine-induced cardioacceleration and myocardial blood flow in subjects with and without coronary artery disease. *Am J Cardiol* 33:327, 1974.

72. Koch-Weser J: Drug therapy: bretylium. *N Engl J Med* 300:473, 1979.

73. Koch-Weser J: Pharmacokinetics of procainamide in man. *Ann NY Acad Sci* 179:370, 1971.

74. Koltmeier CA, Gravenstein JS: The parasympathomimetic activity of atropine and atropine methylbromide. *Anesthesiology* 29:1125, 1968.

75. Koo CC, Allen JD, Pantridge JF: Lack of effect of bretylium on electrical defibrillation in a controlled study. *Cardiovasc Res* 18:762, 1984.

76. Kosnik JW, Jackson RE, Keats S, et al: Dose-related response of centrally administered epinephrine on the change in aortic diastolic pressure during closed chest massage in dogs. *Ann Emerg Med* 14:204, 1985.

77. Koster RW, Dunning AJ: Intramuscular lidocaine for prevention of lethal arrhythmias in the prehospital phase of acute myocardial infarction. *N Engl J Med* 313:1105, 1985.

78. Kupersmith J: Electrophysiological and antiarrhythmic effects of lidocaine in canine acute myocardial ischemia. *Am Heart J* 97:360, 1979.

79. Lawson NW, Butler GH III, Roy CT: Alkalosis and cardiac arrhythmias. *Anesth Analg* 52:951, 1973.

80. Lown B, Vassaux C: Lidocaine in acute myocardial infarction. *Am Heart J* 76:685, 1968.

81. Mace SE: Effect of technique of administration on plasma lidocaine levels. *Ann Emerg Med* 15:552, 1986.

82. Mark LC, Kayden HJ, Steele JM, et al: The physiological disposition and cardiac effects of procainamide. *J Pharmacol Exp Ther* 102:5, 1951.

83. Markis JE, Koch-Weser J: Characteristics and mechanisms of inotropic and chronotropic actions of bretylium tosylate. *J Pharmacol* 178:94, 1971.

84. Mattar JA, Weil MH, Shubin H, et al: Cardiac arrest in the critically ill: II. Hyperosmolar states following cardiac arrest. *Ann J Med* 56:162, 1974.

85. Michael JR, Guerci AD, Koehler RC, et al: Mechanisms by which epinephrine augments cerebral and myocardial perfusion during cardiopulmonary resuscitation in dogs. *Circulation* 69:822, 1984.

86. Minuck M, Sharma GP: Comparison of THAM and sodium bicarbonate in resuscitation of the heart after ventricular fibrillation in dogs. *Anesth Analg* 56:38, 1977.

87. Mitchell JH, Wildenthal D, Johnson LR Jr. The effects of acid-base disturbance on cardiovascular and pulmonary function. *Kidney Int* 1:375, 1972.

88. Narang PK, Adir J, Josselson J, et al: Pharmacokinetics of bretylium in man after intravenous administration. *J Pharmacokinet Biopharm* 8:363, 1980.

89. Newton DW, Fung EF, Williams DA: Stability of five

catecholamines and terbutaline sulfate in 5% dextrose injection in the absence and presence of aminophylline. *Am J Hosp Pharm* 38:1314, 1981.

90. Niemann JT, Criley JM, Rosborough JP, et al: Predictive indices of successful cardiac resuscitation after prolonged arrest and experimental cardiopulmonary resuscitation. *Ann Emerg Med* 14:521, 1985.

91. Niemann JT, Haynes KS, Garner D, et al: Post countershock pulseless rhythms: response to CPR, artificial cardiac pacing and adrenergic agonists. *Ann Emerg Med* 15:112–120, 1985.

92. Niemann JT, Rosborough JP: Effects of academia and sodium bicarbonate therapy in advanced cardiac life support. *Ann Emerg Med* 13(part 2):781, 1984.

93. Niemann JT, Rosborough JP, Ung S, et al: Hemodynamic effects of continuous abdominal binding during cardiac arrest and resuscitation. *Am J Cardiol* 53:269, 1984.

94. Nishimura M, Wantanabe Y: Membrane action and catecholamine release action of bretylium tosylate in normoxic and hypoxic canine Purkinje fibers. *J Am Coll Cardiol* 2:287, 1983.

99. Oldson DW, Thompson BM, Dairn JL, et al: A randomized comparison study of bretylium tosylate and lidocaine in resuscitation of patients from out of hospital ventricular fibrillation in a paramedic system. *Ann Emerg Med* 13:807, 1984.

96. Ornato JP, Bryson BL, Farqualharson RR, et al: Measurement of ventilation during cardiopulmonary resuscitation. *Crit Care Med* 11:79, 1983.

97. O'Rourke GW, Greene NM: Autonomic blockade and the resting heart rate in man. *Am Heart J* 80:469, 1970.

98. Ostrea EM, Odell GB: The influence of bicarbonate administration on blood pH in a "closed system": clinical implications. *J Pediatr* 80:671, 1972.

99. Otto CW, Yakaitis RW: The role of epinephrine in CPR: a reappraisal. *Ann Emerg Med* 13(part 2):840, 1984.

100. Otto CW, Yakaitis RW, Blitt CD: Mechanism of action of epinephrine in resuscitation from asphyxial arrest. *Crit Care Med* 9:321, 1981.

101. Patterson E, Lucchesi BR: Bretylium: a prototype for future development of antidysrhythmic agents. *Am Heart J* 106:426, 1983.

102. Raehl CL: Endotracheal drug therapy in cardiopulmonary resuscitation. *Clin Pharmacol* 5:573, 1986.

103. Ralston SH, Tacker WA, Showen L, et al: Endotracheal versus intravenous epinephrine during electromechanical dissociation with CPR in dogs. *Ann Emerg Med* 14:1044, 1985.

104. Ralston SH, Voorhees WD, Showen L, et al: Venous and arterial blood gases during and after cardiopulmonary resuscitation in dogs. *Am J Emerg Med.* 3:132, 1985.

105. Redding JS, Pearson JW: Resuscitation from ventricular fibrillation: drug therapy. *JAMA* 203:255, 1968.

106. Romhilt DW, Bloomfield SS, Lipicky RJ, et al: Evaluation of bretylium tosylate for the treatment of premature ventricular contractions. *Circulation* 45:800, 1972.

107. Roos A, Boron WF: Intracellular pH. *Physiol Rev.* 61:296, 1981.

108. Rosetti VA, Thompson BM, Aprahamian C, et al: Difficulty and delay in intravascular access in pediatric patients. *Ann Emerg Med* 13:406, 1984.

109. Rosetti VA, Thompson BM, Miller J, et al: Intraosseous infusion: an alternative route of pediatric intravascular access. *Ann Emerg Med* 14:885, 1985.

110. Sanders AB, Ewy GA, Taft TV: Prognostic and therapeutic importance of the aortic diastolic pressure in resuscitation from cardiac arrest. *Crit Care Med* 12:871, 1984.

111. Sanna G, Arcidiacono R: Chemical ventricular fibrillation of the human heart with bretylium tosylate. *Am J Cardiol* 32:982, 1973.

112. Schleien CL, Dean JM, Koehler RC, et al: Effect of epinephrine on cerebral and myocardial perfusion in an infant animal preparation of cardiopulmonary resuscitation. *Circulation* 73:809, 1986.

113. Scott B, Martin FG, Matchett J, Whites S: Canine cardiovascular responses to endotracheally and intravenously administered atropine, isoproterenol and propranolol. *Ann Emerg Med* 16:1/17, 1987.

114. Shechter JA, Caine R, Friehling T, et al: Effect of procainamide on dispersion of ventricular refractoriness. *Am J Cardiol* 52:279, 1983.

115. Shensa TD, Gilbert CJ, Schmidt DH, et al: Procainamide and retrograde atrioventricular nodal conduction in man. *Circulation* 65:355, 1982.

116. Singer DH, Strauss HC, Hoffman BF: Biphasic effects of procainamide on cardiac conduction. *Bull NY Acad Med* 43:1194, 1968.

117. Singh BN, Vaughn Williams EM: Local anesthetic and antiarrhythmic actions of alprenolol relative to its effect on intracellular action potentials and other properties of isolated cardiac muscle. *Br J Pharmacol* 38:749, 1970.

118. Sobel BE, Braunwald E: The management of acute myocardial infarction. In Braunwald E (ed): *Heart Disease: A Textbook of Cardiovascular Medicine*, ed 2. Philadelphia, WB Saunders, 1984, vol 2, p 1308.

119. Spear JR, Moore EN, Gerstenblith G: Effect of lidocaine on the ventricular fibrillation threshold in the dog during acute ischemia and premature ventricular contractions. *Circulation* 46:65, 1972.

120. Standards and guidelines for cardiopulmonary resuscitation and emergency cardiac care. *JAMA* 255:2841, 1986.

121. Stargel WW, Shand DG, Routledge PA, et al: Clinical comparison of rapid infusion and multiple injection methods for lidocaine loading. *Am Heart J* 102:872, 1981.

122. Steenbergen C, Deleeuw G, Rich T, et al: Effects of acidosis and ischemia on contractility and intracellular pH of rat heart. *Circ Res* 41:849, 1977.

123. Steuven HA, Thompson B, Aprahamian C, et al: The effectiveness of calcium chloride in refractory electromechanical dissociation. *Ann Emerg Med* 14:626, 1985.

124. Steuven HA, Thompson B, Aprahamian C, et al: Lack of effectiveness of calcium chloride in refractory asystole. *Ann Emerg Med* 14:630: 1985.

125. Steuven HA, Tonsfeldt DJ, Thompson BM, et al: Atropine in asystole: human studies. *Ann Emerg Med* 13(part 2):815, 1984.

126. Stulz PM, Scheidegger D, Drop LJ, et al: Ventricular pump performance during hypocalcemia. *J Thorac Cardiovasc Surg* 78:185, 1979.

127. Tacker WA, Niebauer MJ, Babbs CR, et al: The effect of newer antiarrhythmic drugs on defibrillation threshold. *Crit Care Med* 8:177, 1980.

128. Telivuo L, Maamies T, Siltanen P, et al: Comparison of alkalizing agents in resuscitation of the heart after ventricular fibrillation. *Ann Chir Gynaecol Fenn* 57:221, 1968.

129. Thomson PD, Melmon K, Richardson JA, et al: Lidocaine pharmacokinetics in advanced heart failure, liver disease, and renal failure in humans. *Ann Intern Med* 78:872, 1973.

130. Vatner SR, Baig H: Comparison of the effects of ouabain and isoproterenol on ischemic myocardium of conscious dogs. *Circulation* 58:654, 1978.

131. Vaughan, Williams EM: Classification of antiarrhythmic drugs. In Sandoe E, et al (eds): *Arrhythmias*. Sweden, Sodertalje, 1970, p 449.

132. Volpi A, Maggioni A, Franzosi MG, et al: In-hospital prognosis of patient with acute myocardial infarction complicated by primary ventricular fibrillation. *N Engl J Med* 317:257, 1987.

133. Voorhees WD, Jaeger CS, Babbs CR, et al: Regional

blood flow during cardiopulmonary resuscitation in dogs. *Crit Care Med* 8:134, 1980.

134. Vyden JK, et al: The effect of lidocaine on peripheral hemodynamics. *J Clin Pharmacol* 15:506, 1975.

135. Ward JT Jr: Endotracheal drug therapy. *Ann J Emerg Med* 1:71, 1983.

136. Weil MH, Afifi AA: Experimental and clinical studies on lactate and pyruvate as indicators of the severity of acute circulatory failure (shock). *Circulation* 41:989, 1970.

137. Weil MH, Rackow EC, Trevino R, et al: Difference in acid-base state between venous and arterial blood during cardiopulmonary resuscitation. *N Engl J Med* 315:153, 1986.

138. Weiner N: Atropine, scopolamine, and related antimuscarinic drugs. In Gilman AG, Goodman LS, Rall TW, Murad F (eds): *Goodman and Gilman's, The Pharmacologic Basis of Therapeutics.* New York, Macmillan, 1985, pp 130–144.

139. Weiner N: Norepinephrine, epinephrine and the sympathomimetic amines. In Gilman AC, Goodman LS, Rall TW, Murad F (eds): *Goodman and Gilman's, The Pharmacological Basis of Therapeutics.* New York, Macmillan, 1985, pp 160–161.

140. Wellens, JJH, Durrer DL: Effect of procaine amide, quinidine and ajmaline in the Wolff-Parkinson-White syndrome. *Circulation* 50:114, 1974.

141. Woosely RL, Reele SB, Roden DM, et al: Pharmacologic reversal of hypotensive effect complicating antiarrhythmic therapy with bretylium. *Clin Pharmacol Ther* 32:313, 1982.

142. Wortsman J, Frank S, Cryer PE: Adrenomedullary response to maximal stress in humans. *Am J Med* 77:779, 1984.

143. Yakaitis RW, Otto CW, Blitt CD: Relative importance of alpha and beta adrenergic receptors during resuscitation. *Crit Care Med* 7:293, 1979.

144. Zoll PM, Zoll RH, Falk RH, et al: External noninvasive temporary cardiac pacing: clinical trials. *Circulation* 71:937, 1985.

7

Colloids and Crystalloids

Thomas G. Rainey, M.D.
James F. English, M.D.

In this chapter we review the use of colloids and crystalloids in the therapy of shock. Controversy exists as to the changes in body compartment composition in critical illness. Some investigations show depletion of extracellular fluid in shock from hemorrhage (with intravascular and interstitial fluid volumes both depleted) and an increase in intracellular water secondary to cell membrane and sodium-potassium pump dysfunction (25, 142–144). On the other hand, in surgical patients post trauma, extracellular fluid is found not to be decreased but actually increased, whereas intravascular volume is depleted (42, 135). Despite this controversy, one thing is agreed upon—intravascular volume is depleted in many types of critical illness. Prompt restoration of intravascular volume depletion is essential to reestablish cellular perfusion and accomplish successful resuscitation.

A thorough knowledge of the distribution and pharmacokinetics of plasma expanders allows the clinician to promptly and efficiently resuscitate patients in shock from various causes, including trauma, sepsis, hemodilution, and burns. An understanding of this pharmacologic subject helps the physician to minimize side effects associated with overaggressive volume resuscitation (respiratory failure, peripheral edema) or inadequate resuscitation (renal failure, refractory shock). The chapter begins with a discussion of the general principles of fluid distribution within the body, and then reviews the pharmacology of common plasma volume–expanding agents and their application in various clinical situations.

BODY FLUID DISTRIBUTION BY COMPARTMENTS

The total body water (TBW) ranges from 45% to 65% of total body weight in the human adult. The average adult man's TBW equals 60% of total body weight (55, 104) or 48 liters for an 80-kg man (125) (Table 7.1). Body water is distributed into two main compartments, the intracellular fluid (ICF) space, and the extracellular fluid (ECF) space. Two-thirds (32 liters) of the TBW resides in the ICF space and one-third (16 liters) in the ECF space (Fig. 7.1). The ECF space is further subdivided into the intravascular space and the interstitial space. Normally, approximately one-fourth of ECF resides in the intravascular compartment (4 liters) and three-fourths in the interstitial compartment (12 liters). The membranes separating these compartments are freely permeable to water, which moves under the force of osmotic drive until the osmolality in each compartment is equivalent.

When water is added into one compartment it distributes evenly throughout the TBW, and the amount of volume added to any given compartment is proportional to its fractional representation of TBW. As an example, if 3 liters of "free" water (no osmotically active particles) is added to the intravascular space (assuming none of that water exists in the body), the compartment volumes change from 16 to 17 liters in the ECF space and 32 to 34 liters in the ICF space (Fig 7.2). Note that 3

Table 7.1
Total Body Water as Percentage of Body Weight[a]

| Build | Total Body Water (% of Body Weight) | |
	Male	Female
Thin	65	55
Average	60	50
Obese	55	45

[a] Modified from Scribner BH (ed): *University of Washington Teaching Syllabus for the Course on Fluid and Electrolyte Balance.* Seattle, University of Washington Press, 1969.

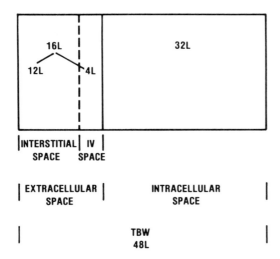

Figure 7.1 Distribution of total body water *(TBW)* in an 80-kg man. *IV,* intravascular.

liters of free water placed in the intravascular space results in a net increase of only 250 ml in the intravascular volume after equilibration takes place. Approximately 30 minutes after a rapid volume infusion, less than one-tenth of the volume infused remains in the intravascular space (156)! If the 3 liters of infused solution is isotonic with plasma (Ringer's lactate, normal saline), a different fluid distribution occurs (Fig. 7.3). Since there is no difference in osmolality between the infused fluid and the body fluids, there is no driving force to cause water to diffuse into the intracellular compartment. The intact membrane between the interstitial space and the intravascular space is permeable to ions and small particles, whereas the membrane surrounding the ICF space functionally is not. Consequently, the ECF space is the distribution space for isotonic fluids such as normal saline and Ringer's lactate. Note also that knowledge of the distribution space for isotonic fluid has important practical applications for resuscitation. Only one-fourth of the volume of isotonic fluid infused remains in the intravascular space after 30 minutes.

Application of these basic concepts allows one to predict the space of distribution for any standard intravenous solution since they are all some combination of free water and isotonic fluid. For example, 1000 ml of 0.45% saline can be thought of as 500 ml of normal (0.9%) saline plus 500 ml of free water. The portion that is isotonic (saline) distributes through the ECF space, and the portion that is

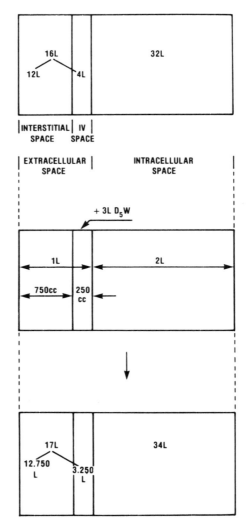

Figure 7.2. Distribution of 3 liters of free water (5% dextrose in water, *D₅W*) in an 80-kg man with total body water of 48 liters. *IV,* intravascular.

water distributes through the TBW. If one tries to expand the intravascular volume of a hypotensive patient by giving 1000 ml of 0.45% saline over 1 hour, the resultant increase in intravascular volume is only 165 ml! After distribution, the 500 ml of free water adds only 40 ml and the 500 ml of normal saline adds approximately 125 ml to the intravascular volume. What initially appears to be a large volume of fluid adds very little to the intravascular volume of 4–5 liters. Writing intravenous fluid prescriptions and predicting the outcome of therapy becomes simple when fluid balance and distribution are thought of in these terms.

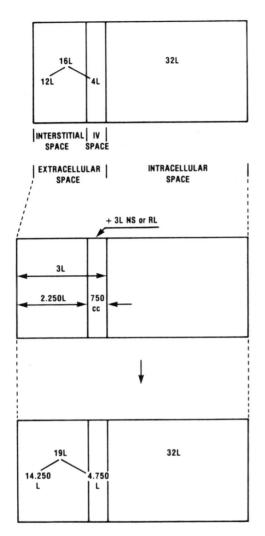

Figure 7.3. Distribution of 3 liters of normal saline *(NS)* or Ringer's lactate *(RL)* in an 80-kg man with total body water of 48 liters, *IV,* intravascular.

CRYSTALLOIDS

The term crystalloid as used here refers to solutions, isotonic with human plasma, that contain sodium as their major osmotically active particle. Ringer's lactate and normal saline are the only solutions considered.

Physiology and Pharmacokinetics

As described in the previous section, isotonic fluids such as Ringer's lactate and normal saline distribute evenly throughout the extracellular space. In normal healthy adults, approximately one-fourth of the volume infused remains in the intravascular space after 1 hour. Equilibration with the extracellular space occurs within 20–30 minutes after infusion. In the critically ill or injured patient, only one-fifth (54) or less (23) may remain in the circulation 1–2 hours after infusion. The "dwell time" in the circulation is the same in shock as in nonshock states (54).

In experimental acute blood loss leading to circulatory collapse, plasma volume becomes reduced and returns to normal over 3–4 days. As this equilibration occurs, hematocrit progressively falls. It takes 24 hours or longer for the hematocrit to stabilize as intravascular volume is restored at the expense of interstitial and ICF volume. By 2 hours, 14–36% of the ultimate change in hematocrit occurs; 36–50% occurs in 8 hours and 63–77% in 24 hours (40). When any plasma expander, including crystalloid, is infused (exogenous fluid), a more immediate fall in hematocrit occurs. However, as redistribution of resuscitation fluid out of the intravascular space occurs, the hematocrit again rises. The apparently erratic changes in serial hematocrit values seen during large-volume crystalloid resuscitations are often the result of these fluid shifts rather than repeated episodes of bleeding.

The total serum protein levels show similar changes. Endogenous restoration of depleted intravascular volume occurs through movement of interstitial fluid into the intravascular space. Catecholamines mediate arteriolar vasoconstriction, which diminishes capillary bed hydrostatic pressure favoring influx of interstitial fluid into the vascular tree distal to the arteriolar constriction. Subsequently, lymphatic flow returns plasma proteins to the intravascular space. Increases in interstitial pressure caused by crystalloid distribution into the interstitial space may augment lymphatic flow and thus the "protein-refill" mechanism (81). This process, combined with increased albumin synthesis and spontaneous diuresis secondary to volume repletion, explains the return of serum protein levels to normal within days after crystalloid resuscitation (143, 166).

Normal saline and Ringer's lactate can be used interchangeably (see prescribing information). The lactate load in Ringer's lactate solution does not potentiate the lactic acidemia associated with shock (161). Rather, as circulating blood volume is restored, diminished lactic acid production and decreased serum lactate levels are found (22, 115). The use of Ringer's lactate does not alter the reliability of blood lactate measurements (85).

The theoretical concern that large volumes of normal saline produce a "dilution acidosis" is not a problem clinically. Normal saline, like Ringer's lactate, causes no acidosis when studied in traumatic shock for which large volumes are administered (85). Saline resuscitation provides an excess of circulating chloride ion, which is normally excreted by the kidney without problem. In patients with acidosis caused by an organic acid (ketoacidosis or lactic acidosis), hyperchloremic acidosis may be seen during the postresuscitation period (101). However, this acidosis is due to loss of the bicarbonate substrate (ketones) in the urine rather than secondary to the administered chloride load.

Indications

Crystalloid solutions are indicated for plasma volume expansion (84, 96). They are inexpensive (Table 7.2), readily available, easily stored, reaction free, and help to correct extracellular electrolyte and volume deficits. In hemorrhagic shock, crystalloids can be used to replace plasma volume immediately (while blood is being crossmatched) and can limit the total amount of blood required for resuscitation. Crystalloids decrease blood viscosity as the blood volume is expanded. In the oliguric patient, a diagnostic "volume challenge" with crystalloid may safely help to distinguish between intravascular volume depletion and acute renal failure.

Side Effects

Crystalloid solutions are nontoxic and free from side effects if used appropriately. Excessive crystalloid administration may cause peripheral and pulmonary edema.

PERIPHERAL EDEMA

Edema is expected from crystalloid use since three-quarters or more of the volume administered distributes in the interstitial compartment of the extracellular space. Edema can be limited by appropriate monitoring of the adequacy of resuscitation to prevent volume overload.

PULMONARY EDEMA

Crystalloid resuscitation lowers colloid oncotic pressure by reducing the serum protein concentrations (53, 166). Whether the reduction in plasma proteins and consequent lowering of plasma colloid oncotic pressure decreases lung function is a controversial issue (54, 57, 112, 123, 136, 142, 167). "Edema safety factors," such as increased lymphatic flow, diminished pulmonary interstitial oncotic pressure, and increased interstitial hydrostatic pressure, limit the effect of lowered colloid oncotic pressure to increase fluid transudation from the vascular space (81). When the total crystalloid volume administered is controlled to prevent volume overload, there is no difference in lung function in resuscitation of shock using crystalloid or colloid solutions (54, 84, 96, 98, 166). The development of the adult respiratory distress syndrome (ARDS) is associated more closely with the presence of sepsis than with the type of fluid used in shock resuscitation.

Table 7.2
Comparative prices of Volume-Expanding Agents[a]

Agent	Amount (ml)	Average Cost ($)	Cost per 400–500 ml of i.v. Expansion ($)
Albumin 5%	500	130.00	130.00
Albumin 25%	100	125.00	125.00
Hydroxyethyl starch	500	41.11	
Dextran 40	500	33.00	15.00–30.00
Dextran 70	500	21.00	10.00–20.00
Ringer's lactate	1000	4.50	6.00–12.00
Normal saline	1000	3.35	4.40– 8.80

[a] Adapted from Knipping WJ (ed): *Drug Topics Redbook*, ed 90. Oradell, NJ, Medical Economics, 1986.

Recommendations for Use

SHOCK

Crystalloid solutions are used in shock of various etiologies for the restoration of intravascular volume and repletion of interstitial water and electrolyte deficits (98, 130, 154, 166). The volume of crystalloid required to attain adequate volume repletion varies from three (37, 54, 98, 144) to 12 (34) times the volume of colloid solution required to reach the same hemodynamic endpoint. The patient in shock, whether from trauma, hemorrhage, or sepsis, should receive immediate volume replacement with crystalloid solutions during evaluation of the clinical situation. Two to three liters administered promptly may restore blood pressure and peripheral perfusion. If the hematocrit is greater than 30% and hemodynamic stability remains, further aggressive fluid resuscitation may be unnecessary. Acute blood loss of 10–20% of the blood volume may be adequately replaced with crystalloid if given in a quantity of three to four times the blood lost (13, 161, 166). If continued fluid resuscitation is required and the hematocrit remains above 30%, the authors recommend the use of crystalloid in conjunction with 5–10% colloid solutions in a ratio of 4:1 (crystalloid: colloid by volume). If the hematocrit falls below 30%, packed red blood cells should be transfused. If the serum albumin level falls below 2–2.5 g/dl, albumin or another colloid should be added to maintain the colloid oncotic pressure. Other blood components should be administered as necessitated by serial measurement of platelet count, prothrombin time, and partial thromboplasin time.

The major pitfall to avoid in crystalloid resuscitation is inadequate fluid administration. Five liters of crystalloid may be needed to replenish a 1-liter blood loss (134). Edema is to be expected and should not be interpreted as intravascular volume overload. Adequacy of intravascular volume repletion must be assessed by the usual parameters that indicate adequacy of peripheral perfusion—stable mean arterial pressure of 70–80 torr, heart rate less than 100 beats/min, warm extremities with good capillary refill, adequate CNS function, urine volume of 0.5–1 ml/kg/hr, and absence of advancing acidosis. In massive resuscitation or other critical situations, pulmonary artery wedge pressure, cardiac output, mixed venous oxygen content, and arteriovenous oxygen concentration difference ($AVDo_2$) must supplement these other parameters in guiding fluid administration. A more detailed discussion of hemodynamic monitoring in resuscitation of shock may be found elsewhere (134).

DIAGNOSIS OF OLIGURIA

Oliguria (urine output <0.5 ml/kg/hr) may indicate prerenal hypoperfusion due to intravascular volume depletion or congestive heart failure (CHF). In the critically ill patient (often with underlying chronic obstructive pulmonary disease, ARDS, edema due to large volume resuscitation, hypoproteinemia, or sepsis with capillary leak) it may be impossible to distinguish volume depletion from CHF by physical examination. A volume challenge (500 ml over 5 minutes) with crystalloid solution can be helpful. If after an adequate volume challenge the patient's urine output increases, the diagnosis of intravascular volume depletion is confirmed and subsequent fluid management can be appropriately altered. If the oliguria is not due to intravascular volume depletion, no increase in urine output occurs with volume challenge. Since crystalloid fluids distribute out of the intravascular space rapidly, only a transient increase in intravascular volume results from a fluid challenge, and the patient with CHF does not experience a prolonged increase in vascular volume.

An adequate fluid challenge consists of no less than 500 ml of Ringer's lactate or normal saline given over 5 minutes. A smaller volume or a longer time for infusion will not expand the intravascular volume significantly. Only 100–150 ml of the 500 ml administered will remain in the intravascular space after 30 minutes. If the volume challenge is given over 30 minutes, the intravascular volume (5 liters for a 70-kg man) would be expanded by a trivial 100–150 ml, thereby providing no information on the etiology of the oliguria since the intravascular volume was never expanded. Similarly, increasing the infusion rate of an oliguric patient from 100 ml/hr to 200 or 300 ml/hr provides no answer to the question of etiology of the oliguria, nor does it adequately treat volume depletion.

Prolonged prerenal hypoperfusion can lead to renal failure. The timely diagnosis and treatment of oliguria secondary to volume depletion is essential to avoid this disastrous consequence. If crystalloid volume challenge does not provide the answer, invasive diagnosis with a pulmonary artery catheter may be required. Colloid solutions should not be used to differentiate between intravascular volume depletion and CHF since their dwell time in the intravascular space is much longer and osmotic diuresis occurs immediately with some preparations (dextran, hydroxyethyl starch).

Prescribing Information

The contents of normal saline and Ringer's lactate solutions are shown in Table 7.3, and their costs in relation to other volume-expanding agents are listed in Table 7.2.

Ringer's lactate contains 28 mEq of lactate, which must undergo hepatic metabolism to bicarbonate to release 28 mEq of free base per liter of solution. In patients with renal failure, this bicarbonate source may be useful as an acid buffer; however, when hyperkalemia is a problem, use of normal saline avoids the 4 mEq/liter potassium content of Ringer's lactate. Similarly, normal saline is preferred in hypercalcemic or hyponatremic states. In the presence of established hyperchloremic metabolic acidosis, Ringer's lactate is preferred to provide a bicarbonate source and to diminish the administered chloride load.

ALBUMIN

Human serum albumin is effective in restoring blood volume in intravascular volume depletion (147). Its clinical indications are controversial, and it costs more than other plasma volume–expanding agents.

Pharmacology and Pharmacokinetics

ENDOGENOUS ALBUMIN

Albumin is produced in the liver and represents 50% of hepatic protein production (119). Its molecular weight is 65,000 (range, 66,300–69,000) (163). In health, approximately 12–14 g/day or 130–200 mg/kg/day are produced by the body (82, 119, 164). Albumin is the major oncotically active plasma protein, contributing about 80% of the plasma colloid oncotic pressure (81, 156). A 50% reduction of the serum albumin concentration decreases the colloid oncotic pressure to one-third of normal (156). Albumin binds cations and anions despite its strong negative charge and is a major transport protein for metals, drugs, fatty acids, hormones, and enzymes (163).

In the adult, 4–5 g of albumin per kilogram of body weight is available in the extracellular space, and 30–40% is present in the intravascular compartment. Albumin is secreted directly from the hepatocyte into the sinusoidal plasma. The final serum concentration of 3.5–5.0 g/dl results from the combination of albumin secretion, volume of distribution, rate of loss from the intravascular space, and ultimate degradation. In cirrhosis with portal hypertension, a large portion of the albumin produced enters directly into the peritoneal space (ascites) rather than the intravascular space, contributing to hypoproteinemia despite a normal or even elevated synthetic rate.

Approximately 50–60% of endogenous albumin is in the interstitial space. Some is tissue-bound and unavailable to the circulation. Free interstitial space albumin returns to the intravascular compartment by lymphatic drainage. This return of non–tissue-bound al-

Table 7.3
Ionic Composition of Various Volume-Expanding Agents

Agent	Component (mEq/liter)				
	Na$^+$	Cl$^-$	K$^+$	Ca^{2+}	Lactate
Ringer's lactate	130	109	4	3	28
Normal saline	154	154	—	—	—
Albumin 5%	130–160	130–160	<1	—	—
Albumin 25%	130–160	130–160	<1	—	—
Dextran 40					
10% in normal saline	154	154	—	—	—
10% in water	0	0	—	—	—
Dextran 70					
6% in normal saline	154	154	—	—	—
6% in water	0	0	—	—	—
Hydroxyethyl starch (hetastarch)	154	154	—	—	—

bumin increases during intravascular volume depletion, as does the synthesis and secretion of new albumin (82, 142). Interstitial space albumin that is tissue-bound is subsequently incorporated into the intracellular space where it is metabolized to amino acids, which return to the liver in a cycle similar to the Cori cycle (136). Catabolism increases albumin metabolism, perhaps accounting for part of stress-induced hypoalbuminemia. Decreases in the degradation of albumin and increases in its distribution in the interstitial space help to compensate for hypoalbuminemia due to loss (nephrotic syndrome, hemorrhage, bowel ob-

Table 7.4
Potential Albumin Losses in Pathologic States

Fluid	Albumin
Edema	
Congestive heart failure	1 g/dl
Renal disease	
Cirrhosis	
Lymphedema	>2 g/dl
Ascites	1–2 g/dl
Urine—nephrosis[a]	Usually 100–400 mg/kg/day, but may be more or less

[a] Requires proteinuria of ≥3 g/24 hours.

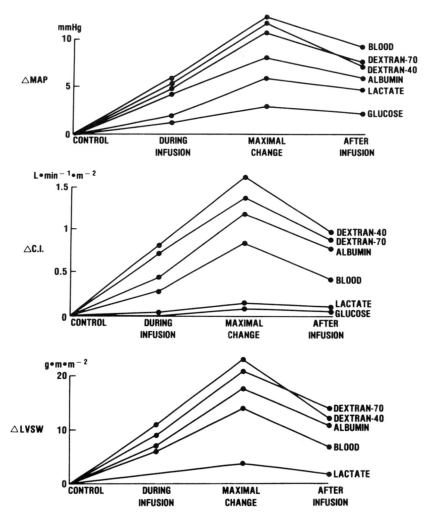

Figure 7.4. Hemodynamic effects of 500 ml of whole blood, 5% albumin, 10% dextran 40, dextran 70, and 1000 ml of 5% glucose or Ringer's lactate all infused over 1 hour. *MAP,* mean arterial pressure; *C.I.,* cardiac index; *LVSW,* left ventricular stroke work. (Modified from Shoemaker WC: Comparison of the relative effectiveness of whole blood transfusions and various types of fluid therapy in resuscitation. *Crit Care Med* 4:71–78, 1976.)

struction) or diminished production (starvation) (61, 116, 119). In injury or stress, albumin synthesis falls acutely whereas the production and serum levels of acute phase reactants (such as globulins, fibrinogen, haptoglobin) increase. In such situations, a 50% depletion of albumin can be corrected by translocation of interstitial albumin into the intravascular space (97). Subsequently, albumin synthesis can increase if hepatic function and the supply of nutrients are adequate (116). For instance, albumin synthesis increases after hemorrhage and burns,

although acutely, serum levels and synthesis fall (119). When appropriate nutrients are provided, albumin synthesis increases in the critically ill patient (116, 144). Albumin synthesis is increased by thyroid hormone and cortisone (81, 117) through stimulation of RNA production, is decreased by malnutrition, and is finely regulated by the oncotic environment of the hepatocytes (119). The serum albumin level exerts no feedback control on albumin synthesis except through albumin's contribution to colloid oncotic pressure (119).

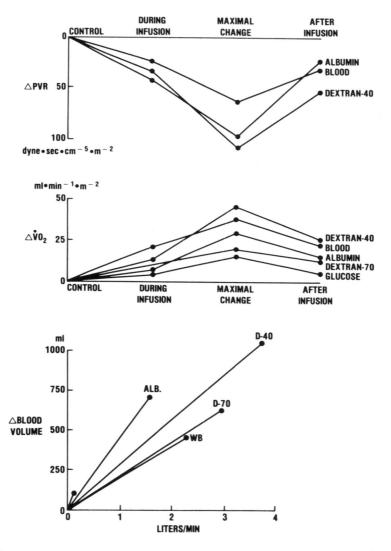

Figure 7.5 Hemodynamic effects of 500 ml of whole blood, 10% dextran 40, dextran 70, and 1000 ml of 5% glucose or Ringer's lactate all infused over 1 hour, *PVR,* pulmonary vascular resistance; *VO₂,* oxygen consumption. (Modified from Shoemaker WC: Comparison of the relative effectiveness of whole blood transfusions and various types of fluid therapy in resuscitation. *Crit Care Med* 4:71–78, 1976.)

Albumin loss can occur through various body fluids (Table 7.4).

EXOGENOUS ALBUMIN

The major clinical use of albumin is as a plasma volume expander, and there are 50 years of experimental evidence to document its effectiveness. The reader is referred elsewhere for specific data concerning albumin use in human shock, trauma, or major surgery (6, 19, 32, 54, 70–74, 103, 127, 133, 143, 166) and animal shock (20, 34, 36, 37, 57, 58, 97, 105, 106). The increase in plasma volume resulting from infusion of albumin solutions is associated with hemodynamic improvement (133) (Figs. 7.4 and 7.5).

Administered albumin distributes itself throughout the extracellular space. It is a commonly held, but false, assumption that albumin distributes solely in the intravascular space. It is only a transient passenger in this compartment, although its length of stay is long compared with that of crystalloid fluids. The plasma half-life of albumin is 16 hours, the same as that of endogenously produced albumin. After 2 hours, 90% remains in the intravascular space. In health, the half-life of albumin in the body is approximately 20 days (81). One gram of intravascular albumin binds

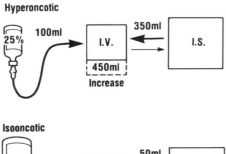

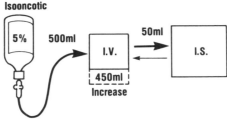

Figure 7.6. schematic drawing of the influence of albumin solutions on the distribution of water to the intravascular *(I.V.)* and interstitial *(I.S.)* fluid compartments of the body. (Modified from Lamke LO, Liljedahl SO: Plasma volume expansion after infusion of 5%, 20%, and 25% albumin solutions in patients. *Resuscitation* 5:85–92, 1976.)

18 ml of water by its oncotic activity (57, 81, 123).

Albumin is clinically available as a 5% or 25% solution in isotonic saline. When 100 ml of 25% albumin solution (25 g albumin) are infused, an increase in the intravascular volume occurs over 30–60 minutes to a final volume of 450 ml (54). The intravascular volume is expanded by the translocation of 350 ml of interstitial fluid into the intravascular space (Fig. 7.6). In the face of extracellular volume depletion, this equilibration is not sufficiently brisk or complete unless supplemental isotonic fluid is provided as part of the resuscitation regimen (81, 82, 174). A 500-ml solution of 5% albumin contains 25 g of albumin and increases the intravascular space by 450–500 ml; however, in this instance the albumin is administered in conjunction with the fluid to be retained.

Indications

Albumin is most widely used for its oncotic properties in the resuscitation of patients with an acutely diminished intravascular volume. It has beneficial effects on viscosity and is used for pump-priming in cardiopulmonary bypass and hemodialysis. Its properties as a transport protein have been used advantageously in binding bilirubin during therapy of hemolytic disease of the newborn.

Side Effects

PULMONARY EDEMA

The "colloid-crystalloid debate" has produced conflicting animal and human studies, some showing adverse effects (32, 60, 70, 86, 87, 140, 170) and others showing beneficial effects of albumin (19, 24, 46, 71–74, 84, 96, 97, 105, 127, 143, 166). The method of resuscitation, overall volume used, and the presence or absence of sepsis affects pulmonary function to a far greater extent than does the type of resuscitation fluid used (43, 105, 168).

DEPRESSED IONIZED CALCIUM LEVELS

Albumin may lower the serum ionized calcium concentration, producing a negative inotropic effect on the myocardium (32, 70, 86, 87, 170) and coagulopathy (28); however, these data are controversial.

ANAPHYLAXIS

The incidence of albumin-induced anaphylaxis is between 0.47% and 1.53% (119). Such reactions are short-lived and include urticaria, chills, fever, and very rarely hypotension. Purified protein fraction has an increased incidence of associated hypotension (compared with albumin), perhaps secondary to the presence of kinins or prekallikrein activator (4, 15, 30, 52).

HEPATITIS RISK

There is no hepatitis risk with albumin. The preparations are heated during processing to 60°C for 10 hours—sufficient time to inactivate the hepatitis virus.

AIDS RISK

There is no known risk of acquired immune deficiency syndrome with albumin.

COST

Albumin is expensive. Hospital units have shown albumin to account for 10–30% of pharmacy budgets (164). The cost per liter of albumin is more than for other colloid solutions and 30 times the cost for the intravascular volume—equivalent amount of crystalloid solution (Table 7.2).

Recommendations for Use

In 1975 a National Institutes of Health task force examined the appropriate use of albumin in the light of increasing cost and apparent indiscriminate use (163). The authors' recommendations for albumin utilization are similar (Table 7.5). Albumin is used for its oncotic activity in the resuscitation of shock. In shock therapy, a major goal is prompt repletion of the intravascular volume in order to restore tissue perfusion. For major volume resuscitation (replacement of greater than 30% of the blood volume) colloids such as albumin or hydroxyethyl starch should be used as part of the resuscitation regimen. If colloids are used early, peripheral perfusion may be restored more promptly than with crystalloid alone. Blood component therapy is dictated by the

Table 7.5
Appropriate Albumin Utilization

Clinical Situations	Guidelines for Use (See Text)
1. Acute intravascular volume depletion, including hemorrhage, trauma, acute hemodilution, acute vasodilation.	In conjunction with crystalloid to limit edema from massive crystalloid volume resuscitation in the elderly or in patients with cardiopulmonary impairment or acute blood loss of >30% blood volume. To keep serum albumin >2.5 g/dl in acute resuscitation. Albumin 5% if patient is not edematous. Albumin 25% if patient is edematous.
2. "Third space" fluid loss, including acute peritonitis, mediastinitis, postoperative radical surgery.	Same guidelines as above.
3. Burns.	Greater than 50% surface area burn. Use after first 24 hours when capillary leak has diminished. Maintain serum albumin >2.5 g/dl. Use in conjunction with hyperalimentation.
4. Chronic disease (cirrhosis, nephrotic syndrome) associated with acute volume depletion (post paracentesis, dialysis, or overaggressive diuresis).	For acute intravascular volume resuscitation. Same guidelines as #1 above.
5. Post cardiopulmonary bypass with hemodilution.	Albumin ≥2.5 g/dl.
6. Adult respiratory distress syndrome.	Maintain lowest PAW that provides a CO adequate for tissue perfusion. Use only after capillary leak has resolved. Albumin >2.5 g/dl. T protein ≥5 g/dl. Colloid osmotic pressure >20 mm Hg. To correct intravascular volume depletion associated with diuretic use.

coagulation profile, hemoglobin concentration, and platelet count. The total volume of crystalloid administered, and thus the potential interstitial space fluid distribution, can be limited by using 5% albumin solution as part of the resuscitation treatment. If the patient is edematous, 25% albumin should be used to mobilize the patient's own interstitial volume. A solution of 100 ml of 25% albumin becomes 400–500 ml of intravascular volume over the course of 30–60 minutes. The greatest problem with its use is avoiding unintentional volume overload and pulmonary edema. Because of albumin's long "dwell time" in the intravascular space, volume overload persists unless diuresis or preload reduction is instituted.

A colloid osmotic pressure (COP) of ≥20 mm Hg, a serum albumin of ≥2.5 g/dl, or a total serum protein of ≥5 g/dl indicates adequate plasma oncotic activity in most situations. Large volumes of crystalloid fluids decrease COP whereas colloids (including albumin) increase COP (53). "Edema safety factors" limit the effect of decreased COP on the development of pulmonary edema; these factors include decreased interstitial oncotic pressure, increased lymphatic flow, and increased interstitial tissue pressure. The importance of decreased COP in pulmonary edema development remains unsettled (121, 136, 167).

Shock is associated with loss of capillary wall integrity ("capillary leak"), especially in the lung with subsequent development of ARDS. The use of albumin in the presence of capillary leak (ARDS, sepsis, intestinal obstruction) must be limited, since albumin crosses the capillary wall and exerts its oncotic influence in the interstitial rather than the intravascular space. The authors recommend that colloid use during capillary leak be minimized. Crystalloid fluids should be used until the capillary leak has resolved. Colloids, including albumin, may then be useful in supporting plasma volume during spontaneous or forced diuresis. Unfortunately, determining when capillary leak is present or has resolved is difficult. In burns (119) and intestinal obstruction (121) capillary integrity is restored after approximately 24 hours. In sepsis or ARDS the "leak" may persist.

In ARDS, as in shock, it is skillful fluid management rather than the type of fluid used that is important. In the complicated post-shock patient with ARDS, the goal of supportive therapy is to minimize further fluid accumulation in the lung while perfusing body tissues. To do this requires adequate monitoring with pulmonary artery, arterial, and bladder catheters. A cardiac output adequate to support tissue perfusion must be obtained, but at the lowest possible capillary hydrostatic pressure to minimize fluid extravasation into the lung. In the presence of a capillary leak, the higher the capillary hydrostatic pressure, the greater the loss of fluid from the intravascular space into the interstitium of the lung.

There are a few clinical situations in which albumin is commonly but inappropriately used. Infusion of albumin to normalize a marginally lowered serum albumin concentration in the face of chronic disease such as malnutrition, cirrhosis, or nephrotic syndrome is unjustified. The serum albumin level is simply an indicator of some more basic underlying problems, and infusing albumin does not solve the problem. Rosenoer and associates (116) make this analogy: "If one's gas gauge points to empty, one simply need smash the glass and move the indicator up to full." Appropriate nutrition, even in cirrhosis, replenishes albumin stores more efficiently than does albumin infusion. Using albumin as a protein nutrient source is inefficient and more expensive than other forms of parenteral nutrition. Albumin does not contain all the essential amino acids (118, 144), and those it does have are unavailable for immediate protein synthesis because of albumin's long half-life (81).

In cirrhosis, infused albumin equilibrates with ascites and may decrease endogenous albumin synthesis (81). In nephrosis, endogenous albumin synthesis is increased, and there is no evidence that chronic edema or the underlying disease is improved by albumin infusion. Rather, infused albumin is lost in the urine. Although inappropriate for chronic use in each of these situations, the use of albumin for plasma volume support is appropriate, e.g., post paracentesis, dialysis, acute blood loss, and diuretic-induced hypotension.

Prescribing Information

Albumin is provided as three distinct preparations (Table 7.6) (12): normal serum albumin (NSA), 5% and 25%, and purified protein fraction (PPF). None of these products contains coagulation components, and hemodilution of the cellular and protein components of blood occurs with albumin use in large volume. Red blood cells and fresh frozen plasma should be added as appropriate to the resuscitation fluids. NSA has a shelf life of 3–

Table 7.6
Human Serum Albumin Products for Clinical Use[a]

Normal serum albumin (human)(NSA)
$25 \pm 1.5\%$ protein
or
$5 \pm 0.3\%$ protein

Purity:	At least 96% of the total protein in the final product must be albumin
pH:	6.9 ± 0.5
Sodium:	25% NSA: not more than 160 mEq/liter
	5% NSA: 130–160 mEq/liter
Dating:	When stored at 2–10°C: 5 years
	When stored at room temperature, no warmer than 37°C: 3 years

Plasma protein fraction (human) (PPF)
$5 \pm 0.3\%$ protein

Purity:	At least 83% of the total protein in the final product must be albumin; no more than 17% shall be globulins; no more than 1% of globulins shall be γ-globulin
pH:	7.0 ± 0.3
Sodium:	100–160 mEq/liter
Potassium:	No more than 2 mEq/liter
Dating:	When stored at 2–8°C: 5 years
	When stored at no warmer than 30°C: 3 years

Applicable to NSA and PPF
Heated at $60°C \pm 0.5°C$ for 10 hours
No preservatives
Pass standard tests for sterility and for pyrogenic substances

Stabilizers:	0.16 mmol sodium acetyltryptophanate
	or 0.08 mmol sodium acetyltryptophanate and
	0.08 mmol sodium caprylate

[a] From Barker LF: *Proceedings of the Workshop on Albumin,* February 12–13, 1975. Washington, DC, Department of Health, Education and Welfare, DHEW Publication No. (NIH) 76-925, 1976.

5 years, depending on the storage conditions. A 25% solution of NSA is hyperoncotic with an osmolality of 1500 mosm, resulting in its expansion to four to five times the administered volume (of 18 ml/g albumin). A 5% solution of NSA is isotonic with plasma. The protein content of NSA preparations is 96% albumin. PPF preparations contain only 83% albumin, with the remainder being α- and β-globulins. PPF is associated with an increased incidence of hypotension, thought to be secondary to kinins or prekallikrein activator activity present among these other proteins (4, 15, 30, 52).

A 25% albumin solution is often referred to as "salt-poor" albumin. This terminology dates from World War II when albumin preparations had to be stabilized with a "salt-rich" Na^+ content of 300 mEq/liter. Improved stabilization methods have now reduced the Na^+ content of all albumin preparations to 145 ± 15 mEq/liter (12). The "salt-poor" label has persisted although "salt-rich" solutions are no longer made (52). Selection among the albumin solutions can alter the amount of Na^+ a patient receives. Expansion of the intravascular space by 500 ml can be accomplished by using 100 ml of 25% albumin, adding 14.5 mEq of Na^+ (100 ml of a solution with 145 mEq/liter), or 500 ml of 5% albumin, adding 72.5 mEq of Na^+ (500 ml of a solution with 145 mEq/liter).

DEXTRAN

Dextran is a large glucose polymer, isolated originally from sugar beets contaminated with bacteria. In its native form it is a branched polysaccharide of 200,000 glucose units (Fig. 7.7). Partial hydrolysis produces polysaccharides of smaller size, which are available commercially as preparations having average molecular weights of 40,000 (dextran 40; D-40) or 70,000 (dextran 70; D-70). Dextran is

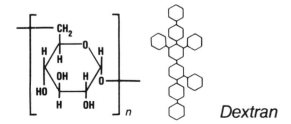

Figure 7.7 Dextran: glucose subunit and polymer.

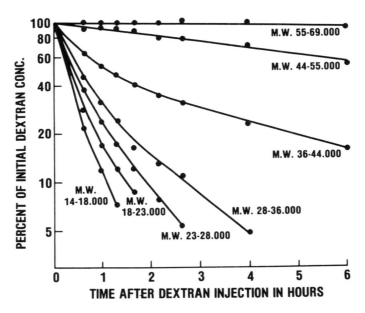

Figure 7.8 The disappearance rate of dextrans of different molecular weights from plasma. (From Arthurson G: *Scand J Clin Lab Invest* 16:76–80, 1964.)

used clinically as a volume-expanding agent; however, it is also used in the prevention of thromboembolism and to increase peripheral blood flow.

Pharmacology and Pharmacokinetics

Dextran molecules distribute in the extracellular space, mainly in the intravascular compartment. The particle size of the various dextrans affects the "dwell time" in the intravascular space and the duration of volume expansion accomplished. The major route of loss of dextran from the intravascular space is through the kidney. Smaller particles (<15,000 molecular weight) are rapidly filtered, not reabsorbed, and lost in the urine; however, while in the circulation, they exert osmotic activity. Larger particles remain in the circulation longer but exert less osmotic activity. D-40 and D-70 contain particles with molecular weights ranging from 10,000 to 80,000 (33) and 40,000 to 100,000, respectively. The circulating half-life of dextran varies with its particle size (37). The half-life for particles with molecular weights of 14,000–18,000 is 15 minutes, whereas for those greater than 55,000 it is several days (Fig. 7.8). Sixty to seventy percent of D-40 and 30–40% of D-70 is cleared in 12 hours (160). Since smaller particles are

cleared more rapidly than larger ones, and D-40 contains smaller particles than does D-70, D-40 is lost from the circulation faster than D-70. As a general rule, only 20% of D-40 dose and 30% of a D-70 dose remains in the circulation after 24 hours, and accumulation of large particles occurs over days of administration. For each preparation, after 24 hours the particles that accumulate have an average molecular weight of more than 80,000. With renal impairment small species accumulate. The larger particles are taken up by the reticuloendothelial system and are eventually metabolized to carbon dioxide and water. Other particles cross into the interstitial space and are recirculated through the lymphatic system.

Indications

VOLUME EXPANSION

Dextran has ideal properties as a plasma volume expander: a long dwell time and ultimate biodegradability. In shock, dextran increases survival (34, 36, 37, 139, 142, 153) and improves hemodynamic parameters (29, 35, 75, 113, 133). Dextran infusion is associated with increased renal plasma flow and a fall in plasma antidiuretic hormone levels when used in hypovolemia (160). It has favorable hemodynamic effects in restoring intravascular volume in shock when compared with other volume expanders (94, 133) (Figs. 7.4 and 7.5).

The reported degree of dextran-induced volume expansion varies, based on the type and concentration of solution used and the experimental setting. Dextran infusion increases the intravascular volume by an amount greater than or equal to that infused; however, the subsequent osmotic diuresis limits the duration of the volume expansion. One gram of dextran obligates 20–30 ml of water to the intravascular space (37, 50, 160). A 500-ml bolus of D-40 produces a 750-ml expansion of intravascular volume at 1 hour and 1050 ml at 2 hours (133). Some volume expansion may persist up to 8 hours in hypovolemic patients. (69). Studies of shock in dogs show similar volume expansion, with 47% of the bolus infused remaining in the intravascular space after 4 hours (37). Four to six hours after the infusion of either D-40 or D-70, the degree of intravascular volume expansion is similar and approximately equal to the amount infused (160).

PROMOTION OF PERIPHERAL BLOOD FLOW

In addition to increasing plasma volume, dextran has other effects on blood flow that potentiate flow in the microvasculature (5). By coating endothelial surfaces, dextran reduces interaction with the cellular elements in blood (160). Sludging and cellular aggregation seen in shock are reduced by reduction of blood viscosity (29) and coating of cellular elements. Altered platelet function, including diminished adherence and degranulation, limits thrombus formation and activation of the clotting cascade mechanism (1, 80, 171). Dextran is also reported to copolymerize with fibrin monomer, resulting in a less stable clot that is more susceptible to endogenous lysis (1).

PREVENTION OF THROMBOEMBOLISM

Dextran is effective in reducing the incidence of thromboembolic disease (115, 122). It is beneficial, compared with controls, for the prevention of deep venous thrombosis in general surgery patients and following total hip replacement. However, data for use of heparin in this same group are as good or better (47, 61), without the attendant risks of dextran.

OTHER USES

Dextran has been used in the therapy of ichemic ulceration of the skin, arterial occlusion, frostbite, and stroke, and in cell harvest in plasmapheresis and priming for extracorporeal circulation.

Side Effects

RENAL FAILURE

Dextran-induced renal failure may occur (45, 89, 90), especially in the face of unrecognized hypovolemia. The mechanism for the renal failure is tubular obstruction secondary to concentration and precipitation of dextran in the tubules with cast formation (26). Three conditions are necessary to cause this side-effect: (a) decreased renal perfusion pressure, (b) dextran in the tubule, and (c) a continued stimulus for water reabsorption. Unfortunately, these conditions exist in intravascular volume depletion and its resuscitation with dextran.

ANAPHYLAXIS

The incidence of anaphylactic reactions to dextran is between 1% (111) and 5.3% (156). Reactions occur early, within one-half hour after the infusion is begun, and may include urticaria, rash, nausea, bronchospasm, shock, and death. Dextran is a potent antigen and has cross-reactivity with bacterial polysaccharide antigens. Patients with *Streptococcus pneumoniae* or *Salmonella* infections may therefore be more prone to dextran reactions. Gut flora make endogenous dextran from dextrose, and a small portion of the patient population has never received dextran yet has circulating precipitins to the dextran molecule.

OSMOTIC DIURESIS

As previously noted, osmotic diuresis occurs almost immediately on infusion of any dextran preparation as smaller species are filtered and not reabsorbed. The effect is greater with D-40 than D-70 because of the prevalence of small species in D-40. In the face of this obligate osmotic diuresis, urine volume cannot serve as a guide to the adequacy of intravascular volume repletion. If blood volume is inadequately restored in the patient receiving dextran, the stage is set for all the conditions to be met to produce renal failure.

BIOCHEMICAL ALTERATIONS

Blood glucose levels can be falsely elevated in patients receiving dextran if the glucose measurement is done by analysis using acid, which converts dextran to dextrose. Dextran may also cause false elevations of the total protein concentration. Total protein measurements can be checked using a refractometer. The refractometer reading is within 1 g/dl of the true value.

Dextran can interfere with the cross-matching of blood. The coating action of dextran on red blood cells causes cells to aggregate, mimicking a (nonexistent) cross-match problem. This is a problem especially when blood is drawn from a site proximal to the dextran intravenous infusion site, and is simply handled by drawing blood prior to dextran infusion or notifying the blood bank that the patient is receiving dextran. Other biochemical alterations include false elevation of the serum bilirubin level and alteration of colloid oncotic pressure measurements (52).

BLEEDING DIATHESIS

Dextran inhibits erythrocyte aggregation in vivo (29). It adheres to vessel walls and cellular elements of the blood (16, 80); decreases platelet adhesiveness (80, 172), serum fibrinogen, and other factor levels (33); and increases Ivy bleeding time and incisional bleeding (156). In dogs, clinical bleeding is not observed until 80% replacement of plasma volume has been achieved (154). At doses less than 1.5 g/kg/day, clinical bleeding is not encountered (160).

RETICULOENDOTHELIAL BLOCKADE

Dextran temporarily impairs reticuloendothelial system function (76), and by so doing may diminish immune competence.

Recommendations for Use

Dextran is an effective agent for intravascular volume expansion and has some specific beneficial effects on blood flow through the microvasculature that makes its use in shock very attractive. In addition, it is ultimately biodegradable. Its side effects, as described above, are noteworthy in the critically ill population. Dextran can cause a bleeding diathesis and interfere with blood cross-matching in a patient suffering from hemorrhagic shock. Its use can produce renal failure whenever renal perfusion is impaired, i.e., in any shock situation. Dextran causes an immediate osmotic diuresis, which if misinterpreted may potentiate volume depletion and ultimately renal failure, especially in critically ill patients with underlying diseases such as diabetes mellitus.

Prescribing Information

PREPARATIONS

Dextran 40 is commercially available as a 10% solution in normal saline or 5% dextrose in water. Dextran 70 is commercially available as a 6% solution in normal saline or 5% dextrose in water or in 10% invert sugar. These preparations require no mixing and can be "hung" just as supplied.

DOSAGE

To avoid bleeding diathesis, the total administered dosage should remain less than 1.5 g/kg/day of D-40 and 2 g/kg/day of D-70. For restoration of blood volume in shock, this amount (approximately 1000 ml of 10% D-40 for a 70-kg man) may be given acutely in conjunction with crystalloid, packed red blood cells, and plasma as necessary. The *Medical Letter on Drugs and Therapeutics* recommends using less than 1000 ml/day of D-40 (3). For use in prophylaxis of thromboembolic disease or peripheral vascular disease, dosage should be increased to 50 ml/hr in 5 ml increments of D-40, with monitoring of urine output and specific gravity. Infusion should be discontinued for specific gravity greater than 1.030 and urine volume less than 0.5 ml/kg/hr (155).

HYDROXYETHYL STARCH

Hydroxyethyl starch is a synthetic starch molecule closely resembling glycogen. Its development is the result of a concerted effort to find a colloidal volume-expanding agent that is free from the toxicities of previously developed plasma expanders. Its similarity to glycogen may account for its relative freedom from immune reactions (Fig. 7.9).

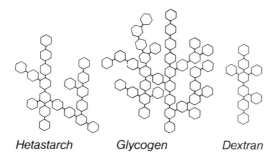

Hetastarch   *Glycogen*   *Dextran*

Figure 7.9 Two-dimensional representations of hydroxyethyl starch (hetastarch), glycogen, and dextran molecules. (Modified from Thompson WL: Proceedings from a Symposium: Hespan (Hetastarch): Historical Perspective and Development. Toronto, February 1982.)

Physiology and Pharmacokinetics

Hydroxyethyl starch (hetastarch) is available for clinical use as a 6% solution in normal saline. The average molecular weight of the particles is 69,000, with a range of 10,000–1,000,000. Glucose subunits are linked in α-1,4 and α-1,6 linkages to form a polymer that is more branched than dextran and is globular rather than linear. In addition, hydroxyethyl groups are substituted on the glucose subunits, which slows degradation in vivo (Figs. 7.9 and 7.10).

After intravenous infusion there is an almost immediate appearance of smaller particles in the urine (molecular weight, 50,000) (93). Studies in normal human volunteers show that 46% of an administered dose is excreted in the urine by 2 days and 64% by 8 days (108, 176). Larger particles remain in the circulation longer. Their rate of disappearance depends on their absorption by tissues (notably liver and spleen), gradual return to the circulation, uptake by the reticuloendothelial system, and subsequent degradation to smaller particles cleared through urine and bile. Blood α-amylase also degrades larger particles to smaller species. The rate of amylase degradation of hetastarch is slow compared with the rate for naturally occuring starches, probably because of the presence of hydroxyethyl groups substituted on 70% of the glucose subunits. Less than 1% of infused hetastarch can be recovered as exhaled CO_2.

As with dextran, the half-life of hetastarch represents a composite of the half-lives of various sized particles. Ninety percent of a single infusion of hetastarch leaves the circulation in 42 days, with a half-life of 17 days (176). The remaining 10% has a half-life of 48 days. Small amounts of hetastarch have been measured in the circulation as long as 17 weeks after a single infusion. The uptake of hetastarch molecules by the cells of the reticuloendothelial system has caused concern that the immune function of the patient could be compromised. However, clinically significant reticuloendothelial system dysfunction has not been demonstrated (78, 128, 149).

Plasma volume expansion after infusion of hetastarch is equal to or greater than that produced by D-70 (79, 92, 146, 154, 157, 158) or 5% albumin. Studies in humans show an increase in blood volume from 2.3 liters/m² to

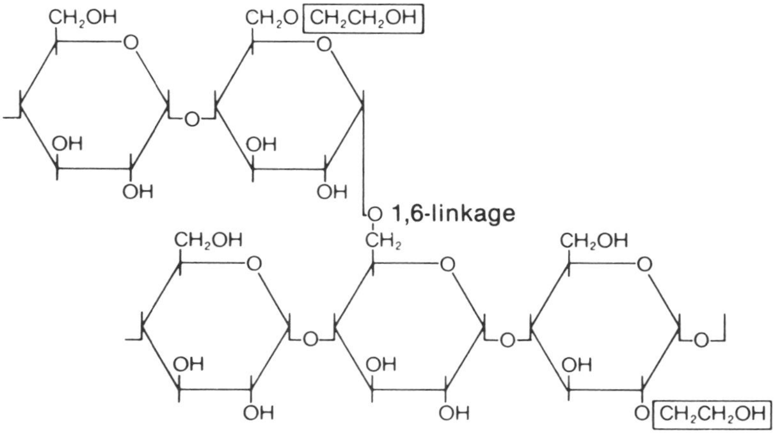

Figure 7.10 The hydroxyethyl starch molecule. Note the α-1,6-linkage and hydroxyethyl groups in *boxes*. (Modified from *Answers to Frequently Asked Questions About Hespan (Hetastarch)*. McGraw Park, IL, American Critical Care Publications, 1981, p. 1.

2.9 liters/m^2, with a duration of at least 3 hours (77). Although there is some variability, infusions of hetastarch increase intravascular volume by an amount equal to or greater than the volume infused (11, 62, 75, 77, 92, 146, 159). The increase in intravascular volume is associated with improvement in hemodynamic parameters in critically ill patients (38, 63, 77, 88, 108, 129). The increase in colloid pressure is similar to that seen with albumin (53, 63).

Indications

Hydroxyethyl starch is indicated for use as a plasma volume–expanding agent in shock from hemorrhage, trauma, sepsis, or burns. It has adjunctive application in leukapheresis, and as a pump prime and volume expander in cardiopulmonary bypass.

Side Effects

COAGULOPATHY

Hetastarch is associated with minor alterations in laboratory measurements, but not with clinical bleeding when used in doses below 1500 ml/day (79, 145); doses greater than 1500 ml/day have been administered without bleeding complications (129). Dilutional effects on cellular and protein elements of the blood clotting cascade are produced secondary to the blood volume–expanding effect. However, the laboratory abnormalities are not explained by dilution alone. Coagulation profile discrepancies include a transient decrease in platelet count, prolonged prothrombin and partial thromboplastin times, and a decrease in the tensile clot strength (114, 145, 150–152, 169). In clinical series bleeding is a problem in only a small minority of cases (79, 145). Experience with hetastarch in leukapheresis is extensive, with bleeding complications occurring only rarely (44, 148).

PULMONARY EDEMA

Hetastarch has been used successfully in critically ill patients with various forms of shock without production of pulmonary edema or change in pulmonary function (77, 108).

ANAPHYLAXIS

The incidence of anaphylactic reactions to hetastarch (molecular weights > 16,000) in-

fusions is less than 0.085%. The incidence of severe reactions including shock or cardiopulmonary arrest is 0.008% (111). Hetastarch is not immunogenic (91, 112) and does not induce histamine release (83).

HYPERAMYLASEMIA

Serum amylase levels are elevated following hetastarch administration (67). Complexes of amylase and hetastarch molecules create macroamylase particles, which undergo urinary excretion at a much slower rate than the solitary amylase molecule. Serum amylase levels commonly reach twice normal after hetastarch infusion. There is no alteration of normal pancreatic function.

Recommendations for Use

Hetastarch may be used whenever colloid is required to restore plasma volume. Its properties as a volume-expanding agent are similar to those of 5% albumin solutions. At doses of 1500 ml/day or less, bleeding complications are avoided; doses greater than 1500 ml/day have been administered without bleeding complications (129). Hetastarch, like other colloid solutions, does not carry oxygen and must be administered in conjunction with packed red blood cells to maintain adequate oxygen content of the blood. Although rare, clinical bleeding has been associated with its use. Fresh frozen plasma and platelets should be replaced as indicated by clinical bleeding and the results of serial coagulation profiles. Hetastarch should be used with extreme caution in the presence of a known bleeding diathesis.

Adequate monitoring for detection of volume overload is crucial in hetastarch as with infusion of all other volume expanders. Volume overload pulmonary edema may be unwittingly produced despite careful monitoring of left heart filling pressures as the osmotic action of the infused hetastarch draws interstitial space water into the circulation. The immediate osmotic diuresis associated with its use protects somewhat from this phenomenon. Urine volume must be expected to increase acutely secondary to the osmotic diuresis, and this must not be misinterpreted as a sign of adequate peripheral perfusion. Patients with renal impairment are particularly subject to initial volume overload and to accumulation of hetastarch in the circulation and tissues with repeated administration. In these patients, initial volume resuscitation accomplished with hetastarch should be maintained with another plasma volume expander such as albumin or crystalloid.

Serum amylase values will be approximately twice normal after hetastarch infusion and are not indicative of pancreatitis. When serum amylase measurements are important (as in pancreatitis, bowel obstruction, parotitis), serum levels should be measured prior to infusion of hetastarch. Elevations of serum amylase may persist for 5 days postinfusion.

Hetastarch costs about one-fourth as much as an equivalent amount of 5% albumin (Table 7.2). Although dextran preparations cost even less than hetastarch, their use is associated with more side effects, such as anaphylactoid reactions, interference with blood typing and cross-matching, antigenicity, coagulopathy, and renal failure.

Prescribing Information

PREPARATIONS

Hetastarch is available as a 6% solution of 0.9% sodium chloride. The pH is 5.5 and the osmolarity 310 mosm/liter. It is bottled ready for infusion in 500-ml bottles.

DOSAGE

Usual total dosage is 20 ml/kg/day, but this is not an absolute upper limit. The total volume may be administered over 1 hour if the clinical situation demands adequate volume resuscitation.

For leukapheresis, 250–700 ml may be infused in the ratio of 1:8 with venous blood. Ten repetitions over the course of 5 weeks have been reported to be safe; however, hetastarch accumulation in the tissues will occur. Safety beyond this duration and frequency of administration is not known.

References

1. Aberg M, Hedner V, Bergentz S: Effect of dextran on factor VIII and platelet function. Ann Surg 189:243–247, 1979.
2. Abramowicz M (ed): Hetastarch (Hespan) a new plasma expander. Med Lett Drugs Ther 23(4):16, 1981.
3. Abramowicz M (ed): Med Lett Drugs Ther 10(1):3,1968.
4. Alving BM, Hojima Y, Pisano JJ: Hypotension associated with prekallikrein activator (Hageman-factor fragments) in plasma protein fraction. N Engl J Med 299:66–70, 1978.
5. Amundson B. Jennische E, Haljamae H: Skeletal muscle microcirculatory and cellular metabolic effects of whole blood. Ringer's acetate and dextran-70 infusions in hemorrhagic shock. Circ Shock 7:111–120, 1980.
6. Appel PL, Shoemaker WC: Evaluation of fluid therapy in adult respiratory failure. Crit Care Med 9:862–869, 1981.
7. Arthurson G. Granath K, Thoren L, Wallenius G: The renal excretion of LMW dextran. Acta Clin Scand 127:543–551, 1964.
8. Arthurson G, Wallenius G: The renal clearance of dextran of different molecular sizes in normal humans. Scand J Clin Lab Invest 16:81–86, 1964.
9. Atik M: Dextran-40 and dextran-70, a review. Arch Surg 94:664–672, 1967.
10. Atik M: The uses of dextran in surgery: a current evaluation. Surgery 65:548–562, 1969.
11. Ballinger WF: Preliminary report on the use of hydroxyethyl starch solution in man. J Surg Res 6:180–183, 1966.
12. Barker LF: Albumin products and the Bureau of Biologics. In Proceedings of the Workshop on Albumin, February 12–13, 1975. Washington, DC, Department of Health, Education and Welfare, DHEW Publication No. (NIH) 76–925, 1976, pp 22–27.
13. Baue AE, Tragus ET, Wolfson SK: Hemodynamic and metabolic effects of Ringer's lactate solution in hemorrhagic shock. Ann Surg 166:29–38, 1967.
14. Bergentz SE: Dextran prophylaxis of pulmonary embolism. World J Surg 2:19–24, 1978.
15. Bland JHL, Laver MB, Lowenstein E: Vasodilation effect of commercial 5% plasma protein fraction solutions. JAMA 224:1721–1724, 1973.
16. Bloom WL, Harmer J, Bryant MF: Coating of blood vessel surfaces and blood cells: a new concept in the prevention of intravascular thrombosis. Proc Soc Exp Biol Med 115:384–386, 1964.
17. Bogan RK, Gale GR, Walton RP: Fate of ^{14}C labelled hydroxyethyl starch in animals. Toxicol Appl Pharmacol 15:206–211, 1969.
18. Boon JC, Jesch F, Ring J, Messmer K: Intravascular persistence of hydroxyethyl starch in man. Eur Surg Res 8:497–503, 1976.
19. Boutros AR, Ruess R, Olson L: Comparison of hemodynamic, pulmonary and renal effects of use of 3 types of fluid after major surgical procedures on abdominal aorta. Crit Care Med 7:9–13, 1979.
20. Brinkmeyer DO, Safar P, Motoyama E: Superiority of colloid over electrolyte solution for fluid resuscitation (severe normovolemic hemodilution). Crit Care Med 9:369–371, 1981.
21. Browse NL, Clemeson G, Bateman NT: Effect of IV dextran-70 and pneumatic leg compression on incidence of post-op pulmonary embolism. Br Med J 2:1281–1284, 1976.
22. Canizaro PC, Prager MC, Shires GT: The influence of Ringer's lactate solution during shock: changes in lactate, excess lactate and pH. Am J Surg 122:494–501, 1971.
23. Carey JS, Scharschmidt BF, Culliford AT: Hemodynamic effectiveness of colloid and electrolyte solutions for replacement of simulated operative blood loss. Surg Gynecol Obstet 131:679–686, 1970.
24. Carey LC, Lowery BD, Cloutier CT: Hemorrhagic shock. Curr Probl Surg 1:3–48, 1971.
25. Carrico CJ, Canizaro PC, Shires GT: Fluid resuscitation following injury; rationale for the use of balanced salt solutions. Crit Care Med 4:46–54, 1976.
26. Chinitz JL: Pathophysiology and prevention of dextran-40 induced anuria. J Lab Clin Med 77:76–87, 1971.
27. Christensen EI, Moundsback AB: Effects of dextran on lysosomal ultrastructure and protein digestion in renal proximal tubule. Kidney Int 16:301–311, 1979.
28. Coghill TH, Moore EE, Dunn EI: Coagulation changes after albumin resuscitation. Crit Care Med 9:22–26, 1981.

29. Cohn JN, Luria MH, Daddario RC: Studies in clinical shock and hypotension. V. Hemodynamic effects of dextran. *Circulation* 35:316–326, 1967.

30. Coleman RW: Paradoxical hypotension after volume expansion with plasma protein fraction. *N Engl J Med* 299:97–98, 1978.

31. Coller FA, Iob B, Vaughn HH, Kalder NM, Moyer CA: Translocation of fluid produced by intravenous administration of isotonic salt solutions in man postoperatively. *Ann Surg* 122:663–677, 1945.

32. Dahn MS, Lucas CE, Ledgerwood AM: Negative inotropic effect of albumin resuscitation for shock. *Surgery* 86:235–241, 1979.

33. Data JL, Nies AS: Dextran 40. *Ann Intern Med* 81:500–504, 1974.

34. Dawidson I, Eriksson B: Statistical evaluations of plasma substitutes based on 10 variables. *Crit Care Med* 10:653–657, 1982.

35. Dawidson I, Eriksson B, Gelin LE: Oxygen consumption and recovery from surgical shock in rats: a comparison on the efficacy of different plasma substitutes. *Crit Care Med* 7:460–465, 1979.

36. Dawidson I, Gelin LE, Haglind E: Plasma volume, intravascular protein content, hemodynamic and oxygen transport changes during intestinal shock in dogs. Comparison of relative effectiveness of various plasma expanders. *Crit Care Med* 8:73–80, 1980.

37. Dawidson I, Gelin LE, Hedman L: Hemodilution and recovery from experimental intestinal shock in rats: a comparison of the efficacy of three colloids and one electrolyte solution. *Crit Care Med* 9:42–46, 1981.

38. Diehl JT, Lester JL, Cosgrove DM: Clinical comparison of hetastarch and albumin in postoperative cardiac patients. *Ann Thor Surg* 34:674–679, 1982.

39. Diomi P: Studies on renal tubular morphology and toxicity after large doses of dextran-40 in the rabbit. *Lab Invest* 22:355–360, 1970.

40. Ebert RV, Stead EA Jr, Gibson JG: Response of normal subjects to acute blood loss with special reference to the mechanism of restoration of blood volume. *Arch Intern Med* 68:578–590, 1941.

41. Elkington JR, Danowski TS: *The Body Fluids: Basic Physiology and Practical Therapeutics.* Baltimore, Williams & Wilkins, 1955.

42. Elwyn DH, Bryan-Brown CW, Shoemaker WC: Nutritional aspects of body water dissociations in postoperative and depleted patients. *Ann Surg* 182:76–85, 1975.

43. Esrig BC, Fulton RL: Sepsis, resuscitated hemorrhagic shock and "shock lung." An experimental correlation. *Ann Surg* 182:218–227, 1975.

44. Farrales FB, Belcher C, Summers T, Bayer WL: Effect of hydroxyethyl starch on platelet function following granulocyte collection using the continuous flow cell separator. *Transfusion* 17:635–637, 1977.

45. Feest TG: Low molecular weight dextran: a continuing cause of acute renal failure. *Br Med J* 2:1300, 1976.

46. Gaisford WD, Pandey D, Jensen CG: Pulmonary changes in hemorrhagic shock. II. Ringer's solution vs. colloid infusion. *Am J Surg* 124:738–743, 1972.

47. Gallus AS, Hirsch J, O'Brien SE: Prevention of venous thrombosis with small, subcutaneous doses of heparin. *JAMA* 235:1980–1984, 1976.

48. Gelin LE, Solvell L, Zederfeldt B: Plasma volume expanding effect of low viscous dextran and macrodex. *Acta Chir Scand* 122:309–322, 1961.

49. Granger DN, Gabel JC, Drahe RE, Taylor AD: Physiologic basis for the clinical use of albumin solutions. *Surg Gynecol Obstet* 146:97–104, 1978.

50. Gruber VF, Messmer K: Colloids for blood volume support. *Prog Surg* 15:49–76, 1977.

51. Guyton AC: *Textbook of Medical Physiology,* ed 4. Philadelphia, WB Saunders, 1971.

52. Habel M: Critical care update. *Crit Care Med* 8:14–21, 1981.

53. Haupt MT, Rackow EC: Colloid osmotic pressure and fluid resuscitation with hetastarch, albumin and saline solutions. *Crit Care Med* 10:159–162, 1982.

54. Hauser CJ, Shoemaker WC, Turpin I: Oxygen transport responses to colloids and crystalloids in critically ill surgical patients. *Surg Gynecol Obstet* 150:811–816, 1980.

55. Hays RM: Dynamics of body water and electrolytes. In Maxwell MH, Kleeman CR (eds): *Clinical Disorders of Fluid and Electrolyte Metabolism.* New York, McGraw-Hill, 1972.

56. Heye JT, Janeway CA: The use of human albumin in military practice. *US Navy Med Bull* 40:785–791, 1942.

57. Holcroft JW, Trunkey DD: Extravascular lung water following hemorrhagic shock in the baboon: comparison between resuscitation with Ringer's lactate and plasmanate. *Ann Surg* 180:408–417, 1974.

58. Holcroft JW, Trunkey DD: Pulmonary extravasation of albumin during and after hemorrhagic shock in baboons. *J Surg Res* 18:91–97, 1979.

59. Janeway CA, Gibson ST, Woodruff LM: Albumin in the treatment of shock. *J Clin Invest* 23:465–475, 1944.

60. Johnson D, Lucan CE, Gerrick SJ: Altered coagulation after albumin supplements for treatment of oligemic shock. *Ann Surg* 114:379–383, 1979.

61. Kakkar VV: International multicenter trial: prevention of fatal postoperative pulmonary embolism by low doses of heparin. *Lancet* 2:45–51, 1975.

62. Kilian J, Spilker D, Borst R: Effect of 6% hydroxyethyl starch, 4.5% dextran 60 and 5.5% oxypolygelatine on blood volume and circulation in human volunteers. *Anaethesist* 24:193–197, 1975.

63. Kirklin JK, Lell WA, Kouchoukos NT: Hydroxyethyl starch vs. albumin for colloid infusion following cardiopulmonary bypass in patients undergoing myocardial revascularization. *Ann Thorac Surg* 37:40–46, 1984.

64. Klapp D, Harrison WL: Evaluation of albumin use by medical audit. *Am J Hosp Pharm* 36:1205–1209, 1979.

65. Knipping WJ (ed): *Drug Topics Redbook,* ed 90. Oradell, NJ, Medical Economics, 1986.

66. Knopp R, Claypool R, Leonardi D: Use of the tilt test in measuring acute blood loss. *Ann Emerg Med* 9(2):29–32, 1980.

67. Kohler H, Kirch W, Horstmann HJ: Hydroxyethyl starch–induced macroamylasemia. *Int J Clin Pharmacol* 15:428–431, 1977.

68. Kohler H, Kirch W, Klein H: The effect of 6% hydroxyethyl starch 450/0.7, 10% dextran 40 and 3.5% gelatin on plasma volume in patients with terminal renal failure. *Anaesthesist* 24:193–197, 1975.

69. Kohler H, Zschiedrich H, Clasen R: Blutvolumen, kolloidosmotischer Druck un Nierenfunktion von Probanden nach Infusion Mittelmolekularer 10% Hydroxyethylstarke 200/0.5 und 10% Dextran 40. *Anaesthesist* 31:61–67, 1982.

70. Kovalik SG, Ledgerwood AM, Lucas CE: The cardiac effect of altered calcium homeostasis after albumin resuscitation. *J Trauma* 21:275–279, 1981.

71. Laks H, O'Connor NE, Anderson W, et al: Crystalloid versus colloid hemodilution in man. *Surg Gynecol Obstet* 142:506–512, 1976.

72. Laks H, Pilon RN, Anderson W: Intraoperative prebleeding in man: effect of colloid hemodilution on blood volume, lung water, hemodynamics and oxygen transport. *Surgery* 78:130–137, 1975.

73. Laks H, Pilon RN, Anderson W, et al: Acute normovolemic hemodilution with crystalloid vs colloid replacement. *Surg Forum* 25:21–22, 1974.

74. Laks H, Pilon RN, Klovekorn WP: Acute hemodilution; its effects on hemodynamics and oxygen transport in anesthetized man. *Ann Surg* 180:103–109, 1974.

75. Lamke LO, Liljedahl SO: Plasma volume changes after infusion of various plasma expanders. *Resuscitation* 5:93–102, 1976.

76. Lamke LO, Liljedahl SO: Plasma volume expansion after infusion of 5%, 20%, and 25% albumin solutions in patients. *Resuscitation* 5:85–92, 1976.

77. Lazrove S, Waxman K, Shippy C: Hemodynamic blood volume and oxygen transport responses to albumin and hydroxyethyl starch infusions in critically ill post operative patients. *Crit Care Med* 8:302–306, 1980.

78. Lenz G, Hempel V, Jurger H, Worle H: Effect of hydroxyethyl starch, oxypolygelatin and human albumin on the phagocytic function of the reticuloendothelial system in healthy subjects. *Anaesthesist* 35:423–428, 1986.

79. Lee WH, Cooper N, Weidner MG: Clinical evaluation of a new plasma expander; hydroxyethyl starch. *J Trauma* 8:381–393, 1968.

80. Lewis JH, Szetol LF, Beyer WL: Severe hemodilution with hydroxyethyl starch and dextrans. *Arch Surg* 93:941–950, 1966.

81. Lewis RT: Albumin: role and discriminative use in surgery. *Can J Surg* 23:322–328, 1980.

82. Liljedahl JO, Rieger, A: Blood volume and plasma protein. IV. Importance of thoracic duct lymph in restitution of plasma volume and plasma proteins after bleeding and immediate substitution in splenectomized dogs. *Acta Chir Scand [Suppl]* 379:39–51, 1967.

83. Lorenz W, Dolniche A, Freund M: Plasma histamine levels in man following infusion of hydroxyethyl starch: a contribution to the question of allergic or anaphylactoid reactions following administration of a new plasma substitute. *Anesthesist* 24:228–230, 1975.

84. Lowe RJ, Moss GS, Jilek J, et al: Crystalloid vs. colloid in the etiology of pulmonary failure after trauma; a randomized trial in man. *Surgery* 81:676–683, 1977.

85. Lowery BD, Cloutier CT, Carey LC: Electrolyte solutions in resuscitation in human hemorrhagic shock. *Surg Gynecol Obstet* 133:273–284, 1971.

86. Lucas CE, Ledgerwood AM, Higgins RF: Impaired pulmonary function after albumin resuscitation from shock. *J Trauma* 20:446–451, 1980.

87. Lucas CE, Weaver D, Higgins RF: Effects of albumin vs. nonalbumin resuscitation on plasma volume and renal excretory function. *J Trauma* 18:564–570, 1978.

88. Maggio RA, Rha CC, Somberry ED, Praeger PI, Pasley RW, Reed GE: Hemodynamic comparison of albumin and hydroxyethyl starch in post operative cardiac surgery patients. *Crit Care Med* 11:943–945, 1983.

89. Mailoux L, Swartz CD, Capizzi R, et al: Acute renal failure after administration of LMW dextran. *N Engl J Med* 277:1113–1118, 1967.

90. Matheson NA, Diomi P: Renal failure after the administration of dextran-40. *Surg Gynecol Obstet* 131:661–668, 1970.

91. Maurer PH, Berardinelli B: Immunologic studies with hydroxyethyl starch (HES). *Transfusion* 8:265–268, 1968.

92. Metcalf W, Papadopoulos A, Talano R: Clinical physiologic study of hydroxyethyl starch. *Surg Gynecol Obstet* 131:255–267, 1970.

93. Mishler JM, Borberg H, Emerson PM: Hydroxyethyl starch, an agent for hypovolemic shock treatment. II. Urinary excretion in normal volunteers following three consecutive daily infusions. *Br J Pharmacol* 4:591–595, 1977.

94. Modig J: Effectiveness of dextran 70 vs. Ringer's acetate in traumatic shock and adult respiratory distress syndrome. *Crit Care Med* 14:454–457, 1986.

95. Moore FD, Daher FJ, Boyden CM: Hemorrhage in normal man. I. Distribution and dispersal of saline infusions following acute blood loss; clinical kinetics of blood volume support. *Ann Surg* 163:485–504, 1966.

96. Moss GS, Lower RJ, Jilek J, et al: Colloid or crystalloid in the resuscitation of hemorrhagic shock. A controlled clinical trial. *Surgery* 89:434–438, 1981.

97. Moss GS, Proctor JH, Homer LD: A comparison of asanguinous fluids and whole blood in the treatment of hemorrhagic shock. *Surg Gynecol Obstet* 129:1247–1257, 1969.

98. Moss GS, Siegel DC, Cochin A, et al: Effects of saline and colloid solutions on pulmonary function in hemorrhagic shock. *Surg Gynecol Obstet* 133:53–58, 1971.

99. Muller N, Popov-Cenic S, Kladetzky RG: The effect of hydroxyethyl starch on the intra and postoperative behavior of haemostasis. *Bibl Anat* 16:460–462, 1977.

100. Nilsson E, Lamke LO, Liljedahl SO: Is albumin therapy worthwhile in surgery for colorectal cancer? *Acta Chir Scand* 146:619–622, 1980.

101. Oh MS, Carroll HT, Goldstein DA: Hyperchloremic acidosis during the recovery phase of diabetic ketosis. *Ann Intern Med* 89:925–927, 1978.

102. O'Riordan JP: Current concepts in utilization and provision of human albumin. *Haematologia* 13:175–184, 1980.

103. Paul K, Schlesinger RG, Schanfield MS: Reaction to albumin (letter to editor). *JAMA* 245:234–235, 1981.

104. Pitts RF: Volume and composition of the body fluids. In *Physiology of the Kidney and Body Fluids.* Chicago, Year Book, 1974.

105. Poole GV, Meredity JW, Pernell T, et al: Comparison of colloids and crystalloids in resuscitation from hemorrhagic shock. *Surg Gynecol Obstet* 154:577–586, 1982.

106. Proctor HJ, Moss GS, Homer LD, et al: Changes in lung compliance in experimental shock and resuscitation. *Ann Surg* 169:82–92, 1969.

107. Puri VK, Howard M, Paidipaty B: Comparative studies of hydroxyethyl starch and albumin in hypovolemia (abstract). *Crit Care Med* 10:230, 1982.

108. Puri VK, Paidipaty B, White L: Hydroxyethyl starch for resuscitation of patients with hypovolemia in shock. *Crit Care Med* 9:833–837, 1981.

109. Reynolds M: Cardiovascular effects of large volumes of isotonic saline infused intravenously into dogs following severe hemorrhage. *Am J Physiol* 158:418–428, 1949.

110. Rice CL, Moss GS: Blood and blood substitutes: current practice. *Adv Surg* 13:93–114, 1979.

111. Ring J, Messmer K: Incidence and severity of anaphylactoid reactions to colloid volume substitutes. *Lancet* 1:466–469, 1977.

112. Ring J, Siefert J, Messmer K: Anaphylactoid reactions due to hydroxyethyl starch infusion. *Eur Surg Res* 8:389–399, 1976.

113. Risberg B, Miller E, Hughes J: Comparison of the pulmonary effects of rapid infusion of a crystalloid and a colloid solution. *Acta Chir Scand* 147:613–618, 1981.

114. Rock G, Wise P: Plasma expansion during granulocyte procurement. Cumulative effects of hydroxyethyl starch. *Blood* 53:1156–1163, 1979.

115. Rose SD: Prophylaxis of thromboembolic disease. *Med Clin North Am* 63:1205–1224, 1979.

116. Rosenoer VM, Skillman JJ, Hastings PR: Albumin synthesis and nitrogen balance in postoperative patients. *Surgery* 87:305–312, 1980.

117. Rothschild MA, Bauman A, Yalow RS: The effect of large doses of desiccated thyroid on the distribution and metabolism of albumin ^{131}I in euthyroid subjects. *J Clin Invest* 36:422–428, 1957.

118. Rothschild MA, Oratz M, Schreiber SS: Albumin metabolism *Gastroenterology* 64:324–337, 1973.

119. Rothschild MA, Oratz M, Schreiber SS: Albumin synthesis. *N Engl J Med* 286:748–756, 816–820, 1972.

120. Rothschild MA, Schreiber SS, Oratz M: The effects of adrenocortical hormones on albumin metabolism studies with albumin [131]I. *J Clin Invest* 37:1229–1235, 1958.

121. Rowe MI, Arango A: Colloid vs. crystalloid resuscitation in experimental bowel obstruction. *J Pediatr Surg* 11:635–643, 1976.

122. Sasahara AA, Sharma GV, Parisi AF: New develop-

ments in the detection and prevention of venous thromboembolism. *Am J Cardiol* 43:1214–1224, 1979.

123. Scattchard G, Batchelder AC, Brown A: Chemical, clinical and immunological studies on the products of human plasma fraction. VI. The osmotic pressure of plasma and serum albumin: *J Clin Invest* 23:458–464, 1944.

124. Schildt B, Bouvang RM, Sollenberg M: Plasma substitute induced impairment of the reticuloendothelial system function. *Acta Chir Scand* 141:7–13, 1975.

125. Scribner BH (ed): *University of Washington Teaching Syllabus for the Course on Fluid and Electrolyte Balance.* Seattle, University of Washington Press, 1969.

126. Sgouris JT, Rene A (eds): *Proceedings of the Workshop on Albumin,* February 12–13, 1975. Washington, DC, Department of Health, Education and Welfare, DHEW Publication No. (NIH) 76–925, 1976.

127. Shah DM, Browner BD, Dutten RE: Cardiac output and pulmonary wedge pressure, use for evaluation of fluid replacement in trauma patients. *Arch Surg* 112:1161–1164, 1977.

128. Shatney CH, Chaudry IH: Hydroxyethyl starch administration does not depress reticuloendothelial function or increase mortality from sepsis. *Circ Shock* 13:21–26, 1984.

129. Shatney CH, Deapiha K, Militello PR. Majerus TC, Dawson RB: Efficacy of hetastarch in the resuscitation of patients with multisystem trauma and shock. *Arch Surg* 118: 804–809, 1983.

130. Shires GT, Canizaro PC: Fluid resuscitation in the severely injured. *Surg Clin North Am* 53:1341–1366, 1973.

131. Shires T, Cohn D, Carrico J: Fluid therapy in hemorrhagic shock. *Arch Surg* 88:688–693, 1964.

132. Shires GT, Williams J, Brown F: Acute changes in extracellular fluids associated with major surgical procedures. *Ann Surg* 154:803–810, 1961.

133. Shoemaker WC: Comparison of the relative effectiveness of whole blood transfusions and various types of fluid therapy in resuscitation. *Crit Care Med* 4:71–78, 1976.

134. Shoemaker WC: Fluids and electrolyte problems in the adult. In Shoemaker WC, Thompson WL: *Critical Care State of the Art.* Fullerton, CA, Society of Critical Care Medicine, 1982.

135. Shoemaker WC, Bryan-Brown CW, Quigley L: Body fluid shifts in depletion and post-stress states and their correction with adequate nutrition. *Surg Gynecol Obstet* 136:371–374, 1973.

136. Shoemaker WC, Hauser CJ: Critique of crystalloid vs colloid therapy in shock and shock lung. *Crit Care Med* 7:117–124, 1979.

137. Shoemaker WC, Montgomery ES, Kaplan E: Physiologic patterns in surviving and nonsurviving shock patients. *Arch Surg* 106:630–636, 1973.

138. Shoemaker WC, Schluchter M, Hopkins JA: Comparison of the relative effectiveness of colloids and crystalloids in emergency resuscitation. *Am J Cardiol* 142:73–84, 1981.

139. Shoemaker WC, Schluchter M, Hopkins JA: Fluid therapy in emergency resuscitation; clinical evaluation of colloid and crystalloid regimens. *Crit Care Med* 9:367–368, 1981.

140. Siegel SC, Moss GS, Cochin A: Pulmonary changes following treatment for hemorrhagic shock; saline vs. colloid infusion. *Surg Forum* 21:17–19, 1970.

141. Skillman JJ: The role of albumin and oncotically active fluids in shock. *Crit Care Med* 4:55–61, 1976.

142. Skillman JJ, Hassan AK, Moore FD: Plasma protein kinetics of the early transcapillary refill after hemorrhage in man. *Surg Gynecol Obstet* 125:983–996, 1967.

143. Skillman JJ, Restall DS, Salzman EW: Randomized trial of albumin vs. electrolyte solutions during abdominal aortic operations. *Surgery* 78:291–303, 1975.

144. Skillman JJ, Rosenoer VM, Smith PC: Improved albumin synthesis in postoperative patients by amino acid infusion. *N Engl J Med* 295:1037–1040, 1976.

145. Solanke TF: Clinical trial of 6% hydroxyethyl starch (a new plasma expander). *Br Med J* 3:783–785, 1968.

146. Solanke TF, Khwaja MS, Madojemu EI: Plasma volume studies with four different plasma volume expanders. *J Surg Res* 11:140–143, 1971.

147. Stead EA Jr, Ebert RV: Studies on human albumin. In Mudd S, Thaliver W (eds): *Blood Substitutes and Blood Transfusion.* Springfield, IL, Charles C Thomas, 1942.

148. Strauss RG, Koepke JA, McGuire LC, et al: Clinical and laboratory effects on donors in intermittent flow centrifugation platelet-leukopheresis performed with hydroxyethyl starch and citrate. *Clin Lab Haematol* 2:1–11, 1980.

149. Strauss RG, Snyder EL, Stuber J, Fick RB: Ingestion of hydroxyethyl starch by human leukocytes. *Transfusion* 26:88–90, 1986.

150. Strauss RG, Stump DC, Henrikson RA: Hydroxyethyl starch accentuates von Willebrand's disease. *Transfusion* 25:235–237, 1985.

151. Strauss RG, Stump DC, Henrikson RA, Saunders R: Effects of hydroxyethyl starch on fibrinogen, fibrin clot formation and fibrinolysis. *Transfusion* 25:230–234, 1985.

152. Stump DC, Strauss RG, Henrikson RA, Peterson RE, Saunders R: Effects of hydroxyethyl starch on blood coagulation, particularly factor VIII. *Transfusion* 25:349–354, 1985.

153. Takaori M, Safar P: Acute severe hemodilution with lactated Ringer's solution. *Arch Surg* 94:67–73, 1967.

154. Takaori M, Safar P: Treatment of massive hemorrhage with colloid and crystalloid solutions. *JAMA* 199:297–302, 1967.

155. Thomas JM, Silva JR: Dextran 40 in the treatment of peripheral vascular diseases. *Arch Surg* 106:138–141, 1973.

156. Thompson WL: Rational use of albumin and plasma substitutes. *Johns Hopkins Med J* 136:220–225, 1975.

157. Thompson WL, Britton JJ, Walton RP: Persistence of starch derivatives and dextran when infused after hemorrhage. *J Pharmacol Exp Ther* 136:125–132, 1962.

158. Thompson WL, Fukushima T, Rutherford RB, et al: Intravascular persistence, tissue shortage and excretion of hydroxyethyl starch. *Surg Gynecol Obstet* 131:965–972, 1970.

159. Thompson WL, Walton RP: Circulatory responses to intravenous infusions of hydroxyethyl starch solutions. *J Pharmacol Exp Ter* 146:359–364, 1964.

160. Thoren L: The dextrans–clinical data. Joint WHO/IABS symposium on the standardization of albumin plasma substitutes and plasmaphoresis, Geneva 1980. *Dev Biol Stand* 48:157–167, 1981.

161. Trinkle JK, Rush BF, Eiseman B: Metabolism of lactate following major blood loss. *Surgery* 63:782–787, 1968.

162. Trudnowski RJ, Goel SB, Lam FT, Evers JT: Effect of Ringer's lactate solution and sodium bicarbonate on surgical acidosis. *Surg Gynecol Obstet* 125:807–814, 1967.

163. Tullis JL: Albumin. I. Background and use. *JAMA* 237:355–360, 1977.

164. Tullis JL: Albumin. 2. Guidelines for clinical uses. *JAMA* 237:460–463, 1977.

165. Virgilio RW: Crystalloid vs. colloid resuscitation (reply to letter to editor). *Surgery* 86:515, 1979.

166. Virgilio RW, Rice CL, Smith DE: Crystalloid vs colloid resuscitation: is one better? A randomized clinical study. *Surgery* 85:129–139, 1979.

167. Virgilio RW, Smith DE, Zarino DK: Balanced electrolyte solutions: experimental and clinical studies. *Crit Care Med* 7:98–106, 1979.

168. Vito L, Dennis RC, Weisel RD: Sepsis presenting as

acute respiratory insufficiency. *Surg Gynecol Obstet* 138:896–900, 1974.

169. Weatherbee L, Spencer HH, Knopp CT: Coagulation studies after the transfusion of hydroxyethyl starch protected frozen blood in primates. *Transfusion* 14:109–115, 1974.

170. Weaver DW, Ledgerwood AM, Lucas CE: Pulmonary effects of albumin resuscitation for severe hypovolemic shock. *Arch Surg* 113:387–392, 1978.

171. Weil MH, Henning RJ, Puri VK: Colloid oncotic pressure: clinical significance. *Crit Care Med* 7:113–116, 1979.

172. Weiss HJ: The effect of clinical dextran on platelet aggregation, adhesion and ADP release in man: in vivo and in vitro studies. *J Lab Clin Med* 69:37–46, 1967.

173. Weissler AM, Roehill JR, Peeler RG: Effect of posture on the cardiac response to increased peripheral demand. *J Lab Clin Med* 59:1000–1007, 1962.

174. Woodruff LM, Gobsin ST: Use of human albumin in military medicine. Clinical evaluation of human albumin. *US Navy Med Bull* 40:791–796, 1942.

175. Wong PY, Carroll RE, Lipinski TL: Studies on the renin-angiotensin-aldosterone system in patients with cirrhosis and ascites: effect of saline and albumin infusion. *Gastroenterology* 77:1171–1176, 1979.

176. Yacobi A, Stoll RG, Sum CY: Pharmacokinetics of hydroxyethyl starch in normal subjects. *J Clin Pharmacol* 22:206–212, 1982.

8

Thrombolytic Therapy

Paul R. Eisenberg, M.D., M.P.H.
Allan S. Jaffe, M.D.

Thrombolytic agents have been investigated extensively for the treatment of thrombotic disorders since the initial observations by Tillet and Garner in 1933 (126) that filtrates of β-hemolytic streptococci had fibrinolytic activity. However, because of the potential for bleeding and the lack of adequate documentation of benefit, the indications for the use of thrombolytic agents have been limited. Recently, enthusiasm for thrombolytic therapy has increased because of the development of agents with greater clot specificity, and the demonstration that prompt reperfusion of coronary arteries occluded by thrombi in patients with acute myocardial infarction leads to a reduction in mortality (49, 68, 114) and preservation of ventricular function (97, 112, 113). As a result, the optimum means for induction of fibrinolysis and indications for its use are now being extensively redefined.

OVERVIEW OF THE FIBRINOLYTIC SYSTEM

The fibrinolytic system is an enzymatic system present in blood that induces clot dissolution via the formation of the enzyme, plasmin. Plasmin is derived from the circulating zymogen, plasminogen, by the action of agents known as plasminogen activators. Once generated, plasmin degrades fibrin as well as fibrinogen, prothrombin, factor V, factor VIII, prekallikrein, several components of the complement system, and other circulating proteins (2). The proteolytic activity of plasmin is controlled by rapid interactions with several circulating inhibitors in blood (19).

Plasminogen is a single-chain glycoprotein that exists in several forms. Native plasminogen has a glutamic acid at the amino terminus, and is referred to as "glu-plasminogen" (141). Limited plasmin digestion of plasminogen during activation results in a modified glycoprotein with lysine, alanine, or methionine at the amino terminus, referred to collectively as "lys-plasminogen." Within the plasminogen molecule are sites referred to as the lysine-binding sites, which serve as the points of interaction for the binding of plasminogen to fibrin or to its inhibitor, α-2-antiplasmin (19, 147). Lys-plasminogen has a higher affinity for fibrin than does glu-plasminogen and is also more rapidly converted to plasmin by the plasminogen activator, urokinase (18, 95).

MECHANISM OF ACTION OF PLASMINOGEN ACTIVATORS

Plasminogen can be activated by a number of mechanisms. It is activated by factor XII, prekallikrein, high molecular weight kininogen, and possibly other plasma constituents of the kallikrein system (66). The physiologic importance of this type of activation (intrinsic) is undetermined. The significance of activation due to the secretion of plasminogen activators from tissue or endothelium is better understood (extrinsic activation). Tissue-type plasminogen activator has been extensively studied and is probably identical to blood plasminogen activator and vascular plasminogen activator (101). It has very little plasminogen activator activity in isolation; however, in the presence of fibrin, activation of plasminogen increases markedly (58). Thus, in physiologic systems, tissue-type plasminogen activator converts only fibrin-bound plasminogen to plasmin, providing a localized mechanism for clot dissolution (21).

Urokinase is a two-chain serum protease that has been isolated from human urine and cultured kidney cells (91, 151). It exists in both a high and low molecular weight form (145). Two-chain urokinase activates plasminogen by lysis of a single arginine-valine bond (102). A single-chain proenzyme form of urokinase (scu-PA) also has been isolated and has plasminogen activator activity even without conversion to the two-chain form (22, 50).

Streptokinase, in contrast, activates plasminogen indirectly. It first forms an equimolar complex with plasminogen, which exposes an active site on plasminogen and transforms it into an activator complex (16, 85). Streptokinase-plasminogen complexes have been modified by the synthesis of derivatives containing acyl groups at the active site (116). In the circulation, acylation prevents plasminogen activation. These derivatives are deacylated slowly, and active streptokinase-plasmin(ogen) activator complexes result. The less pronounced induction of systemic plasminogen activation and the potential for deacylation in the vicinity of clot allows for slightly greater clot specificity than with streptokinase alone.

Once generated, plasmin is rapidly inhibited by the formation of an equimolar complex with α-2-antiplasmin (146). Plasmin interacts with fibrin at the enzyme's lysine-binding site. Plasmin that is bound to fibrin is protected from rapid inhibition by α-2-antiplasmin since the lysine-binding site is occupied by fibrin. α-2-Macroglobulin also inhibits plasmin, though more slowly (19).

CLINICAL PHARMACOLOGY OF FIBRINOLYTIC AGENTS

Streptokinase

Because streptokinase (SK) is derived from a common bacterial species, antibodies to it are present in most patients. Although allergic reactions can occur, a well-documented case of anaphylaxis with currently available preparations has not been reported. When streptokinase is administered systemically, an initial large dose is used to overcome the inhibitory effect of high antibody titers. The administration of 250,000 units overcomes antibody resistance and induces a systemic lytic state in more than 90% of patients (55). The maintenance dose used subsequently varies, but in theory must be sufficient to generate enough plasmin to overcome circulating inhibitors. On the other hand, an excessive dose of streptokinase could consume or complex all of the available plasminogen, leaving none for further activation. Thus, both insufficient and/or

excessive doses may result in failure to achieve a lytic state.

The half-life of streptokinase in vivo has not been precisely delineated. After an injection of radiolabeled streptokinase, an initial α-distributive half-life of 18 minutes has been observed, followed by a β-distributive half-life of 83 minutes (37). However, the clearance of functionally active SK-plasminogen complexes has been estimated to be only 23 minutes (86). Nonetheless, plasmin activity can be demonstrated for up to 4 hours after administration of streptokinase, documenting persistent fibrinolytic activity despite clearance of active complexes from plasma (35).

Since streptokinase activates both circulating plasminogen and plasminogen bound to fibrin, both local and systemic effects are observed after its administration. Degradation of circulating fibrinogen, plasminogen, and coagulation factors is the most significant hemostatic alteration (111). Formation of fibrinogen degradation products may exacerbate the tendency toward bleeding induced by the low levels of circulating fibrinogen and other coagulation factors by inhibiting thrombin and fibrin polymerization (76, 83). Low-dose local infusions of streptokinase have been used to limit these adverse systemic effects.

Urokinase

Urokinase (UK) has also been used extensively as a fibrinolytic agent. Since urokinase is not antigenic in humans and is a direct activator of plasminogen, the dose-response relationships of this activator are less complex. After administration, urokinase is cleared with a half-life of 14 ± 6 minutes. Since urokinase activates both circulating plasminogen and plasminogen bound to fibrin, intravenous administration results in systemic effects similar to those observed after streptokinase (38). Local infusions of urokinase have also been used to minimize these effects. In general, the effects of urokinase and those of streptokinase are similar but urokinase is considerably more expensive.

Tissue Plasminogen Activator

Human tissue-type plasminogen activator (t-PA) has recently become available for clinical use. Initial studies using a product isolated from a human melanoma cell line demonstrated successful thrombolysis in both dogs and humans (11, 134). More recently t-PA has become available in large quantities through the use of recombinant gene technology (25, 133). This product is functionally similar to that derived from cell culture. Tissue-type plasminogen activator exists as either a one-chain or two-chain form (140). Both forms have similar fibrinolytic activity in purified systems; however, in plasma, one-chain t-PA is converted to two-chain t-PA during fibrinolysis (100). After a bolus injection, t-PA is cleared from plasma with a half-life of approximately 6 minutes (88). However with larger infusions, a β half-life of 1.3 hours has been documented for one preparation of the recombinant product (138). More recent preparations have a slightly shorter half-life (43). Lytic activity after administration of t-PA persists for many hours after clearance of activator (35).

Unlike urokinase or streptokinase, t-PA has little systemic effect at low doses (24, 134). The markedly enhanced activation of plasminogen by t-PA in the presence of fibrin should result in clot lysis without significant systemic plasminogen activation. However, the selectivity for plasminogen bound to fibrin is only relative, and in the presence of very high concentrations of t-PA, circulating plasminogen is degraded as well (117, 125). Thus, in clinical trials in patients with acute myocardial infarction, higher doses (100–150 mg) of t-PA produce some systemic plasminogen activation and fibrinogen breakdown (20). Nonetheless, systemic effects are less with t-PA than with other activators.

Trials of recombinant t-PA (Genentech, Inc., San Francisco, CA) in patients with acute myocardial infarction have utilized intravenous administration in order to permit treatment at the earliest possible instance. However, infusions into the coronary artery and peripheral arteries have also been employed, and offer the advantage of a significantly lower dose with similar beneficial effects (25, 47) when the early administration of treatment is less critical. Heparin competes with t-PA for fibrin binding (5, 90); thus, the concomitant use of heparin may increase the plasminogenolytic activity of t-PA and reduce its fibrin specificity.

Acylated Streptokinase/Plasminogen Complex Derivatives

The acylated streptokinase-plasminogen complex chosen for clinical trials, BRL-26921 (ASPAC), in experimental models induces clot lysis, while inducing less systemic lytic activity than streptokinase (115). Deacylation occurs with a half-life of 40 minutes; subsequently, clearance is similar to that of unmodified streptokinase-plasminogen complexes. In humans there is little systemic fibrinogenolytic activity when 7–12 mg is administered as an intravenous bolus (93, 119). However, at higher doses, progressive systemic lytic activity has been observed (56, 67). In recent trials, bolus doses of 30 mg were required to induce rapid coronary thrombolysis (9, 82, 139). In this dose range, significant systemic lytic activity is observed.

Single-Chain Urokinase Plasminogen Activator

Single-chain urokinase plasminogen activator (scu-PA) directly activates plasminogen to plasmin. Circulating scu-PA is converted to the two-chain form of urokinase, resulting in still further plasminogen activation (26, 80). In plasma, activation of plasminogen by scu-PA is limited by competition with a specific inhibitor (80), which is thought to be inactivated in the presence of fibrin. The half-life of scu-PA in experimental models is similar to that of urokinase. Preliminary trials with scu-PA demonstrate greater clot selectivity in humans than with urokinase (135). Whether therapeutic doses will be as selective as those observed with t-PA is undetermined. Synergism with t-PA has been demonstrated (23).

MONITORING OF THE COAGULATION SYSTEM DURING FIBRINOLYSIS

Ideally, laboratory monitoring of coagulation during treatment with fibrinolytic agents should provide precise information regarding the effect of the activator on coagulation and hence the intensity of fibrinolytic activity, the extent of clot dissolution, and the potential for bleeding. Conventional assays of coagulation can only document the presence of a systemic lytic state when it is induced, and do not distinguish between the effects of the activators and those of heparin (111). With the newer, more clot-selective plasminogen activators, monitoring has focused primarily on detection of systemic lytic activity as an index of excessive dosage. Once the lytic state has waned, assays of coagulation are used to titrate heparin administration.

Conventional laboratory monitoring of thrombolytic therapy may include assays of thrombin time, activated partial thromboplastin time, prothrombin time, fibrinogen, fibrinogen degradation products, and euglobulin lysis time. An understanding of each test and how it is affected by plasminogen activation is essential to proper interpretation of assay results (111).

The *thrombin time* (TT) is critically dependent on the concentration of fibrinogen in plasma and is extremely sensitive to heparin and fibrinogen degradation products in the sample (61). The thrombin time is prolonged after administration of fibrinolytic agents if fibrinogen is depleted and/or fibrin(ogen) degradation products are formed. When heparin has been administered, the addition of protamine sulfate to the plasma sample reverses the effects of heparin, thus allowing for detection of the consequences of systemic lytic activity alone.

The *activated partial thromboplastin time* (aPTT) assesses the activity of the coagulation factors other than factors VII and XIII, and is used primarily to monitor the effects of heparin (92). It is affected by decreased fibrinogen and elevated fibrinogen degradation products, but to a lesser extent than the thrombin time. Once the systemic lytic state has resolved, the aPTT is the best presently available coagulation test for monitoring and titrating heparin.

The *prothrombin time* (PT) measures the activity of factors V, VII, and X, prothrombin, and fibrinogen. It is affected to an even lesser extent than the aPTT by low levels of fibrinogen and/or fibrin(ogen) degradation products.

Determination of *fibrinogen* degradation is one of the most common criteria for documenting systemic plasminogen activation. Several methods are available for measurement of fibrinogen. The Clauss procedure measures the kinetics of clot formation and hence clottable fibrinogen. This assay is sensitive to the presence of fibrin(ogen) degradation products that are not clottable or inhibit polymerization of fibrin, and is inaccurate when fibrinogen levels are extremely low (generally less than 55 mg/dl) as is frequently the case after intravenous administration of conventional activators (e.g., SK). The Ellis method of measuring fibrinogen is an endpoint assay that measures the total amount of fibrinogen clotted after prolonged incubation. This assay is less affected by fibrin(ogen) degradation products and generally yields higher values for fibrinogen than those obtained from the Clauss method, particularly when the fibrinogen level is very low. Large amounts of heparin in the sample can lead to spuriously low values. Reversal of the effects of heparin with protamine sulfate corrects for this effect. Precipitation procedures and most immunologic methods generally do not differentiate fibrinogen from large nonclottable fibrinogen degradation products.

The most commonly used procedure for measurement of *fibrin(ogen) degradation products* utilizes antifibrinogen antibody–coated latex particles. This method and most others detect products of both fibrinogen and fibrinolysis (122).

The euglobulin fraction of plasma does not contain inhibitors of plasmin. Thus, the *euglobulin lysis time* measures the functional activity of plasminogen activators in plasma (75). Enhanced lytic activity in the euglobulin fraction on plasma clots or fibrin plates or on clots in other systems is evidence of the presence of functional plasmin activity in vivo.

With conventional activators such as streptokinase, monitoring generally should include baseline and posttreatment measurements of the aPTT, TT, fibrinogen, and/or fibrin(ogen) degradation products to document induction of the lytic state (111). Reduction of the fibrinogen to 50% of baseline values or less can be considered evidence of systemic lytic activity. When very low levels of fibrinogen are present, the Ellis assay is more likely to be accurate. Subsequently, a normal protamine-corrected TT can be used to document the absence of residual effects due to plasminogen activation. Once the systemic lytic state has resolved, the aPTT may be used to titrate heparin. With newer, more clot-specific activators such as t-PA that may not induce systemic plasminogen activation, a shortened euglobulin lysis time may be the only evidence of circulating plasminogen activator, since fibrinogen degradation and other alterations of coagulation may only be present after large doses.

Fibrinopeptide A (FPA) is a 16 amino acid polypeptide cleaved from fibrinogen by thrombin as part of the formation of fibrin. Elevated levels of FPA in plasma are common in patients with acute transmural myocardial infarction early after the onset of symptoms (34). Thus, this assay detects the thrombotic state associated with acute transmural myocardial infarction. When streptokinase is given, FPA decreases markedly when recanalization occurs (33). In patients in whom recanalization does not occur, FPA increases markedly, suggesting that continued thrombin activity is competing with thrombolysis and is an important determinant of the lack of recanalization (33). Increased levels of FPA are observed even 4 hours after the administration of streptokinase, but rapidly decrease in response to heparin. Thus, measurement of FPA may provide a useful index of the intensity of thrombin activity in vivo during therapy and may provide a criterion for the success or failure of treatment. In addition, since FPA directly measures thrombin activity, it may facilitate titration of heparin.

Several new assays have been developed recently to distinguish fibrin from fibrinogen degradation products (41, 107, 144). These assays have been used to show that fibrin dissolution (following tissue plasminogen activator and streptokinase) persists for many hours after these activators are cleared from the circulation (35). In the future these assays may permit both sensitive and specific quantitative detection of fibrin dissolution in vivo, allowing for more precise titration of thrombolysis.

CLINICAL APPLICATIONS OF THROMBOLYSIS

Deep Venous Thrombosis

The traditional objective of therapy for lower extremity venous thrombosis was to prevent pulmonary embolism and its often catastrophic complications (28, 63, 70). Treatment with heparin usually does not result in dissolution of the thrombus by itself. As a consequence of residual thrombosis, morbidity due to venous valvular insufficiency with lower extremity edema, aching, stasis dermatitis, and ulceration (postphlebitic syndrome) may occur, especially after extensive proximal venous thrombosis (13, 150). As many as 80% of patients treated with heparin for venous thrombosis ultimately develop signs and/or symptoms of the postphlebitic syndrome (89). Fibrinolytic agents have the potential to more thoroughly dissolve occlusive thrombi. If residual clot is the etiology of the "postphlebitic syndrome," this therapy should reduce its incidence.

RANDOMIZED TRIALS COMPARING STREPTOKINASE WITH HEPARIN

Nine randomized trials have compared the efficacy of clot lysis induced by streptokinase with that induced by heparin as assessed by

Table 8.1
Results of Trials Comparing Thrombolysis with Heparin Therapy for Deep Venous Thrombosis

Study	Venographic Improvement (% of patients)[a]	
	Streptokinase	Heparin
Anreson et al (6)	71 (15/21)	14 (3/21)
Beiger et al (10)	NA[b]	NA[b]
Elliot et al (36)	65 (17/26)	0 (0/25)
Kakkar et al (64)	78 (8/9)	22 (2/9)
Marder et al (84)	58 (7/12)	25 (3/12)
Robertson et al (103)	66 (6/9)	29 (2/7)
Rosch et al (105)	45 (10/22)	27 (7/26)
Tsapogas et al (130)	53 (10/19)	7 (1/15)
Watz and Savidge (142)	67 (12/18)	36 (6/17)
Average (totals)	62 (84/136)	20 (26/132)

[a] Number of patients in parentheses.
[b] Only late venograms were performed in this study.

venography (6, 10, 36, 64, 84, 103, 105, 130, 142). In six, long-term end-points also were assessed (7, 27, 36, 64, 65, 130). In response to streptokinase, generally administered as a bolus of 250,000 units followed by an intravenous infusion of 100,000 units/hr for 24–72 hours, improved venous patency was observed in 62% of patients (Table 8.1). Only 20% of patients treated with heparin demonstrated similar improvement. Bleeding complications after streptokinase occurred in up to 26% of patients. Despite the improved efficiency of clot lysis with streptokinase, the short-term clinical response was similar with either regimen in most series.

Long-term clinical benefit was also evident in those patients treated with streptokinase (Table 8.2). Approximately 60% of the patients who received streptokinase had normal or only minor abnormalities on follow-up venography at intervals from 2 to 6½ years; 74% were asymptomatic. In contrast, only 20% of the patients treated with heparin alone demonstrated similar findings by venography, and more than 70% had symptomatic postphlebitic syndrome. Thus, fibrinolytic therapy results in more rapid and more complete resolution of deep venous thrombosis acutely, and less morbidity chronically.

TRIALS WITH OTHER PLASMINOGEN ACTIVATORS

More recent trials have employed acylated plasminogen-streptokinase complex (BRL-26921) and t-PA activator to treat deep venous thrombosis in the hope that less systemic fi-

Table 8.2
Late Results of Trials Comparing Thrombolysis with Heparin Therapy for Deep Venous Thrombosis

Study	Follow-up	Normal Venogram (% of patients)[a]	
		Streptokinase	Heparin
Anreson et al (7)	6.5 yr	56 (9/16)	33 (6/18)
Beiger et al (10)	3–4 months	40 (2/5)	20 (1/5)
Elliot et al (36)	3 months	60 (12/20)	0
Kakkar et al (65)	6–12 months	57 (4/7)	12 (1/8)
Rosch et al and Common et al (27, 105)	7 months	40 (6/15)	8 (1/12)
Watz and Savidge (142)	1–2 months	92 (11/12)	13 (1/8)
Average (totals)		59 (44/75)	20 (10/51)

[a] Number of patients in parentheses.

brinogen degradation would be induced thus reducing bleeding. BRL-26921 is effective (116); however, at doses higher than 5 mg/day, significant fibrinogen degradation occurs (67). In two patients treated with a low dose of melanoma-derived t-PA, complete lysis of deep venous thrombi occurred without systemic plasminogen activation (143). Preliminary results from ongoing trials suggest that t-PA will be effective and may be safer. Thus, t-PA may become the therapy of choice for deep venous thrombosis once optimal regimens for its use are defined.

SUMMARY

Thrombolytic therapy of deep venous thrombosis is beneficial. The more complete dissolution of thrombi prevents venous valvular damage and venous hypertension, reducing the incidence of the postphlebitic syndrome. Thrombolytic therapy should be considered in well-selected younger patients with extensive proximal venous thrombosis, who are free of contraindications to treatment (Table 8.3). After treatment, patients should receive heparin titrated to maintain the aPTT at approximately twice normal, followed by long-term Coumadin. The availability of agents with greater clot selectivity such as t-PA may enhance the safety of therapy and ultimately make fibrinolytic agents the treatment of choice for deep venous thrombosis.

Pulmonary Embolism

The use of heparin for the treatment of pulmonary embolism has markedly reduced mortality from recurrent emboli (8). Once treatment has been initiated, mortality is approximately 8% and often is secondary to associated illness (30). Nonetheless, patients with severe reduction in the cross-sectional area of the pulmonary artery (greater than 50%) frequently have right ventricular failure and shock, and have a poor prognosis despite heparin treatment.

Several controlled trials have attempted to show that more rapid clot lysis induced by fibrinolytic agents improves prognosis. The largest trial, sponsored by the National Institutes of Health, was performed in two phases. In the first phase, the effects of a 12-hour infusion of urokinase were compared with the effects of heparin alone (Urokinase Pulmonary Embolism Trial, PET) (131). In the second,

Table 8.3
Contraindications to Thrombolytic Therapy

Absolute contraindications
  Active bleeding
  Cerebrovascular accident within 2 months, or active intracerebral process
Major relative contraindications
  Major recent surgery, organ biopsy, or invasive vascular procedure within 10 days
  Active malignancy
  Recent serious trauma, including prolonged cardiopulmonary resuscitation
  Severe hypertension (systolic ≥ 170 mm Hg or diastolic ≥ 110 mm Hg)
Other relative contraindications
  Chronic or acute renal failure
  Endocarditis
  Pregnancy or immediate postpartum state
  Age > 75 yr
  Diabetic hemorrhagic retinopathy
  Chronic therapeutic anticoagulation
  Inflammatory bowel disease
  Cutaneous ulcerations
  Chronic liver disease
  Disorders of hemostasis
  History of cerebrovascular accident

Table 8.4
Resolution of Lung Scan Defects in the National Institutes of Health Trials with Thrombolytic Agents

Protocol	Lung Scan Resolution (%)				
	1 day	2 days	5 days	14 days	3 months
UPET					
Urokinase (12 hr)[a]	6.2	8.0	11.3	14.9	—
Heparin only	2.7	4.9	9.3	14.7	—
USPET					
Urokinase (12 hr)[a]	9.0	—	—	—	28.6
Urokinase (24 hr)[a]	11.6	—	—	—	26.0
Streptokinase (24 hr)[a]	7.0	—	—	—	21.6

[a] All patients received heparin after infusion of the fibrinolytic agent.

12- and 24-hour infusions of urokinase and a 24-hour infusion of streptokinase were compared (Urokinase-Streptokinase Pulmonary Embolism Trial, USPET) (132). In both studies, patients subsequently received heparin for 5 days, then Coumadin for 14 days (Table 8.4). Both of these trials, as well as several smaller series, demonstrated that fibrinolytic therapy accelerated the dissolution of pulmonary emboli.

In the 333 patients randomized in UPET and USPET, resolution of emboli, judged by perfusion scans and pulmonary angiography, was more complete during the first 24 hours after fibrinolytic agents (Table 8.4). This rapid resolution was associated with a more rapid decrease of mean pulmonary artery pressure and pulmonary vascular resistance, and modest improvements in cardiac index (Table 8.5). However, by 5 days or more after treatment, the degree of lung scan resolution was similar after urokinase or heparin (UPET). Mortality was similar in patients who presented in shock (5–6%), whether or not they received thrombolytic agents. Bleeding was more common

following thrombolytic therapy: 45% of the patients given urokinase compared with 27% who received heparin.

In addition to the NIH trials, two smaller randomized controlled trials have compared the effects of streptokinase with those of heparin in patients with massive pulmonary emboli (81,124). In both, streptokinase was administered for 72 hours at a rate of 100,000 units/hr. Streptokinase resulted in more rapid and complete dissolution of emboli than heparin alone. Bleeding complications occurred in 30% of the patients who received streptokinase and 18% of those who received heparin alone. Thus, the more rapid dissolution of emboli appears to be associated with an improved clinical course in patients with massive insult; however, enthusiasm for fibrinolytic therapy has been blunted by the greater incidence of bleeding.

Recent studies suggest that use of t-PA for pulmonary embolism may be associated with fewer bleeding complications. In a case report, nearly complete dissolution of a massive pulmonary embolus occurred after a 90-minute

Table 8.5
Hemodynamic Response to Thrombolysis in the National Institutes of Health Trials[a]

Protocol	PA Mean (mm Hg)		Cardiac Index (liters/min/m²)		Total Pulmonary Resistance (dyne/sec/cm⁻⁵)	
	Pre	Post	Pre	Post	Pre	Post
UPET						
Urokinase (12 hr)	26.3	20.7	3.2	3.3	330.3	244.7
Heparin only	26.0	24.8	3.1	3.0	365.0	395.7
USPET						
Urokinase (12 hr)	27.4	20.1	2.9	3.0	403.4	298.9
Urokinase (24 hr)	27.5	20.0	2.6	2.9	365.0	244.7
Streptokinase (24 hr)	26.2	20.9	2.8	3.6	181.3	121.5

[a] Measurements made before (pre) and 24 hours after (post) start of infusion of the fibrinolytic agent. Urokinase 12-hour group had been on heparin for 12 hours at time of posttreatment measurements. PA, pulmonary artery pressure.

infusion of 30 mg of recombinant t-PA (12). A larger clinical trial (35 patients) demonstrated marked resolution of pulmonary emboli in 67% of patients and moderate to slight dissolution in an additional 23% after an intravenous dose of 50 mg of t-PA over 2 hours followed by an additional 40 mg over the next 4 hours (46). Heparin was given prior to and after treatment with t-PA. Major bleeding occurred in two patients and "minor bleeding" sufficient to halt administration of t-PA (usually at puncture sites) occurred in five. If the optimal doses of activator can be determined and the need for invasive procedures reduced, clot-selective activators may become the preferred treatment for patients with pulmonary emboli.

At present, thrombolytic therapy should be considered when pulmonary embolism is massive and complicated by right ventricular failure, hypotension, or obstruction of 50% or more of a major pulmonary artery. Therapy with streptokinase or urokinase (the only presently available activators) should be given for 24 hours or less. Streptokinase is generally given as an intravenous bolus of 250,000 units over 15–30 minutes, followed by infusion of 100,000 units/hr. For urokinase, a bolus of 300,000 units followed by infusion of 2,000 units/kg/hr is as efficacious as higher doses (4,400 units/kg/hr) (48). Prior to and during therapy, meticulous management to avoid bleeding due to vascular trauma is essential. Pulmonary artery catheters for monitoring or angiography should be placed through antecubital fossa venous cut down rather than percutaneously in noncompressible vessels (i.e., large central veins). Arterial blood gases should be obtained only if essential with a 23-gauge needle from the radial artery. The artery should then be compressed for a minimum of 15 minutes. Whenever possible, noninvasive monitoring of oxygen saturation is preferred.

Acute Myocardial Infarction

Much of the recent enthusiasm for thrombolytic therapy has been stimulated by the demonstration of improved outcome in acute myocardial infarction after treatment with fibrinolytic agents. When coronary reperfusion occurs within 2 hours after the onset of acute transmural myocardial infarction, regional left ventricular wall motion often improves and mortality is reduced, particularly in patients with anterior infarction. (49, 74, 97, 113, 114). When treatment is started later, benefit is of lesser magnitude and less consistent (3, 4, 68, 69, 71, 99, 104, 109). Thus, with acute myocardial infarction time is the most critical parameter.

The use of thrombolytic therapy for acute myocardial infarction was first reported in 1958 (39, 40). However, until recently the data demonstrating a benefit for such therapy were not sufficiently persuasive to justify its use in view of the potential for serious hemorrhage. In addition, during the 1970s, skepticism regarding the role of coronary thrombosis in acute myocardial infarction further discouraged the use of antithrombotic and fibrinolytic agents. The rediscovery of the importance of coronary thrombosis in transmural infarction can be attributed to DeWood and associates (31), who demonstrated total coronary occlusion in 87% of 126 patients studied within the first 4 hours of the onset of infarction, and nearly total obstruction in an additional 10%. In patients studied later (12–24 hours) the incidence of total occlusion decreased to 65%. These data, coupled with the retrieval of thrombus during subsequent emergent coronary revascularization in a large subset (51 patients), conclusively established the presence of coronary thrombosis early during the evolution of acute myocardial infarction. Although Chazov and coworkers (17) were the first to report pharmacologic coronary fibrinolysis, Rentrop and associates (98) popularized the concept that coronary reperfusion could be achieved by guide-wire fragmentation followed by intracoronary streptokinase. Subsequently it has been demonstrated that intracoronary administration of streptokinase elicits recanalization in approximately 70% of cases (Table 8.6).

Initially, intracoronary administration of fibrinolytic therapy was thought preferable since lower doses could be administered, systemic lytic effects were thought to be minimal, and the results of therapy could be immediately

Table 8.6
Recanalization Rates in Trials of Intracoronary Streptokinase for Coronary Thrombosis

Study	Recanalization Rate	
	No. of Patients	%
Anderson et al (4)	15/20	75
Khaja et al (71)	12/20	60
Kennedy et al (68)	73/108	83
Leibhoff et al (78)	15/22	68
Rentrop et al (98)	17/20	85
Rentrop et al (99)	32/43	74

appreciated. However, rapid mixing of the activator in the systemic circulation occurs after intracoronary administration and results in systemic activation of plasminogen and induction of a systemic lytic state (29, 106). In addition, the time needed to perform coronary angiography prior to the initiation of treatment results in a delay often as long as 90 minutes, during which the magnitude of potential benefit from reperfusion is diminishing. The relatively late initiation of therapy due to this obligatory time delay in most trials of intracoronary streptokinase may explain why consistent improvement in global left ventricular function has not been demonstrated in many randomized studies. However, when ventriculographic analysis of regional left ventricular wall motion (defined angiographically) is performed, improvement in regional performance can be documented in 82% of patients in whom recanalization is induced within 2 hours of the onset of symptoms (112, 113). Regional wall motion improvement is less consistent in those in whom recanalization occurs later.

Several studies also have documented reduced mortality in patients with acute myocardial infarction treated with intracoronary streptokinase. In the Western Washington trial, 134 patients who received intracoronary streptokinase were compared with 116 patients treated conventionally (68). Patients were eligible for randomization if they presented during the first 12 hours of acute infarction. The mean time to presentation was 4.7 ± 2.5 hours. Thirty-day mortality was dramatically reduced for those who received intracoronary streptokinase (3.7%) compared with controls (11.6%, $P<0.02$). Patients with anterior infarction were more likely to benefit. However, mortality at 1 year was no longer significantly different between the two groups, in large part because of patients with no reperfusion, less than "complete reperfusion," or inferior infarction (68). In the Interuniversity Cardiology Institute Randomized Study, the mean time to reperfusion was 200 minutes after treatment with intracoronary streptokinase alone, in some instances preceded by intravenous streptokinase. The reduction in mortality in this trial was similar to that in the Western Washington study (114). At 28 days, 6% of the patients given streptokinase had died, compared with 12% of the control patients ($P=0.03$). Improved survival was still evident at 12 months. Despite the encouraging results of these trials, not all of the studies employing intracoronary streptokinase for treatment of acute myocardial infarction have shown benefit, likely because of the delays inherent in its initiation.

Intravenous administration of fibrinolytic agents has the advantage of permitting more prompt institution of therapy and simpler logistics. Although prior to 1980 several studies documented the benefits of treatment with intravenous streptokinase for evolving acute myocardial infarction, others did not and the reported benefits did not seem to justify the risk of bleeding, which was substantial (120). However, because of the delays inherent with intracoronary streptokinase, there was renewed interest in intravenous administration of fibrinolytic agents. In comparison with intracoronary streptokinase, intravenous streptokinase leads to recanalization less often (1, 42, 108, 118). In studies in which preinterventional coronary angiograms have been acquired, the success rate of intravenous streptokinase is approximately 45%, whereas it is approximately 70% with intracoronary administration (Table 8.7) (96). Studies in which preinterventional angiography was not performed suggested rates of recanalization of 70% or higher; however, this result reflected the inclusion of some patients without total thrombotic occlusion (5–21%). Nonetheless, early administration of intravenous streptokinase significantly decreases mortality in patients with acute myocardial infarction. In the largest study thus far (GISSI), 5,630 patients were treated with intravenous streptokinase at the time of admission to the emergency room and their course compared with 5,852 patients

Table 8.7
Recanalization Rate in Trials of Intravenous Streptokinase for Acute Myocardial Infarction

Study	Recanalization Rate	
	No. of Patients	%
Preinterventional angiogram performed		
Rogers et al (104)	7/16[a]	44
Schroeder et al (108)	11/21	52
Alderman et al (1)	8/13	62
Spann et al (118)	21/44[b]	48
Preinterventional angiogram not performed		
Ganz et al (42)	65/68	96
Schroeder et al (108)	42/52	84
Taylor et al (121)	99/121	82
Anderson et al (3)	16/22	73

[a] Patients given dose of 1,000,000 IU.
[b] Includes patients given 850,000 IU and those given 1,500,000 IU.

treated conventionally (49). No adjunctive therapy (including heparin) was given and the patients did not subsequently undergo coronary angiography. Nonetheless, mortality was less at 21 days in patients given streptokinase (10.7%) than in those treated conventionally (13%, P<0.002). The reduction in mortality was most marked in those patients treated within the first 3 hours of infarction (9.2% compared with 12% in controls). A modest but significant improvement in mortality was also observed for those patients treated 3–6 hours after onset of symptoms. On further analysis, it appeared that only those patients less than 65 years of age or those with anterior infarction were likely to benefit. In a smaller study, intravenous streptokinase was administered to 53 patients within 4 hours of the onset of symptoms, in some cases in a mobile care unit at the patient's home (74). Patients treated within 1.5 hours of the onset of infarction were found to have a significantly better left ventricular ejection fraction after infarction than those treated later.

When used for coronary thrombolysis, streptokinase is given in a dose of 750,000–1,500,000 units/hr intravenously. The intravenous dose for urokinase is 2,000,000 units/hr. Heparin is usually given prior to treatment or at the end of the infusion, and titrated to keep the aPTT at greater than 1.5–2 times normal.

OTHER PLASMINOGEN ACTIVATORS IN MYOCARDIAL INFARCTION

Tissue-type plasminogen activator has been the most extensively studied of the more recently developed activators for clinical use. Initial data demonstrated the ability of very low doses of intravenous t-PA to induce coronary thrombolysis in patients with acute myocardial infarction (25, 134). In a dose-finding study, t-PA given intravenously in a dose of 0.5 mg/kg produced reperfusion in 76% of patients by 90 minutes, results similar to those achievable with intracoronary streptokinase (25). Subsequently, the NIH-sponsored Thrombolysis in Myocardial Infarction Trial (TIMI) found that t-PA induced recanalization in 66% of patients given recombinant t-PA intravenously, compared with only 36% of those patients given intravenous streptokinase (123). These results have been confirmed by the European Cooperative Study, which reported a 70% rate of recanalization with t-PA, compared with 55% for streptokinase (137). Intravenous t-PA clearly has an efficacy similar to

that of intracoronary streptokinase, and by virtue of the greater degree of clot selectivity, intravenous t-PA is safer and can be administered without the delays inherent in a catheterization procedure. Recent studies suggest that prolonged low-dose infusion of t-PA may result in more complete thrombolysis and reduce the incidence of coronary reocclusion (44). Whether similar results might occur without adjunctive therapy with heparin is unknown but of potential importance, since bleeding has not been decreased in trials that have used t-PA, perhaps due to the effects of heparin (137).

Single-chain urokinase (scu-PA) type plasminogen activator was also highly effective in inducing recanalization in acute myocardial infarction in two small clinical trials (135, 136). Coronary reperfusion was induced in patients with acute myocardial infarction at a rate similar to that observed for t-PA. However, complete thrombolysis requires a high dose (70 mg), which is associated with a fairly marked degree of systemic lytic activity in approximately half of the patients. Since the half-life of scu-PA is relatively short (approximately 8 minutes), a continuous infusion is required as for t-PA. At the present time, the therapeutic:toxic ratio seems to be less favorable than that demonstrated for t-PA. A recent preliminary report suggests that low doses of t-PA and scu-PA may be synergistic and both more potent and more selective than higher doses of either activator alone (23).

Acylated streptokinase plasminogen complexes (BRL-26921, ASPAC) have been used to induce coronary thrombolysis in a number of studies (9, 49, 50, 82, 119). Because deacylation to the active streptokinase plasminogen activator complex is relatively slow, the agent can be administered as an intravenous bolus. Optimal rates of recanalization appear to require a dose of at least 30 mg, which results in significant systemic lytic activity. In a recent large trial, recanalization after treatment with ASPAC did not appear to be as frequent as in most trials using t-PA (9). In addition, ASPAC resulted in far more systemic fibrinogen depletion. The primary advantage of ASPAC at the present time appears to be the ability to administer it as an intravenous bolus.

ADDITIONAL CONSIDERATIONS AFTER CORONARY THROMBOLYSIS

After successful coronary thrombolysis a high-grade residual stenosis generally persists.

Since this stenosis is a potential site for reocclusion and reinfarction, aggressive management of the residual stenosis is recommended by many. In most centers, if a high-grade residual stenosis is documented, coronary angioplasty (PTCA) is performed in order to improve flow to the injured region (32, 45, 57, 77, 110, 128, 129, 149). In the hands of experienced operators angioplasty can be safely performed even in the presence of a systemic lytic state. Urgent coronary artery bypass surgery has also been employed in selected patients; however, the presence of a systemic lytic state increases the potential for morbidity with this procedure.

Patients who have been given intravenous streptokinase should undergo coronary angiography if recanalization appears to have occurred. Clinical indicators of successful coronary recanalization include a rapid rise and early peaking of MB creatine kinase, evidence for reperfusion arrhythmias, rapid resolution of ST segment elevation, and rapid resolution of chest discomfort after administration of plasminogen activators. None of these findings is definitive; however, when they are used in concert, the clinician is often able to correctly predict the occurrence or failure of recanalization. Recurrent chest discomfort following the timely administration of plasminogen activators is often an indication of impending reocclusion after coronary recanalization.

The timing of coronary angiography and PTCA is controversial. In general, the bias has been that patients at high risk (i.e., those with extensive anterior infarction, previous infarction, recurrent pain or arrhythmia, congestive heart failure, or hypotension with or without shock) who cannot tolerate further loss of myocardium should have immediate or at least expeditious procedures, whereas those who are stable clinically and at lower risk can undergo angiography electively. If a high-grade residual stenosis is identified, angioplasty or coronary artery bypass surgery, depending on the overall coronary anatomy and the clinical condition of the patient, is recommended. Recent data have indicated that PTCA need not be done emergently unless the patient is unstable (127). In addition, prolonged infusions of t-PA may result in sufficient remodeling to reduce the need for PTCA in many patients (4).

β-Adrenergic blockers (54, 59) and to a lesser extent intravenous nitroglycerin (15, 60) have been reported to reduce infarct size and improve survival in patients with acute myocardial infarction. Recent data suggest that such agents may also be useful in conjunction with thrombolysis. Ongoing research suggests that calcium channel blockers (53, 72, 73), α-adrenergic blockers (148), β-adrenergic blockers (51), and oxygen free-radical scavengers (14, 62, 87, 94) may enhance the salvage of myocardium following thrombolysis. However, until the results of ongoing clinical trials are available these agents should not be used because of the potential for deleterious effects.

Heparin has been used almost universally following administration of fibrinolytic agents. Its use is predicated on the need to avoid recurrent coronary thrombosis. Reocclusion after coronary recanalization with streptokinase is common, occurring in 20–43% of patients despite use of heparin (52, 78). With t-PA, 20% of patients manifested reocclusion within 30 minutes of completion of the infusion despite use of heparin. However, reocclusion was prevented by a longer infusion of t-PA (44). It is prudent to administer heparin to patients following fibrinolytic therapy, at least for 72 hours. If bleeding develops, heparin may be discontinued, and subsequent angiography planned should recurrent symptoms develop. Although the logic for the use of heparin is compelling, little direct data support its use, and a substantial reduction in mortality was documented in the GISSI trial without it (49). In view of the possibility that heparin may exacerbate bleeding, more data are needed to define its importance.

SUMMARY

When coronary reperfusion is accomplished within 1–2 hours after the onset of symptoms, patients benefit, especially those with anterior wall myocardial infarction. When treatment is initiated later, benefit is less consistent. Thus, the decision to employ thrombolytic therapy more than 2 hours after the onset of infarction depends on consideration of both the risk and potential benefit for the individual patient. Since rapid initiation of therapy is essential, intravenous fibrinolytic agents appear to be the treatment of choice. Streptokinase is the most widely available fibrinolytic agent, but t-PA will likely become the preferred agent in the near future. The development of still newer types of plasminogen activators should ultimately make efficacious and safe therapy possible. (See Editor's note on p. 167).

References

1. Alderman EL, Jutzky KR, Berte LE, et al: Randomized comparison of intravenous versus intracoronary streptokinase for myocardial infarction. *Am J Cardiol* 54:14, 1984.
2. Alkjaersig N, Fletcher AP, Sherry S: The mechanism of clot dissolution by plasmin. *J Clin Invest* 38:1086, 1959.
3. Anderson JL, Marshall HW, Askens JC, et al. A randomized trial of intravenous and intracoronary streptokinase in patients with acute myocardial infarction. *Circulation* 70:606, 1983.
4. Anderson JL, Marshall HW, Bray BE, et al: A randomized trial of intracoronary streptokinase in treatment of acute myocardial infarction. *N Engl J Med* 308:1312, 1983.
5. Andrade-Gordon P, Strickland S. Interaction of heparin with plasminogen activators and plasminogen: effects on the activation of plasminogen. *Biochemistry* 25:403, 1986.
6. Arneson H, Heilo A, Jakobsen E, et al. A prospective study of streptokinase and heparin in the treatment of deep vein thrombosis. *Acta Med Scand* 203:457, 1978.
7. Arneson H, Hoiseth A, Ly B. Streptokinase or heparin in the treatment of deep venous thrombosis. *Acta Med Scand* 211:65, 1982.
8. Barritt DW, Jordan SC. Anticoagulant drugs in the treatment of pulmonary embolism. A controlled trial. *Lancet* 1:1309, 1960.
9. Been M, de Bona DP, Muir AL, et al. Coronary thrombolysis with intravenous anisoylated plasminogen streptokinase complex BRL26921. *Br Heart J* 53:253, 1985.
10. Beiger R, Boehout-Mussert RJ, Hohmann F. Is streptokinase useful in the treatment of deep venous thrombosis? *Acta Med Scand* 199:81, 1976.
11. Bergmann SR, Fox KAA, Ter-Pogossian MM, et al. Clot selective coronary thrombolysis with tissue-type plasminogen activator. *Science* 220:1181, 1983.
12. Bounameaux HM, Vermylen J, Collen D. Thrombolytic treatment with recombinant tissue-type plasminogen activator in a patient with massive pulmonary embolism. *Ann Intern Med* 103:64, 1985.
13. Browse NL, Clemenson G, Lea Thomas ML. Is the postphlebitic leg always postphlebitic? Relationship between phlebographic appearances of deep-vein thrombosis and late sequelae. *Br Med J.* 281:1167, 1980.
14. Burton KP. Superoxide dismutase enhances recovery following myocardial ischemia. *Am J Physiol* 248:H637, 1985.
15. Bussman W, Passek D, Seidel E. Reduction of CK and CK-MB indices of infarct size by intravenous nitroglycerine. *Circulation* 63:615, 1981.
16. Castellino FJ. A unique enzyme-protein substrate modifier reaction: plasmin/streptokinase interaction. *Trends Biochem Sci* 4:1, 1979.
17. Chazov EL, Mateeva LS, Mazaev AV, et al. Intracoronary administration of fibrinolysin in acute myocardial infarction *Ter Arkh* 48:8–19, 1976.
18. Claeys H., Vermylen J. Physico-chemical and proenzyme properties of NH_2-terminal lysine human plasminogen. Influence of 6-aminohexanoic acid. *Biochim Biophys Acta* 342:351, 1974.
19. Collen D. On the regulation and control of fibrinolysis. *Thromb Haemost* 45:77, 1981.
20. Collen D, Bounameaux H, De Cock F, et al. Analysis of coagulation and fibrinolysis during intravenous infusion of recombinant human tissue-type plasminogen activator in patients with acute myocardial infarction. *Circulation* 73:511, 1986.
21. Collen D, Lijnen HR. The fibrinolytic system in man. An overview. In Collen D, Lijnen HR, Verstraete M.

(eds): *Thrombolysis: Biological and Therapeutic Properties of New Thrombolytic Agents.* Edinburgh, Churchill Livingstone, 1985.
22. Collen D, Stassen JM, Blaber M, et al. Biological and thrombolytic properties of the proenzyme and active forms of human urokinase. III. Thrombolytic properties of natural and recombinant urokinase in rabbits with experimental jugular vein thrombosis. *Thromb Haemost* 52:26, 1984.
23. Collen D, Stassen J, Stump DC, et al. Synergism of thrombolytic agents in vivo. *Circulation* 74:838, 1986.
24. Collen D, Stassen JM, Verstraete M. Thrombolysis with human extrinsic (tissue-type) plasminogen activator in rabbits with experimental jugular vein thrombosis. Effect of molecular form and dose of activator, age of thrombus, and route of administration. *J Clin Invest* 71:1012, 1984.
25. Collen D, Topol EJ, Tiefenbrunn AJ, et al. Coronary thrombolysis with recombinant human tissue-type plasminogen activator: a prospective, randomized, placebo-controlled trial. *Circulation* 70:1012, 1984.
26. Collen D, Zamarron C, Lijnen HR, et al. Activation of plasminogen by pro-urokinase. 2. Kinetics. *J Biol Chem* 261:1259, 1986.
27. Common HH, Seaman AJ, Rosch J, et al. Deep vein thrombosis treated with streptokinase or heparin. *Angiology* 27:645, 1976.
28. Coon WW, Willis PW, Symons MJ. Assessment of anticoagulant treatment of venous thromboembolism. *Ann Surg* 170:559, 1969.
29. Cowley MJ, Hastillo A, Vetrovec GW. Effects of intracoronary streptokinase in acute myocardial infarction. *Am Heart J* 102:1149, 1981.
30. Dalen JE, Alpert JS. Natural history of pulmonary embolism. *Prog Cardiovasc Dis* 17:259, 1975.
31. DeWood MA, Spores J, Notske RN, et al. Prevalence of total coronary occlusion during the early hours of transmural myocardial infarction. *N Engl J Med* 303:897, 1980.
32. Dodge HT, Sheehan FH, Mathey DG, et al. Usefulness of coronary artery bypass graft surgery or percutaneous transluminal angioplasty after thrombolytic therapy. *Circulation* 72(part 2):39, 1984.
33. Eisenberg PR, Sherman LA, Rich M, et al. Importance of continued activation of thrombin reflected by fibrinopeptide A to the efficacy of thrombolysis. *J Am Coll Cardiol* 7:1255, 1986.
34. Eisenberg PR, Sherman LA, Schechtman K, et al. Fibrinopeptide A: a marker of acute coronary thrombosis. *Circulation* 71:912, 1985.
35. Eisenberg PR, Sherman LA, Tiefenbrunn AJ, et al. Sustained fibrinolysis after t-PA in man. *Thromb Haemost* 57:35, 1987.
36. Elliot MS, Immelman EJ, Jeffrey P, et al. A comparative randomized trial of heparin versus streptokinase in the treatment of acute proximal venous thrombosis: an interim report of a prospective trial. *Br J Surg* 66:838, 1979.
37. Fletcher AP, Alkjaersig N, Sherry S. The clearance of heterologous protein from the circulation of normal and immunized man. *J Clin Invest* 37:1306, 1959.
38. Fletcher AP, Alkjaersig N, Sherry S, et al. The development of urokinase as a thrombolytic agent. Maintenance of a sustained thrombolytic state in man by its intravenous infusion. *J Lab Clin Med* 65:713, 1965.
39. Fletcher AP, Alkjaersig N, Smyrniotis FE, et al. The treatment of patients suffering from early myocardial infarction with massive and prolonged streptokinase therapy. *Trans Assoc Am Physicians* 71:287, 1958.
40. Fletcher AP, Sherry S, Alkjaersig N, et al. The maintenance of a sustained thrombolytic state in man. II. Clinical observations on patients with myocardial infarction and other thromboembolic disorders. *J Clin Invest* 38:111, 1959.
41. Gaffney PJ, Perry MJ. Unreliability of current serum

fibrin degradation product (FDP) assays. *Thromb Haemost* 53:310, 1984.

42. Ganz W, Geft I, Lew AS, et al. Intravenous streptokinase in evolving acute myocardial infarction. *Am J Cardiol* 53:1209, 1984.

43. Garabedian HD, Gold HK, Leinbach RC, et al. Comparative properties of two clinical preparations of recombinant human tissue-type plasminogen activator in patients with acute myocardial infarction. *J Am Coll Cardiol* 9:599, 1987.

44. Gold HK, Leinbach RC, Garabedian HD, et al. Acute coronary reocclusion after thrombolysis with recombinant human tissue-type plasminogen activator: prevention by a maintenance infusion. *Circulation* 73:347, 1986.

45. Goldberg S, Urban PL, Greenspon A, et al. Combination therapy for evolving myocardial infarction: intracoronary thrombolysis and percutaneous transluminal angioplasty. *Am J Med* 72:994, 1982.

46. Goldhaber SZ, Vaughn DE, Markis JE, et al. Acute pulmonary embolism treated with tissue plasminogen activator. *Lancet* 2:886, 1986.

47. Graor RA, Risius B, Young JR, et al. Peripheral artery and bypass graft thrombolysis with recombinant human tissue-type plasminogen activator. *J Vasc Surg* 3:115, 1985.

48. Groupe de Recherche Urokinase-Embolie Pulmonaire: Rapport prepare par B. Charbonnie, Tours. Etude Mulliticentrique sur seux protocoles d'urokinase dans l'embolie pulmonaire grave. *Arch Mal Coeur* 7:773, 1984.

49. Gruppo Italiano per lo Studio della Sreptochinasi nell'Infarcto Miocardio (GISSI): Effectiveness of intravenous thrombolytic treatment in acute myocardial infarction. *Lancet* 1:398, 1986.

50. Gurewich V, Pannell R, Louie S, et al. Effective and fibrin-specific clot lysis by a zymogen precursor form of urokinase (prourokinase). A study *in vitro* and in two animal species. *J Clin Invest* 73:1731, 1984.

51. Hammerman H, Kloner RA, Briggs LL, et al. Enhancement of salvage of reperfused myocardium by early beta-adrenergic blockade (timolol). *J Am Coll Cardiol* 3:1438, 1984.

52. Harrison DC, Ferguson DW, Collin SM, et al. Rethrombosis after reperfusion with streptokinase: importance of geometry of residual lesions. *Circulation* 69:991, 1984.

53. Henry PD, Schuchleib R, Davis J, et al. Myocardial contracture and accumulation of mitochondrial calcium in ischemic rabbit heart. *Am J Physiol* 233:H677, 1977.

54. Herltiz J, Elmfeldt D, Holmberg S, et al. Goteberg Metoprolol Trial: Mortality and causes of death. *Am J Cardiol* 53:9D, 1984.

55. Hirsch J, O'Sullivan EF, Martin M. Evaluation of a standard dosage schedule with streptokinase. *Blood* 35:341, 1970.

56. Hoffman JJML, van Rey FJW, Bonnier JJRM. Systemic effects of BRL 26921 during thrombolytic treatment of acute myocardial infarction. *Thromb Res* 37:567, 1985.

57. Holmes DR Jr, Smith HC, Vlietstra RE, et al. Percutaneous transluminal coronary angioplasty, alone or in combination with streptokinase therapy, during acute myocardial infarction. *Mayo Clin Proc* 60:449, 1985.

58. Hoylaerts M, Rijken DC, Lijnen HR, et al. Kinetics of the activation of plasminogen by human tissue-type plasminogen activator. Role of fibrin. *J Biol Chem* 257:2912, 1982.

59. ISIS Group: Vascular Mortality after early IV beta blockade in acute myocardial infarction (MI). *Circulation* 72:III, 1985.

60. Jaffe AS, Geltman EM, Teifenbrunn AJ, et al. Reduction of infarct size in patients with inferior infarction with intravenous glyceryl trinitrate. A randomized study. *Br Heart J* 49:452, 1982.

61. Jim RTS. A study of plasma prothrombin time. *J Lab Clin Med* 50:45, 1957.

62. Jolly SR, Kane WJ, Bailie MB, et al. Canine myocardium reperfusion injury, its reduction by the combined administration of superoxide dismutase and catalase. *Circ Res* 54:277, 1984.

63. Kakkar VV, Flank C, Howe CT, et al. Natural history of post-operative deep vein thrombosis. *Lancet* 2:230, 1969.

64. Kakkar VV, Flanc C, Howe CT, O'Shea M, Flute PT. Treatment of deep venous thrombosis. A trial of heparin, streptokinase, and Arvin. *Br Med J* 1:806, 1969.

65. Kakkar VV, Howe CT, Laws JW, et al. Late results of treatment of deep venous thrombosis. *Br Med J* 1:810, 1969.

66. Kaplan AP. Initiation of the intrinsic coagulation and fibrinolytic pathways of man: the role of surfaces, Hagemen factor, prekallekrein, HMW kininogen, and factor XI. *Prog Hemost Thromb* 4:127, 1978.

67. Kasper W, Erbel R, Meinertz T. Intracoronary thrombolysis with an acylated streptokinase plasminogen activator (BRL 26921) in patients with acute myocardial infarction. *J Am Coll Cardiol* 4:357, 1984.

68. Kennedy JW, Ritchie RL, Davis KB, et al. Western Washington randomized trial of intracoronary streptokinase in acute myocardial infarction. *N Engl J Med* 309:1477, 1983.

69. Kennedy JW, Ritchie RL, Davis KB, et al. The Western Washington randomized trial of intracoronary streptokinase: a 12 month follow up. *N Engl J Med* 312:1073, 1985.

70. Kernogan RJ, Todd C. Heparin therapy in thromboembolic disease. *Lancet* 1:621, 1966.

71. Khaja F, Walton JA, Brymer JF, et al. Intracoronary fibrinolytic therapy in acute myocardial infarction: report of a prospective randomized trial. *N Engl J Med* 308:756, 1983.

72. Klein HH, Schobothe M, Nebendahl K, et al. The effects of two different diltiazem treatments on infarct size in ischemic reperfused porcine hearts. *Circulation* 69:1000, 1984.

73. Knabb RM, Rosamond TI, Fox KAA, et al. Enhanced salvage of reperfused ischemic myocardium by diltiazem. *J Am Coll Cardiol* 8:861, 1986.

74. Koren G, Weiss AT, Hasin Y, et al. Prevention of myocardial damage in acute myocardial ischemia by early treatment with intravenous streptokinase. *N Engl J Med* 313:1384, 1985.

75. Kowalski E, Kopec M, Niewiarowski S. An evaluation of the euglobulin method for determination of fibrinolysis. *J Clin Pathol* 12:215, 1959.

76. Larrieu MJ, Rigollot C, Marder VJ. Comparative effects of fibrinogen degradation products D and E on coagulation. *Br J Haematol* 72:719, 1973.

77. Lee G, Low RI, Takeda P, et al. Importance of follow-up medical and surgical approaches to prevent reinfarction, reocclusion, and recurrent angina following intracoronary thrombolysis with streptokinase in acute myocardial infarction. *Am Heart J* 104:921, 1982.

78. Leibhoff RH, Katz RJ, Wasserman AG, et al. A randomized angiographically controlled trial of intracoronary streptokinase in acute myocardial infarction. *Am J Cardiol* 53:404, 1984.

79. Lew AS, Laramee P, Cercek B, et al. The hypotensive effect of intravenous streptokinase in patients without mycardial infarction. *Circulation* 72:1321, 1985.

80. Lijnen HR, Zamarron C, Blaber M, et al. Activation of plasminogen by pro-urokinase. I. Mechanism. *J Biol Chem* 261:1253, 1986.

81. Ly B, Anreson H, Eie H, et al. A controlled trial of streptokinase and heparin in the treatment of major pulmonary embolism. *Acta Med Scand* 1203:465, 1978.

82. Marder VJ, Rothbard RL, Fitzpatrick PG, et al. Rapid lysis of coronary artery thrombi with anisoylated plas-

minogen:streptokinase activator complexes. *Ann Intern Med* 104:304, 1986.

83. Marder VJ, Shulman NR. High molecular weight derivatives of human fibrinogen produced by plasmin. *J Biol Chem* 244:2120, 1969.

84. Marder VJ, Soulen BL, Atichartakarn V, et al. Quantitative venographic assessment of deep vein thrombosis in the evaluation of streptokinase and heparin therapy. *J Lab Clin Med* 89:1018, 1977.

85. McKlintock DK, Bell PH. the mechanism of activation of human plasminogen by streptokinase. *Biochem Biophys Res Commun* 43:694, 1971.

86. Mentzer RL, Budynski AZ, Sherry S. High-dose, brief duration intravenous infusion of streptokinase in acute myocardial infarction: description of effects on the circulation. *Am J Cardiol* 57:1220, 1986.

87. Myers ML, Bolli R, Lekich RF, et al. Enhancement of recovery of myocardial function by oxygen free-radical scavengers after reversible regional ischemia. *Circulation* 72:915, 1985.

88. Nilsson T, Wallen P, Mellbring G. Turnover of human extrinsic (tissue-type) plasminogen activator in man. *Haemostasis* 14:90, 1984.

89. O'Donnell TF, Browse NL, Burnand KG, et al.: The socioeconomic effects of an iliofemoral venous thrombosis. *J Surg Res* 22:483, 1977.

90. Paques EP, Stohr HA, Heimburger N. Study on the mechanism of action of heparin and related substances on the fibrinolytic systems: relationship between plasminogen activator and heparin. *Thromb Res* 42:797, 1986.

91. Ploug J, Kheldgaard NO. Urokinase: an activator of plasminogen from urine. I. Isolation and properties. *Biochim Biophys Acta* 24:282, 1957.

92. Proctor RR, Rapaport SI. The partial thomboplastin time with kaolin. *Am J Clin Pathol* 6:212, 1963.

93. Prowse CW, Davies J, Lane DA. Proteolysis of fibrinogen in healthy volunteers following major and minor *in vivo* plasminogen activation. *Thromb Res* 27:91, 1982.

94. Przyklenk K, Kloner RA. Superoxide dismutase plus catalase inprove contractile function in the canine model of "stunned myocardium." *Circ Res* 58:148, 1986.

95. Rakoczi I, Wiman B, Collen D. On the biological significance of the specific interaction between fibrin, plasminogen, and antiplasmin. *Biochim Biophy Acta* 1540:295, 1978.

96. Rentrop KP. Thrombolytic therapy in patients with acute myocardial infarction. *Circulation* 71:627, 1985.

97. Rentrop P, Blanke H, Karsch KR, et al. Changes in left ventricular function after intracoronary streptokinase infusion in clinical evolving myocardial infarction. *Am Heart J* 102:1188, 1981.

98. Rentrop P, Blanke H, Karsch KR, et al. Selective intracoronary thrombolysis in acute myocardial infarction and unstable angina pectoris. *Circulation* 63:307, 1981.

99. Rentrop KP, Feit F, Blanke H, et al. Effects of intracoronary streptokinase and intracoronary nitroglycerine infusion on coronary angiographic patterns and mortality in patients with acute myocardial infarction. *N Engl J Med* 311:1457, 1984.

100. Rijken DC, Hoylaerts M, Collen D. Fibrinolytic properties of one-chain and two chain human extrinsic (tissue-type) plasminogen activator. *J Biol Chem* 257:2920, 1982.

101. Rijken DC, Wijngaards G, Collen D. Tissue-type plasminogen activator from human tissue and cell cultures and its occurrence in plasma. In Collen D, Lijnen HR, Verstraete M (eds:) *Thrombolysis: Biological and Therapeutic Properties of New Thrombolytic Agents.* Edinburgh, Churchill Livingstone, 1985.

102. Robbins KC. The human plasma fibrinolytic system: regulation and control. *Mol Cell Biochem* 20:149, 1978.

103. Robertson BR, Nilsson IM, Nylander G. Thrombolytic

effect of streptokinase as evaluated by phlebography of deep venos thrombi of the leg. *Acta Chir Scand* 136:173, 1970.

104. Rogers WJ, Mantle, JA, Hood WP: Prospective randomized trial of intravenous and intracoronary streptokinase in acute myocardial infarction. *Circulation* 68:1051, 1983.

105. Rosch J, Dotter CT, Seaman AJ, Porter JM, et al. Healing of deep venous thrombosis: Venographic findings in a randomized study comparing streptokinase and heparin. *AJR* 127:553, 1976.

106. Rothbard RL, Fitzpatrick PG, Francis CW, et al. Relationship of the lytic state to successful reperfusion with standard and low dose intracoronary streptokinase. *Circulation* 71:562, 1985.

107. Rylatt DB, Blake AS, Cottis LE, et al. An immunoassay for human D dimer using monoclonal antibodies. *Thromb Res* 31:767, 1983.

108. Schroeder R, Biamino G, Von Leitner ER, et al Intravenous short-term infusion of streptokinase in acute myocardial infarction. *Circulation* 67:536, 1983.

109. Schroeder R, Neuhaus KL, Leizorovicz A, et al. A prospective placebo-controlled double-blind multicenter trial of intravenous streptokinase in acute myocardial infarction (ISAM): long-term mortality and morbidity. *J Am Coll Cardiol* 9:197, 1987.

110. Serruys PW, Wijns W, van den Brand M, et al. Is transluminal coronary angioplasty mandatory after successful thrombolysis? Quantitative coronary angiographic study. *Br Heart J* 50:257, 1983.

111. Shafer KE, Santoro SA, Sobel BE, et al. Monitoring of fibrinolytic agents. A therapeutic challenge. *Am J Med* 76:879, 1984.

112. Sheehan FH, Detley GM, Schofer J, et al. Effect of interventions in salvaging left ventricular function in acute myocardial infarction: a study of intracoronary streptokinase. *Am J Cardiol* 52:431, 1983.

113. Sheehan FH, Mathey DS, Schofer J, et al. Factors that determine recovery of left ventricular function after thrombolysis in patients with acute myocardial infarction. *Circulation* 71:1121, 1985.

114. Simmons ML, Brand M, de Zwaan C, et al. Improved survival after early thrombolysis in acute myocardial infarction. *Lancet* 2:578, 1985.

115. Smith RAG, Dupe RJ, English PD, et al. Acyl-enzymes as thrombolytic agents in a rabbit model of venous thrombosis. *Thromb Haemost* 47:269, 1982.

116. Smith RAG, Dupe RJ, English PD, et al. Fibrinolysis with acyl-enzymes: a new approach to thrombolytic therapy. *Nature* 290:505, 1981.

117. Sobel BE, Gross RW, Robison AK. Thrombolysis, clot selectivity, and kinetics. *Circulation* 70:160, 1984.

118. Spann JF, Sherry S, Carabello BA, et al. Coronary thrombolysis by intravenous streptokinase in acute myocardial infarction: acute and follow-up studies. *Am J Cardiol* 53:655, 1984.

119. Stainforth DH, Smith RAG, Hibbs M. Streptokinase and anisoylated streptokinase plasminogen complex. Their action on haemostasis in human volunteers. *Eur J Pharmacol* 24:751, 1983.

120. Stampfer MJ, Goldhaber SZ, Yusef S, et al. Effect of intravenous streptokinase on acute myocardial infarction. Pooled results from randomized trials. *N Engl J Med* 307:1180, 1982.

121. Taylor GJ, Mikell SL, Moses HW, et al: Intravenous versus intracoronary streptokinase therapy for acute myocardial infarction in community hospitals. *Am J Cardiol* 54:256, 1984.

122. Thomas D, Niewiarowski S, Meyers AR, et al. A comparative study of four methods for detecting fibrinogen degradation products in patients with various diseases. *N Engl J Med* 283:663, 1970.

123. The Thrombolysis in Myocardial Infarction (TIMI) Trial: phase I findings. *N Engl J Med* 312:932, 1985.

124. Tibbutt DA, Davies JA, Anderson JA, et al. Comparison

by controlled clinical trial of streptokinase and heparin in treatment of life-threatening pulmonary embolism. *Br Med J* 1:343, 1974.

125. Tiefenbrunn AJ, Robison AK, Kurnik PB, et al. Clinical pharmacology in patients with evolving myocardial infarction of tissue-type plasminogen activator produced by recombinant DNA technology. *Circulation* 71:110, 1985.

126. Tillet WS, Garner RL. The fibrinolytic activity of hemolytic streptococci. *J Exp Med* 58:485, 1933.

127. Topol EJ, Califf RM, George BS, et al. A multicentered randomized trial of intravenous recombinant tissue plasminogen activator and emergency coronary angioplasty for acute myocardial infarction: preliminary report from the TAMI study. *Circulation* 74:II-74, 1986.

128. Topol EJ, O'Neill WW, Langburd AB, et al. A randomized, placebo-controlled trial of intravenous recombinant tissue-type plasminogen activator and emergency coronary angioplasty in patients with acute myocardial infarction. *Circulation* 75:420, 1987.

129. Topol EJ, Weiss JL, Brinker JA, et al. Regional wall motion improvement after coronary thrombolysis with recombinant tissue plasminogen activator: importance of coronary angioplasty. *J Am Coll Cardiol* 6:426, 1985.

130. Tsapogas MJ, Peabody RA, Wu KT, et al. Controlled trial of thrombolytic therapy in deep vein thrombosis. *Surgery* 74:973, 1973.

131. Urokinase Pulmonary Embolism Trial, phase 1 results. *JAMA* 214:2163, 1970.

132. Urokinase-Streptokinase Pulmonary Embolism Trial, phase 2 results. *JAMA* 229:1606, 1974.

133. Van de Werf F, Bergmann SR, Fox KAA, et al. Coronary thrombolysis with intravenously administered human tissue-type plasminogen activator produced by recombinant DNA technology. *Circulation* 69:605, 1984.

134. Van de Werf F, Ludbrook PA, Bergmann SR, et al. Coronary thrombolysis with intravenously administered human tissue-type plasminogen activator in patients with acute myocardial infarction. *N Engl J Med* 311:609, 1984.

135. Van de Werf F, Nobuhara M, Collen D. Coronary thrombolysis with human single-chain urokinase-type plasminogen activator (prourokinase) in patients with acute myocardial infarction. *Ann Intern Med* 104:345, 1984.

136. Van de Werf F, Vanhaecke J, de Geest H, et al. Coronary thrombolysis with recombinant single-chain urokinase type plasminogen activator in patients with acute MI. *Circulation* 74:1066, 1986.

137. Verstraete M, Bory M, Collen D, et al. Randomized trial of intravenous recombinant tissue-type plasminogen activator versus intravenous streptokinase in acute myocardial infarction, *Lancet* 1:842, 1985.

138. Verstraete M, Bounameoux H, De Cock F, et al. Pharmacokinetics and systemic fibrinogenolytic effects of recombinant human tissue-type plasminogen activator (rt-PA) in humans. *J Pharmacol Exp Ther* 235:506, 1985.

139. Walker ID, Davidson JR, Rae AP, et al. Acylated streptokinase-plasminogen complex in patients with acute myocardial infarction. *Thromb Haemost* 51:204, 1984.

140. Wallen P, Bergsdorf N, Ranby M. Purification and identification of two structural variants of porcine tissue plasminogen activator by affinity adsorption of fibrin. *Biochim Bioplys Acta* 719:318, 1982.

141. Wallen P, Wiman B. Characterization of human plasminogen. II. Separation and partial characterization of different molecular forms of human plasminogen. *Biochim Biophys Acta* 257:122.

142. Watz R, Savidge GF. Rapid thrombolysis and preservation of valvular function in high deep venous thrombosis. *Acta Med Scand* 205:293, 1979.

143. Weimar W, Stibbe AJ, van Seyen AJ, et al. Specific lysis of an iliofemoral thrombus by administration of extrinsic (tissue type) plasminogen activator. *Lancet* 2:1018, 1980.

144. Whitaker AN, Elms NJ, Masci PP. Measurement of crosslinked fibrin derivatives in plasma an immunoassay using monoclonal antibodies. *J Clin Pathol* 37:882, 1984.

145. White WF, Barlow GH, Mozen MN. The isolation and characterization of plasminogen activators (urokinase) from human urine. *Biochemistry* 5:2160, 1966.

146. Wiman B, Collen D. On the kinetics of the reaction between human antiplasmin and plasmin. *Eur J Biochem* 84:573, 1978.

147. Wiman B, Collen D. Purification and characterization of human antiplasmin, the fast-acting plasmin inhibitor in plasma. *Eur J Biochem* 78:19, 1977.

148. Yamada K, Saffitz JE, Sobel BE, et al. Enhanced salvage of reperfused ischemic myocardium by alpha-adrenergic blockade. *J Am Coll Cardiol* 7:54, 1986.

149. Yasuno M, Saito Y, Ishida M, et al. Effects of percutaneous transluminal coronary angioplasty: intracoronary thrombolysis with urokinase in acute myocardial infarction. *Am J Cardiol* 53:1217, 1984.

150. Young AE, Lea Thomas M, Browse NL. Comparison between sequelae of surgical and medical treatment of venous thromboembolism. *Br Med J* 4:127, 1974.

151. Zammarron C, Lijnen HR, Van Hoef B, et al. Biological and thrombolytic properties of proenzyme and active forms of human urokinase. 1. Fibrinolytic and fibrinogenolytic properties in human plasma *in vitro* of urokinases obtained from human urine or by recombinant DNA technology. *Thromb Haemost* 52:19, 1984.

Editor's note added in proof: After submission of this chapter, tissue plasminogen was approved by the FDA for the treatment of acute myocardial infarction.

9

Antiarrhythmics

John P. DiMarco, M.D., Ph.D.

The introduction of cardiac defibrillation and the development of pharmacologic agents with potent antiarrhythmic activity have made possible the successful reversal and prevention of many forms of cardiac arrhythmia. Optimal antiarrhythmic therapy requires a knowledge of the basic pathophysiology for a patient's arrhythmia. Frequently, if the etiology of the arrhythmia can be identified and reversed, the use of agents with specific electrophysiologic effects may be avoided. Particularly in the setting of the critical care unit where such factors are common, the first step in evaluation of the patient with an arrhythmia should be a search for reversible causes of the arrhythmia such as hypoxia, myocardial ischemia, abnormal intracardiac pressures, acid-base imbalance, or electrolyte abnormalities. However, in many situations antiarrhythmic drugs will be required either as temporary measures to permit stabilization of a patient's rhythm until reversible factors may be normalized, or continuously in those patients whose underlying cardiac disease makes them chronically susceptible to paroxysmal arrhythmias.

During the last several decades progress in both clinical and basic investigation has greatly enhanced our understanding of the mechanisms responsible for cardiac arrhythmias and for the actions of antiarrhythmic drugs. In the basic research laboratory, investigators have described the effects of antiarrhythmic agents on the various ionic currents that determine the electrical activities of cardiac cells. The parallel development of techniques for intracardiac stimulation and recording has allowed many clinical arrhythmias to be studied under controlled laboratory conditions. It has become apparent from these studies that therapy for each patient's arrhythmia must be individualized since electrocardiographically similar arrhythmias in different patients may require totally different forms of therapy.

CELLULAR ELECTROPHYSIOLOGY

The electrical properties of cardiac cells have been extensively studied and excellent reviews are available (8, 13, 69, 80, 124, 135, 153). Only a brief review of current concepts is presented in this section.

Electrically active myocardial cells at rest maintain a potential difference between their cytoplasm and the surrounding extracellular fluid. When excited, these cells manifest a characteristic sequence of transmembrane potential changes called the action potential, which has traditionally been divided into five phases (Fig. 9.1). When the diastolic potential spontaneously reaches or is brought to a certain level, termed the threshold potential, a rapid depolarization occurs with a transient reversal of polarity (phase 0). Repolarization is then accomplished in three stages: a brief but rapid repolarization (phase 1), a plateau period during which there is little change in the transmembrane potential (phase 2), and a final period of repolarization back to the maximal diastolic potential (phase 3). Cells of the specialized conduction system, but not normal working atrial or ventricular myocytes, possess an intrinsic capacity for spontaneous depolarization during diastole (phase 4) that will continue until either the threshold potential is reached or the cell is brought to threshold by a conducted or exogenous stimulus. The action potential differs in various tissues within the heart depending on the relative activities of the currents discussed below in each tissue.

The action potential is produced by a complex interplay of a number of ionic currents (Table 9.1), which are, in turn, regulated by changes in the selected permeabilities of the cellular membrane. At rest, the cell membrane is permeable to potassium and highly impermeable to sodium, chloride, and calcium. Thus, the resting transmembrane potential ap-

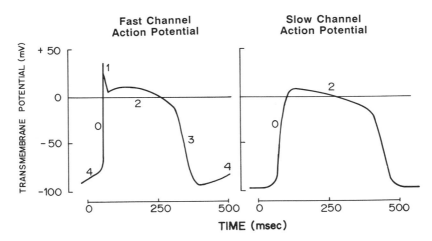

Figure 9.1. Representative cardiac action potentials from tissues dependent on either fast response (Na$^+$ channels) or slow response (Ca^{2+} channels) for action potential generation.

proximates the equilibrium potential for K$^+$ predicted by the Nernst equation for the transmembrane K$^+$ concentration gradient (K$^+$ concentration is approximately 4 mM in the extracellular space and 150 mM intracellularly). As a result, at the maximal point of repolarization in diastole, the transmembrane potential of a myocardial Purkinje fiber will be between -75 and -95 mV. If the threshold potential is reached, a dramatic change in membrane permeability and ionic currents take place. Sodium ion permeability increases and an inward Na$^+$ current (i_{Na}) is rapidly activated, pushing the transmembrane potential toward the equilibrium potential for Na$^+$ (approximately $+70$ mV). This change in membrane Na$^+$ conductance is probably due to the activation of molecular gates or channels that control the flow of specific ions through the membrane. Current theory describes a model in which each ionic channel is a protein that spans the lipid bilayer membrane (Fig. 9.2)

(68–70). In this model, an activation gate, called the "m gate," opens during phase 0 permitting an influx of Na$^+$ into the cell, which results in depolarization. An inactivation gate, termed the "h gate," then closes the Na$^+$ channel in a voltage-dependent manner before the full Na$^+$ equilibrium potential is reached. The kinetics of activation and inactivation of the channel are rapid, and the duration of the Purkinje fiber action potential upstroke is only 1 or 2 msec. For the remainder of the cardiac cycle the Na$^+$ channel remains in a resting state, closed but available for activation. Presumably by similar molecular mechanisms, the other ionic channels described below contribute to the full cardiac action potential.

During phase 1 of the action potential, inactivation of i_{Na} is completed and a Cl$^-$ current (i_{qr}) is activated leading to a transient period of rapid repolarization.

Phase 2 of the action potential, the plateau phase, involves the interactions of several fac-

Table 9.1
Ionic Currents Responsible for the Action Potential

Symbol[a]	Ion(s) Responsible	Activity
i_{Na}	Na$^+$	Activation produces phase 0 rapid depolarization
i_{qr}	Cl$^-$	Contributes to rapid repolarization (phase 1)
i_{si}	Ca^{2+}	Produces plateau phase and action potential in sinus and atrioventricular nodes
i_{x1}	K$^+$	Repolarizes fiber in phase 3
i_{bi}	Na$^+$	Contributes to phase 4 depolarization
i_{K1}	K$^+$	Background K$^+$ current
i_f	Na$^+$(K$^+$)	Pacemaker current in sinoatrial node
i_{K2}	K$^+$(Na$^+$)	Pacemaker current in Purkinje fiber

[a]The symbols used to denote specific currents have not been standardized and vary widely in discussions by different authors.

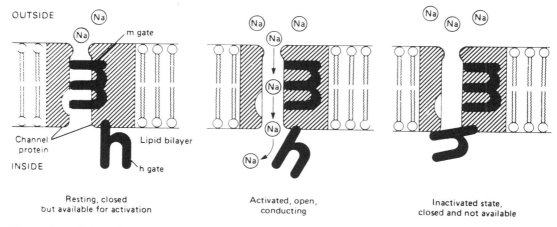

Figure 9.2. Schematic representation of the cardiac sodium channel. Shown is a protein *(shaded area)* spanning the bilayered lipid membrane with m and h gates. At rest, the m gate is closed but the h gate is open. With activation, the m gate opens and current flow is possible. Sodium current flow ceases with the rapid closing of the h gate ending phase 0. (From Hondeghem LM, Mason JW: Agents used in cardiac arrhythmias. In Katzung BG (ed): *Basic and Clinical Pharmacology.* Norwalk, CT, Appleton & Lange, 1987, pp. 151–167.)

tors. An outward background K$^+$ current, i_{K1}, is present throughout the action potential and it is balanced by an inward current (i_{si}) carried by Ca^{2+}, and to a lesser extent by Na$^+$, that is slowly activated by membrane depolarization in phase 0 and then slowly decays during the plateau period.

As i_{si} decays, more rapid repolarization occurs as a transient outward K$^+$ current (i_{x1}) is activated and the combined actions of i_{x1} and i_{K1} drive the transmembrane potential toward full diastolic depolarization.

The electrophysiologic characteristics of the action potential in sinus and atrioventricular (AV) nodal cells are quite different from those observed in Purkinje fibers. In the former, maximum negative diastolic potential is only −40 to −60 mV, and phase 0 of the action potential is not generated by the fast Na$^+$ channel but rather by a slow channel dependent on Ca^{2+} (Fig. 9.1). During phase 0, these cells exhibit a much slower rate of depolarization and a lower action potential amplitude and lack the overshoot seen in Purkinje fibers. Since conduction velocity is proportional to the rate of phase 0 depolarization, conduction in cells dependent on slow channel action potentials is also markedly slower.

The ionic mechanisms responsible for spontaneous diastolic depolarization remain incompletely understood. Early experiments in Purkinje fibers suggested that decay of an outward K$^+$ current in association with the constant effects of two time-independent background currents, i_{bi} and i_{K1}, led to diastolic depolarization. More recent experiments have suggested that a time-dependent inward current (i_f) carried by K$^+$ and Na$^+$ may be the primary mechanism for phase 4 depolarization. However, in sinus node cells, K$^+$ background currents, i_{si}, and electrogenic sodium pumping also may play a role in determining spontaneous activity.

DEFINITIONS: AUTOMATICITY, EXCITABILITY, REFRACTORINESS, RESPONSIVENESS, AND CONDUCTION

Effects of pharmacologic agents on the electrophysiologic characteristics of cardiac cells are often described in terms of several basic properties. Automaticity refers to the frequency of spontaneous impulse formation. Normally, it depends on three factors: the level of maximum diastolic depolarization, the rate of depolarization, and the level of the threshold potential. Excitability describes the strength of a stimulus required to initiate a new action potential at any given point during the action potential cycle. Refractoriness is the period during which the cell remains unexcitable after an action potential. Its most commonly used measure is the effective refractory period (ERP), the minimal interval between two propagated action potentials using an exciting stimulus of fixed intensity. In Purkinje fibers and working atrial and ventricular myocytes, the ERP is a function chiefly of the duration of the action potential. In cells located in the sinus and AV node, however, refractorineses is prolonged well after recovery of full diastolic depolarization. Membrane responsiveness describes the characteristics of a transmembrane potential response produced by an exciting stimulus. It has been demonstrated that the maximum rate of rise of the transmembrane potential ($\dot{V}_{max}$) during phase 0 may be used an an appropriate measure of the state of activation of the fast sodium channel and thus of sodium conductance. $\dot{V}_{max}$ in turn is related to the degree of membrane depolarization, and the relationship of the two has been termed the membrane responsiveness. Conduction occurs when an exciting stimulus brings a section of tissue to its threshold and the action potential generated serves as source of depolarizing current enabling adjacent sections to also reach threshold. The speed of conduction will depend on the passive electrical properties (cable properties) of the fiber and the membrane responsiveness.

MECHANISMS OF ARRHYTHMIAS

In broad terms, arrhythmias may be thought of as secondary to disorders of impulse formation (automaticity), impulse conduction, or a combination of the two (Table 9.2).

Arrhythmias Due to Abnormal Automaticity

In the normal heart, the cells of the sinoatrial (SA) node exhibit the most rapid rate of depolarization during diastole and reach thresh-

Table 9.2
Mechanisms for Arrhythmias

I. Disorders of automaticity
  A. Normal mechanisms—abnormal rate
    1. Sinus bradycardia or tachycardia
    2. Irregular sinus rhythm
  B. Abnormal mechanisms
    1. Enhanced spontaneous depolarization
    2. Early afterdepolarizations
    3. Late afterdepolarizations
    4. Triggered activity
II. Disorders of conduction
  A. Blocked normal impulse (sinoatrial exit block, AV block, etc.)
  B. Unidirectional block and reentry
    1. Random over multiple pathways (fibrillation)
    2. Organized over single pathway

old first. Cells in the distal AV junction and the His-Purkinje system also possess intrinsic automaticity, but because they manifest a slower rate of phase 4 depolarization, they normally are only latent or subsidiary pacemakers. The primary role of the SA node, the pacemaker for the rest of the heart, is reinforced by the phenomenon known as "overdrive suppression." Repetitive depolarization of a pacemaker cell by a stimulus from another source results in increased activity of the Na^+-K^+ exchange pump, thus generating a hyperpolarizing current. As a result, should a transient alteration in frequency of impulses from the SA node occur, a period of recovery is required before subsidiary pacemaker activity becomes manifest. Overdrive suppression enables the SA node to change rate modestly without competition from lower pacemakers and forms the basis for several clinical tests used to assess sinus node function.

The normal sinus node is highly responsive to alterations in autonomic nervous system output and in its biochemical surroundings. Increased adrenergic innervation produces major changes in ionic current activity in SA nodal cells. Catecholamine stimulation increases i_{si}, i_{x1}, and i_f, leading to a shorter action potential duration and an increase in the spontaneous rate of diastolic depolarization. Vagal stimulation and endogenous purines such as adenosine increase outward K^+ currents, thus hyperpolarizing the cells and inhibiting depolarization. In some cases, latent pacemakers may be more subject to the increase in adrenergic tone, and increased AV nodal or His-Purkinje automaticity induced by catecholamines may be responsible for the clinical occurrence of arrhythmias such as nonparoxysmal junctional tachycardia. In other situations, capacity for spontaneous depolarization may be induced by disease in working atrial or ventricular myocytes that would normally manifest a stable diastolic potential.

Other mechanisms for arrhythmias due to abnormal impulse formation are also possible. Under certain conditions, most notably intracellular calcium overload, oscillations, termed afterdepolarizations, in the transmembrane potential may be recorded either during phase 3 (early afterdepolarizations) or during the early part of phase 4 (late afterdepolarizations). Should these afterdepolarizations reach threshold, a new action potential will be generated and under appropriate conditions, propagated to adjacent cells (Fig. 9.3). Early and late afterdepolarizations may be observed

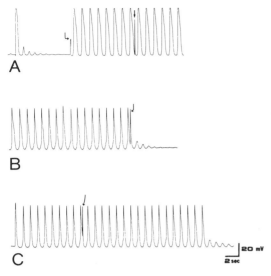

A

B

C

|20 mV
|2 sec

Figure 9.3. Triggered automaticity in an isolated superfused guinea pig myocyte. **A, B,** and **C** depict action potential recordings obtained from an impaled myocyte in the presence of isoproterenol, 10 μM. **A,** The first action potential is followed by several delayed afterdepolarizations that fail to achieve threshold. At the *arrow,* an applied stimulus initiates sustained rhythmic activity. **B,** A single extrastimulus terminates the arrhythmia. Subthreshold delayed afterdepolarizations are again observed. As shown in **C,** triggered activity may also terminate spontaneously. (Courtesy of Dr. L. Belardinelli, University of Virginia.)

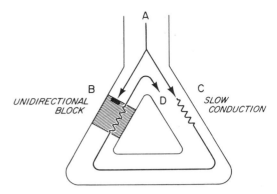

Figure 9.4. Diagram of the requirements for reentry. A premature impulse from some proximal point arrives at a branch point *(A)* with unequal conduction in the two branches. On side *B,* the tissue is still refractory and antegrade conduction block occurs. On side *C,* the impulse is slowed but traverses the area. It can then conduct around to point *B,* which has sufficiently recovered to permit retrograde conduction. If the tissue at *D* has recovered excitability, the reentry loop is completed and may continue.

in response to hypothermia, electrolyte imbalance, catecholamine excess, or stretch. Late afterdepolarizations may also be of particular importance in some of the arrhythmias due to digitalis intoxication.

Disorders of Impulse Conduction

Many cardiac arrhythmias are probably due to a recirculation or reentry of impulses within circuits of conducting cells. This concept may be described as follows. An impulse reaches a branch point in the cardiac conduction system and is conducted unequally down the two limbs available for conduction (Fig. 9.4). On one side, antegrade conduction is blocked and the area distal to the site of block remains inactivated. On the opposite side, impulse conduction is delayed but the impulse still traverses the region of delay. The impulse can now complete the loop and under appropriate conditions traverse the area of the original antegrade block in the retrograde direction. If

the conduction velocity through the pathway has been slow enough so that the tissue encountered by the reentrant impulse distal to the region of block has recovered excitability, reactivation may occur and the process repeated. Thus, in this model, for reentry to occur, there must be an inhomogeneity of electrical properties within the circuit such that delayed conduction, unidirectional block, and the recovery of excitability simultaneously coexist during one or multiple cycles.

Conduction velocity in normal atrial or ventricular myocardium is so rapid relative to the duration of refractoriness that reentry could not occur unless very long pathways were involved. Conduction in the sinus and AV nodes and in fibers that have been damaged by disease, and are therefore partially depolarized, is quite slow, however, and reentry over anatomically feasible circuits becomes possible. The classic example of a reentrant arrhythmia is paroxysmal supraventricular tachycardia in patients with extranodal accessory pathways. In these patients an exact sequence of activation of various parts of the heart by the reentrant impulse can be measured. In other cases in which reentry pathways are thought to occur either within atrial or ventricular muscle or within the AV node, such clear-cut evidence for the presence of reentry is, however, lacking; nonetheless, the reentry model has still provided an adequate explanation for many types of clinically important arrhythmias.

MECHANISM OF ANTIARRHYTHMIC DRUG ACTION

Antiarrhythmic drugs exert their effects by means of interactions with ion channels. As shown in Figure 9.5, these drugs usually have a high affinity for open channels and inactive channels, but low affinity for channels in the resting state. When channels are in the drug-bound state, conductance of the ion regulated by that channel is inhibited.

Several phenomena observed to be associated with antiarrhythmic drugs may be explained using this modulated receptor hypothesis. Since at faster rates cells will spend less time in the resting or drug-insensitive state, antiarrhythmic drugs will typically produce greater effects at faster rates (68, 111). This phenomenon is called use or frequency dependence. Also, the increased activity of many drugs on damaged cells is explained by the fact that loss of resting potential results in many inactivated channels that will show an increased sensitivity to drugs. Finally, the relative kinetics of association and dissociation of the channel in each state may be used to explain the differences between the various drugs' effects on the action potential. Although the modulated receptor hypothesis has been most extensively tested for the interaction of drugs with sodium channels, it is likely that other ionic channels behave similarly.

DRUG CLASSIFICATION

Over the years, various schemes have been proposed for the classification of antiarrhythmic drugs. These classifications are all limited in their ability to predict the efficacy of an individual antiarrhythmic drug in a given clinical situation, but they do allow a grouping of agents into classes with similar mechanisms of action and potential clinical spectrum (Table 9.3). The most widely used classification groups antiarrhythmic drugs into four major classes based on their predominant effects on the electrophysiologic properties of isolated normal cells (141).

Class I agents are local anesthetic agents that have as their predominant effect a depression of sodium conductance during phase 0 of the action potential. These drugs produce depression of $\dot{V}_{max}$, slow conduction velocity, and decrease excitability. Most of the drugs in class I also affect potassium repolarization currents and suppress automaticity in ectopic pacemakers. Recently it has been proposed that class I agents should be further divided into several subclasses (141). Class Ia agents, such as quinidine, procainamide, and disopyramide, produce a moderate depression of sodium conductance during phase 0 of the action potential, thereby depressing $\dot{V}_{max}$, slowing conduction velocity, and decreasing excitability. These drugs also depress K^+ cur-

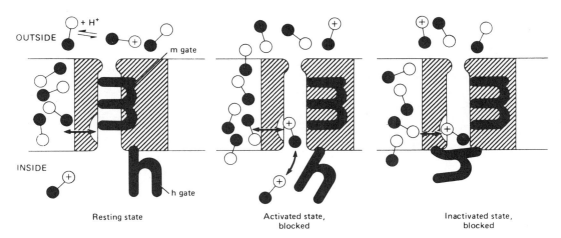

Figure 9.5. Interactions between antiarrhythmic drugs and the sodium channel. The *unshaded semicircular area* on the channel represents a hypothetical binding for the antiarrhythmic agent. In the resting state, closure of the m gate interferes with drug access and binding. In the activated and inactivated states, access is possible and the drug can bind to the receptor, blocking the channels. The kinetics of drug association and dissociation and the frequency of use of the channel all influence drug activity. (From Hondeghem LM, Mason JW: Agents used in cardiac arrhythmias. In Katzung BG (ed): *Basic and Clinical Pharmacology.* Norwalk, CT, Appleton & Lange, 1987, pp 151–167.)

Table 9.3
Classification of Antiarrhythmic Drugs

Class	Major Action	ECG Effects	Examples
I	Na$^+$ channel blockade	Ia: moderate ↓ conduction; moderate ↑ repolarization	Quinidine, procainamide, disopyramide
		Ib: mild ↑ conduction; little effect on repolarization	Lidocaine, mexiletine, tocainide, phenytoin
		Ic: marked ↓ conduction; little effect on repolarization	Encainide, flecainide, propranolol
II	β-Adrenergic blockade	Antagonizes endogenous catecholamines	Propafenone, metoprolol, many others
III	Variable and mixed	Prolongs action potential duration	Bretylium, amiodarone, sotalol
IV	Ca^{2+} channel blockade	Slows conduction in AV node; inhibits triggered activity	Verapamil, diltiazem

rents and prolong repolarization. Class Ib agents have minimal effects on sodium conductance and may actually shorten repolarization in normal fibers, but have more typical class I actions in partially depolarized fibers. Class Ic agents produce marked effects on sodium conductance and conduction velocity in normal and depolarized cells but have relatively little effect on repolarization.

Class II agents act by blocking β-adrenergic receptor stimulation. Some of these agents may produce class I–type effects at high concentrations, but their principal actions are to depress phase 4 depolarization in the sinus node, slow AV nodal conduction, and block catecholamine-induced changes in other electrophysiologic properties of cardiac tissues.

Class III agents are so grouped because they produce in vitro a marked prolongation of the action potential duration. Bretylium, sotalol, and amiodarone are placed in class III, but these drugs differ markedly in their clinical utility, and the mechanisms by which they exert their antiarrhythmic effects remain poorly understood.

Class IV agents depress the activity of the calcium-dependent slow channel and as a result are often referred to as "calcium blockers." These agents have been most useful clinically in the management of supraventricular arrhythmias that utilize the AV node for antegrade conduction, but may also prove to be of value in arrhythmias due to triggered automaticity.

There are numerous limitations to this classification scheme. The groupings are made on the basis of the single major effect of a drug on the action potential. Effects on other ionic channels or on the autonomic nervous system that may provide important contributions to a drug's overall antiarrhythmic effects are ignored. The classification is often based on ex-perimental data obtained using normal tissues in vitro, but these observations may not accurately describe a drug's effect in a diseased tissue. Metabolites of a drug may be effective and may produce different electrophysiologic actions than the parent compound. Finally, since the mechanisms responsible for a given arrhythmia may differ from patient to patient, it is frequently not possible to predict accurately a drug's effectiveness based solely on this classification. Despite these limitations, however, this classification schema is widely used and does provide a rough guide on which to base therapy.

INDIVIDUAL ANTIARRHYTHMIC AGENTS

The pharmacokinetic properties of the antiarrhythmic drugs discussed in this text are listed in Table 9.4. Table 9.5 provides a brief index of the major side effects that may be expected to occur during therapy.

Quinidine

Quinidine, one of the cinchona alkaloids, has been used to treat cardiac arrhythmias for almost 200 years. Early in this century, Frey (41) reported on its efficacy in the management of atrial fibrillation, and it has subsequently been used to treat other atrial and ventricular arrhythmias.

ELECTROPHYSIOLOGIC AND ECG EFFECTS (61, 64, 77)

In clinically relevant concentrations, quinidine depresses fast channel sodium conductance, thus decreasing $\dot{V}_{max}$ and the amplitude

Table 9.4
Pharmacokinetic Properties of Antiarrhythmic Drugs

Drug	Class	Oral Absorption	Systemic Bioavailability (%)	Estimated Volume of Distribution (Steady State) (liters/kg)	Amount Protein-Bound (%)	Mode of Elimination	Estimated Elimination Half-life (hr)	Effective Serum Concentration	Comments
Quinidine	Ia	Good	60–90	2.0–3.0	90	Hepatic, renal	4.0–8.0	1.5–4 µg/ml	Concentration ranges vary with different assays currently in use; range quoted here is for quinidine-specific assays only
Procainamide	Ia	Good	70–90	2.5–3.5	15	Renal	2.0–4.0	4–16 µg/ml	Active metabolite may accumulate, especially with renal failure
Disopyramide	Ia	Good	80–90	1.0–1.5	5–65 (see text)	Renal	6.0–8.0	2–4 µg/ml	Protein binding decreases at high serum levels
Lidocaine	Ib	Good	<30	1.5 (see text)	50	Hepatic	1.5–2.5	1–5 µg/ml	Elimination dependent on hepatic blood flow
Phenytoin	Ib	Good	90	0.6	90	Hepatic	18.0–30.0	10–20 µg/ml	Elimination half-life highly variable
Mexiletine	Ib	Good	80–90	6.0–8.0	30–50	Hepatic	10.0–24.0	0.5–2 µg/ml	
Tocainide	Ib	Good	90–100	1.5–3.0	50	Hepatic, renal	10.0–15.0	6–12 µg/ml	
Encainide	Ic	Variable	Variable	1.0	70	Hepatic	<2.0	See comment	Major metabolites with longer half-lives accumulate during therapy and may account for therapeutic effects
Flecainide	Ic	Good	90–100	1.0–2.0	40	Hepatic, renal	14.0–20.0	400–800 ng/ml	
Propafenone	Ic	Good	Nonlinear	2–3	95	Hepatic	6–13	See comment	Active metabolites contribute to effects
Bretylium	III	Poor	10–30	3.0–5.0	Low	Renal	8.0–13.0	Unknown	
Amiodarone	III	Poor	10–30	>20	>95	Unknown	Weeks	0.5–2 µg/ml	
Verapamil	IV	Good	10–30	4.0	90	Hepatic	3.0–6.0	70–200 ng/ml	
Diltiazem	IV	Good	30–40	NA	80	Hepatic	3.0–4.0	50–200 ng/ml	

Table 9.5
Major Extracardiac Side Effects of Antiarrhythmic Drugs

Drug	Gastrointestinal	Hematologic	Ocular	CNS	Dermatologic	Other
Quinidine	Nausea, vomiting, diarrhea, hepatitis	Thrombocytopenia, anemia			Rash	Fever, cinchonism, anaphylaxis, increased serum digoxin levels
Procainamide	Anorexia, nausea	Agranulocytosis, leukopenia			Rash	Fever, lupus-like syndrome
Disopyramide	Constipation, nausea		Blurred vision, glaucoma			Dry mouth, urinary retention
Lidocaine				Dizziness, dysarthria, convulsions		
Phenytoin		Lymphadenopathy, neutropenia		Drowsiness, ataxia, nystagmus	Rash	Gingival hyperplasia, disorders of calcium metabolism
Mexiletine	Nausea, vomiting			Tremor, dizziness, paresthesias, ataxia		
Tocainide	Nausea	Agranulocytosis		Headache, tremor, paresthesias	Rash	Pulmonary fibrosis
Encainide[a]	Nausea, vomiting			Dizziness, ataxia, tremor	Rash	
Flecainide[a]	Dysgeusia		Blurred vision	Dizziness, vertigo		
Propafenone[a]	Gastrointestinal upset, dysgeusia		Blurred vision	Dizziness		
Bretylium	Nausea, vomiting, parotitis (late)					Hypotension, often severe
Sotalol[a]				Fatigue		
Amiodarone[a]	Nausea, vomiting, constipation, and elevated hepatic enzymes		Corneal deposits	Peripheral neuropathy, myopathy	Bluish discoloration, photosensitivity	Pulmonary infiltrates and thyroid dysfunction
Verapamil	Constipation			Vertigo		

[a] Experience with new or investigational agents is limited and additional side effects may be noted in the future.

of phase 0 of the action potential. Conduction in Purkinje fibers is thereby slowed. Quinidine also slows the rate of phase 4 depolarization in isolated Purkinje fibers and makes the threshold potential less negative, thus decreasing normal automaticity. There is little effect on early or late afterpotentials or on the slow channel-mediated automaticity of depolarized fibers. The duration of the action potential is mildly increased and the ERP is prolonged as a function of increasing quinidine concentration. The normal sinus node shows little direct influence from quinidine, but in patients with intrinsic sinus node dysfunction, marked sinus slowing is occasionally noted.

Quinidine has mixed effects on AV nodal conduction. The direct depressant effect seen in isolated preparations is often overcome clinically by a vagolytic acceleration of AV nodal conduction. Accessory pathways, which resemble atrial or ventricular muscle in their response to quinidine, display slowed conduction and prolonged refractoriness. When studied in patients undergoing clinical electrophysiologic studies, quinidine increases the HV interval and the ERP of atrial and ventricular muscle, while minimally decreasing the AH interval and the antegrade refractory period of the AV node. The PR interval usually remains unchanged, whereas small dose-related increases in the QRS duration and larger increases in the QT_c interval are noted. At toxic concentrations, a widened QRS, AV block, and marked prolongation of the QT interval may occur. When quinidine is given to patients with atrial flutter or atrial fibrillation, its vagolytic effects on AV nodal conduction may produce dangerous increases in ventricular rate. This is a particular problem in atrial flutter in which the vagolytic effect in conjunction with a quinidine-induced increase in atrial cycle length may allow 1:1 AV conduction. Ventricular arrhythmias may also be aggravated by quinidine and this aggravation may occur even at usual plasma concentrations. The emergence of these arrhythmias is often but not always preceded by a marked prolongation of the QT interval.

PHARMACOKINETICS (49)

Quinidine is most commonly used orally, although intravenous infusions may be used safely in appropriate settings. The drug is well absorbed after oral administration but does undergo some first pass hepatic metabolism. This results in a systemic bioavailability of between 60% and 90%, depending on the preparation used. After intravenous administration, quinidine distributes rapidly (distribution half-life < 5 minutes) into a volume of distribution of approximately 2–3 liters/kg. The drug is highly bound (85–95%) to plasma proteins.

Hepatic metabolism is the principal method of elimination of quinidine. The major metabolites are (3S)-3-hydroxyquinidine and quinidine-N-oxide, and smaller quantities of 2'-oxoquinidine and O-desmethylquinidine may also be detected. The elimination half-life is between 6 and 8 hours. Quinidine metabolism is accelerated if the drug is administered in conjunction with a compound known to induce oxidative enzymes in hepatic microsomes. The clinical significance of this effect has been demonstrated during coadministration with either phenytoin or phenobarbital. The rate of quinidine metabolism is decreased in patients with congestive heart failure and in the elderly.

Renal excretion of unchanged quinidine accounts for only about 10–20% of drug elimination. However, azotemic patients on hemodialysis manifest decreased hepatic clearance and a decreased volume of distribution, and the dosage should be titrated in renal failure based on serum quinidine concentrations.

A variety of analytic techniques have been used in reports correlating plasma concentrations of quinidine and clinical efficacy. The older protein precipitation methods measured inactive or weakly active metabolites, and a therapeutic range of 4–8 μg/ml was usually reported. Plasma levels, measured either fluorometrically after extraction of metabolites or with more specific chromatographic assays, are considerably lower. When serum levels are measured by these latter techniques, serum concentrations in effectively treated patients will usually be between 1.5 and 4 μg/ml.

DIGOXIN-QUINIDINE INTERACTIONS (12, 89)

An interaction between quinidine and digoxin was first reported in 1978 (89) and the initial observations have been subsequently confirmed and extended in many studies. Initiation of quinidine therapy in a patient receiving a stable dose of digoxin decreases the volume of distribution of digoxin and decreases renal and possibly nonrenal clearance of digoxin. As a result, the serum digoxin concentration will gradually rise over 4–8 days, and with therapeutic doses of quinidine, a 1.5- to 3-fold increase in serum digoxin level is produced. A smaller rise in serum digitoxin level also occurs after initiation of quinidine therapy.

HEMODYNAMIC EFFECTS

During oral therapy, adverse hemodynamic effects from quinidine are rarely seen. When given intravenously, however, quinidine produces an α-sympatholytic effect that commonly causes hypotension and reflex tachycardia. This effect has limited the use of intravenous quinidine to special situations.

SIDE EFFECTS

In addition to the hemodynamic and ECG toxicity that may be associated with the drug, other side effects are commonly observed in patients treated with quinidine. Gastrointestinal intolerance is the most common side effect associated with quinidine therapy. Nausea, vomiting, and diarrhea are frequently seen and may preclude further therapy. Such reactions are common, occurring in up to one-third of those treated even if plasma concentrations are monitored within the "therapeutic range" (114).

Cinchonism is a syndrome that includes tinnitus, hearing loss, visual problems, and gastrointestinal upset caused by dose-related toxicity to quinidine or other cinchona alkaloids.

Immunologic reactions to quinidine include fever, thrombocytopenia, and anaphylaxis. Quinidine occasionally produces hemolytic anemia mediated either by a red cell antigen or by glucose-6-phosphate dehydrogenase deficiency. Blood cell counts should be monitored for several weeks after quinidine therapy has been initiated.

CLINICAL USE

Quinidine is useful in a variety of atrial arrhythmias. It may suppress ectopic atrial contractions that precipitate reentrant arrhythmias, convert established atrial flutter or atrial fibrillation to normal sinus rhythm, and by slowing conduction in accessory AV nodal pathways and in the "fast pathway" of patients with dual AV nodal pathways, can prevent or terminate some paroxysmal supraventricular tachycardias.

Ventricular arrhythmias may also be treated successfully with quinidine. Premature ventricular beats in the setting of acute myocardial infarction and in patients with chronic ventricular ectopy may be suppressed by quinidine. During electrophysiologic testing, quinidine suppresses the initiation of ventricular tachycardia with programmed ventricular stimulation in about one-third of patients studied (27). If ventricular tachycardia is not suppressed, the effect on tachycardia cycle length is somewhat variable, but the tachycardia in most patients shows cycle length prolongation. gation.

DOSAGE AND ADMINISTRATION

Quinidine is available for oral administration in several forms. A 200-mg tablet of quinidine sulfate contains 165 mg of quinidine base, and a 324-mg tablet of quinidine gluconate contains 206 mg of quinidine base. A 275-mg tablet of quinidine polygalacturonate is equivalent to 200 mg of quinidine sulfate. The gluconate and polygalacturonate are more slowly, but also more variably, absorbed than is the sulfate salt. The useful dose range is usually 800–2000 mg of quinidine sulfate daily in three or four divided doses, but plasma concentration monitoring should be used to guide therapy. Intramuscular administration of quinidine causes local irritation and should be discouraged. Quinidine gluconate may be given by a slow intravenous infusion if arterial pressure is carefully monitored. The usual initial intravenous loading dose is between 600 and 1000 mg (approximately 10 mg/kg) administered over 30–60 minutes.

Procainamide

First introduced in 1951, procainamide remains an important antiarrhythmic agent.

ELECTROPHYSIOLOGIC AND ECG EFFECTS (64, 75)

The electrophysiologic and ECG effects of procainamide are essentially the same as those produced by quinidine. In contrast to quinidine, however, procainamide has little anticholinergic activity. Procainamide, therefore, will widen the QRS, lengthen the QT interval, and prolong the HV interval while having little effect on AV nodal conduction. Sinus node function is usually not affected except in patients with sinus node disease. The ERPs of atrial and ventricular muscle and of many extranodal bypass tracts are prolonged by procainamide, thus procainamide given during a tachycardia often produces a dose-related prolongation of tachycardia cycle length and may eventually terminate the arrhythmia and block its reinitiation.

PHARMACOKINETICS (43, 44)

Procainamide may be used orally or parenterally. When administered orally, the drug is readily absorbed from the small intestine with a systemic bioavailability of 70–90%. Peak serum concentrations are achieved within 30–120 minutes of ingestion. The volume of distribution is approximately 1.5–2.5 liters/kg. Only about 15% of circulating procainamide is bound to plasma proteins.

The major mode of elimination of procainamide is renal tubular excretion of the unchanged compound. Procainamide also undergoes acetylation in the liver to N-acetylprocainamide. The rate of acetylation is variable, with patients separable into slow and fast acetylator subgroups (150). N-Acetylprocainamide has some antiarrhythmic activity and may contribute to the overall antiarrhythmic effect of procainamide. The elimination half-life for procainamide in normal subjects is approximately 3 hours. In patients with renal failure, renal elimination of procainamide and its metabolite are markedly prolonged and high levels of N-acetylprocainamide may accumulate.

The therapeutic range for procainamide plasma concentrations is broad. Little effect is seen below 4 μg/ml. Recent studies have shown that increased efficacy may be achieved with plasma concentrations up to 20 μg/ml (53), but this may often not be of clinical value (104). Different conditions may require different serum concentrations. However, toxicity is more frequent as plasma levels increase and may limit aggressive therapy in many patients.

HEMODYNAMIC EFFECTS

In high concentrations, procainamide may depress myocardial performance. Rapid intravenous infusion may lower peripheral resistance and blood pressure, but the latter effect is less commonly seen and is usually less marked than the hypotension associated with an electrophysiologically equivalent intravenous dose of quinidine.

SIDE EFFECTS

Side effects are uncommon during the first few days of procainamide therapy if low serum concentrations ($\leq$ 10 μg/ml) are maintained. With increasing doses, nausea, vomiting, and anorexia become increasingly prominent and may limit therapy. These gastrointestinal side effects may be seen even after parenteral administration.

Procainamide produces a variety of immunologically mediated reactions that limit its clinical use. Fever, leukopenia, and agranulocytosis may occur during the first days to weeks of therapy. The most common immunologic side effect, however, is development of a clinical syndrome resembling systemic lupus erythematosus (150). During chronic therapy about 60–70% of patients develop positive antinuclear antibodies. With continued therapy, some of these patients will develop a clinical syndrome characterized by arthralgia, fever, and serositis. Lupus erythematosus cell preparations may be positive. The syndrome is reversible if procainamide is discontinued, but recovery may be prolonged and persistent symptoms may require treatment with salicylates or corticosteroids.

The development of this syndrome is more common in slow acetylators, and a plasma concentration–related exposure to procainamide itself seems to be required for its development. Procainamide-induced lupus has not been observed during treatment with only N-acetylprocainamide. Since N-acetylprocainamide (NAPA) has electrophysiologic activity, trials with this compound have been performed. However, although ventricular premature beat suppression in some patients treated with NAPA has been shown, results in patients with chronic ventricular tachycardia have been disappointing.

CLINICAL USE

The ease of its oral or parenteral administration and its relative freedom from early side effects at moderate serum concentrations have made procainamide a popular choice in the treatment of many atrial and ventricular arrhythmias. Its clinical spectrum is similar to that of quinidine, although the latter has been more commonly used for termination of, or prophylaxis against, atrial flutter or fibrillation. The recent introduction of sustained-release preparations (44) has obviated the need for short dosing intervals, and patients who reliably absorb these preparations may often be managed on only three or four daily doses. The development of hypersensitivity reactions during chronic therapy remains a major problem.

DOSAGE AND ADMINISTRATION

Procainamide may be given either intravenously, orally, or intramuscularly. Intravenous infusion should be given cautiously and slowly to avoid marked hypotension. A loading dose of 10–20 mg/kg should be given by intermittent bolus injection of 100 mg every 1–3 minutes or as an infusion over 30–45 minutes. Careful blood pressure and rhythm monitoring are mandatory during intravenous loading. Intramuscular injections of procainamide may be used since the drug is well absorbed from intramuscular injection sites and does not cause tissue necrosis. Oral therapy with procainamide requires multiple daily doses because of the drug's short elimination half-life. The introduction of sustained-release preparations has improved this situation, but oral absorption of these preparations is more variable and monitoring of plasma concentrations is essential. The usual dose of procainamide needed to achieve adequate serum concentrations is 3–6 g/day. Occasionally, patients may respond to still larger doses but the risk of toxicity becomes substantial.

Disopyramide

Disopyramide was approved for clinical use in the United States in 1977. Its antiarrhythmic activity was first reported in 1963 and it became available in some European countries in 1969 (84). Since it has electrophysiologic effects similar to those of quinidine and procainamide, it was initially hoped that it might effectively substitute for these drugs, with a decreased incidence of side effects. With several years clinical experience, however, an increased incidence of toxicity has been noted and chronic therapy with disopyramide is not feasible in many patients.

ELECTROPHYSIOLOGIC AND ECG EFFECTS (58, 84)

The direct electrophysiologic effects of disopyramide are similar to those of quinidine and procainamide. It depresses the rate of phase 0 depolarization, prolongs the duration of the action potential, and increases the ERP of atrial and ventricular muscle. In Purkinje fibers, conduction velocity is delayed and the slope of spontaneous diastolic depolarization is decreased. Disopyramide has significant anticholinergic properties and these tend to cancel out a direct depressant effect on atrioventricular conduction. Although sinus node testing in normal subjects shows few effects from disopyramide, the drug may produce marked depression of the sinus node in patients with a clinical history of sinus node dysfunction. Disopyramide prolongs the HV interval and in rare patients may precipitate AV block. During routine clinical usage, disopyramide at usual concentrations produces little change in sinus cycle length and PR interval, a minor prolongation of QRS duration, and a moderately prolonged QT_c interval.

PHARMACOKINETICS (58)

Disopyramide may be administered either orally or intravenously, but only the oral preparation is currently available for use in the United States. The drug is well absorbed orally and reaches a peak serum concentration approximately 1–2 hours after ingestion. The drug's volume of distribution after an intravenous bolus is about 1.0–1.5 liters/kg and is decreased in patients with acute myocardial infarction, congestive heart failure, or renal failure.

Renal excretion of unchanged drug is the major mode of elimination for disopyramide. The compound also undergoes N-dealkylation to a mono-N-dealkylated inactive metabolite. In normal volunteers, the elimination half-life is approximately 6–8 hours. Elimination is prolonged in renal failure and doses must be adjusted according to serum concentration. The effects of hemodialysis on disopyramide metabolism are variable, but resin or charcoal hemoperfusion has been used in the emergency treatment of poisoning with the drug.

Protein binding of most antiarrhythmic drugs remains constant within the therapeutic range. In contrast, the degree of protein binding for disopyramide decreases markedly with increasing total concentrations within the usually observed range of plasma concentrations of 2–4 mg/ml (102). This fact has potential clinical significance since most clinical laboratories report only total drug concentrations, and a small increase in total concentration may represent a large increase in active drug.

HEMODYNAMIC EFFECTS

Disopyramide has markedly negative inotropic effects that complicate its use in patients with congestive heart failure. Disopyramide has been reported to lower cardiac output, raise systemic vascular resistance, and depress left ventricular function. In one clinical series, symptomatic congestive heart failure was exacerbated or precipitated by disopyramide in 16 of 100 patients (119). This event occurred in 50% of the treated patients with a prior history of congestive heart failure. As a result of these observations, disopyramide therapy should be initiated in patients with congestive heart failure with great caution and only if no suitable alternative is available.

SIDE EFFECTS

Disopyramide has potent anticholinergic activity in many organ systems and produces dry mouth, urinary hesitancy, and constipation. Acute urinary retention may occur in patients with prostate enlargement or diabetes mellitus. The drug may also precipitate acute glaucoma. Rare cases of hepatitis have been reported.

DOSAGE AND ADMINISTRATION

At the present time, disopyramide is available for administration in the United States only as capsules containing 100 or 150 mg of the drug and as sustained-release capsules of the same size. The usual loading dose is 300 mg, with subsequent doses of 100–200 mg every 6 or 8 hours for the regular capsules. The interval between doses should be decreased in the presence of renal failure.

Lidocaine

Lidocaine is readily administered intravenously and has few side effects at therapeutic serum concentrations; its effects dissipate rapidly after an infusion is terminated. For these and other reasons, it has gained acceptance as the drug of choice for the short-term treatment of many acute ventricular arrhythmias (128).

ELECTROPHYSIOLOGIC AND ECG EFFECTS

Although lidocaine is grouped with quinidine and procainamide as a class I antiarrhythmic drug, there are marked differences in its electrophysiologic effects. Lidocaine depresses fast channel sodium conductance, but its effects are more prominent in partially depolarized fibers (3, 131). In normal fibers, lidocaine shortens the action potential duration, shortens the ERP, and decreases spontaneous automaticity. Conduction velocity shows little change. In depolarized fibers or in fibers damaged by ischemia, however, lidocaine prolongs the action potential and slows conduction. When given to normal subjects, lidocaine has little effect on sinus cycle length, PR interval, QRS duration, or QT interval. The AH and HV intervals usually remain normal. Lidocaine may rarely produce AV block in patients with severe preexisting intraventricular conduction disorders.

PHARMACOKINETICS (129, 151)

Lidocaine is well absorbed orally, but extensive first pass hepatic metabolism makes oral administration unreliable and the drug is used only parenterally. After intravenous administration, lidocaine distributes rapidly into a central compartment with a volume of distribution of approximately 0.5 liter/kg. The size of the central compartment is decreased in patients with heart failure or shock. With prolonged infusion of lidocaine, peripheral tissues become saturated and the steady state volume of distribution is approximately 1.5 liters/kg. In the blood, about 50% of the total lidocaine is bound to plasma proteins, principally albumin. Intramuscular lidocaine is also well tolerated and has been used in an emergency setting before hospital admission.

Lidocaine is eliminated chiefly via hepatic metabolism with the metabolic rate proportional to hepatic blood flow. A variety of metabolites have been detected. The major pathway is oxidative N-deacylation to monoethylglycinexylidide, an active metabolite, with subsequent hydrolysis to 2,6-xylidine. A number of other hydroxylated metabolites may also be found. In congestive heart failure, the volume of distribution in the central compartment is decreased and hepatic blood flow may be decreased if cardiac output is depressed. Hepatic failure slows clearance rate but does not affect the volume of distribution. Since less than 10% of lidocaine is excreted unchanged in the urine, little adjustment is required in renal failure. The elimination half-life after short-term infusion averages 1.5–2.5 hours, but is often prolonged in critically ill patients or in patients who have had prolonged courses of therapy.

The desired serum concentration of lidocaine should be 1–5 μg/ml. Toxicity begins to appear at a serum concentration between 5 and 10 μg/ml and a severe toxicity is common at higher levels.

HEMODYNAMIC EFFECTS

At the concentrations normally employed clinically, lidocaine produces few adverse hemodynamic changes.

SIDE EFFECTS

The principal side effects associated with lidocaine therapy are concentration-related and are manifest clinically as disturbances of central nervous system function. These effects may be quite subtle and are commonly overlooked in the critical care setting. The side effects are more frequent in elderly patients and those with compromised cardiac output in whom the volume of distribution is usually decreased. In such patients, lidocaine toxicity may be mistakenly thought to be due to the patient's overall condition and drug toxicity not suspected. Dysarthria is often the first warning of lidocaine toxicity, with paresthesias, disorientation, and agitation also frequent complaints. At higher concentrations, seizures and respiratory arrest may occur. These latter side effects are most commonly seen in patients with reduced central volumes of distribution due to age or heart failure in whom bolus injection may transiently produce marked elevations in serum concentrations.

CLINICAL USE

Lidocaine has been used chiefly for treating ventricular arrhythmias. Its ease of parenteral administration has made it the most common drug chosen for the initial therapy of acute arrhythmias in the critical care setting. Controlled data concerning lidocaine efficacy in most clinical situations are unfortunately lacking. In the absence of such data, however, the relative safety of lidocaine and its ease of use justify its traditional role.

The use of prophylactic lidocaine in cases of acute myocardial infarction remains controversial since conflicting data have been reported from equally well-designed studies (Table 9.6) (33, 87, 91, 115, 140). A decision as to whether lidocaine should be administered to patients with known or suspected myocardial infarction must continue to be made on an individualized basis.

DOSAGE AND ADMINISTRATION

Lidocaine may be used intramuscularly or intravenously, but the intravenous route is most commonly used. The initial loading dose of 1.5–2.5 mg/kg should be given in two injections separated by 20–30 minutes or as a continuous infusion over 30 minutes. Maintenance therapy may require infusion rates of 1–4 mg/min, but plasma level monitoring should be used if long-duration, high-dose infusions are used. The decreased central volume of distribution seen in congestive heart failure and shock requires that both loading and maintenance doses be lowered. In particular, caution is required when bolus injections of lidocaine are given to severely ill patients already on a maintenance infusion. In such situations it is often safer to switch to a second agent rather than risk major toxicity while attempting to achieve a maximal lidocaine effect.

Mexiletine

Mexiletine was first developed as an anticonvulsant, but subsequent studies indicated significant antiarrhythmic activity. It has been

Table 9.6
Prophylactic Lidocaine in Suspected Acute Myocardial Infarction[a]

Authors	Lidocaine Dose	Period of Evaluation (hr)	No. of Patients				
			Total	Sustained VT or VF		Asystole or CHB	
				Lidocaine	Placebo	Lidocaine	Placebo
Lie et al (91)	100 mg i.v. +3 mg/min	48	212	2	15	NR	NR
O'Brien et al (115)	75 mg i.v. +2.5 mg/min	48	300	18	18	7	2
Valentine et al (140)	300 mg i.m.	2	269	3	7	NR	NR
Koster and Dunning (87)	400 mg i.m.	1	6024	8	17	26	13
Dunn et al (33)	300 mg i.m. +100 mg i.v.	1	402	3	3	3	1

[a] CHB, complete heart block; NR, not reported; VT, ventricular tachycardia; VF, ventricular fibrillation.

widely used for a number of years in Europe and Great Britain and was released in the United States in 1986. It is usually classified as a class Ib agent.

ELECTROPHYSIOLOGIC AND ECG EFFECTS (127)

Mexiletine is structurally similar to lidocaine and its electrophysiologic effects are similar. In usual clinical concentrations, mexiletine produces no change in AH or HV intervals or in sinus or AV nodal function. The effect on the ERP in ventricular muscle is somewhat variable but most patients will manifest no change in sinus rate, PR, QRS, or QT_c intervals.

PHARMACOKINETICS (17)

Mexiletine is well absorbed orally, with peak concentrations achieved 30–90 minutes after a dose. After intravenous administration, the volume of distribution is large (6–8 liters/kg) reflecting extensive tissue binding. Thirty to 50% of the drug in plasma is protein bound. The major mode of elimination is hepatic transformation via oxidation or reduction to a variety of metabolites. The antiarrhythmic activities of these metabolites are unknown. Only a small fraction of the dose is excreted as unchanged drug in the urine. Although the urinary excretion is increased at lower urinary pH, this fact is of limited clinical significance. The elimination half-life of mexiletine is about 10 hours in normal volunteers, but is increased to 10–24 hours in patients with cardiac disease. The useful plasma therapeutic range for mexiletine appears to be about 0.5–2.0 μg/ml.

HEMODYNAMIC EFFECTS

Mexiletine has few or no clinically important hemodynamic effects during chronic oral therapy (136). Mild or moderate depression of left ventricular function has been reported after intravenous infusion. These effects have been similar to those observed with therapeutic doses of lidocaine.

SIDE EFFECTS (17)

The clinical use of mexiletine is limited by a high incidence of gastrointestinal and central nervous system reactions. Nausea, vomiting, and gastrointestinal upset are frequently seen. In some patients, these toxic effects may be prevented by administering small doses in association with meals. Neurologic toxicity is also prominent. Tremor, dizziness, confusion, and ataxia are often seen and may require discontinuation of therapy. These side effects may occur with plasma levels well within the useful range described above. Hypotension and increased AV block are not usually seen.

CLINICAL USE

Although mexiletine has been evaluated in a variety of clinical settings, no consensus about its current role in antiarrhythmic therapy exists. It does provide symptomatic relief in some patients with palpitations due to ventricular premature beats and nonsustained ventricular tachycardia. Mexiletine, however, has not proven to be consistently effective as single therapy in patients with a history of sustained ventricular tachycardia (26, 144), or in postinfarct patients (19, 73). The use of mexiletine in combination with a second antiarrhythmic drug or with a β-adrenergic blocker has seemed more promising, however, in patients with sustained arrhythmias (31).

DOSAGE AND ADMINISTRATION

The normal dosage range of mexiletine is 300–900 mg daily in three or four divided doses. Occasional patients may tolerate a twice-a-day dosage schedule.

Tocainide

Tocainide is another compound structurally related to lidocaine that has similar electrophysiologic properties. Its chief advantage over lidocaine is its long elimination half-life and its ability to be taken orally.

ELECTROPHYSIOLOGIC AND ECG EFFECTS (95)

The effects of tocainide on electrophysiologic parameters parallel those of lidocaine and mexiletine. After intravenous infusion, the drug produces only minor changes in sinus rate or in the PR, QRS or QT_c intervals. The AH and HV intervals and the ERPs of the His-Purkinje system and right ventricular muscle show no change. When given to some patients with ventricular tachycardia, tocainide may paradoxically shorten the tachycardia cycle length and cause degeneration to ventricular fibrillation (34).

PHARMACOKINETICS (95)

Tocainide is rapidly absorbed orally with almost 100% bioavailability. Peak serum levels are seen 1–2 hours are oral ingestion. About 50% of the drug is bound to plasma proteins at clinically relevant plasma concentrations. The volume of distribution is about 1–2 liters/kg. The drug is eliminated both by hepatic metabolism and by renal filtration. The principal metabolites detected in urine are the glucuronide conjugate of N-carboxytocainide and lactylxylide. The elimination half-life is between 10 and 15 hours. Antiarrhythmic effects are noted at plasma concentrations of 5–12 μg/ml.

HEMODYNAMIC EFFECTS

Only limited information is available on the hemodynamic actions of tocainide. Tocainide probably produces only minor changes in systolic function even in patients with heart failure.

SIDE EFFECTS

Central nervous system toxicity is a frequent complication of tocainide therapy, with tremors, headache, visual disturbances, dizziness, and paresthesia observed frequently with plasma levels below 10 μg/ml. Nausea, vomiting, dyspepsia, and anorexia are seen in approximately 10–25% of patients. Other rare adverse reactions include an allergic rash, leukopenia, and pulmonary fibrosis.

CLINICAL USE

Tocainide has been shown to suppress ventricular premature beats in 40–70% of patients with stable, asymptomatic arrhythmias (95). The response rate to tocainide for patients with sustained ventricular tachycardia or ventricular fibrillation is much lower, however, and like mexiletine, it should probably not be used as a single agent in therapy of sustained ventricular tachyarrhythmias. Tocainide has not been shown to be of significant benefit during acute myocardial infarction (18).

Encainide

Encainide is a benzanilide derivative that has recently been released for use in the United States. It is considered to be a class Ic antiarrhythmic agent.

ELECTROPHYSIOLOGIC AND ECG EFFECTS (126, 148)

In Purkinje fibers, encainide depresses $\dot{V}_{max}$ during phase 0 of the action potential, shortens action potential duration, prolongs the ERP relative to the action potential duration, and decreases the rate of spontaneous phase 4 depolarization. Conduction velocity in Purkinje fibers is markedly reduced. Normal sinus node function and AV nodal conduction are only slightly affected by intravenous encainide, but the HV interval is markedly prolonged. During chronic therapy, however, accumulation of active metabolites may cause prolongation of the AH interval. The ECG of patients during chronic therapy will usually show a prolonged PR interval and a widened QRS, but the JT_c interval will only rarely be lengthened.

PHARMACOKINETICS (143, 149)

Encainide is rapidly and well absorbed after oral administration, but in approximately 90% of the North American population, extensive first pass hepatic extraction and metabolism occur before the drug reaches the systemic circulation. Two major metabolites, O-desmethylencainide (ODE) and 3-methoxy-O-desmethylencainide (MODE), and a third, minor metabolite, N-desmethylencainide, have been identified. The former two compounds are both pharmacologically active, producing electrophysiologic effects similar to those of encainide itself (125). In patients who possess the capacity to metabolize encainide rapidly, the parent compound itself has an elimination half-life of only 1–2 hours, but ODE and MODE have elimination half-lives of approximately 11 and 24 hours, respectively, with final elimination occurring via conjugation and renal excretion. Thus, in these patients most of the clinically apparent effects are produced by the metabolites.

Approximately 6–10% of the North American population genetically lacks the ability to metabolize encainide readily (143). In these patients much higher plasma concentrations of encainide are seen; the parent compound itself has an elimination half-life of about 12 hours and is responsible for any antiarrhythmic activity.

Since the effects of encainide are due to the combined actions of several compounds, no firm guidelines for using plasma concentrations to guide therapy have been described.

HEMODYNAMIC EFFECTS (139)

Encainide has not produced significant acute changes in left ventricular function even in patients with moderate congestive heart failure, but long-term data concerning this question are not available.

SIDE EFFECTS

Encainide causes dose-related side effects that limit therapy in about 25% of patients treated with the drug. The most common adverse reactions reported are dizziness, blurred vision, ataxia, tremor, headache, and gastrointestinal upset. The nature of the relationships between these side effects and the individual plasma concentrations of encainide and its major metabolites is unknown.

Encainide, like flecainide and other similarly acting drugs, has a potential for producing proarrhythmic effects without warning. In the most severe form, these arrhythmias are sustained ventricular tachycardia with unusually wide QRS complexes that may be resistant to cardioversion attempts (147).

CLINICAL USE

Encainide is a generally safe and effective agent for suppressing ventricular premature beats and nonsustained ventricular tachycardia in patients without important structural heart disease. Results in patients with a history of sustained arrhythmias are less predictable (99). In addition, since antiarrhythmic effects in each patient are the sum of effects of the parent compound and the active metabolites, a standardized range of plasma concentrations to guide therapy is not available. In patients with sustained ventricular tachycardia, encainide at lower doses usually results in a slower tachycardia if the arrhythmia recurs.

Encainide may be useful in patients with supraventricular arrhythmias. If relatively high doses (150–200 mg/day) are used, encainide can markedly prolong the ERP of, or even block conduction in, accessory pathways (1, 121). The role of encainide in patients with paroxysmal atrial flutter or fibrillation has not been thoroughly investigated.

DOSAGE AND ADMINISTRATION

Encainide therapy is usually initiated at a dose of 25 mg three times daily, and this dose may be cautiously increased every 3–4 days up to a maximum dose of 200 mg daily. Rapid loading should be avoided because of the risk of overshooting the desired effects and either adversely affecting AV conduction or producing proarrhythmic effects. Although the population may be divided into two genetically determined groups based on their ability to metabolize encainide, phenotyping is unnecessary since the clinical results of therapy are similar in both groups.

Flecainide

Flecainide acetate was first synthesized in 1975 and was recognized to have significant antiarrhythmic activity in early preclinical and clinical trials. It was released for general use in the United States in 1986. Flecainide is classified as a type Ic antiarrhythmic agent.

ELECTROPHYSIOLOGIC AND ECG EFFECTS (66, 108)

Flecainide is a potent inhibitor of fast sodium channel activity and thus markedly depresses the upstroke of the action potential during phase 0. Conduction velocity in Purkinje fibers and both atrial and ventricular muscle is slowed. Normal sinus node automaticity is usually not changed, but Purkinje fiber automaticity is inhibited. Conduction velocity in the AV node is also decreased. During electrophysiologic studies, flecainide prolongs both the AH and HV intervals, prolongs or blocks conduction times in accessory pathways, and produces minor increases in atrial and ventricular refractoriness.

During chronic flecainide therapy, increases in the PR interval and QRS duration may be seen. Increases in QRS duration of more than 25% are related to elevated plasma concentrations and indicate toxicity.

PHARMACOKINETICS (23)

Oral flecainide is well absorbed, with 90–95% of an oral dose bioavailable. There is no alteration of bioavailability by food or antacids. Little first pass hepatic extraction occurs. The degree of plasma protein binding is approximately 40%. The steady state volume of distribution is 7–9 liters/kg. There are two major hepatic metabolites: *meta-O*-dealkylated flecainide and the *meta-O*-dealkylated lactan. These compounds do not have clinically relevant antiarrhythmic activity. During chronic therapy, about 40–60% of flecainide is excreted in the urine as unchanged drug. The average elimination half-life is between 12 and 24 hours, but this time may be prolonged in patients with congestive heart failure or renal insufficiency. Careful monitoring is required to maintain plasma concentrations within the desired range. For the reasons discussed below, this desired range requires adjustment from patient to patient to avoid toxicity. Therapeutic effects begin to be seen at concentrations over 200 ng/ml. Plasma concentrations should be maintained below 600 ng/ml in patients with congestive heart failure. Concentrations up to 1000 ng/ml may be tolerated by patients with normal ventricular function and may yield increased antiarrhythmic activity.

HEMODYNAMIC EFFECTS (76)

Flecainide has important negative inotropic effects in both animal and clinical studies. After intravenous administration, flecainide decreases left ventricular ejection fraction, cardiac index, and stroke work index and increases left and right ventricular filling pressures. During chronic oral therapy, 5–15% of patients treated with flecainide will either develop new congestive heart failure or a worsening of preexisting failure. This is a particularly difficult problem, since as heart failure develops, flecainide elimination is prolonged leading to further depression of ventricular function or to drug-induced arrhythmias if the dose is not reduced.

SIDE EFFECTS

The prevalence of adverse reactions during flecainide therapy is highly dependent on the patient population studied. In stable patients with normal ventricular function, minor extracardiac side effects including dizziness, dysgeusia, blurred vision, nausea, and headache may be seen. These adverse reactions are usually associated with plasma concentrations above 800 ng/ml and are manageable with dosage adjustments (39).

In contrast, patients with more serious cardiac disease are susceptible to several life-threatening forms of cardiac toxicity. Flecain-ide has been associated with a 10–15% incidence of worsened arrhythmias when given to patients with a history of sustained ventricular tachycardia or cardiac arrest (110, 118). This proarrhythmic effect often presents as sustained ventricular tachycardia with a very wide, poorly defined QRS complex that despite a relatively long cycle length may not support a blood pressure. This rhythm may be resistant to attempts at DC cardioversion and may prove fatal despite immediate and appropriate resuscitation attempts. In most but not all cases, this phenomenon has been associated with elevated plasma concentrations (>600 ng/ml) that occurred either during the first few days of therapy or after a change in dosage or metabolism.

Complete AV block may also be seen if flecainide is used in patients with preexisting AV conduction system disease. Worsened congestive heart failure is also common, as discussed above.

CLINICAL USE

In a large number of clinical trials, flecainide has been shown to suppress frequent and complex ventricular ectopy in over 80% of clinically stable patients (6, 37, 63). Results in patients with a history of sustained ventricular tachycardia and structural heart disease have not been as promising and further data are required (4, 38, 146). In these patients, response rates of 20–30% may be expected in previously untreated subjects. A history of prior failure of one or more agents may be expected to lower this rate of response.

Flecainide has also been reported to be effective in patients with several types of supraventricular arrhythmias (60, 79). Since the drug affects the AV node as well as atrial and ventricular muscle, it has shown promise in the treatment of both paroxysmal atrial fibrillation and paroxysmal supraventricular tachycardia. Patients with the Wolff-Parkinson-White syndrome and antegrade preexcitation may manifest greater increases in bypass tract refractoriness with well-tolerated doses of flecainide than may be achievable with quinidine or procainamide therapy.

At present, flecainide seems a reasonable first choice drug in patients with normal ventricular function and symptomatic sustained or nonsustained atrial and ventricular arrhythmias. Although it may be used in patients with compromised ventricular function, this approach requires caution and careful monitoring to prevent the appearance of adverse cardiac reactions.

DOSAGE AND ADMINISTRATION

Since cardiac toxicity to flecainide has been commonly seen during the first few days of therapy, rapid loading with flecainide is not recommended. In stable patients without congestive heart failure, the initial dose should be 100 mg twice daily, with increases up to 200 mg twice daily possible after steady state plasma concentrations have been measured. In patients with heart failure, 50 mg twice daily is a more appropriate initial dose, and upward increments should be made with caution. During chronic therapy, plasma concentrations should be monitored at frequent intervals since flecainide elimination may vary over time. Because of its potential for producing life-threatening adverse reactions, it is usually unwise to increase dosage aggressively in hopes of maximizing antiarrhythmic effects.

Propafenone

Propafenone is an antiarrhythmic agent that has been readily available in Europe for a number of years.

ELECTROPHYSIOLOGIC AND ECG EFFECTS (21, 22)

Propafenone depresses sodium conductance and results in a depression in $\dot{V}_{max}$ during phase 0 of the action potential. Conduction velocity in the His-Purkinje system in atrial and ventricular muscle is slowed. In cardiac tissues that display spontaneous automaticity, the rate of phase 4 depolarization is also decreased. In electrophysiologic studies, propafenone has variable effects on the sinus node recovery time; lengthens the refractorial periods of the atrium, AV node, and ventricle; and slows intraatrial, AV nodal, His-Purkinje, and intraventricular conduction. The PA, AH, and HV intervals are all prolonged. The surface ECG shows a modest increase in the PR interval and QRS duration but little change in the JT_c interval.

Propafenone also produces a mild degree of β-adrenergic blockage with a potency of about $\frac{1}{40}$ that of propranolol. The clinical significance of this latter effect remains undefined.

PHARMACOKINETICS (22, 132)

Propafenone is well absorbed (>95%) after oral ingestion, but undergoes extensive first pass hepatic metabolism before reaching the systemic circulation. This extraction system is partially saturable, thus first pass clearance decreases with larger single doses and during chronic therapy. Peak plasma concentrations are seen 2–3 hours after oral dosing. The steady state volume of distribution is between 0.7 and 1.1 liters/kg. Propafenone is highly (>95%) protein bound in the circulation.

Propafenone is extensively metabolized in most subjects, unchanged propafenone excretion accounting for less than 1% of total elimination. The rate of metabolism is at least partially genetically determined, with patients known to be slow metabolizers of debrisoquine having a correspondingly slow metabolism. During propafenone therapy, several metabolites including 4-hydroxypropafenone, hydroxymethoxypropafenone, and various glucuronide and sulfate conjugates have been identified. It is known that at least the 4-hydroxy metabolite has significant antiarrhythmic activity and contributes to propafenone's activity during clinical usage. Since oxidative metabolism of propafenone is genetically determined, the measured elimination half-life may vary greatly from patient to patient, with a range of 1.8–32 hours reported. Thus, the antiarrhythmic effects seen during propafenone therapy are due to the combined actions of the parent compound and its metabolites, and a practical "therapeutic range" for all patients is difficult to define. In rapid metabolizers, however, plasma propafenone concentrations are usually between 0.5 and 1.5 μg/ml.

HEMODYNAMIC EFFECTS (9)

Propafenone has been demonstrated to produce negative inotropic effects in both preclinical and clinical trials. As with other agents, these effects are most pronounced in subjects with preexisting congestive heart failure.

SIDE EFFECTS

Propafenone is usually well tolerated. Minor extracardiac side effects including dysgeusia, xerostomia, nausea and vomiting, constipation, dizziness, and blurred vision may be seen in up to 20% of patients. These problems are usually dose-related and can often be managed by dosage adjustment. Cardiac toxicity in the form of congestive heart failure, bradycardia due to sinus node suppression or AV block, and aggravation of tachyarrhythmias may occur at any dose and usually require discontinuation of therapy. Like other drugs with similar electrophysiologic effects, propafenone has been associated with a hemodynamically unstable, ventricular tachycardia that is resistant to attempts at cardioversion (109).

CLINICAL USE

Propafenone has been shown to produce antiarrhythmic effects in both ventricular and supraventricular arrhythmias. In studies on patients with chronic, stable ventricular premature beats, between 60% and 75% of patients manifest suppression of the arrhythmias (117, 130); however, when used in patients with sustained ventricular tachycardia, response rates have been much lower (10–40%) (21, 22, 29, 59). Propafenone usually lengthens the tachycardia cycle length in the latter patients, but despite this fact, hypotension during tachycardia may be more profound.

Propafenone appears to be useful for managing a variety of supraventricular arrhythmias (16, 56). In patients with preexcitation, propafenone prolongs the ERP and may cause block even in patients with a short ERP. Successful therapy of paroxysmal atrial flutter or atrial fibrillation and AV nodal reentry has also been reported.

DOSAGE AND ADMINISTRATION

Propafenone therapy is usually initiated at a dosage of 150 mg or 200 mg three times daily. Few patients have been treated with daily doses of over 1200 mg. The appearance of extracardiac side effects, worsened congestive heart failure, or QRS widening is an indication to decrease dosage since plasma level monitoring is unreliable.

Amiodarone

Amiodarone is a heavily iodinated benzofuran derivative that was initially developed as an antianginal agent. During early clinical use in Europe, it was observed to produce powerful antiarrhythmic effects in patients with both supraventricular and ventricular arrhythmias. However, its unusual pharmacokinetic profile and its potential for producing toxicity in many organ systems have limited the drug's overall utility.

ELECTROPHYSIOLOGIC AND ECG EFFECTS (97, 98)

Since amiodarone is virtually insoluble in aqueous media, few reports on its acute, in vitro electrophysiologic effects are available. In preparations taken from animals treated chronically with the drug, action potential duration is prolonged with the major effect apparent during phases 2 and 3. Phase 0 depolarization under baseline conditions is little affected, but a use-dependent depression of sodium channel conductance may be demonstrated. Amiodarone also produces a mild noncompetitive β-blockade and inhibits peripheral conversion of thyroxine (T_4) to triiodothyronine (T_3), thus producing indirect effects as well.

During chronic amiodarone therapy in humans, a number of electrophysiologic changes have been reported. Sinus node automaticity is decreased. AV nodal conduction velocity and refractoriness are both depressed. His-Purkinje conduction intervals are increased, as are the effective and functional refractory periods of atrium and ventricle. In patients with accessory pathways, both antegrade and retrograde refractory periods are increased.

The surface ECG during chronic amiodarone therapy usually shows a moderate sinus bradycardia, a slight prolongation of the PR interval, a marked prolongation in the QT_c, and the appearance of prominent U-waves, particularly in the midprecordial leads.

PHARMACOKINETICS (2, 54, 67)

Amiodarone has variable and unusual pharmacokinetic parameters. Bioavailability after a single oral dose has been reported to range from 22% to 86%, with peak plasma concentrations seen between 2 and 10 hours after ingestion. The volume of distribution is greater than 20 liters/kg, reflecting extensive tissue binding particularly in liver, lung, muscle, and adipose tissue. Elimination kinetics are complex. Plasma levels decline very slowly after discontinuation of chronic therapy, with detectable plasma concentrations present as long as 6–12 months after the last dose.

During chronic amiodarone therapy, an active metabolite, desethylamiodarone, accumulates and eventually achieves plasma concentrations of 60–80% of those of the parent drug. The mechanisms of final elimination of amiodarone and desethylamiodarone from the body are still uncertain.

The value of plasma concentration monitoring to guide therapy with amiodarone has remained controversial (36, 48). During chronic therapy (200–400 mg/day), plasma concentrations of amiodarone usually range between 0.5 and 3.5 μg/ml. Although weak correlations between dose and plasma concentrations and between electrophysiologic effects and plasma concentrations can be demonstrated, there is wide interindividual variability and the correlations are not of clinical value. In addition, significant toxicity from amiodarone may occur at all clinically useful doses and over a wide range of plasma concentrations.

HEMODYNAMIC EFFECTS (86)

Since steady state amiodarone effects cannot be practically achieved with short courses of administration, the direct hemodynamic effects of amiodarone remain uncertain. There seems to be little change in left ventricular ejection fraction or cardiac output during chronic oral therapy, but some patients may not tolerate the sinus bradycardia usually seen during therapy. Acute intravenous infusion of amiodarone has been reported to lower vas-

cular smooth muscle tone and to produce a modest negative inotropic effect.

SIDE EFFECTS

Chronic amiodarone therapy commonly produces at least minor toxicity, the majority of patients treated for several years experiencing one or more adverse reactions (48, 97). Adverse reactions may be seen at all clinically useful dosage levels, but are more common with higher doses and with increased durations of exposure.

The most dangerous side effect associated with amiodarone therapy is pulmonary infiltrates (134). This reaction has been reported in up to 10–20% of patients treated with amiodarone for several years. It may appear at any point during therapy. Patients with amiodarone pulmonary toxicity usually present with dyspnea and a nonproductive cough. Pyrexia may also occur. The chest x-ray shows diffuse interstitial infiltration (Fig. 9.6). Arterial blood gases show marked hypoxemia with a low or normal P_{CO_2}. Pulmonary function tests show restrictive lung volumes but no new obstruc-

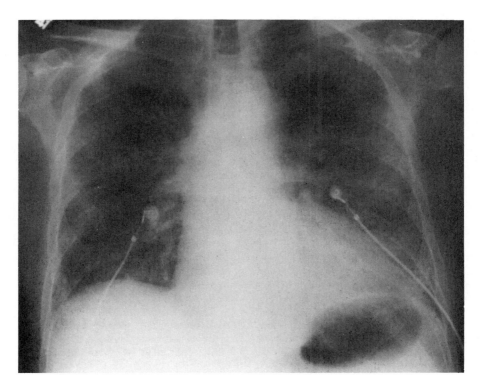

Figure 9.6. Radiologic findings in amiodarone-induced pulmonary toxicity. Diffuse interstitial infiltrates that may be difficult to distinguish from those seen with infection or heart failure characterize this syndrome.

tive defect. Diffusion capacity is usually markedly reduced.

Amiodarone pulmonary toxicity may develop gradually, but more commonly presents after a short course of rapid deterioration. The differential diagnosis at presentation often includes aggravated congestive heart failure and pulmonary infection. Catheterization of the right side of the heart and gallium scanning may be used to distinguish drug toxicity from these conditions. In equivocal cases, lung biopsy may be helpful. Biopsies show thickened alveolar septa and fibrosis with macrophages and other inflammatory cells in the alveoli. The macrophages contain lipid-containing lysosomal inclusion bodies.

Therapy of amiodarone pulmonary toxicity requires discontinuation of the drug, support of respiratory function, and control of arrhythmias. Although steroid therapy is frequently recommended, no conclusive evidence of its benefit has been shown. Amiodarone pulmonary toxicity, once clinically evident, usually takes weeks to resolve, and infection, respiratory failure, and recurrent arrhythmias often intervene to produce an overall mortality that may reach 20–40%.

Almost all patients receiving amiodarone chronically develop corneal microdeposits. Although these are readily visible during a slit lamp examination, they only rarely affect visual activity (74). However, approximately 10% of patients report visual blurring or halo vision.

Amiodarone has several interactions with thyroid hormone metabolism (15, 96). Each 200-mg tablet contains 75 mg of organic iodine. Iodine-induced hypothyroidism or hyperthyroidism may be seen, with the relative prevalence dependent on the dietary iodine content of the population studied. Amiodarone also inhibits conversion of T_4 to T_3. In patients who remain euthyroid, plasma concentrations of T_4 and reverse T_3 are elevated, whereas T_3 and thyroid-stimulating hormone concentrations should remain normal. Supplementation with thyroxine will prevent clinical symptoms of hypothyroidism without affecting antiarrhythmic activity; the development of hyperthyroidism is frequently signalled by arrhythmia recurrence.

Dermatologic toxicity is common after therapy with amiodarone and may present in two forms (152). Up to 50% of patients develop increased photosensitivity to UVA waveband light sources. In a smaller percentage of patients, bluish-gray skin discoloration on sun-

exposed areas may develop because of an accumulation of lipofuscin granules in dermal macrophages. All patients treated with amiodarone should be instructed to use photoprotective topical therapy and clothing during periods of sun exposure.

Neuromuscular toxicity is commonly seen during amiodarone therapy, particularly in older patients treated with doses over 200 mg/day (20). Proximal muscle weakness, tremor, and peripheral neuropathy are the most frequent presentations. Other symptoms include distal paresthesias and numbness, muscle weakness and wasting, and areflexia. Other forms of neurologic reactions, including ataxia and sleep disturbance, are also common, particularly during the first weeks of treatment. All of these neurologic reactions appear to respond, albeit slowly, to reduction in dosage.

Liver function abnormalities may be detected in approximately one-third of patients receiving amiodarone. The usual finding is a minor (< 2-fold) elevation of serum glutamic-oxaloacetic transaminase (SGOT), glutamic-pyruvic transaminase (SGPT), and lactic dehydrogenase (LDH) that may be either persistent or transient. A few cases of hepatitis or hepatic failure have been reported. Nausea, vomiting, and constipation have also been re-

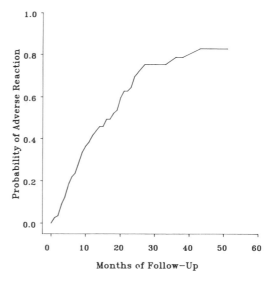

Figure 9.7. Expected incidence of adverse reactions during amiodarone therapy. (From Greenberg ML, Lerman BB, Shipe JR, et al: Relation between amiodarone and desethylamiodarone plasma concentrations and electrophysiologic effects, efficacy and toxicity. *J Am Coll Cardiol* 9:1148–1155, 1987.)

ported, but rarely limit therapy except during high-dose oral loading (50).

Bradycardias due to either sinus node suppression or drug-induced AV block are frequently encountered during long-term amiodarone therapy. Because of the long period that would be required for drug elimination, permanent pacing is often required.

Because of the frequent and serious adverse reactions produced by amiodarone, careful surveillance during long-term treatment is required. Blood tests for liver function and thyroid function abnormalities should be obtained, and periodic chest x-rays are also recommended. Such routine testing, along with a careful interim history and physical examination, is necessary to minimize the risk to any individual patient.

Amiodarone has a number of important drug interactions. It raises serum digoxin concentrations and interferes unpredictably with warfarin therapy (97, 105). The plasma levels of many other drugs also rise during amiodarone therapy.

CLINICAL USE

Although it has not been subjected to rigorous, placebo-controlled trials, amiodarone is undoubtedly an extremely potent antiarrhythmic agent. Most studies have dealt almost exclusively with patients who had previously failed one or more antiarrhythmic drug trials (40, 50, 72, 97, 101, 145). Nevertheless, long-term efficacy rates of 75–90% in patients with supraventricular arrhythmias and 45–75% in patients with ventricular arrhythmias have commonly been achieved. Amiodarone is highly effective in patients with recurrent atrial flutter and with paroxysmal supraventricular tachycardia due to either AV nodal reentry or reentry involving an accessory AV pathway. Paroxysmal atrial fibrillation also responds in many cases to amiodarone.

In patients with sustained ventricular tachycardia, amiodarone will often either eliminate or decrease the frequency of episodes. The rate of the tachycardia, should it recur, is usually significantly slowed (78). Although early reports suggested that programmed electrical stimulation was of little value for guiding amiodarone therapy (55, 107, 145), more recent reports have shown that ventricular stimulation can be used to define those at low risk of recurrence and to predict the characteristics of a potentially recurrent arrhythmia (72, 101).

DOSAGE AND ADMINISTRATION

Because of its great potential for producing toxicity and its unusual pharmacokinetics, amiodarone must be administered cautiously. In stable patients with supraventricular arrhythmias, an initial dose of 600 mg/day for 2–3 weeks followed by a maintenance dose of 200 mg/day is usually employed. In patients with serious ventricular arrhythmias, the usual starting dose of 1200–1800 mg/day is continued for 7–14 days and then decreased to 200–400 mg/day. There is no agreement on whether a gradual tapering of dosage after the early load is necessary, and clinical judgment is required. Chronic doses of over 400 mg/day are associated with significant morbidity and should only be used if no alternatives exist.

Amiodarone has also been used with success intravenously in unstable patients. The usual reported dose has been 600–1800 mg/day for 2–3 days (83). Intravenous amiodarone, however, causes severe phlebitis and only infusion into a central vein should be used.

β-Adrenergic Blockers

A large number of β-adrenergic blocking agents are now available for clinical use for a variety of cardiac indications. Used alone as antiarrhythmic drugs, they are useful in arrhythmias that depend on increased sympathetic tone and for their depressant effect on AV nodal conduction. However, β-adrenergic blockers are frequently helpful during antiarrhythmic therapy either to potentiate the effects of other antiarrhythmic agents or to indirectly affect the etiologic factors (e.g., ischemia, catecholamine excess) responsible for the arrhythmia.

Although significant differences have been described between β-adrenergic blocking drugs in terms of β_1 selectivity, membrane-stabilizing activity, and intrinsic sympathomimetic activity, the practical value of these variables for selecting the optimal β-blocking drug for treating arrhythmias in most situations has not been defined (42). Sotalol is an unusual drug with β-blocking and antiarrhythmic properties.

ELECTROPHYSIOLOGIC AND ECG EFFECTS

β-Adrenergic blockers decrease the slope of phase 4 depolarization in the sinus node and in Purkinje fibers. Phase 0 of the action potential is unchanged. At moderate concentrations, the effects of isoproterenol to shorten the refractory period of atrial and ventricular muscle and to lower the threshold for ventricular fibrillation are blocked. The other major effects of clinical relevance are increases in conduction time and refractoriness in AV nodal tissue.

Patients on β-adrenergic blocking agents without intrinsic sympathomimetic activity usually have a modest sinus bradycardia with normal PR, QRS, and QT_c intervals. Exercise-related or stress-related sinus tachycardia is usually blunted. Significant bradycardias may be precipitated in patients with sinus node dysfunction, autonomic dysfunction, or AV conduction system disease.

PHARMACOKINETICS (42)

β-Adrenergic blocking agents with a wide range of pharmacokinetic properties are currently available. Agents such as propranolol and metoprolol that are highly lipid soluble tend to be well absorbed, undergo extensive first pass hepatic extraction, and have a relatively short elimination half-life. Agents such as nadolol and atenolol are relatively water soluble, are incompletely absorbed, are cleared by renal excretion, and have longer elimination half-lives. Other agents exhibit properties between these extremes. The properties of some of these agents are summarized in Table 9.7.

HEMODYNAMIC EFFECTS

The hemodynamic effects of β-adrenergic blocking drugs are dependent on the level of intrinsic adrenergic activity and on the functional reserve of the heart. In general, β-adrenergic blockers lower heart rate and arterial blood pressure, decrease indices of myocardial contractility, and lower cardiac output.

SIDE EFFECTS

The side effects of β-adrenergic blocking agents are related to their effects on adrenergic receptors in various organs. Bronchospasm may be seen in patients with asthma and chronic obstructive pulmonary disease, and this risk is not totally eliminated by the use of relatively selective β_1-antagonists. Heart failure, hypotension, and bradycardia may be produced in susceptible patients. Some patients on β-blockers complain of fatigue, sleep disturbance, or impotence.

CLINICAL USE

β-Adrenergic drugs share several common uses. They may be used to increase AV nodal refractoriness and therefore control ventricular rate in atrial fibrillation and prevent episodes of paroxysmal supraventricular tachycardia. They also may act synergistically with other antiarrhythmic drugs whose actions to prolong conduction and increase refractoriness in atrial

Table 9.7
Selected Properties of β-Adrenergic Blocking Drugs[a]

Drug	Relative β_1 Selectivity	ISA	MSA	Absorption (%)	Bioavailability (%)	Elimination Half-life	Major Route of Elimination	Usual Intravenous Dose	Usual Oral Dose (mg)
Acebutolol	+	+	+	70	50	3–4 hr	Renal	—	200–600 b.i.d.
Atenolol	+	–	–	50	40	6–9 hr	Renal	—	50–100 q.d.
Esmolol	+	–	–	—	—	9–10 min	Hepatic	500 µg/kg load, then 100–300 µg/kg/min	—
Metoprolol	+	–	–	90	50	3–4 hr	Hepatic	5 mg × 3 over 10 min	25–100 b.i.d. or t.i.d.
Nadolol	–	–	–	30	30	14–24 hr	Renal	—	20–80 q.d.
Pindolol	–	+ +	+	90	90	3–4 hr	Renal, hepatic	—	5–20 b.i.d.
Propranolol	–	–	+ +	90	30	3–4 hr	Hepatic	5–10 mg at 1 mg/2–3 min	40–80 q.i.d.
Sotalol	–	–	–	70	60	8–10 hr	Renal	—	80–320 b.i.d.
Timolol	–	–	–	90	75	4–5 hr	Renal, hepatic	—	2.5–10 b.i.d.

[a] ISA, intrinsic sympathomimetic activity; MSA, membrane stabilizing activity.

or ventricular muscle are antagonized by adrenergic stimulation.

A number of studies have described a beneficial effect when β-blocking drugs are administered prophylactically to patients recovering from myocardial infarction (11, 62, 113). The precise mechanism by which this effect is achieved remains controversial.

Esmolol is a β-adrenergic blocking agent with an extremely brief elimination half-life (<10 minutes) and is available only for intravenous use. Because of this fact it is of particular value in the intensive care unit since it permits rapid intravenous titration of dosage and thus rapid control of ventricular rate in atrial arrhythmias. It appears to be of particular value in patients with postoperative atrial flutter and fibrillation (35, 45).

Sotalol is a β-adrenergic drug with mixed antiarrhythmic properties (90, 106). In addition to possessing about one-third the β-blocking potency per milligram of propranolol, it also has direct effects on the action potential similar to those produced by amiodarone. It has been successfully used to treat both supraventricular and ventricular arrhythmias. Sotalol produces QT prolongation, and when used in the setting of hypokalemia has been associated with the induction of polymorphic ventricular tachycardias.

Bretylium

Bretylium tosylate is a benzyl quaternary ammonium compound that was first introduced as an antihypertensive during the 1950s. The development of more effective and less toxic agents for blood pressure control prevented its widespread use for this purpose. It was subsequently reintroduced as an antiarrhythmic drug for parenteral use in 1974.

ELECTROPHYSIOLOGIC AND ECG EFFECTS (85, 93)

The majority of bretylium's electrophysiologic effects are due to its complex interactions at sympathetic nerve terminals. Early after acute administration of this drug, norepinephrine is released from the presynaptic nerve endings of postganglionic adrenergic neurons. Subsequently, bretylium accumulates in the nerve ending, produces depletion of norepinephrine stores, inhibits norepinephrine release, and blocks reuptake of catecholamines. These lat-

ter effects require 3–6 hours to become apparent.

After initial administration, bretylium causes a transient increase in sinus rate, AV conduction, and ventricular automaticity, effects presumably due to intramyocardial catecholamine release. Chronically, bretylium prolongs the ventricular action potential duration and ERPs without changing $\dot{V}_{max}$ and conduction velocity. In animal models, bretylium increases ventricular fibrillation threshold, particularly during myocardial ischemia (65).

PHARMACOKINETICS (5, 32)

Bretylium is poorly absorbed after oral administration and is usually administered intravenously or more rarely, intramuscularly. The apparent volume of distribution is 3–5 liters/kg and the drug is not bound to plasma proteins. Bretylium is not metabolized in the body and is excreted in unchanged form by the kidney. Bretylium is highly bound in tissues, and plasma concentrations are not accurate indicators of antiarrhythmic activity. The half-life of elimination is 8–13 hours, but elimination kinetics are not linear and are not accurately described using a two-compartment model. Since bretylium has two phases of activity, initial responses are not predictive of more chronic efficacy. No useful "therapeutic range" of effective plasma concentrations has been described.

HEMODYNAMIC EFFECTS

The initial positive chronotropic and inotropic effects of bretylium are related to the sympathetic discharge seen immediately after administration. Hypertension may be seen initially after bretylium administration is started, but with continued therapy, severe hypotension is commonly observed. The hypotension is aggravated by postural changes, but may persist even if the patient remains supine. Cardiac index is usually maintained unless adverse effects are produced by the hypotension.

SIDE EFFECTS

The immediate toxicity associated with bretylium is mediated via its effects on the sympathetic nervous system. Transient hypertension, increased automaticity in either the sinus node or in ectopic foci, and an increase in myocardial oxygen demand may all produce deleterious effects. With prolonged intravenous treatment, severe hypotension is the major side effect. Pretreatment with tricyclic antidepressants may block uptake of bretylium into adrenergic nerve terminals, but this has not been of practical clinical value. An analogue, bethanidine, which is well absorbed orally, has undergone testing for the chronic suppression of ventricular arrhythmias. In these studies, bethanidine has been administered along with the tricyclic antidepressant, protriptyline. Unfortunately, bethanidine has not been shown to be a particularly effective antiarrhythmic agent, and hypotension associated with its use has been particularly severe.

Rapid intravenous infusion of bretylium frequently produces nausea and vomiting. This may be ameliorated if the drug is given by slow injection over 8–10 minutes. Chronic oral therapy with bretylium has also been associated with parotitis.

CLINICAL USE (57, 116)

The role of bretylium in the treatment of ventricular arrhythmias requires continued assessment. The immediate and delayed antiarrhythmic effects of bretylium are presumably mediated by different mechanisms and data from clinical trials are difficult to analyze. Since it has electrophysiologic properties that are strikingly different from those of other conventionally available antiarrhythmic agents, bretylium may well prove useful in a different spectrum of arrhythmias and data obtained in traditional models may not be relevant. At present, it seems to be of sufficient potential efficacy to warrant consideration for the short-term control of ventricular fibrillation only. Antiarrhythmic effects may be delayed, and a trial of at least 6–8 hours of therapy seems indicated before bretylium can be considered a failure. Unfortunately, since the chief clinical experience with bretylium has been in cases of cardiac arrest or in the management of patients with multiple factors contributing to their arrhythmias, an objective analysis of bretylium's clinical efficacy even in cardiac arrest patients is not possible based on the current data (57, 116). There are no convincing data that bretylium is effective for hemodynamically stable ventricular tachycardia outside the setting of acute myocardial infarction, and considerable experience shows that the hypotension it causes can be harmful (10, 51).

DOSAGE AND ADMINISTRATION

Bretylium is available in 10-ml ampules containing 500 mg of bretylium tosylate. Except in cardiopulmonary resuscitation, when it is usually injected as a bolus of 5 mg/kg, the drug should be diluted with either 5% dextrose or saline to a concentration of 10 mg/ml and infused slowly over 8–10 minutes. The initial loading dose should be 5 mg/kg. A second dose of 5 mg/kg may be administered if the first is ineffective. Maintenance therapy, for those rare cases in which it is indicated, usually requires 5–10 mg/kg every 6–8 hours or 1–2 mg/min by continuous infusion. Intramuscular therapy is possible and requires no dosage adjustment if peripheral circulation is intact. Careful monitoring of arterial blood pressure is mandatory and intraarterial monitoring is often necessary. Dosage should be reduced in patients with reduced renal function.

Verapamil

Verapamil is the prototype for a class of agents that selectively affect calcium transport. These "calcium blockers" have potential clinical utility in a variety of clinical situations: hypertension, variant and typical angina, and hypertrophic myopathies as well as for the treatment of various arrhythmias.

ELECTROPHYSIOLOGIC AND ECG EFFECTS
(7, 94, 133)

Verapamil produces its electrophysiologic effects by altering the kinetics of activation, inactivation, and recovery of the calcium-dependent slow channel. At high concentrations, verapamil has local anesthetic activity, but this activity is absent at clinically relevant drug concentrations. Verapamil depresses action potentials dependent on slow channel activity in normal cells of the sinus and AV nodes and those slow action potentials seen in partially depolarized fibers. Conduction velocity in these cells is selectively depressed, whereas fibers in which the action potential is mediated by fast channel currents are relatively unaffected. Verapamil also suppresses triggered activity via its influence on intracellular calcium concentrations.

During electrophysiologic studies, verapamil may produce depression of sinus node function, particularly in patients with sinus node disease. Verapamil prolongs the AH interval and the refractory period of the AV node, but has no effect on the ERPs of atrial or ventricular muscle. The refractory period for antegrade conduction over accessory bypass tracts may either show no effect or actually shorten, but the latter effect may be reflex mediated. The ECG may show slight prolongation of the PR interval whereas the QRS and QT_c usually remain unchanged.

PHARMACOKINETICS (81, 100)

Verapamil may be administered either orally or intravenously. After intravenous administration, the drug initially distributes into a central compartment with a volume of distribution of approximately 2 liters/kg. At steady state, the volume of distribution is about 4 liters/kg. When administered orally, the drug is well absorbed but undergoes substantial first pass hepatic degradation. The system for hepatic extraction and metabolism is saturable so that initial doses and lower doses are more completely cleared. The systemic bioavailability of the drug is only 10–30%. Ninety percent of the drug in plasma is protein-bound. Verapamil elimination is via hepatic metabolism. The principal metabolite, norverapamil, accumulates in plasma to a concentration greater than that of the parent compound during chronic therapy. Norverapamil has measurable antiarrhythmic activity, but is much less potent than verapamil. The elimination half-life for verapamil is about 3–6 hours. Elimination is prolonged in cirrhosis and in conditions of decreased hepatic blood flow. If hepatic blood flow is decreased, however, the fractional transhepatic extraction increases, partly compensating for the decreased flow. Effective serum concentrations during chronic oral therapy for arrhythmias have not been reported, but serum concentrations observed during verapamil therapy for hypertrophic cardiomyopathy are 30–150 ng/ml. In patients who receive 0.075 mg/kg intravenously for the termination of reentrant supraventricular tachycardias, concentrations ranging from 72 to 195 ng/ml have been seen (138).

HEMODYNAMIC EFFECTS (138)

Verapamil has marked negative inotropic effects and produces relaxation of vascular smooth muscle. In most patients, the decrease in blood pressure after intravenous verapamil is principally due to peripheral vasodilation, but left ventricular end-diastolic pressure increases and the drug may precipitate congestive heart failure. In many patients with mild or moderate heart failure, however, the improvement in afterload and attenuation of ischemia may al-low the negative inotropic effects to be well compensated. Verapamil and other calcium channel blockers are also useful in angina, hypertension, and other disorders.

SIDE EFFECTS

The principal extracardiac side effect reported with oral verapamil is constipation. Nausea, vomiting, vertigo, headache, and nervousness have also been reported. After intravenous administration, hypotension and bradycardia may be seen. Ventricular asystole has been reported in patients who previously received intravenous β-adrenergic blocker. Verapamil causes a rise in serum digoxin concentrations in patients previously taking digoxin. The magnitude of the increase is less than that seen with quinidine.

CLINICAL USE (137, 138)

Verapamil administered intravenously at a dose of 0.075 or 0.15 mg/kg (5–10 mg total) terminates most episodes of reentrant supraventricular tachycardia in which the AV node is involved in the reentry loop. In atrial flutter or fibrillation, conduction through the AV node is delayed and a stable ventricular rate may be achieved. Reflex adrenergic stimulation in response to hypotension seen after verapamil injection may blunt these effects in unstable patients. Verapamil has no predictable effect on ventricular arrhythmias except in rare cases, and the hypotension it causes may prove dangerous. When given to patients with Wolff-Parkinson-White syndrome conducting antegradely over an accessory pathway, verapamil may actually speed antegrade conduction and increase ventricular rates. As a general rule, verapamil should never be given to a patient with a wide complex tachycardia of unknown mechanism.

Chronic oral verapamil is useful in the chronic prophylaxis of recurrent paroxysmal supraventricular tachycardia. It also can provide a stable ventricular rate in selected patients with chronic atrial fibrillation. The optimal dose ranges for these purposes are not firmly established, but therapy is usually initiated with 80–120 mg three or four times daily.

Other Calcium Antagonists

Several other calcium channel antagonists are now available in the United States. Nifedipine and nitrendepine have no electrophysiologic effects and therefore no potential as antiarrhythmic agents. Diltiazem has electrophysiologic actions similar to those of verapamil and may be of potential use as an antiarrhythmic drug. Further studies to characterize the antiarrhythmic actions and dose requirements of diltiazem are necessary, however, before it can be recommended as a substitute for verapamil in treating arrhythmias.

Other Antiarrhythmic Drugs

There has been an explosive growth in the number of pharmacologic agents that may be used for treating cardiac arrhythmias. The role of many of the more recently developed agents has not as yet been fully defined and these agents are not discussed in detail in this chapter. However, some relevant properties of selected new agents are listed in Table 9.8.

PACING AND CARDIOVERSION

Electrical pacing of the heart may be useful in the prevention or termination of many arrhythmias. The earliest uses of pacing were for treating bradycardia-dependent arrhythmias. Some arrhythmias are triggered by late diastolic premature beats. In bigeminal rhythms, the long pause after the premature beat can prolong repolarization after the subsequent normal beat and lead to an "R-on-T" phenomenon. In these two instances, overdrive pacing at faster rates may prove effective in preventing arrhythmias. In patients having a relative bradycardia associated with hemodynamic compromise that causes a secondary arrhythmia, either atrial, ventricular, or dual chamber pacing may help prevent further episodes. Unfortunately, for the long-term management of most arrhythmias, overdrive pacing by itself is only occasionally successful.

Pacing techniques, however, may be extremely valuable for the termination of an acute arrhythmia. This fact has been particularly true in patients after cardiac surgery in whom temporary epicardial pacing wires are often implanted, thus facilitating the procedure. As new technologies become available, implantable pacing units with antitachycardia capabilities may become more common.

The arrhythmia most commonly treated with pacing is atrial flutter (47). The delivery of bursts of atrial stimuli at cycle lengths shorter than the atrial cycle lengths results in atrial capture and a change in the flutter wave on the ECG, and in most cases will either terminate flutter or accelerate it to atrial fibrillation. If atrial capture can be reliably achieved, most episodes of atrial flutter can be terminated in this fashion. Even if atrial fibrillation is produced, it is often easier to control the ventricular rate with medications with resultant hemodynamic improvement. Reentrant supraventricular tachycardias may also be terminated in this manner. Atrial fibrillation, multifocal atrial tachycardia, and automatic atrial or junctional tachycardias do not respond.

Ventricular tachycardia may also be terminated with pacing. Single or double extrastimuli or bursts of rapid pacing terminate a

Table 9.8
Investigational Antiarrhythmic Drugs—Preliminary Data

Agent	Action	Elimination Half-life	Major Side Effects	Possible Future Use
Adenosine (28)	Slows AV nodal conduction	1–3 sec	Dyspnea	Termination of paroxysmal supraventricular tachycardia
Cibenzoline (88)	Ic and III	4 hr	Nausea, vomiting, headache	Ventricular arrhythmia
Clofilium (52)	III	?	Flushing	Ventricular arrhythmia
Indecainide (112)	Ic	6–12 hr	Dizziness, blurred vision	Ventricular arrhythmia
Lorcainide (82)	Ic	7–9 hr	Sleep disturbance, tremor	Ventricular arrhythmia
Meobentine (30)	Ic and III	11–27 hr	Hypotension, dyspnea	Ventricular arrhythmia
Moricizine (120)	Ib ?	6–14	Nausea, vomiting, rash	Ventricular arrhythmia
Pirmenol (123)	Ia	4–15 hr	Flushing, dysgeusia, constipation	Ventricular arrhythmia
Recainam (24)	Ic	7–12 hr	Nausea	Ventricular arrhythmia

majority of relatively slow, recurrent ventricular tachycardias and may decrease the need for frequent cardioversions. There is a substantial risk of producing acceleration of the tachycardia or inducing ventricular fibrillation, however, and the operator should be prepared for emergency resuscitation. This potential for arrhythmia acceleration has limited the introduction of automatic antitachycardia pacemakers for recurrent sustained ventricular tachycardia.

Direct current countershock is the treatment of choice for any arrhythmia that is associated with hemodynamic collapse or with severe angina in a patient with coronary artery disease, or one that is resistant to other forms of treatment. When used to treat supraventricular arrhythmias or a well-tolerated ventricular tachycardia, the DC countershock delivery should be synchronized with the peak of the QRS complex to avoid precipitating ventricular fibrillation by delivering the shock during the T wave. Digitalis toxicity should be excluded, if possible, prior to elective cardioversion since digitalis toxicity may lead to irreversible ventricular fibrillation after countershock.

The automatic internal cardioverter defibrillator was approved for general use in the United States in 1986 (103). This fully implantable device continually senses the heart's rhythm and is set to deliver shocks from internal electrodes in response to rapid or disorganized ventricular rhythms. As this technology develops, further modifications can be expected to improve arrhythmia detection, add antitachycardia pacing capability, eliminate the need for thoracotomy, and miniaturize the components. When such advances are realized, devices, probably in conjunction with drugs, may become the standard treatment for the more life-threatening forms of ventricular arrhythmias.

ASSESSMENT OF ANTIARRHYTHMIC THERAPY

When choosing to initiate therapy with an antiarrhythmic drug, the physician must balance the indication for treatment against the potential for toxicity associated with each agent. The goals of antiarrhythmic therapy may include termination of an acute arrhythmia, modification of an acute or chronic arrhythmia so that adverse hemodynamic effects are eliminated, or prophylaxis against the future oc-

Table 9.9
Goals of Antiarrhythmic Therapy

I. Short-term therapy
   A. Termination of an acute arrhythmia
   B. Modification of an arrhythmia to minimize hemodynamic effects
   C. Prevention of a life-threatening arrhythmia
II. Chronic Therapy
   A. Prevention of sudden cardiac death
   B. Elimination of symptomatic arrhythmia

currence of a life-threatening or symptomatic arrhythmia (Table 9.9). The likelihood of achieving these goals must be weighed against the potential adverse reactions and the cost of therapy. Arrhythmias that are not associated with symptoms and do not indicate a substantial risk for a life-threatening arrhythmia seldom require therapy.

The optimal methods for assessing antiarrhythmic therapy remain controversial. Except when arrhythmia termination provides an easily assessed therapeutic objective, the physician is often forced to use intermediate endpoints for assessing the efficacy of antiarrhythmic therapy. The endpoint selected, however, may vary depending on the clinical circumstances in which therapy is considered. Whatever the endpoint used to evaluate therapy, it should correlate with the ultimate goal of treatment.

It is essential to determine the optimal method for evaluating intermediate endpoints beginning chronic therapy when a treatment failure would result in an arrhythmia with life-threatening potential. Ventricular arrhythmias not associated with transmural myocardial infarction are responsible for the majority of sudden cardiac deaths, and prevention of these arrhythmias has become an important therapeutic challenge. The optimal method for the selection of chronic therapy for preventing sporadic sustained ventricular arrhythmias has not been determined, but several approaches are currently in use.

When coronary care units were first introduced, it was observed that some patients who later developed an episode of ventricular fibrillation would develop so-called "warning arrhythmias" before the event. Lown and Wolf (92) proposed a grading system for ventricular premature beats (VPBs) that ranked them in five grades of severity (Table 9.10). Although the maximum grade achieved is strongly related to the frequency of total VPBs and the concept of warning arrhythmias has been

Table 9.10
Lown-Wolf Grading System for Ventricular
Premature Beats (VPBs)

Grade 0	No VPBs
Grade 1	Occasional VPBs (<20/hr, <1/min)
Grade 2	Frequent VPBs (≥30/hour)
Grade 3	More than one ECG morphology
Grade 4	Repetitive VPBs
4A	Paired VPBs
4B	Three or more consecutive VPBs
Grade 5	R-on-T VPBs

questioned, the basic Lown-Wolf grading system has been widely used to assess the prognostic significance of asymptomatic arrhythmias in certain populations and to evaluate responses to antiarrhythmic therapy. The various criteria for VPB suppression used in clinical studies have not been subjected to rigorous validation, but are based either on reduction of total VPB count or on both a reduction in VPB total and elimination of higher grade VPBs during ambulatory or, in some studies, exercise ECG. Such an approach has recently been reported to predict accurately the chronic efficacy of antiarrhythmic therapy in patients with a prior history of malignant ventricular arrhythmias (46). This method is limited, however, in that as many as 30–40% of patients with a history of sustained ventricular tachycardia or fibrillation will not have enough spontaneous VPBs to guide therapy, and is also limited by the extreme variability of VPB frequency and grade over time. In addition, some of the newer antiarrhythmic drugs are extremely potent suppressors of VPBs but do not prevent sustained ventricular tachycardia or fibrillation over the long term.

A second approach for the selection of chronic antiarrhythmic therapy has also been advocated. Electrode catheters are placed within the heart and the response to premature extrastimuli determined. In many patients, arrhythmias that have been observed clinically may be reproduced by these techniques, and if the ability to initiate the arrhythmia with stimulation is abolished by medical or surgical therapy, long-term efficacy of that therapy is accurately predicted. Therapy based on this electrophysiologic approach is useful in many patients with both ventricular and supraventricular arrhythmias (25, 122). Since electrophysiologic testing was first used in patients with ventricular arrhythmias, many questions about its value have been answered but some problems still remain. The technique works best in patients with coronary artery disease and prior myocardial infarction. In these patients, electrophysiologic testing is essential for guiding surgical or device-based therapy, and drugs likely to prove highly effective are readily identified. Unfortunately, 40–50% of patients may not achieve "control" by electrophysiologic criteria yet may remain arrhythmia-free. In patients with cardiac diagnoses other than coronary artery disease, the results of electrophysiologic testing are less reliable and further studies are required for reproducing arrhythmias and defining drug therapy.

PROARRHYTHMIC EFFECTS OF ANTIARRHYTHMIC DRUGS

The ability of antiarrhythmic drugs to induce or exacerbate arrhythmias has been appreciated for many years. A number of different mechanisms may be responsible. Most antiarrhythmic drugs produce changes in conduction and under appropriate conditions, might facilitate rather than abolish reentrant arrhythmias. This phenomenon may be seen with subthreshold doses of a drug that may be effective if higher concentrations are maintained. Many agents prolong repolarization and may result in a drug-induced long QT syndrome in which the prolonged and nonuniform recovery of excitability makes the tissue susceptible to the initiation of fibrillation by a critically timed premature beat. Some drugs may produce deleterious hemodynamic effects or conduction abnormalities that secondarily precipitate arrhythmias. Aggravation of arrhythmia has been reported during therapy with almost every antiarrhythmic agent, but the exact frequency of the reaction has only recently been appreciated. Current estimates based on data from both invasive and noninvasive studies suggest that proarrhythmic effects occur during approximately 10% of drug trials in patients with sustained ventricular arrhythmias (14, 71, 142). Therefore, it is important to suspect a proarrhythmic effect whenever an arrhythmia is seen in a patient receiving an "antiarrhythmic" drug.

MANAGEMENT OF SPECIFIC ARRHYTHMIAS

The usual therapies of some common arrhythmias are listed in Table 9.11.

Table 9.11
Therapy of Specific Arrhythmias

Arrhythmia	Maneuvers or Agents	
	Acute Termination	Chronic Prophylaxis
Paroxysmal supraventricular tachycardia (AV node or AV reentry)	Vagal maneuvers, verapamil, adenosine	Digoxin, β-blockers, Ca^{2+} blockers, Ia, Ic
Atrial flutter	Rapid atrial pacing, cardioversion, procainamide	Ia, Ic(?), amiodarone, sotalol
Atrial fibrillation	Cardioversion, rate control, Ia antiarrhythmics	Ia, Ic(?), amiodarone, sotalol
Nonparoxysmal junctional tachycardia	Reverse etiology	Atrial pacing (?)
Multifocal atrial tachycardia	Reverse etiology	Verapamil (?)
Sustained ventricular tachycardia	Cardioversion, lidocaine, procainamide	See text
Ventricular fibrillation	DC shock	See text

Sinus Tachycardia

Sinus tachycardia is characterized by normal P waves with 1:1 AV conduction usually at rates between 100 and 220 beats/min. In most cases, sinus tachycardia is an appropriate physiologic response to an acute stress and does not require specific therapy. Therefore, therapy should be directed at improving the underlying condition. However, if sinus tachycardia causes symptoms or contributes to an increased myocardial oxygen demand with resultant ischemia, it may require treatment. β-Adrenergic blockers are the usual drugs of choice.

Paroxysmal Supraventricular Tachycardia

Paroxysmal supraventricular tachycardia (PSVT) may be due to several mechanisms. Atrioventricular reentry, either with manifest preexcitation or in patients with concealed bypass tracts that function in retrograde fash-

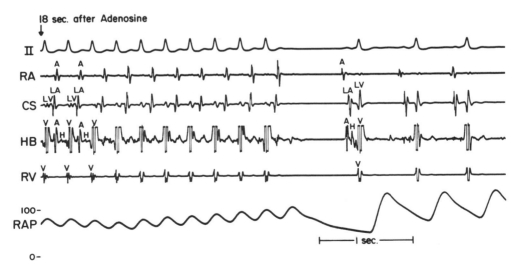

Figure 9.8. Termination of supraventricular tachycardia by adenosine. The tracings represent surface ECG leads II and intracardiac recordings from the right atrium *(RA)*, coronary sinus *(CS)*, bundle of His *(HB)*, and right ventricle *(RV)*, and a radial artery pressure *(RAP)*. With arrival of the adenosine bolus at the heart 21 seconds after injection, AV nodal conduction is blocked and sinus rhythm and a normal blood pressure are restored. (From DiMarco JP, Sellers TD, Lerman BB, et al: Diagnostic and therapeutic use of adenosine in patients with supraventricular tachyarrhythmias. *J Am Coll Cardiol* 6:417–425, 1985.)

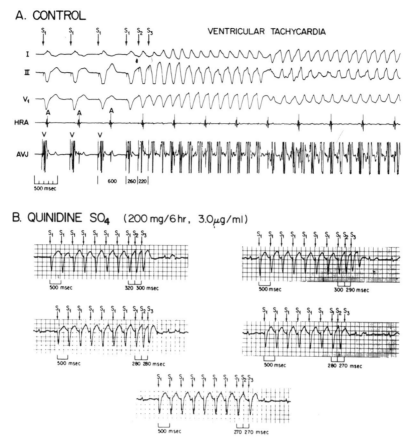

Figure 9.9. Electrophysiologic testing in a patient with cardiac arrest. **A,** Surface ECG leads I, II, and V_1 and intracardiac recordings from the high right atrium *(HRA)* and the AV junction *(AVJ)*. Two extrastimuli with coupling intervals of 260 and 220 msec initiated a rapid ventricular tachycardia that required countershock for termination. **B,** Repeat testing on quinidine shows that no arrhythmia is inducible. (From DiMarco JP, Garan H, Ruskin JN: Quinidine for ventricular arrhythmias: value of electrophysiologic testing. *Am J Cardiol* 51:90–95, 1983.)

ion only, or AV nodal reentry are the most common mechanisms. Intraatrial and sinus node reentry may also be seen. Automatic atrial tachycardia is a relatively rare chronic arrhythmia in adults, but may be more common in critically ill patients in whom increased adrenergic influences may unmask ectopic automatic atrial foci.

Since the majority of episodes of PSVT involve the AV node as part of the reentry pathway, initial attempts to terminate the arrhythmia usually involve maneuvers or agents that slow AV nodal conduction. Vagal maneuvers (e.g., Valsalva, carotid sinus massage) are often effective and some patients with repeated episodes are able to use them to self-terminate their arrhythmias. If drug therapy is required, the most effective agent for acute termination

is intravenous verapamil; the usual dose is 5 or 10 mg.

Recently, the electrophysiologic properties of the endogenous nucleoside adenosine have been described (28). Adenosine depresses AV nodal conduction and is cleared from the circulation within seconds after a bolus injection. When administered to patients with PSVT due to AV nodal or AV reentry, adenosine terminates the tachycardia by producing block within the AV node within 30 seconds after injection (Fig. 9.9). Individual dosage titration is usually required, the average dose being approximately 100 μg/kg.

Intravenous digoxin, propranolol, and edrophonium (Tensilon) were traditionally used in attempts to terminate PSVT prior to the availability of verapamil and adenosine. At the present time, however, they should be considered as second choice agents for acute therapy. The use of pressor agents is not recommended.

The chronic prophylaxis of PSVT must be individualized for each patient. Some patients respond best to agents that slow antegrade AV nodal conduction (digoxin, verapamil, and β-blocking drugs), whereas others respond better to agents that either suppress the premature beats that trigger the arrhythmias or depress retrograde atrioventricular conduction (class Ia or Ic agents, β-blockers, or amiodarone). Electrophysiologic studies are often helpful in drug selection in patients with severe symptoms during PSVT who have not responded to digoxin, propranolol, or verapamil.

Atrial Flutter and Atrial Fibrillation

Atrial flutter is characterized by repetitive atrial activity at an atrial rate of 250–350 beats/min. The QRS is normal. A second form of atrial flutter ("type II") has been described, but this latter arrhythmia is managed more like atrial fibrillation. In atrial flutter, the discrete atrial impulses bombard the AV conduction system at regular intervals and in most patients, 2:1 conduction due to alternating conduction and block is seen. Since the alternate impulse arrives during the absolute refractory period of the AV node, no part of the node is depolarized and it therefore can fully recover by the arrival of the next impulse 200 msec later. Smooth control of ventricular rate in atrial flutter is therefore difficult since major changes in AV nodal refractoriness would have to be produced and changes in rate would occur suddenly with fixed increments.

Atrial flutter is thought to involve intraatrial reentry and therefore is unlikely to terminate following administration of agents selective for the AV node. Quinidine has traditionally been used as the drug of choice if chemical cardioversion is to be attempted, but procainamide is probably equally effective. Unfortunately, only about 20–30% of patients with stable atrial flutter undergo successful cardioversion within 48 hours after starting one of these agents. During the start of therapy the patient's ventricular rate should be monitored since both quinidine and procainamide may slow the atrial rate, and quinidine by its vagolytic action may facilitate AV nodal conduction, thus resulting in 1:1 AV conduction at rates in excess of 200 beats/min. Quinidine raises serum digoxin concentrations, and since digoxin is the usual drug chosen to block this vagolytic effect, careful monitoring of the patient's condition is required. In the majority of patients either atrial pacing or cardioversion must be employed to terminate atrial flutter, since chemical conversion is usually unsuccessful and ventricular rates may be difficult to control.

In atrial fibrillation there is chaotic or very rapid atrial electrical activity and an irregularly irregular ventricular rate. Multiple impulses reach the AV node and either conduct, partially penetrate the node, or are totally blocked. Those that partially penetrate the node reset the refractory period of the penetrated nodal tissue and thereby affect the conduction of subsequent impulses. Agents that prolong AV nodal refractoriness cause a higher degree of partial penetration, and thus a relatively weak drug effect can produce major changes in ventricular rate in atrial fibrillation.

The usual initial approach to the patient with new onset atrial fibrillation is control of ventricular rate. Digoxin, verapamil, or β-adrenergic blockers are all effective and each may have advantages in certain patients. Patients with grossly enlarged atria or those who cannot be maintained in sinus rhythm on chronic drug therapy, may be successfully managed long-term with these drugs to control ventricular rates.

Conversion of the first episode of atrial fibrillation should always be attempted if the rhythm persists after treatment of reversible causes and if the atria are normal or only moderately enlarged. Twenty to 30% of patients undergo successful cardioversion with type Ia or Ic antiarrhythmic agents, and new agents such as sotalol or amiodarone may be more effective. Patients who do not respond to medications alone should undergo transthoracic cardioversion after a 2- to 3-week period of anticoagulation to reduce the small risk of thromboembolism. In patients with new and highly symptomatic atrial fibrillation, cardioversion may be performed emergently without chronic anticoagulation.

Nonparoxysmal Junctional Tachycardia

Nonparoxysmal junctional tachycardia (NPJT) is an automatic tachycardia arising from AV junctional tissue above the bifurcation of the bundle of His. The ECG shows a tachycardia with normal QRS at rates between 60 and 150 beats/min. Either AV dissociation or 1:1 AV conduction may be seen. NPJT usually arises in the setting of simultaneous sinus node depression and catecholamine stimulation. Drug toxicity (lithium, lidocaine, digoxin, etc.) and cardiac surgery are the most common precipitating factors.

Like other automatic arrhythmias, NPJT is difficult to manage. Efforts should be directed to reverse the causes for sympathetic overactivity and to stop drugs that may have depressed the sinus node. Atrial pacing at a faster rate may provide hemodynamic improvement. No specific drug therapy is likely to be effective.

Multifocal Atrial Tachycardia

Multifocal atrial tachycardia (MAT) is produced by enhanced automaticity in multiple atrial foci. The ECG will show three or more discrete P wave morphologies with an average rate of between 120 and 190 beats/min. There is usually 1:1 AV conduction. This arrhythmia is most commonly seen in patients with severe acute illness, especially in those with chronic obstructive pulmonary disease. Excess catecholamine stimulation or methylxanthine toxicity are frequent causes. MAT cannot be terminated acutely either with antiarrhythmic drugs or with electrical countershock. Treatment of the underlying etiology of the arrhythmia is the only effective means of therapy.

The ECG of the patient in MAT may superficially resemble atrial fibrillation and may lead to therapy with digoxin or another cardiac glycoside. In MAT, however, toxic concentrations of digoxin are required before a reduction in ventricular rate is observed, and digitalis-induced arrhythmias may occur. Propranolol is usually contraindicated when MAT is seen. Verapamil may slow the atrial rate in milder forms of MAT, but its use might aggravate the more critically ill patient's hemodynamic status. In most cases, MAT must be tolerated until the factors that precipitated it can be reversed.

Ventricular Tachycardia and Ventricular Fibrillation

The acute management of the patient with cardiac arrest is discussed elsewhere in this text. The elective treatment of ventricular tachycardia that is hemodynamically well tolerated remains largely empiric. Episodes in a small number of patients may be terminated rapidly by intravenous administration of a class I antiarrhythmic agent, usually either lidocaine or procainamide. In tachycardias with long cycle lengths, increasing intravenous doses of procainamide can produce gradual prolongation of the cycle length and may eventually terminate the arrhythmia. Acute drug therapy is often ineffective and either ventricular pacing or cardioversion is usually the treatment of choice for terminating ventricular tachycardia. If the patient is already on an antiarrhythmic drug at the time of the arrhythmia, knowledge of the plasma concentration of that agent is helpful when future prophylactic therapy is designed.

The best approach for selecting prophylactic therapy against ventricular arrhythmias remains controversial. However, clinical experience has shown that there is substantial variability among patients in response to the different antiarrhythmic agents and therapy must be individualized. At the present time, no single agent possesses such obvious clinical advantages that it should be recommended over all the other drugs currently in use. Each drug should be selected for trial and its results evaluated in systematic fashion. A better understanding of the mechanisms responsible for ventricular arrhythmias will allow a more rational approach to therapy in the future.

References

1. Abdollah H, Brugada P, Green M, et al: Clinical efficacy and electrophysiologic effects of intravenous and oral encainide in patients with accessory atrioventricular pathways and supraventricular arrhythmias. *Am J Cardiol* 54:544–549, 1984.
2. Adams PC, Holt DW, Storey GCA, et al: Amiodarone and its desethyl metabolite: tissue distribution and morphologic changes during long-term therapy. *Circulation* 72:1064–1075, 1985.
3. Allen JD, Brennan FJ, Wit AL: Actions of lidocaine on transmembrane potentials of subendocardial Purkinje fibers surviving in infarcted canine hearts. *Circ Res* 43:470–481, 1978.
4. Anderson JL, Lutz JR, Allison SB: Electrophysiologic and antiarrhythmic effects of oral flecainide in patients with inducible ventricular tachycardia. *J Am Coll Cardiol* 2:105–14, 1983.
5. Anderson JL, Patterson E, Wagner JG, et al: Clinical pharmacokinetics of intravenous and oral bretylium tosylate in survivors of ventricular tachycardia or fibrillation: clinical application of a new assay for bretylium. *J Cardiovasc Pharmacol* 3:485–499, 1981.
6. Anderson JL, Stewart JR, Perry BA, et al: Oral flecainide acetate for the treatment of ventricular arrhythmias. *N Engl J Med* 305:473–477, 1981.
7. Antman EM, Stone PH, Muller JE, et al: Calcium channel blocking agents in the treatment of cardiovascular

disorders. Part I: Basic and clinical electrophysiologic effects. *Ann Intern Med* 93:875–885, 1980.

8. Arnsdorf MF: Basic understanding of the electrophysiologic actions of arrhythmic drugs. Sources, sinks, and matrices of information. *Med Clin Am* 68:1247–1280, 1984.

9. Baker BJ, Dihn H, Kroskey D, et al: Effect of propafenone on left ventricular ejection fraction. *Am J Cardiol* 54:20D–22D, 1984.

10. Bauernfreind RA, Hoff JV, Swiryn S, et al: Electrophysiologic testing of bretylium tosylate in sustained ventricular tachycardia. *Am Heart J* 105:973–980, 1983.

11. β-Blocker Heart Attack Trial Research Group: A randomized trial of propranolol in patients with acute myocardial infarction. I. Mortality results. *JAMA* 247:1707–1714, 1982.

12. Bigger JT Jr: The quinidine-digoxin interaction. *Mod Concepts Cardiovasc Dis* 51:73–78, 1982.

13. Bigger JT Jr, Hoffman BF: Antiarrhythmic drugs. In Goodman, Gilman (eds): *The Pharmacological Basis of Therapeutics*, ed 5. New York, Macmillan, 1985, pp 748–791.

14. Bigger JT Jr, Sahar DI: Clinical types of proarrhythmic response to antiarrhythmic drugs. *Am J Cardiol* 59:2E–9E, 1987.

15. Borowski GD, Garofano CD, Rose LI: Effect of long-term amiodarone therapy on thyroid hormone levels and thyroid function. *Am J Med* 78:443–450, 1985.

16. Breithardt G, Borggrefe M, Wiebringhaus E, et al: Effect of propafenone in the Wolff-Parkinson-White syndrome: electrophysiologic findings and long-term follow-up. *Am J Cardiol* 54:29D–39D, 1984.

17. Campbell RWF: Drug therapy: mexiletine. *N Engl J Med* 36:29–34, 1987.

18. Campbell RWF, Hutton I, Elton RA, et al: Prophylaxis of primary ventricular fibrillation with tocainide in acute myocardial infarction. *Br Heart J* 49:557–563, 1983.

19. Chamberlain DA, Jewiit DE, Julian DG, et al: Oral mexiletine in high-risk patients after myocardial infarction. *Lancet* 2:1227, 1980.

20. Charness ME, Morady F, Scheinman MM: Frequent neurologic toxicity associated with amiodarone therapy. *Neurology* 34:669–671, 1984.

21. Chilson DA, Heger JJ, Zipes DP, et al: Electrophysiologic effects and clinical efficacy of oral propafenone therapy in patients with ventricular tachycardia. *J Am Coll Cardiol* 5:1407–1413, 1985.

22. Connolly SJ, Kates RE, Lebsack CS, et al: Clinical efficacy and electrophysiology of oral propafenone for ventricular tachycardia. *Am J Cardiol* 52:1208–1213, 1983.

23. Conrad GJ, Ober RE: Metabolism of flecainide. *Am J Cardiol* 53:41B–51B, 1984.

24. Davies RF, Lineberry MD, Echt DS, et al: Dose titration and pharmacokinetics of recainam, a new antiarrhythmic drug (abstract). *Circulation* 74:II-103, 1987.

25. DiMarco JP: Intracardiac electrophysiology in cardiac catheterization and angiography. In Grossman W (ed): ed 3. Philadelphia, Lea & Febiger, 1986, pp 339–358.

26. DiMarco JP, Garan H, Ruskin JN: Mexiletine for refractory ventricular arrhythmias: results using serial electrophysiologic testing. *Am J Cardiol* 47:13–38, 1981.

27. DiMarco JP, Garan H, Ruskin JN: Quinidine for ventricular arrhythmias: value of electrophysiologic testing. *Am J Cardiol* 51:90–95, 1983.

28. DiMarco JP, Sellers TD, Lerman BB, et al: Diagnostic and therapeutic use of adenosine in patients with supraventricular tachyarrhythmias. *J Am Coll Cardiol* 6:417–425, 1985.

29. Doherty JU, Waxman HL, Kienzle MG, et al: Limited role of intravenous propafenone hydrochloride in the treatment of sustained ventricular tachycardia: electrophysiologic effects and results of programmed ventricular stimulation. *J Am Coll Cardiol* 4:378–381, 1984.

30. Duff HJ, Oates JA, Roden DM, et al: The antiarrhythmic activity of meobentine sulfate in man. *J Cardiovasc Pharmacol* 6:650–656, 1984.

31. Duff HJ, Roden D, Primm RK, et al: Mexiletine in the treatment of resistant ventricular arrhythmias. Enhancement of efficacy and reduction of dose-related side effects by combination with quinidine. *Circulation* 67:1124–1128, 1983.

32. Duff HJ, Roden DM, Yacobi A, et al: Bretylium: relations between plasma concentrations and pharmacologic actions in high-frequency ventricular arrhythmias. *Am J Cardiol* 55:395–401, 1985.

33. Dunn HM, McComb JM, Kinney CD, et al: Prophylactic lidocaine in the early phase of suspected myocardial infarction. *Am Heart J* 110:353–362, 1985.

34. Engler RL, LeWinter M: Tocainide-induced ventricular fibrillation. *Am Heart J* 101:494–496, 1981.

35. The Esmolol vs Placebo Multicenter Study Group: Comparison of the efficacy and safety of esmolol, a short-acting beta blocker, with placebo in the treatment of supraventricular tachyarrhythmias. *Am Heart J* 111:42–48, 1986.

36. Falik R, Flores BT, Shaw L, et al: Relationship of steady-state serum concentrations of amiodarone and desethylamiodarone to therapeutic efficacy and adverse effects. *Am J Med* 82:1102–1108, 1987.

37. The Flecainide-Quinidine Research Group: Flecainide versus quinidine for treatment of chronic ventricular arrhythmias. A multicenter clinical trial. *Circulation* 67:1117–1123, 1983.

38. Flecainide Ventricular Tachycardia Study Group: Treatment of resistant ventricular tachycardia with flecainide acetate. *Am J Cardiol* 57:1299–1304, 1986.

39. Flowers D, O'Gallagher D, Torres V, et al: Long-term treatment using a reduced dosing schedule. *Am J Cardiol* 55:79–83, 1985.

40. Fogoros RN, Anderson KP, Winkle RA, et al: Amiodarone: clinical efficacy and toxicity in 95 patients with recurrent, drug-refractory arrhythmias. *Circulation* 68:88–94, 1983.

41. Frey W: Weitere erfahrunger mit clinidin bei absoluter nezunregelin assigkeit. *Wien Klin Wochenschr* 55:849–853, 1918.

42. Frishman WH, Teicher M: Beta-adrenergic blockade. An update. *Cardiology* 72:280–296, 1985.

43. Giardina E-GV, Dreyfuss J, Bigger JT Jr, et al: Metabolism of procainamide in normal and cardiac subjects. *Clin Pharmacol Ther* 19:339–351, 1975.

44. Graffner C, Johnson G, Sjogren J: Pharmacokinetics of procainamide intravenously and orally as conventional and slow release tablets. *Clin Pharmacol Ther* 17:414–423, 1974.

45. Gray RJ, Bateman TM, Ozer LSC, et al: Esmolol: a new ultrashort-acting beta-adrenergic blocking agent for rapid control of heart rate in postoperative supraventricular tachyarrhythmias. *J Am Coll Cardiol* 5:141–56, 1985.

46. Grayboys TB, Lown B, Podrid PJ, et al: Long-term survival of patients with malignant ventricular arrhythmias treated with antiarrhythmic drugs. *Am J Cardiol* 50:437–443, 1982.

47. Greenberg ML, Kelly TA, Lerman BB, et al: Atrial pacing for conversion of atrial flutter. *Am J Cardiol* 58:95–99, 1986.

48. Greenberg ML, Lerman BB, Shipe JR, et al: Relation between amiodarone and desethylamiodarone plasma concentrations and electrophysiologic effects, efficacy and toxicity. *J Am Coll Cardiol* 9:1148–1155, 1987.

49. Greenblatt DJ, Pfeifer HJ, Ochs JR, et al: Pharmacokinetics of quinidine in humans after intravenous, intramuscular and oral administration. *J Pharmacol Exp Ther* 202:365–377, 1977.

50. Greene HL, Graham EL, Werner JA, et al: Toxic and therapeutic effects of amiodarone in the treatment of cardiac arrhythmias. *J Am Coll Cardiol* 2:1114–1128, 1983.

51. Greene HL, Werner JA, Gross BW, et al: Failure of bretylium to suppress inducible ventricular tachycardia. *Am Heart J* 105:717–721, 1983.

52. Greene HL, Werner JA, Gross BW, et al: Prolongation of cardiac refractory times in man by clofilium phosphate, a new antiarrhythmic agent. *Am Heart J* 106:492–501, 1983.

53. Greenspan AM, Horowitz LN, Spielman SR, et al: Large dose procainamide therapy for ventricular tachyarrhythmias. *Am J Cardiol* 46:453–463, 1980.

54. Haffajee CI, Love JC, Canada AT, et al: Clinical pharmacokinetics and efficacy of amiodarone for refractory tachyarrhythmias. *Circulation* 67:1347–1355, 1983.

55. Hamer AW, Finerman WB, Peter T, Mandel WJ: Disparity between the clinical and electrophysiologic effects of amiodarone in the treatment of recurrent ventricular tachyarrhythmias. *Am Heart J* 103:992–1000, 1981.

56. Hammill SC, McLaran CJ, Wood DL, et al: Doubleblind study of intravenous propafenone for paroxysmal supraventricular reentrant tachycardia. *J Am Coll Cardiol* 9:1364–1368, 1987.

57. Haynes RE, Chinn TL, Copass MK, et al: Comparison of bretylium tosylate and lidocaine in management of out-of-hospital ventricular fibrillation: a randomized clinical trial. *Am J Cardiol* 48:353–356, 1981.

58. Heel RC, Brogden RN, Speight TM, et al: Disopyramide: a review of its pharmacological properties and therapeutic use in treating cardiac arrhythmias. *Drugs* 15:331–368, 1978.

59. Heger JJ, Hubbard J, Zipes DP, et al: Propafenone treatment of recurrent ventricular tachycardia: comparison of continuous electrocardiographic recording and electrophysiologic study in predicting drug efficacy. *Am J Cardiol* 54:40D–44D, 1984.

60. Hellestrand KJ, Nathan AW, Bexton RS, et al: Cardiac electrophysiologic effects of flecainide acetate for paroxysmal reentrant junctional tachycardias. *Am J Cardiol* 51:770–776, 1983.

61. Hirschfeld DS, Veda CT, Rowland M, et al: Clinical and electrophysiological effects of quinidine in man. *Br Heart J* 39:309–316, 1977.

62. Hjalmarson A, Elmfeldt D, Herlitz J, et al: Effect on mortality of metoprolol in acute myocardial infarction: a double-blind randomised trial. *Lancet* 2:823–827, 1981.

63. Hodges M, Haugland M, Granrud G, et al: Suppression of ventricular ectopic depolarizations by flecainide acetate, a new antiarrhythmic agent. *Circulation* 65:879–885, 1982.

64. Hoffman BF, Rosen MR, Wit AL: Electrophysiology and pharmacology of cardiac arrhythmias. VII. Cardiac effects of quinidine and procainamide. *Am Heart J* 89:804–808, 1975.

65. Holland K, Patterson E, Lucchesi BR: Prevention of ventricular fibrillation by bretylium in a conscious canine model of sudden coronary death. *Am Heart J* 105:711–717, 1983.

66. Holmes B, Heel RC: Flecainide: a preliminary review of its pharmacodynamic properties and therapeutic efficacy. *Drugs* 29:1–33, 1985.

67. Holt DW, Tucker GT, Jackson PR, et al: Amiodarone pharmacokinetics. *Br J Clin Pract* 40(suppl 4):109–14, 1986.

68. Hondeghem LM: Antiarrhythmic agents: modulated receptor applications. *Circulation* 75:514–520, 1987.

69. Hondeghem LM, Katzung BG: Antiarrhythmic agents: the modulated receptor mechanism of action of sodium and calcium channel–blocking drugs. *Annu Rev Pharmacol Toxicol* 24:387–423, 1984.

70. Hondeghem LM, Mason JW: Agents used in cardiac arrhythmias. In Katzung BG (ed): *Basic and Clinical Pharmacology*, ed 3. Norwalk, CT, Appleton & Lange, 1987, pp 151–167.

71. Horowitz LN, Greenspan AM, Rae AP, et al: Proar-

rhythmic responses during electrophysiologic testing. *Am J Cardiol* 59:45E–48E, 1987.

72. Horowitz LN, Greenspan AM, Spielman SR, et al: Usefulness of electrophysiologic testing in evaluation of amiodarone therapy for sustained ventricular tachyarrhythmias associated with coronary heart disease. *Am J Cardiol* 55:367–371, 1985.

73. Impact Research Group: International mexiletine and placebo antiarrhythmic coronary trial: I. Report on arrhythmia and other findings. *J Am Coll Cardiol* 4:1148–1163, 1984.

74. Ingram DV: Ocular effects in long-term amiodarone therapy. *Am Heart J* 106:902–904, 1983.

75. Josephson ME, Caracta AR, Ricciotti MA, et al: Electrophysiologic properties of procainamide in man. *Am J Cardiol* 33:596–603, 1974.

76. Josephson ME, Kaul S, Hopkins J, et al: Hemodynamic effects of intravenous flecainide relative to the level of ventricular function in patients with coronary artery disease. *Am Heart J* 109:41–45, 1985.

77. Josephson ME, Seides SF, Batsford WP, et al: The electrophysiologic effects of quinidine on the atrioventricular conducting system in man. *Am Heart J* 87:55–64, 1974.

78. Kadish AH, Buxton AE, Waxman HL, et al: Usefulness of electrophysiologic study to determine the clinical tolerance of arrhythmia recurrences during amiodarone therapy. *J Am Coll Cardiol* 10:90–96, 1987.

79. Kappenberger LJ, Fromer MA, Shenasa M, et al: Evaluation of flecainide acetate in rapid atrial fibrillation complicating Wolff-Parkinson-White syndrome. *Clin Cardiol* 8:321–326, 1985.

80. Kass RS: The ionic basis of electrical activity in the heart. In Sperelakis N (ed): *Physiology and Pathology of the Heart*. Boston, Martinus Nijhoff, 1984, pp 63–92.

81. Kates RE: Calcium antagonists. Pharmacokinetic properties. *Drugs* 25:113–24, 1983.

82. Keefe DL, Peters F, Winkle RA: Randomized doubleblind placebo controlled crossover trial documenting oral lorcainide efficacy in suppression of symptomatic ventricular tachyarrhythmias. *Am Heart J* 103:511–518, 1982.

83. Kerin NZ, Blevins RD, Frumin H, et al: Intravenous and oral loading versus oral loading alone with amiodarone for chronic refractory ventricular arrhythmias. *Am J Cardiol* 55:90–91, 1985.

84. Koch-Weser J: Disopyramide. *N Engl J Med* 300:957–962, 1979.

85. Koch-Weser J: Drug therapy—bretylium. *N Engl J Med* 300:473–477, 1979.

86. Kosinski EJ, Albin JB, Young E, et al: Hemodynamic effects of intravenous amiodarone. *J Am Coll Cardiol* 4:565–570, 1984.

87. Koster RW, Dunning AJ: Intramuscular lidocaine for prevention of lethal arrhythmias in the prehospitalization phase of acute myocardial infarction. *N Engl J Med* 313:105–110, 1985.

88. Kostis JB, Krieger S, Moreyra A, et al: Cibenzoline for treatment of ventricular arrhythmias: a double-blind placebo-controlled study. *J Am Coll Cardiol* 4:372–377, 1984.

89. Leahey EB Jr, Reiffel JA, Drusin RE, et al: Interaction between digoxin and quinidine. *JAMA* 240:533–534, 1978.

90. Lidell C, Rehnqvist N, Sjogren A, et al: Comparative efficacy of oral sotalol and procainamide in patients with chronic ventricular arrhythmias: a multicenter study. *Am Heart J* 109:970–975, 1985.

91. Lie KI, Wellens HJ, van Capelle FJ, et al: Lidocaine in the prevention of primary ventricular fibrillation. *N Engl J Med* 291:1324–1326, 1974.

92. Lown B, Wolf M: Approaches to sudden death from coronary heart disease. *Circulation* 4:130–142, 1972.

93. Lucchesi BR, Patterson E: Therapeutic advances in the

management of cardiac arrhythmias: Part II—brety-lium. *Pract Cardiol* 8:101–112, 1982.

94. Lucchesi BR, Patterson E: Therapeutic advances in the management of cardiac arrhythmias: Part III—verapamil. *Pract Cardiol* 8:43–59, 1982.

95. Lynch JJ, Lucchesi BR: New antiarrhythmic agents: Part IV—the pharmacology and clinical use of tocainide. *Pract Cardiol* 11:108–137, 1985.

96. Martino E, Safran M, Aghini-Lombardi F, et al: Environmental iodine intake and thyroid dysfunction during chronic amiodarone therapy. *Ann Intern Med* 101:28–34, 1984.

97. Mason JW: Amiodarone. *N Engl J Med* 316:455–458, 1987.

98. Mason JW, Hondeghem LM, Katzung BG: Block of inactivated sodium channels and of depolarization-induced automaticity in guinea pig papillary muscle by amiodarone. *Circ Res* 55:277–285, 1984.

99. Mason JW, Peters FA: Antiarrhythmic efficacy of encainide in patients with refractory recurrent ventricular tachycardia. *Circulation* 63:670–675, 1981.

100. McAlister RG: Clinical pharmacology of slow channel blocking agents. *Prog Cardiovasc Dis* 25:83–102, 1982.

101. McGovern B, Garan H, Malacoff RF, et al: Long-term clinical outcome of ventricular tachycardia or fibrillation treated with amiodarone. *Am J Cardiol* 53:1558–1563, 1984.

102. Meffin PJ, Roberts EW, Winkle RA, et al: Role of concentration dependent plasma protein binding on disopyramide disposition. *J Pharmacol Kinet Bio Pharm* 7:29–46, 1979.

103. Mirowski, M: The automatic implantable cardioverter-defibrillator: an overview. *J Am Coll Cardiol* 6:461–466, 1985.

104. Morady F, DiCarlo LA Jr, deBuitleir MD, et al: Effects of incremental doses of procainamide on ventricular refractoriness, intraventricular conduction and induction of ventricular tachycardia. *Circulation* 74:135–164, 1986.

105. Moysey JO, Jaggarao NSV, Grundy EN, et al: Amiodarone increases plasma digoxin concentrations. *Br Med J* 282:272–274, 1981.

106. Nademanee K, Feld G, Hendrickson J, et al: Electrophysiologic and antiarrhythmic effects of sotalol in patients with life-threatening ventricular tachyarrhythmias. *Circulation* 72:555–564, 1985.

107. Nademanee K, Hendrickson J, Kannan R, Singh BN: Antiarrhythmic efficacy and electrophysiologic actions of amiodarone in patients with life-threatening ventricular arrhythmias: potent suppression of spontaneously occurring tachyarrhythmias versus inconsistent abolition of induced ventricular tachycardia. *Am Heart J* 103:950–959, 1982.

108. Nathan AW, Hellestrand KJ: Flecainide acetate: a review. *Clin Prog Pacing Electrophysiol* 2:43–53, 1984.

109. Nathan AW, Hellestrand KJ, Bexton RS, et al: Fatal ventricular tachycardia in association with propafenone, a new class IC antiarrhythmic agent. *Postgrad Med J* 60:155–156, 1984.

110. Nathan AW, Hellestrand KJ, Beston RS, et al: Proarrhythmic effects of the new antiarrhythmic agent flecainide acetate. *Am Heart J* 107:222–228, 1984.

111. Nattel S, Zeng F-D: Frequency-dependent effects of antiarrhythmic drugs on action potential duration and refractoriness of canine cardiac Purkinje fibers. *J Pharmacol Exp Ther* 229:283–291, 1984.

112. Nestico PF, Morganroth J, Horowitz LN, et al: Efficacy of oral and intravenous indecainide in ventricular arrhythmias. *Am J Cardiol* 59:1332–1336, 1987.

113. The Norwegian Multicenter Study Group: Timolol-induced reduction in mortality and reinfarction in patients surviving acute myocardial infarction. *N Engl J Med* 304:801–807, 1981.

114. Nygaard TW, Sellers TD, Cook TS, et al: Adverse reactions to antiarrhythmic drugs during therapy for ventricular arrhythmias. *JAMA* 256:55–58, 1986.

115. O'Brien KP, Taylor PM, Croxson RS: Prophylactic linocaine in hospitalized patients with acute myocardial infarction. *Med J Aust* 2:536–537, 1973.

116. Olson DW, Thompson BM, Darin JC, et al: A randomized comparison study of bretylium tosylate and lidocaine in resuscitation of patients from out-of-hospital ventricular fibrillation in a paramedic system. *Ann Emerg Med* 13:807–810, 1984.

117. Podrid P, Lown B: Propafenone: a new agent for ventricular arrhythmia. *J Am Coll Cardiol* 4:117–125, 1984.

118. Podrid PJ, Morganroth J: Aggravation of arrhythmia during drug therapy: experience with flecainide acetate. *Pract Cardiol* 11:55–70, 1985.

119. Podrid PJ, Schoeneberger A, Lown B: Congestive heart failure caused by oral disopyramide. *N Engl J Med* 302:614–617, 1980.

120. Pratt CM, Yepsen SC, Taylor AA, et al: Ethmozine suppression of single and repetitive ventricular premature depolarizations during therapy: documentation of efficacy and long-term safety. *Am Heart J* 106:85–90, 1983.

121. Prystowsky EN, Klein GJ, Rinkenberger RL, et al: Clinical efficacy and electrophysiologic effects of encainide in patients with Wolff-Parkinson-White syndrome. *Circulation* 69:278–287, 1984.

122. Rae AP, Greenspan AM, Spielman SR, et al: Antiarrhythmic drug efficacy for ventricular tachyarrhythmias associated with coronary artery disease as assessed by electrophysiologic studies. *Am J Cardiol* 55:1494–1499, 1985.

123. Reiter MJ, Mann DE, Easley AR: New antiarrhythmic agents: Part VIII—antiarrhythmic properties of pirmenol. *Pract Cardiol* 11:129–137, 1985.

124. Reuter H: Ion channels in cardiac cell membranes. *Annu Rev Physiol* 46:473–484, 1984.

125. Roden DM, Dawson AK, Duff HJ, et al: Electrophysiology of O-demethyl encainide in a canine model of sustained ventricular tachycardia. *J Cardiovasc Pharmacol* 6:588–595, 1984.

126. Roden DM, Reele SB, Higgins SB, et al: Total suppression of ventricular arrhythmias by encainide: pharmacokinetic and electrocardiographic characteristics. *N Engl J Med* 302:877–882, 1980.

127. Roos JC, Paalman ACA, Duxning AJ: Electrophysiological effects of mexiletine in man. *Br Heart J* 38:1262–1271, 1976.

128. Rosen MR, Hoffman BF, Wit AL: Electrophysiology and pharmacology of cardiac arrhythmias. V. Cardiac antiarrhythmic effects of lidocaine. *Am Heart J* 89:52–56, 1975.

129. Routledge PA, Stargel WW, Barchowsky A, et al: Control of lidocaine therapy: new perspectives. *Ther Drug Monit* 4:265–270, 1980.

130. Salerno DM, Granrud G, Sharkey P, et al: A controlled trial of propafenone for treatment of frequent and repetitive ventricular premature complexes. *Am J Cardiol* 53:77–83, 1984.

131. Sanchez-Chapula J, Tsuda Y, Josephson IR: Voltage- and use-dependent effects of lidocaine on sodium current in rat single ventricular cells. *Circ Res* 52:557–565, 1983.

132. Siddoway LA, Roden DM, Woosley RL: Clinical pharmacology of propafenone: pharmacokinetics, metabolism and concentration-response relations. *Am J Cardiol* 54:9D–12D, 1984.

133. Singh BN, Nademanee K, Baky SH: Calcium antagonists. Clinical use in the treatment of arrhythmias. *Drugs* 25:125–153, 1983.

134. Sobol SM, Rakita L: Pneumonitis and pulmonary fibrosis associated with amiodarone treatment: a possible complication of a new antiarrhythmic drug. *Circulation* 65::819–824, 1982.

135. Sperelakis N: Electrical properties of cells at rest and

maintenance of the ion distributions. In Sperelakis N (ed): *Physiology and Pathology of the Heart.* Boston, Martinus Nijhoff, 1984, pp 59–82.

136. Stein J, Podrid P, Lown B: Effects of oral mexiletine on left and right ventricular function. *Am J Cardiol* 54:575–578, 1984.

137. Stone PH, Antman EM, Muller JE, et al: Calcium channel blocking agents in the treatment of cardiovascular disorders. Part II: Hemodynamic effects and clinical applications. *Ann Intern Med* 93:886–904, 1980.

138. Sung RJ, Elser B, McAlister RG: Intravenous verapamil for termination of re-entrant supraventricular tachycardias. *Ann Intern Med* 93:682–689, 1980.

139. Tucker CR, Winkle RA, Peters FA, et al: Acute hemodynamic effects of intravenous encainide in patients with heart disease. *Am Heart J* 104:209–215, 1982.

140. Valentine PA, Frew JL, Mashford MC, et al: Lidocaine in the prevention of sudden death in the pre-hospital phase of acute infarctions. *N Engl J Med* 291:1327–1331, 1974.

141. Vaughn-Williams EM: A classification of antiarrhythmic actions reassessed after a decade of new drugs. *J Clin Pharmacol* 24:129–147, 1984.

142. Velebit V, Podrid P, Lown L, et al: Aggravation and provocation of ventricular arrhythmias by antiarrhythmic drugs. *Circulation* 65:886–894, 1982.

143. Wang T, Roden DM, Wolfenden HT, et al: Influence of genetic polymorphism on the metabolism and disposition of encainide in man. *J Pharmacol Exp Ther* 228:605–611, 1984.

144. Waspe LE, Waxman HL, Buxton AE, et al: Mexiletine for control of drug-resistant ventricular tachycardia: clinical and electrophysiologic results in 44 patients. *Am J Cardiol* 51:1175–1181, 1983.

145. Waxman HL, Groh WC, Marchlinski FE, et al: Amiodarone for control of sustained ventricular tachyarrhythmia: clinical and electrophysiologic effects in 51 patients. *Am J Cardiol* 50:1066–1074, 1982.

146. Webb CR, Morganroth J, Senior S, et al: Flecainide: steady state electrophysiologic effects in patients with remote myocardial infarction and inducible sustained ventricular arrhythmia. *J Am Coll Cardiol* 8:214–220, 1986.

147. Winkle RA, Mason JW, Griffin JC, et al: Malignant ventricular tachyarrhythmias associated with the use of encainide. *Am Heart J* 102:857–864, 1981.

148. Winkle RA, Peters F, Kates RE, et al: Clinical pharmacology and antiarrhythmic efficacy of encainide in patients with chronic ventricular arrhythmias. *Circulation* 64:290–296, 1981.

149. Winkle RA, Peters F, Kates RE, Harrison DC: Possible contribution of encainide to the long-term antiarrhythmic efficacy of encainide. *Am J Cardiol* 51:1182–1188, 1985.

150. Woosley RL, Drayer DE, Reidenberg MM, et al: Effect of acetylator phenotype on the rate at which procainamide induces antinuclear antibodies and the lupus syndrome. *N Engl J Med* 298:1157–1159, 1978.

151. Woosley RL, Echt DS, Roden DM: Effects of congestive heart failure on the pharmacokinetics and pharmacodynamics of antiarrhythmic agents. *Am J Cardiol* 56:25B–33B, 1986.

152. Zachary CB, Slater DN, Holt DW: The pathogenesis of amiodarone-induced pigmentation and photosensitivity. *Br J Dermatol* 110:451–456, 1984.

153. Zipes DP: Genesis of cardiac arrhythmias: electrophysiologic considerations. In Braunwald E (ed): *Heart Disease: A Textbook of Cardiovascular Medicine,* ed 2. Philadelphia, WB Saunders, pp 605–647.

10

Bronchodilators

Marissa Seligman, Pharm.D.

The use of drugs with potent bronchodilator action has proven to be highly effective therapy for the treatment of reversible airway obstruction. In bronchospastic patients, bronchodilator therapy may reverse hypoxia and normalize acid-base abnormalities, thereby helping to improve tissue perfusion and oxygenation. Additionally, these drugs may be used prophylactically to prevent the development of bronchospasm.

Effective use of bronchodilators requires a knowledge of the basic pathophysiology responsible for airway obstruction and the effect of drugs on airway caliber. Clinicians should also employ a systematic approach to the use of the various bronchodilators in patients with reversible airway obstruction.

AIRWAY OBSTRUCTION

Airway caliber and tone are regulated by the parasympathetic and sympathetic divisions of the autonomic nervous system (4, 44). The vagally mediated mechanisms of the parasympathetic nervous system are the primary determinants of bronchomotor tone and bronchial submucosal gland secretion (4, 12, 44). On stimulation of vagal efferent nerves, the neurotransmitter acetylcholine is released from the presynaptic nerve terminal. The acetylcholine then diffuses through the synaptic cleft and binds to muscarinic cholinergic receptors found on postsynaptic tissue cell membranes throughout the respiratory tree. Stimulation of the cholinergic receptors results in an increase in intracellular levels of cyclic guanosine monophosphate (cGMP) in the cytoplasm, thereby increasing the activity of the effector mechanism (44). Acetylcholine receptors are located in or adjacent to the respiratory epithelium, submucosal glands, mast cells, and airway smooth muscle (4, 12, 44). The highest number of receptors is found within the trachea and large bronchi (52). Stimulation of the acetylcholine receptors in the lung causes bronchoconstriction, decreased airway caliber, mast cell degranulation, and increased glandular secretion.

Direct sympathetic nervous system innervation of the respiratory tree is sparse (52). Nevertheless, bronchial smooth muscle cells, especially those located in the smaller airways (52), are well-populated with β_2-adrenergic receptors. β_1-Adrenergic receptors are also found in the lung, but have only a minimal role in lung physiology (27). β_2-adrenergic receptors are stimulated by adrenergic agonists, either endogenous (the presynaptic neurotransmitter norepinephrine, or epinephrine released by the adrenal medulla) or exogenous (drugs). This stimulation results in activation of membrane-bound adenylate cyclase to catalyze the conversion of adenosine triphosphate to cyclic adenosine monophosphate (cAMP) (26). A cascade of enzymatic reactions then progresses, resulting in bronchodilation and possibly increased secretion of mucus (55).

α-Adrenergic receptors are also found in the lung (44). Postsynaptic α_1-receptors are located predominantly in the bronchial and vascular smooth muscle and submucosal glands. Stimulation of these receptors by α-adrenergic agonists such as norepinephrine activates phosphatidylinositol turnover in the cytoplasm (47). The resulting bronchial smooth muscle and submucosal gland tissue responses are bronchoconstriction and increased mucus secretion. In the lung, α_2-receptors are located on the postsynaptic nerve terminal, although they are also located presynaptically elsewhere in the body. Presynaptic α_2-receptors regulate the release of norepinephrine from the presynaptic nerve terminal (47).

To summarize, the primary autonomic innervation of bronchial smooth muscle and the respiratory epithelium is via the parasympathetic (cholinergic) nervous system. This system is excitatory to the lungs; its activation causes bronchial smooth muscle contraction and bronchial gland secretion. This tonic activity is opposed, albeit minimally, by the sympathetic (adrenergic) nervous system. Bronchodilation results from activation of the β_2-receptors of the sympathetic nervous system.

In addition to autonomic nervous system control of airway tone, respiratory tree caliber may be altered by a third neural innervation pathway, the so-called "purinergic" or "nonadrenergic noncholinergic (NANC) nervous system" (1, 4, 12, 52). Stimulation of this pathway produces bronchial smooth muscle contraction. The exact role of the NANC nervous system remains to be defined, but further investigation of this system might eventually lead to novel forms of treatment of airway diseases (45).

Various endogenous substances, e.g., histamine, prostaglandins, and the leukotrienes (the slow-reacting substance of anaphylaxis) also have documented effects on smooth muscle tone (1).

Nonneurogenic factors may alter airway caliber by affecting either airway anatomy or physiology. The most common causes of increased airway resistance are asthma (acute or chronic), emphysema, chronic bronchitis, and cystic fibrosis. Mechanical factors, e.g., tumors, mucous plugging, and foreign bodies, are also frequent causes of airway obstruction (1). Less commonly, airway obstruction develops from inhalation of toxic materials and resultant airway injury, drug-induced bronchoconstriction, infectious bronchitis, or bronchiolitis (1). Acute left ventricular failure may infrequently present as airway obstruction, as can pulmonary emboli. When airway obstruction occurs as a result of immunologic disorders (e.g., collagen-vascular disorders, dust sensitivity) or aspiration, bronchoconstriction is often not involved (1). Accordingly, drug-induced bronchodilation may not reverse the resistance to airflow associated with these conditions.

Clinically, patients with airflow obstruction usually manifest tachypnea, labored respiration with accessory muscle use, pulsus paradoxus, thoracic overinflation, and ventilation-perfusion mismatching (1). Auscultation of the airways commonly demonstrates rales and prolongation of the expiratory phase. Wheezing is a prominent sign but may be absent if airway obstruction is so severe that a wheeze cannot be generated (1). Most patients with airway obstruction demonstrate abnormalities in peak expiratory flow measurements and spirometry. For example, if presenting with an forced expiratory volume in 1 second (FEV-1) of less than 800 ml or a peak expiratory flow rate of less than 100 ml/min, the patient should usually receive aggressive pharmacotherapy (1).

Critically ill patients who are mechanically ventilated may experience airflow obstruction due to abnormalities in lung compliance, thoracic deflation, laryngeal spasm, laryngeal edema, epiglottitis, blunt laryngeal trauma, and tracheal avulsion (1). Thus, when assessing these patients, care should be taken in evaluating artificial airway position and upper airway function.

CLASSIFICATION OF BRONCHODILATOR DRUGS

The classification system used to group bronchodilator drugs is based on their mechanism of action:

a. Direct respiratory smooth muscle relaxants: theophylline and related salts
b. β-Adrenergic agonists: isoetharine, isoproterenol, epinephrine, metaproterenol, albuterol, terbutaline, bitolterol
c. Anticholinergics: atropine, glycopyrrolate, ipratropium

Their sites of action are depicted in Figure 10.1 (48).

Theophylline

Theophylline, a naturally occurring methylxanthine closely related to caffeine and found in tea, has been used to treat bronchospasm for more than 100 years (46). An enormous number of pharmacokinetic and pharmacodynamic data relative to this drug have been generated over the past 20 years. These findings have contributed to renewed interest in theophylline and the introduction of a wide variety of theophylline products into clinical use. Accordingly, theophylline has become one of the most extensively prescribed drugs for the treatment of reversible airway obstruction. In addition, the development of methods to monitor serum theophylline concentrations in patients has contributed to the safe and efficacious clinical use of this drug.

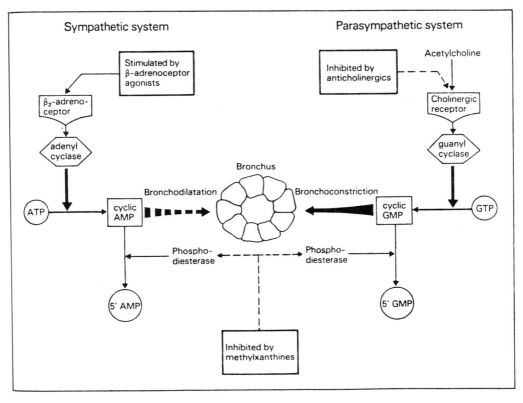

Figure 10.1 Mechanism of action of bronchodilator drugs (Originally published in Kelly HW: Controversies in asthma therapy with theophyline and the beta-2-adrenergic agents. *Clin Pharm* 3:386–395, 1984. Copyright © 1984, American Society of Hospital Pharmacists, Inc. All rights reserved. Reprinted with permission.)

PHARMACOLOGY

The exact mechanism by which theophylline exerts its pharmacologic effects is unclear (21). It is well established that theophylline competitively inhibits the activity of cytoplasmic phosphodiesterase, the enzyme that catalyzes the degradation of cAMP to 5'-AMP (56). This inhibition increases intracellular levels of cAMP, resulting in smooth muscle relaxation. However, this effect can only be demonstrated in vitro using very high concentrations of theophylline (5, 21). Additionally, unlike theophylline, other more potent phosphodiesterase inhibitors do not produce bronchodilation (21). Other postulated mechanisms of action include inhibition of intracellular calcium activity (18), prostaglandin inhibition (17), and increased binding of cAMP to cAMP-binding protein (6, 36). Recently, adenosine receptor antagonism has been proposed as the primary mediator of the pharmacologic and therapeutic actions of methylxanthines (16, 58).

Theophylline is a direct bronchial smooth muscle relaxant (13). If bronchospasm is not present, its effects on air flow and respiratory mechanics are minimal. The drug may also act by decreasing mucosal edema and reducing the production of excessive secretions (13). Other effects of theophylline include direct augmentation of myocardial inotropy and chronotropy (39); stimulation of diaphragmatic contractility (3, 38); dilation of the coronary, pulmonary, renal, and systemic arterioles and veins (2); diuresis (21, 32); stimulation of epinephrine and norepinephrine synthesis and release by the adrenal medulla (46); stimulation of the medullary respiratory center; relaxation of the smooth muscle of the gall bladder and gastrointestinal tract (32); stimulation of gastric acid secretion (18); and decreased cerebral blood flow (58).

SIDE EFFECTS

The most common side effects of theophylline include gastrointestinal effects that are both locally and centrally mediated (32). Frequently reported side effects include nausea, vomiting, and anorexia. Central nervous system effects include headache, irritability, restlessness, nervousness, dizziness, and seizures (5, 14). The incidence and severity of all of these adverse reactions usually decrease with reduction in the daily theophylline dosage (32). Unfortunately, mild side effects such as nausea and vomiting do not necessarily become manifest before serious life-threatening problems such as seizures develop (14, 15, 60). Additionally, theophylline-induced seizures are often unresponsive to standard anticonvulsive therapy, and the mortality rate associated with this problem has been estimated to be as high as 50% (5, 60). Theophylline may cause a number of cardiovascular side effects that are often poorly tolerated by critically ill patients. These effects include palpitations, sinus tachycardia, extrasystoles, and multifocal atrial tachycardia (5). Flushing, hypotension, circulatory collapse, and ventricular arrhythmias have also been reported.

Prior to 1983, the only parenteral form of theophylline was aminophylline. Aminophylline is theophylline compounded with ethylenediamine, which confers water solubility to the insoluble theophylline molecule. By weight, aminophylline is 80% theophylline (e.g., 100 mg of aminophylline is equivalent to 80 mg of theophylline). Interestingly, ethylenediamine contributes to both the efficacy and toxicity of theophylline. Ethylenediamine may augment the respiratory and cardiac stimulant effects of theophylline, but the significance of these effects is questionable (32). More importantly, it is well established that ethylenediamine can induce hypersensitivity reactions characterized by urticaria, generalized pruritus, angioedema, and bronchospasm (32). Recently, a premixed intravenous solution of theophylline in 5% dextrose in water was introduced into clinical use. Although adverse reactions to ethylenediamine occur rarely, theophylline therapy in critically ill patients can be simplified by use of these premixed theophylline solutions.

Because the rapid intravenous injection of aminophylline or theophylline may cause dizziness, palpitations, flushing, hypotension, and profound bradycardia, these drugs must be administered by slow intravenous injection or, preferably, by use of an infusion pump (13, 18). Cardiac arrest may also occur with the rapid administration of aminophylline. Intramuscular injections of theophylline salts are painful and the free drug is slowly and erratically absorbed from the site of administration. Therefore, this route of administration is not recommended (14, 32).

PHARMACOKINETICS

Theophylline is manufactured as a variety of salts for oral, rectal, and parenteral administration (in excess of 150 different products in the United States alone!) (14, 15, 18, 32, 60). Although rectal preparations of theophylline and its related salts are available, their absorption, especially from suppositories, into the systemic circulation is very erratic and unreliable. Use of the suppositories should be avoided in all patients (57). Fixed-dose combinations of theophylline with other drugs such as ephedrine should be avoided (9). The intravenous forms of theophylline are primarily limited to hospitalized patients, particularly those who are critically ill and unable to take oral medications.

The pharmacokinetics of theophylline have been well described (13, 18, 32, 35). Following oral administration, gastric acidity prompts the release of free theophylline from the theophylline salt or compound preparation. The rate of this release and the subsequent absorption of theophylline into the systemic circulation depends on the theophylline product used. For example, theophylline is rapidly absorbed from any of the many available oral solutions and uncoated tablet formulations. Peak serum levels are obtained 1–2 hours after administration. In contrast, extended-release and slow-release tablets are designed to release theophylline over a longer period of time (thereby decreasing the number of required drug doses per day); peak serum levels are usually reached 4 hours after administration. The actual rate of theophylline absorption from slow-release or extended-release formulations varies among formulations and routes of administration (e.g., oral route with or without food).

Theophylline distributes into a volume of distribution of 0.3–0.7 liters/kg in children and adults (14, 16, 32). In premature infants, the volume of distribution increases almost 2-fold. The drug is 56% bound to plasma proteins in children and adults and 36% in premature infants (18, 32, 35).

Hepatic metabolism of theophylline is the principal method of elimination. Eighty-eight to 92% of a theophylline dose is metabolized to three inactive metabolites; 1,3-dimethyluric acid, 1-methyluric acid, and 3-methylxanthine (32). In premature infants, a high percentage of theophylline is metabolized to caffeine. Theophylline and its metabolites are excreted from the body by the kidneys. Small amounts of unchanged theophylline may be excreted in the feces.

The metabolism of theophylline varies widely owing to differing rates of metabolism in different patient populations (18, 19, 32). In otherwise healthy, nonsmoking asthmatic adults, the elimination half-life averages between 7 and 9 hours; in children, between 1.5 and 9.5 hours; and in premature infants, between 15 and 58 hours (18, 32). Patients who are cigarette or marijuana smokers have a much shorter average elimination half-life of 4–5 hours (13). In contrast, patients with congestive heart failure, cor pulmonale, chronic obstructive pulmonary disease, or liver disease may have a markedly prolonged elimination half-life (14, 32).

Because theophylline has a low therapeutic ratio, the drug must be administered by careful dosage titration. Dosages should be calculated by use of lean body weight and consideration of underlying disease states and smoking history (Table 10.1) (14, 18). In addition, a variety of analytic techniques have been used to assess plasma or serum levels of theophylline and assist in reducing clinical toxicity (Table 10.2).

In isolated tracheal and bronchial smooth muscle preparations, theophylline induces bronchodilation in proportion to the log of the serum or plasma concentration over the range of 5–25 μg/ml (21, 37). Based on this relationship, a clinical "therapeutic range" for theophylline has been generated; the most frequently cited range is 10–20 μg/ml (14). Within this range, serious side effects of theophylline, including seizures, are reduced in incidence and severity, while efficacy is maintained. Most patients do not require levels in excess of 25 μg/ml to obtain adequate bronchodilation (35). This therapeutic range only represents the serum levels at which the majority of patients respond to theophylline; some patients respond outside this range. For example, bronchodilation can be produced at the lower end of the therapeutic range, i.e., serum concentrations of 2–10 μg/ml, in chronic asthmatic children (21). However, some patients may require levels in excess of 20 μg/ml (35). Marked interpatient and intrapatient variability exists for the dose-response curves for theophylline (5). Consequently, the ideal use of serum theophylline determinations is as an adjunct for titrating patient response and in determining

Table 10.1
Initial Intravenous Theophylline Maintenance Dosages[a]

Patient Population	Age	Theophylline Infusion Rate[b] (mg/kg/hr)
Neonates	Postnatal age up to 24 days	1 mg/kg q. 12 hours[c]
	Postnatal age above 24 days	1.5 mg/kg q. 12 hours[c]
Infants	6–52 weeks	0.008 × (age in weeks) + 0.21
Young children	1–9 yr	0.8
Older children	9–12 yr	0.7
Adolescents (smokers)	12–16 yr	0.7
Adolescents (nonsmokers)	12–16 yr	0.5[d]
Adults (healthy, smokers)	16–50 yr	0.7[d]
Adults (healthy, nonsmokers)	Above 16 years (including the elderly)	0.4[d]
Adults with cardiac decompensation, cor pulmonale, or liver dysfunction	Above 16 years	0.2[e]

[a]Originally published in Iafrate RP, Massey KL, Hendeles L: Current concepts in clinical therapeutics: asthma. *Clin Pharm* 5:206–227, 1986. Copyright © 1986, American Society of Hospital Pharmacists, Inc. All rights reserved. Reprinted with permission.
[b]Assumes an appropriate loading dose has been given. To achieve a target concentration of 10 μg/ml. Use lean body weight for obese patients. Although these doses are generally safe, many patients will require higher infusion rates as determined by serial serum measurements. These dosages differ from the current FDA recommendations, which include a higher infusion rate for the first 12 hours. Further dosage reductions may be required for patients receiving other drugs that decrease theophylline clearance.
[c]For a target concentration of 7.5 μg/ml (for neonatal apnea).
[d]Not to exceed 900 mg/day unless clinical symptoms and/or serum levels indicate the need for a larger dose.
[e]Not to exceed 400 mg/day unless clinical symptoms and/or serum levels indicate the need for a larger dose.

Table 10.2
Adverse Effects of Theophylline[a]

Serum Concentration	Symptoms	Frequency	Duration	Comments
5–20 μg/ml	Nausea, cramps, insomnia headache	Rare—if dose is slowly titrated over 1–2 weeks	Transient	
		Common—if therapeutic serum concentrations are rapidly attained	Transient	Avoided by dose titration
	Tremor	Rare—with concurrent administration of oral β_2-adrenergic	Unknown	Avoided if β_2-agonist is administered by inhalation
	Excessive gastric acid secretion	Rare		
15–35 μg/ml	Nausea, vomiting, diarrhea, stomach ache, headache, irritability, nervousness, insomnia, sinus tachycardia	Common—at serum concentrations >20 μg/ml	Persistent	Decrease dose
	Hyperglycemia	Rare—may occur in neonates	Persistent	
>35 μg/ml	Seizures, cerebral hypoxia, arrhythmias, cardiorespiratory arrest, death	Common	Persistent	Minor adverse effects often do not precede life-threatening toxicity

[a] Adapted from Hendeles L, Weinberger M: Theophylline: therapeutic use of serum concentration monitoring. In Taylor WJ, Finn AL (eds): *Individual Drug Therapy: Practical Applications of Drug Monitoring*. New York, Gross, Townsend, Frank, Hoffman, 1981, vol 1, pp 32–65. Used with permission of the publishers.

the optimal drug level and drug dosage that are necessary to achieve maximal bronchodilation.

DRUG INTERACTIONS

Theophylline clearance may be altered by a number of disease states and drugs (Table 10.3). Theophylline is reported to augment myocardial sensitivity to digitalis glycosides (32). In addition, theophylline may act synergistically with the β-adrenergic agonists to induce cardiac arrhythmias (21, 32).

CLINICAL USE

The primary role of theophylline is the prevention of bronchospasm in patients with either hyperactive airway disease or chronic obstructive pulmonary disorders (13, 18). For treatment of chronic bronchospasm in patients over 1 year of age, theophylline may be given initially at 16 mg/kg/day or 400 mg/day, whichever is less (14, 15). Depending on patient

response, the dose may be increased up to the following maximum daily doses (14, 15):

Age (yr)	Dosage (mg/kg/day)
1–9	24
9–12	20
12–16	18
>16	13, or 900 mg/day (whichever is less)

Note that in the prophylaxis of chronic bronchospasm, measurement of serum theophylline levels is usually necessary only (a) when these daily dosage recommendations are exceeded, (b) when drug toxicity is suspected, (c) when poor patient compliance to the prescribed regimen is suspected, or (d) to assess why a patient may not be responding to theophylline (e.g., rapid metabolism of the drug) (32, 35). Treatment should be started with an oral preparation of theophylline. The products that should be used are those with consistent 100% bioavailability: uncoated tablets, micro-

Table 10.3
Factors Affecting Theophylline Clearance[a]

Increase theophylline clearance	Decrease theophylline clearance
Smoking (cigarettes or marijuana)	Hepatic cirrhosis
Phenobarbital	Cor pulmonale
High protein/low carbohydrate diet	Congestive heart failure
Charcoal broiled diet	Propranolol
Phenytoin	Allopurinol ($>$600 mg/day)
Carbamazepine	Erythromycin
Rifampin	Cimetidine
	Troleandomycin
	Oral contraceptives

[a]Originally published in Iafrate RP, Massey KL, Hendeles: Current concepts in clinical therapeutics: asthma. *Clin Pharm* 5:206–227, 1986. Copyright © 1986, American Society of Hospital Pharmacists Inc. All rights reserved. Reprinted with permission.

crystalline dosage forms, or oral solutions. Once the patient's response has been demonstrated and dosages titrated, the daily drug dosage may then be converted to an equivalent amount of an extended-release theophylline product (56). For example, if a patient is taking theophylline oral tablets, 100 mg/4 hr, the total daily dose of 600 mg may be given as two 300-mg tablets of an extended-release product and manufacturer's recommendations followed as to the method of administration. Theophylline products should be chosen in accord with patient age and underlying disease state (37). At present a number of extended-release or slow-release theophylline products are available, each with different absorption profiles (18); not all clinicians consider these products to be interchangeable (18).

No theophylline product, oral or intravenous, should be used for the initial treatment of acute bronchospasm. Rather, only if repeated administration of inhaled β-adrenergic agonists, e.g., isoetharine or albuterol, produces a suboptimal effect should theophylline be administered (13, 18). Either intravenous or oral liquid theophylline can be used to treat acute bronchospasm; the former is more commonly used in critically ill patients (13, 14, 18).

Theophylline therapy in an acutely bronchospastic patient (assuming normal volume of distribution) can be initiated as follows (18). If the patient has not received any theophylline during the previous 24 hours, 5 mg/kg of theophylline should be administered as a loading dose over 30 minutes. If the patient has received theophylline within the past 24 hours, the loading dose should be reduced to 2.5 mg/kg. Subsequent intravenous infusion rates should be titrated based on patient response, using the dosing recommendations in Table

10.1. Theophylline levels can be used to maximize therapy, in that each additional 1 mg/kg of theophylline will produce a $2\mu g/ml$ rise in the serum concentration. For example, if a 70-kg bronchospastic patient has a serum concentration of 8 $\mu g/ml$, the administration of an additional 210 mg of theophylline will, in the majority of patients, elevate the serum drug concentration to 14 $\mu g/ml$, well within the "therapeutic range" for theophylline.

β-Adrenergic Receptor Agonists

The value of β-adrenergic agonist therapy in the treatment of reversible airway obstruction was documented at the turn of the century when Solis-Cohen (51) reported the use of desiccated adrenal glands for the treatment of asthma. This discovery was followed by the isolation of ephedrine and the synthesis of isoproterenol. Subsequently, a variety of β-adrenergic agonists have been introduced into clinical use, which vary in affinity for the β_1- and β_2-adrenergic receptors and duration of action. These drugs have become well established as effective medications in the treatment of both acute and chronic reversible airway obstruction.

PHARMACOLOGY

All β-adrenergic receptor agonists act by binding to β_1 and β_2 cell membrane receptors (Fig. 10.1), which results in activation of adenyl cyclase; accordingly, intracellular levels of cAMP are increased (47). This action induces a relaxation of bronchial and vascular smooth muscle. β-Adrenergic agonists may also induce increased mucociliary transport of respiratory secretions (55, 56). Stimulation of β_2-receptors on mast cells inhibits the release of

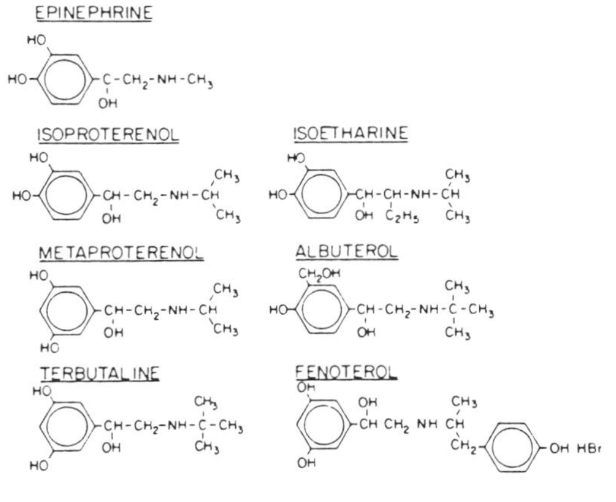

EPINEPHRINE

ISOPROTERENOL   ISOETHARINE

METAPROTERENOL   ALBUTEROL

TERBUTALINE   FENOTEROL

Figure 10.2. Structures of β-adrenergic agonists. (Originally published in Kelly HW: New beta-2-adrenergic agonist aerosols. *Clin Pharm* 4:393–403, 1985. Copyright © 1985, American Society of Hospital Pharmacists, Inc. All rights reserved. Reprinted with permission.)

mediators of bronchospasm, i.e., histamine and slow-reacting substance of anaphylaxis (27).

Distinctions between the β-adrenergic agonists are based on differences in chemistry and selectivity for the β_2-receptor over the β_1-receptor. Chemically, all β-adrenergic agonists are structural derivatives of phenylethylamine (Fig. 10.2). Structural modifications of the phenylethylamine nucleus result in compounds with differing durations of action and receptor activity (Table 10.4).

The catecholamine agents possess adjacent hydroxyl groups on positions 3 and 4 of the benzene ring of the catechol molecule (47). All catecholamines are capable of acting on both β_1- and β_2-adrenergic receptors. Whereas epinephrine and isoproterenol have equal β_1- and β_2-adrenergic receptor activity, isoetharine and bitolterol are reported to have greater affinity for the β_2-receptor than for the β_1-receptor (33). All catecholamines are readily inactivated by the enzymes catechol-O-methyltransferase, found in high concentrations in the liver and kidney, and monoamine oxidase, located in the presynaptic neurons (47). The duration of action of the catecholamines is short because of their rapid metabolism. The exception to this rule among β-agonists is bitolterol (53). Bitolterol is actually a prodrug; hydrolysis by plasma esterases results in the generation of the active drug colterol, which is a catecholamine (18). Because colterol must be generated in the systemic circulation, the duration of action of bitolterol is longer than that of other catecholamines. Catecholamines are usually not administered orally because they are rapidly conjugated and inactivated in the mucosa of the gastrointestinal tract (33).

The substitution of the catecholamine nucleus with resorcinol or saligenin has resulted in the development of drugs with longer durations of action than the catecholamines because they are resistant to the actions of both catechol-O-methyltransferase and monoamine oxidase (18). In addition, they are effective after oral administration and have relatively greater affinity for the β_2-receptor than for the β_1-receptor. The resorcinols include metaproterenol, terbutaline, and the investigational agent fenoterol; the only currently available saligenin is albuterol.

Table 10.4
β-Adrenergic Agents[a]

Drug	Route of Administration			Duration of Action (hr)	Receptor		
	Injection	Inhaled	Oral		β_2	β_1	α
Catecholamines							
Epinephrine	Yes	Yes	No	1–2	+	+	+
Isoproterenol	Yes	Yes	No	2–3	+	+	−
Isoetharine	No	Yes	No	2–3	+ +	+	−
Bitolterol	No	Yes	No	4–6	+ +	+	−
Resorcinols							
Metaproterenol	No	Yes	Yes	3–5	+ +	+	−
Terbutaline	Yes	No	Yes	4–6	+ +	+	−
Fenoterol	No	Yes	No	4–6	+ +	+	−
Saligen							
Albuterol	No	Yes	Yes	4–6	+ +	±	−

[a] Adapted from Iafrate RP, Massey KL, Hendeles L: Current concepts in clinical therapeutics: asthma. *Clin Pharm* 5:206–227, 1986. Copyright © 1986, American Society of Hospital Pharmacists, Inc. All rights reserved. Used with permission.

PHARMACOKINETICS

As previously discussed, the catecholamines are ineffective following oral administration. Accordingly, their only route of enteral administration is oral inhalation, either as a powder in a metered-dose inhaler or as a solution for nebulization. However, the noncatecholamine β-adrenergic agonists, metaproterenol, terbutaline, and albuterol, are also available as oral tablets, and metaproterenol and albuterol are also manufacturered as oral liquids.

Epinephrine, isoetharine, isoproterenol, metaproterenol, albuterol, and bitolterol are the only β-adrenergic agents available for administration by nebulization. The only parenteral β-adrenergic agonists are epinephrine, isoproterenol, and terbutaline; the latter is available for subcutaneous administration only. Not all dosage forms of each drug are marketed in the United States. For example, terbutaline is not approved for use as an aerosol, despite its documented efficacy and the availability in Europe and Canada of an oral solution for nebulization.

Increasingly, the inhaled route of administration is becoming a preferred method of administration for β-adrenergic agonists (18, 22, 33, 40 ,48); nebulization is one of the most common methods of administration used in intensive care units. The reason for this strong interest in oral inhalation of these drugs is 3-fold (22, 40). First, inhalation delivers the drug directly to the site of activity, the airways. Second, administration by inhalation requires a smaller dose of drug to achieve a desired therapeutic response, and the drug is distributed over the large tissue surface area of the lungs, up to 70 m². Third, onset of action is very rapid following oral inhalation and side effects are minimal (40). There are disadvantages to this route of administration, however. In non–mechanically ventilated patients, a great deal of patient cooperation is required to deliver the drug adequately (40). However, spacer devices may improve drug delivery in patients who may have difficulty coordinating the discharge of medication from the inhaler with inhalation (9). Additionally, a high percentage of each drug dose commonly gets trapped in the upper airways or is swallowed; only 13% of a dose from a metered-dose inhaler and 1–5% of a dose administered by nebulization reach the lower respiratory tract (40). Administration by inhalation can result in mouth irritation and dryness. One particular disadvantage occurs in patients with severe bronchospasm: the drug may not be administered to the lower airways where it is needed. In this circumstance, much larger doses of drug are required to achieve a satisfactory response (40).

Few pharmacokinetic data are available on β-adrenergic agonists owing to the very low serum levels of drugs that are achieved after dosing, particularly following inhalation. However, it is well established that most of these drugs have short plasma half-lives and important first pass metabolism (18). For all inhaled catecholamine β-adrenergic agonists (except bitolterol), peak effects occur 5–15 minutes after administration and persist for 1–3 hours. Bitolterol's actions are maximal at 0.5–2 hours after administration and continue for up to 6 hours (22). Metaproterenol has a slow onset of action, up to 30 minutes after administration, and peak effects occur within 1 hour. The duration of action of metaproterenol is usually 3–5 hours. Terbutaline and fenoterol have similar pharmacokinetic profiles (onset of action 5–15 minutes, peak effects in 1–2 hours), and their effects may persist for as long as 6 hours. Like most of the inhaled β-adrenergic drugs, albuterol has a rapid onset of 5–15 minutes after administration, with peak effects in 0.5–2 hours and a persistence of 3–6 hours.

SIDE EFFECTS

The side effects of the β-adrenergic agonists are similar; the majority are transient (22, 28, 40, 43). The most common adverse effects are skeletal muscle tremor, nervousness, insomnia, tachycardia, and palpitations (49). The cardiac effects are primarily due to direct β_1-receptor stimulation. Reflex tachycardia may also result owing to β_2-mediated peripheral vasodilation (18, 22).

Less commonly reported side effects of these drugs include paradoxical bronchoconstriction, skin flushing, headache, and dizziness (43).

Although the incidence of all side effects is very low following inhalation, the oral and parenteral routes commonly induce side effects. The side effects may be so severe that the drugs may have to be discontinued (49). For example, muscle tremor is believed to result primarily from β_2 stimulation and appears to be dose-related (18, 22). In some patients, the tremor can be so serious as to be disabling. Use of oral β-adrenergics should be reserved for patients who are unable or unwilling to use the inhalation dosage forms. Some patients

Table 10.5
β_2-**Adrenergic Aerosol Preparations and Dosages**[a]

Drug	Preparations	Pediatric Dosages	Adult Dosages
Isoproterenol hydrochloride and sulfate			
Various manufacturers	0.25% (1:400) 2.5 mg/ml 0.50% (1:200) 5 mg/ml 1.0% (1:100) 10 mg/ml	0.05–0.1 mg/kg q. 2–4 hr	One to two inhalations of 0.25% solution by hand-bulb nebulizer; via nebulizer q. 2–4 hr

Isuprel Mistometer
  Norisodrine Aerotrol
  Medihaler-Iso
  Norisodrine Sulfate
	131 µg/spray
	120 µg/spray
	80 µg/spray
	110 µg/spray
		One to two inhalations q. 4–6 hr	One to two sprays q. 2–4 hr

Isoetharine			
Isoetharine hydrochloride for inhalation	0.1%, 0.125%, 0.2%	0.1–0.2 mg/kg q. 2–4 hr	3–5 mg undiluted via nebulizer with oxygen at 4–6 liters/min over 15–20 min q. 2–4 hr
Bronkosol	0.25%, 0.5%, 1%		0.5% and 1% solutions diluted 1:3 with 0.9% sodium chloride q. 2–4 hr
Bronkometer	340 µg/spray	One to two sprays q. 4–6 hr	One to two sprays q. 4–6 hr
Metaproterenol			
Alupent	5% (50 mg/ml) solution for nebulization	0.25–0.5 mg/kg q. 2–4 hr (15 mg maximum single dose)	0.3 ml (15 mg) diluted with 2.5 ml of 0.9% sodium chloride nebulized q. 2–4 hr
Metaprel	0.6% (15 mg/2.5 ml)		
Alupent MDI, Metaprel MDI	0.65 mg/puff, powder suspension	One to two puffs q. 4–6 hr and before exercise	Two to three puffs q. 4–6 hr and before exercise
Albuterol			
Ventolin Proventil	90 µg/puff, powder suspension	One to two puffs q. 4–6 hr and before exercise	One to two puffs q. 4–6 hr and before exercise
	0.5% (2.5 mg/ml)	0.05–0.15 mg diluted with 1–2 ml 0.9% normal saline q. 4–6 hr	2.5–5 mg diluted with 0.9% normal saline q. 4–6 hr
Terbutaline			
Brethaire	0.2 mg/puff, powder suspension	One to two puffs q. 4–6 hr and before exercise	One to two puffs q. 4–6 hr and before exercise
Brethine	0.1% (1 mg/ml) (not FDA approved for this use)	0.1–0.3 mg/kg q. 2–6 hr	5–7 mg undiluted q. 4–6 hr
Bitolterol			
Tornalate	0.37 mg/spray	One to three sprays q. 4–6 hr	One to three sprays q. 4–6 hr
Fenoterol hydrobromide[b]			
Berotec	0.16 mg/puff, powder solution	One to two puffs q. 4–6 hr	One to two puffs q. 4–6 hr

[a] Originally published in Kelly HW: New beta-2-adrenergic agonist aerosols. *Clin Pharm* 4:393–403, 1985. Copyright © 1985, American Society of Hospital Pharmacists, Inc. All rights reserved. Used with permission.
[b] Pending FDA approval.

who achieve only suboptimal effects with the inhalant products may benefit from supplementation with an oral β-adrenergic (18).

Because intravenous epinephrine and isoproterenol are associated with myocardial ischemia, infarction, and death (25, 30), their use is generally limited to patients with drug-unresponsive bronchospasm, i.e., status asthmaticus.

Following chronic use of β-adrenergic agonists, decreased responsiveness may develop. Commonly referred to as tolerance or tachyphylaxis, this effect has been documented to occur in both animals and humans (34). Interestingly, although tolerance has been demonstrated to develop to the nonbronchial β-adrenergic responses (e.g., heart rate, tremor), conflicting information exists regarding the bronchial response. Most data indicate that prolonged use of β-adrenergic agonists, either oral or inhaled, can result in a decrease in the duration of drug effect (18, 34).

DRUG INTERACTIONS

β-Adrenergic agonists may act synergistically when administered concurrently either with other β-adrenergic agonists or with theophylline (21, 41). The most important risk of these combinations would be in patients with underlying cardiac disease, with a limited capacity to tolerate high heart rate or arrhythmias (49).

CLINICAL USE

As previously discussed, inhaled β-adrenergic agonists are increasingly considered as the drug therapy of choice for the treatment of acute bronchospasm, particularly in critically ill patients (18). Other indications for their usage include prophylaxis of chronic asthma and exercise-induced asthma (18).

Practically, all of the inhaled β-adrenergics can be considered to be equally effective in treating bronchospasm. However, it has been suggested that metaproterenol and the catecholamines are less effective than albuterol, terbutaline, and isoproterenol (33). Choice of an individual agent reflects both clinician and patient preference, as well as economic factors. In hospitalized patients, isoetharine and metaproterenol are the most commonly used inhaled agents for administration by nebulization (18); an oral solution for nebulization of albuterol has recently been marketed.

DOSING

The dosages of the various β-adrenergic agents are listed in Table 10.5.

Anticholinergic Agents

In the early 1800s, the practice of inhaling burning powders of the anticholinergic alkaloids stramonium and belladonna for the treatment of asthma was introduced to Great Britain by travelers from India (59). Although effective, this practice was accompanied by a high number of adverse effects such as tachycardia, urinary retention, inspissation of secretions, and delirium. Following the development of inhaled bronchodilators, the use of anticholinergic agents for treatment of asthma was abandoned.

Over the last 20 years, interest in the use of anticholinergic drugs for treatment of bronchospasm has been renewed. This interest derives from documentation of the effective use of atropine by inhalation in the treatment of asthma. Additionally, two synthetic anticholinergics have been developed that are much safer and easier to use than atropine: glycopyrrolate and ipratropium.

PHARMACOLOGY

Atropine is a naturally occuring tertiary ammonium alkaloid obtained from plants of the Solanaceae family, including *Atropa belladonna* (deadly nightshade) and *Datura stramonium* (jimson weed) (40, 49). Also known as dl-hyoscyamine, atropine is the prototypic anticholinergic (antimuscarinic) agent. Other antimuscarinic drugs used in the treatment of bronchospasm—glycopyrrolate and the newly marketed compound, ipratropium—are synthetic quaternary ammonium derivatives of atropine (12, 59). Atropine methylnitrate is a quaternary ammonium compound that is available only for investigational use in the United States, but is commercially available in Europe as methylatropine nitrate (59).

All of the antimuscarinic drugs produce their effects by competitively inhibiting the effects of acetylcholine on muscarinic receptors. Specifically, these drugs act by inhibiting the generation of intracellular cGMP (Fig. 10.1) (48). This action results in bronchodilation, especially in the large airways and decreased tracheobronchial secretions. Of these available antimuscarinic agents, only ipratropium is approved by the Food and Drug Administra-

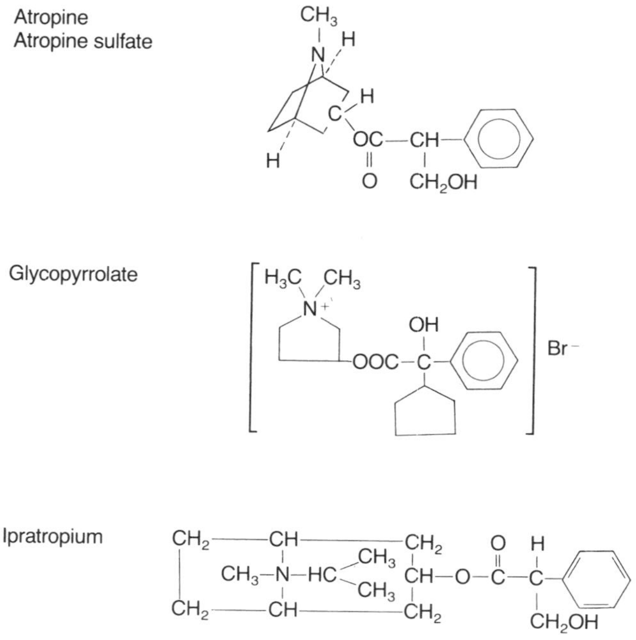

Figure 10.3. Structure of anticholinergic agents.

tion for inhalation in the treatment of bronchospasm.

PHARMACOKINETICS

Atropine is a tertiary ammonium alkaloid (Fig. 10.3), most commonly used as the sulfate salt. Inasmuch as atropine readily crosses epithelial mucosa, it may be administered via the gastrointestinal tract, by inhalation, and parenterally (24, 59). In contrast, atropine methylnitrate, glycopyrrolate, and ipratropium are quaternary ammonium antimuscarinics. The quaternary structure confers an electrical charge on these drugs, resulting in their poor absorption into the systemic circulation following administration by mouth or inhalation (12, 59).

The comparative pharmacokinetics of the inhaled anticholinergic agents are shown in Table 10.6. Following an aerosol dose, onset of action of atropine sulfate is 15–30 minutes; peak effects occur 30–170 minutes after administration. The duration of action of atropine sulfate is 3–5 hours (12, 59). Atropine is widely distributed in the body, including the central nervous system. The plasma half-life is 2–3 hours and the drug is eliminated by hepatic metabolism. About 30–50% of a given dose is metabolized to a variety of inactive metabolites, with the remainder of the dose being eliminated unchanged in the urine. Atropine methylnitrate exhibits a pharmacokinetic profile similar to that of atropine, but has a slightly longer duration of action, 4–6

Table 10.6
Bronchodilator Properties of Anticholinergic Drugs[a]

Drug	Dosages	Route of Administration	Time of Onset (min)	Peak Effect (min)	Duration (hr)
Atropine sulfate	0.025–0.075 mg/kg	Inhalation	15–30	30–170	3–5
	0.4–1 mg	Oral	NA	NA	NA
Atropine methonitrate	1–1.5 mg	Inhalation	15–30	40–60	4–6
Glycopyrrolate	0.0044 mg/kg	Inhalation	15–30	30–45	2–8
		Intramuscular	15–30	30–45	2–7
		Subcutaneous			
	0.2 mg	Intravenous	1	NA	NA
Ipratropium	20–40 µg	Inhalation	3–30	90–120	3–8

[a] Adapted from Ziment I, Au JP: Anticholinergic agents. *Clin Chest Med* 7:355–366, 1986.

hours. In addition, this drug does not diffuse through the pulmonary epithelium nor does it cross the blood-brain barrier (12, 59).

Glycopyrrolate is a quaternary ammonium antimuscarinic, but it is also a complex aminoalcohol ester. Following inhalation, glycopyrrolate, like atropine, has an onset of action of 15–30 minutes; peak effects occur between 30 and 45 minutes after administration (12, 59). The drug has a longer duration of action than atropine, up to 8 hours (59). Like all quaternary ammonium salts, glycopyrrolate does not cross the blood-brain barrier or the pulmonary mucosa.

Ipratropium, also known as N-isopropylnortropine tropic acid ester, is a quaternary methyl derivative of atropine. As with other inhaled antimuscarinic drugs, the onset of action of ipratropium is rapid, 15–30 minutes. Peak effects are noted 90–120 minutes after administration and last for at least 4 hours and up to 6 hours in some patients (59). Systemic absorption is minimal after inhalation, and owing to the drug's quaternary structure, tissue distribution is limited. Ipratropium does not cross the blood-brain barrier (12, 59).

SIDE EFFECTS

As previously discussed, the side effect profile of the antimuscarinics is largely determined by their chemical structure and route of administration. Atropine, being a tertiary ammonium compound, readily crosses the mucosal epithelium into the systemic circulation (24). Accordingly, systemic side effects are common following oral and systemic administration; these effects tend to be dose-related. Because low doses of the drug are used for inhalation, however, side effects are greatly reduced in number and severity with this route of administration (24). Following inhalation of atropine most patients develop mouth dryness. Other possible side effects include flushing, lightheadedness, and slight tachycardia (24, 59). Urinary retention and blurred vision are rare, as are tremors, arrhythmias, and blood pressure changes (59).

For all of the quaternary ammonium compounds, the incidence of systemic side effects is extremely low following inhalation. As previously mentioned, these compounds poorly diffuse across the pulmonary epithelium and therefore have minimal systemic absorption. They do not cross the blood-brain barrier and are therefore devoid of central nervous system effects (12, 59).

Theoretically, the inhaled anticholinergics should alter mucociliary clearance and increase the viscosity of secretions. In practice, these side effects occur most commonly with atropine and not at all with ipratropium (54).

CLINICAL USE

Data are available on the efficacy of atropine (7, 8, 23, 29, 50), but there is only limited information regarding the use of glycopyrrolate as bronchodilator (10, 20, 24). The most information generated concerns the efficacy and safety of ipratropium in the treatment of bronchospasm (42).

Based on controlled and noncontrolled clinical trials, the use of inhaled anticholinergic drugs appears to be primarily as an alternative therapy in the treatment of bronchospastic diseases (12, 34). In contrast to inhaled β-adrenergic drugs, the anticholinergic bronchodilators have been demonstrated to be most effective in decreasing bronchial smooth muscle tone in patients with chronic bronchitis and emphysema. Their efficacy in asthma is inferior to that of β-adrenergic agonists (18). Because the onset of action of inhaled anticholinergics is slower than that of the inhaled β-adrenergics, they should not be used in the treatment of acute bronchospasm. In addition, although they have a longer duration of action than most inhaled β-adrenergics, the anticholinergics produce less bronchodilation and relief of symptoms in asthma (18, 42, 59).

Based on efficacy studies, the use of inhaled anticholinergic drugs should generally be limited to those patients who do not adequately respond to maximal β-adrenergic therapy (18). These patients usually are afflicted with chronic obstructive pulmonary disease, including emphysema and chronic bronchitis. In addition, because of the longer duration of action of these agents, anticholinergics may be found to be useful in special circumstances such as the prevention of nocturnal asthma, but such potential roles remain to be defined.

DOSING

The dosages of anticholinergics by inhalation are listed in Table 10.5.

Acknowledgment

The author thanks Dr. Kenneth Shepherd for his critical review of this chapter.

References

1. Adair NE: Airflow obstruction. In *Current Therapy In Critical Care Medicine.* Philadelphia, BC Decker, 1987, pp 164–169.
2. Andersson KE, Persson CG: Extra-pulmonary effects of theophylline. *Eur J Respir Dis* 61(S109):17–28, 1980.
3. Aubier M, DeTroyer A, Sampson M, et al: Aminophylline improves diaphragmatic contractility. *N Engl J Med* 305:249–252, 1981.
4. Barnes PJ: State of the art: neural control of human airways in health and disease. *Am Rev Respir Dis* 134:1289–1314, 1986.
5. Bergstrand H: Phosphodiesterase inhibition and theophylline. *Eur J Respir Dis* 61(S109):37–44, 1980.
6. Brisson GR, Malaisse-Lagal F, Malaisse-Lagal WJ: The stimulus-secretion coupling of glucose-induced insulin release. 7. A proposed site of action for adenosine 3'5'-cyclic monophosphate. *J Clin Invest* 51:232–241, 1972.
7. Cavanaugh MJ, Cooper DM: Inhaled atropine sulfate: dose-response characteristics. *Am Rev Respir Dis* 114:517–524, 1976.
8. Chick TW, Jenne JW: Comparative bronchodilator response to atropine and terbutaline in asthma and chronic bronchitis. *Chest* 72:719–723, 1977.
9. Drugs used in treatment of asthma. *Med Lett Drugs Ther* 29:11–16, 1987.
10. Gal TJ, Suratt PM, Lu JY: Glycopyrrolate and atropine inhalation: comparative effects on normal airway function. *Am Rev Respir Dis* 129:871–873, 1984.
11. Ginchansky E, Weinberger M: Relationship of theophylline clearance to oral dosage in children with chronic asthma. *J Pediatr* 91:655–660, 1977.
12. Gross NJ, Skorodin MS: The place of anticholinergic agents in the treatment of airways obstruction. *Immunol Allergy Pract* 7:224–231, 1986.
13. Hendeles L, Weinberger M: Theophylline: a state of the art review. *Pharmacotherapy* 3:2–44, 1983.
14. Hendeles L, Weinberger M: Theophylline: therapeutic use of serum concentration monitoring. In Taylor WJ, Finn AL (eds): *Individualizing Drug Therapy: Practical Application of Drug Monitoring.* New York, Gross, Townsend, Frank, Hoffman. 1981, vol 1, pp 32–65.
15. Hendeles L, Weinberger M, Wyatt R: A guide to oral theophylline therapy for treatment of chronic asthma. *Am J Dis Child* 132:876–880, 1978.
16. Holgate ST, Mann JS, Cushey MJ: Adenosine as a bronchoconstriction mediator in asthma and its antagonism by methylxanthines. *J Allergy Clin Immunol* 74:302–306, 1984.
17. Horrobin DF, Manku MS, Franks DJ, et al: Methylxanthine phosphodiesterase inhibitors behave as prostaglandin antagonists in a perfused rat mesenteric artery preparation. *Prostaglandins* 13:33–40, 1977.
18. Iafrate RP, Massey KL, Hendeles L: Current concepts in clinical therapeutics: asthma. *Clin Pharm* 5:206–227, 1986.
19. Jenne JW, Wyze E, Rood FS, MacDonald IM: Pharmacokinetics of theophylline: application to adjustment of clinical dose of aminophylline. *Clin Pharmacol Ther* 13:349–368, 1972.
20. Johnson BE, Suratt PM, Gal TJ, Wilhort SL: Effects of inhaled glycopyrrolate and atropine in asthma precipitated by exercise and cold air inhalation. *Chest* 85:325–328, 1984.
21. Kelly HW: Controversies in asthma therapy with theophylline and the beta-2-adrenergic agonists. *Clin Pharm* 3:386–395, 1984.
22. Kelly HW: New beta-2-adrenergic agonist aerosols. *Clin Pharm* 4:393–403, 1985.
23. Klock LE, Miller TD, Morris AH, et al: A comparative study of atropine sulfate and isoproterenol hydrochloride in chronic bronchitis. *Am Rev Respir Dis* 112:371–376, 1975.

24. Kradjan WA, Lakshminarayan S, Hayden PW, et al: Serum atropine concentration after inhalation of atropine sulfate. *Am Rev Respir Dis* 123:471–472, 1981.
25. Kurland G, Williams J, Lewiston N: Fatal myocardial toxicity during continuous infusion of intravenous isoproterenol therapy for asthma. *J Allergy Clin Immunol* 63:407–411, 1979.
26. Lefkowitz RJ: Clinical physics of adrenoreceptor regulation. *Am J Physiol* 243:E43–E47, 1982.
27. Lofdahl CG, Svedmyr N: Selectivity of beta-adrenergic stimulant and blocking agents. *Eur J Respir Dis* 65(S136):101–113, 1984.
28. Lourenco RV, Eotromanes E: Clinical aerosols II. Therapeutic aerosols. *Arch Intern Med* 142:2299–2308, 1982.
29. Marini JJ, Lakshminarayan S: Inhaled atropine improves airflow in irreversible chronic bronchitis. *Am Rev Respir Dis* 119:148, 1979.
30. Matson JR, Coughlin G, Strunk R: Myocardial ischemia complicating the use of isoproterenol in asthmatic children. *J Pediatr* 92:776–778, 1978.
31. Matthay RA, Berger JH, Loke J, et al: Effects of aminophylline on right and left ventricular performance in chronic obstructive pulmonary disease—noninvasive assessment by radionuclide angiography. *Am J Med* 65:903–910, 1978.
32. McEvoy GK: Theophylline. In McEvoy GK (ed): *AHFS Drug Information 1987.* Bethesda, American Society of Hospital Pharmacists, 1987, pp 1952–1959.
33. McFadden ER Jr: Beta-2 receptor agonist: metabolism and pharmacology. *J Allergy Clin Immunol* 68:91–97, 1981.
34. McFadden ER: Clinical use of beta-adrenergic agonists. *J Allergy Clin Immunol* 76:352–356, 1985.
35. McFadden ER: Introduction: methylxanthine therapy and reversible airway obstruction. *Am J Med* 79(S6A):1–4, 1985.
36. Miech RP, Niedzwick JG, Smith TR: Effect of theophylline on the binding of c-AMP to soluble protein from tracheal smooth muscle. *Biochem Pharmacol* 28:3687–3688, 1979.
37. Mitenko PA, Ogilvie RI: Rational intravenous doses of theophylline. *N Engl J Med* 289:600–603, 1973.
38. Murciano D, Aubier M, Lecocguic Y, Pariente R: Effects of theophylline on diaphragmatic strength and fatigue in patients with chronic obstructive pulmonary disease. *N Engl J Med* 311:349–353, 1984.
39. Nassif EG, Weinberger M, Thompson R, et al: The value of maintenance theophylline in steroid-dependent asthma. *N Engl J Med* 304:71–75, 1981.
40. Newhouse MT, Dolovich MB: Control of asthma by aerosols. *N Engl J Med* 315:870–874, 1986.
41. Nicklas RA, Whitehurst VE, Donohue RF, et al: Concomitant use of beta adrenergic agonists and methylxanthines. *J Allergy Clin Immunol* 73:20–24, 1984.
42. Pakes GE, Brogden RN, Heel TM, et al: Ipratropium bromide: a review of its pharmacologic properties and therapy efficacy in asthma and chronic bronchitis. *Drugs* 20:237–266, 1980.
43. Paterson JW, Woolcock AJ, Shenfield GM: State of the art: bronchodilator drugs. *Am Rev Respir Dis* 120:1149–1188, 1979.
44. Richardson JB, Farguson CC: Neuromuscular structure and function in the airways. *Fed Proc* 38:202–208, 1979.
45. Sackner MA: Effect of respiratory drugs on mucociliary clearance. *Chest* 73:958–966, 1978.
46. Salter H: On some points in the treatment and clinical history of asthma. *Edinburgh Med J* 4:1109–1115, 1858.
47. Seligman M, Chernow B: Use of adrenergic agents in the critically ill patient. *Hosp Formul* 223:348–360, 1987.
48. Shenfield GM: Combination bronchodilator therapy. *Drugs* 24:414–439, 1982.
49. Sly RM, Anderson JA, Bierman CW, et al: Adverse effects and complications of treatment of beta-adrener-

gic agonist drugs. *J Allergy Clin Immunol:* 75:443–449, 1985.

50. Snow RM, Miller WC, Blair HT, et al: Inhaled atropine in asthma. *Ann Allergy* 42:286–289, 1979.

51. Solis-Cohen S: The use of adrenal substance in the treatment of asthma. *JAMA* 34:1164–1168, 1900.

52. Theodore AC, Beer DJ: Pharmacotherapy of chronic obstructive pulmonary disease. *Clin Chest Med* 7:657–671, 1986.

53. Walker SB, Kradgan MA, Bierman CW: Bitolterol mesylate: a beta-adrenergic agent. *Pharmacotherapy* 5:127–137, 1985.

54. Wanner A: Clinical aspects of mucociliary transport. *Am Rev Respir Dis* 116:73–125, 1977.

55. Wanner A: Effects of methylxanthines on airway mucociliary function. *Am J Med* 79(S6A):16–21, 1985.

56. Weinberger M, Hendeles L: Slow-release theophylline: rationale and basis for product selection. *N Engl J Med* 308:760–764, 1983.

57. Weinberger MM, Hendeles L: Theophylline use: an overview. *J Allergy Clin Immunol* 76:277–284, 1985.

58. Winn HR: Methylxanthines, adenosine, and the pulmonary system. *Chest* 91:800–801, 1987.

59. Ziment I, Au JP: Anticholinergic agents. *Clin Chest Med* 7:355–366, 1986.

60. Zwillich CW, Sutton TD, Neft TA, et al: Theophylline-induced seizures in adults: correlations with serum concentration. *Ann Intern Med* 82:784–787, 1975.

11

Pharmacologic Approach to Acute Seizures

Joseph A. Miller, M.D.
John M. Hallenbeck, M.D.

Seizures have been recognized as a major medical problem since the dawn of history, whereas effective therapy has been available only for the last several decades. It is the purpose of this chapter to review current thought regarding diagnostic and therapeutic modalities available for treatment of seizures, particularly in the setting of the intensive care unit (ICU), where extremely complex problems may occur because of coexisting medical and surgical illnesses.

The general area of seizure management in the uncomplicated patient has been exhaustively reviewed in several recent monographs and will be only briefly discussed here; emphasis will be placed on the management of acute seizures, especially status epilepticus, an aspect of seizure control undergoing rapid changes in diagnosis and therapy.

CLASSIFICATION OF SEIZURES

Any discussion of seizures must begin with at least a brief review of the major classification scheme now employed, the International Classification of the Seizures. This classification, which has been in use for nearly 20 years and has been accepted by most authorities in the Western world, has brought a significant degree of order to discussions of seizure disorders, permitting more effective communication about seizures. This has in turn facilitated a more rational approach to recommendations for diagnosis, therapy, and the determination of prognosis. Somewhat revised in 1980, the currently used version is given as Table 11.1.

In addition, a classification of the epilepsies has appeared, aimed at organizing the various recognizable syndromes producing seizures alone or in combination with other neurological and systemic manifestations. It should be recognized that this is only a preliminary clas-

Table 11.1
International Classification of the Seizures[a]

PARTIAL SEIZURES
Simple partial seizures (consciousness preserved)
    Motor
    Somatosensory
    Autonomic
    Psychic
Complex partial seizures (consciousness impaired)
    Beginning as simple partial seizures and
        progressing to impairment of consciousness
        With no other features
        Starting as elementary seizures as in the four types
            of simple partial seizures
        With automatisms
    With impairment of consciousness at onset
Partial seizures evolving to secondarily generalized
    seizures.

GENERALIZED SEIZURES
Absence seizures
    Absence seizures
    Atypical absence seizures
Myoclonic seizures
Clonic seizures
Tonic seizures
Tonic-clonic seizures
Atonic seizures

UNCLASSIFIED SEIZURES
Seizures that cannot be classified because of
    incomplete data.

[a] Abstracted from Commission on Classification and Terminology of the International League Against Epilepsy 1981.

sification and will undoubtedly undergo significant evolution as time progresses. Sufficient time has not passed to allow us to determine whether this is a useful classification.

DIAGNOSIS OF SEIZURE

When approaching any patient with seizures, the clinician must first address this

Table 11.2
Medical Illnesses Resembling Seizures[a]

Processes resembling generalized tonic-clonic
seizures
    Syncope or syncope with myoclonic movements,
      "convulsive syncope"
    Hyperventilation with carpopedal spasm
    Narcolepsy with cataplexy
    Nonepileptic myoclonus
    Psychiatric processes

Processes resembling elementary partial seizures
    Paroxysmal choreoathetosis
    Complicated migraine
    Paroxysmal attacks in multiple sclerosis
    Nonepileptic segmental myoclonus
    Tourette syndrome
    Psychiatric processes

Processes resembling complex partial seizures
    Toxic metabolic encephalopathies
    Transient ischemic attacks
    Transient global amnesia
    Psychiatric processes

[a] This list is not meant to be all inclusive but rather to
serve as an example of the various entities that can
mimic seizures.

Table 11.3
Drugs Reported To Induce Seizures[a]

Aqueous iodinated contrast agents
Anticholinesterases
Antihistamines
Antidepressants
Antipsychotics
Baclofen
β-blockers
Bronchodilators[b]
Camphor
Cefazolin
Chlorambucil
Cocaine
Cycloserine
Cyclosporin A
Ergonovine
Folic acid
General anesthetics (including ketamine, halothane,
    enflurane, propanidid)
Hyperbaric oxygen
Hypoglycemic agents
Hyperosmolar parenteral solutions
Insulin[b]
Isoniazid[b]
Local anesthetics (lidocaine, procaine)[b]
Mefenamic acid
Methylxanthines
Metronidazole
Narcotic analgesics
Penicillins
Phencyclidine
Psychotropic agents[b]
Sympathomimetics

[a] Modified from Messing RO, Closson RG, Simon RP:
Drug-induced seizures: a 10-year experience. *Neurology* 34: 1582–1586, 1984.
[b] Drugs associated with bouts of status.

question: Has the patient actually had a seizure? This is a frequently overlooked issue,
and one that obviously plays a great role in
the outcome of any therapeutic intervention.
It is also a problem that is more vexing than
is apparent at first glance; for example, in one
study of a large number of patients with a
single seizure 30% were ultimately found to
have a cause completely unrelated to seizure
disorder as it is currently understood. Thus, it
is of paramount importance to consider the
various processes that can mimic seizures. It
is only too easy in the stressed circumstances
of the emergency room (ER) or the ICU to
overlook this issue, but perhaps in those areas
it is of greatest importance because of the urgency of the decisions that must be made and
the gravity of their consequences.

There is no simple algorithm for determining whether a patient has had a seizure, and
indeed the question may be difficult to conclusively resolve even under the ideal circumstance of observation. However, several suggestions can be made. First and foremost a
clear history is necessary. Length of history
does not necessarily equate with quality, however, detail is of great importance. Several important areas to cover include questions regarding sensations preceding the suspected
seizure, the patient's level of consciousness
immediately prior to the event, and what the

patient was doing at the time of the seizure.
Questions should also be directed at what time
of day the seizure occurred, how quickly the
seizure developed, what the individual did

Table 11.4
Anticonvulsant Drug Interactions[a]

Anticonvulsant	New Anticonvulsant	Effect on Serum Concentration of Original Anticonvulsant
Valproate	Phenobarbital	Decrease
	Phenytoin	Decrease
Carbamazepine	Phenobarbital	Decrease
	Phenytoin	Decrease
Phenytoin	Phenobarbital	Variable
	Valproate	Decrease
Phenobarbital	Phenytoin	Variable
	Valproate	Increase

[a] Adapted from Penry JK: *Diagnosis and Management of Epilepsy: Monotherapy of Primary Generalized Seizures.* New York, Biomedical Information Corporation, 1986.

during the seizure, and the patient's state after the event. Questions regarding variations in symptoms from spell to spell are useful, particularly when the event in question is a possible recurrent seizure. One must certainly be aware of various medical states that can mimic seizures, for example syncope. A partial list of other diseases that can be associated with seizure-like states is given as Table 11.2. Although it is beyond the scope of this discussion to deal with this subject in greater detail, it must be emphasized that failure to recognize the importance of this aspect of seizure care will doom subsequent efforts in a large number of cases. Finally, seizures triggered by medications represent another frequently neglected diagnostic consideration (3, 4). A partial list of drugs reported capable of at least aiding the induction of seizures is given as Table 11.3. Although about 2% of all seizures appear to be drug induced, it is difficult to determine how much drug induction of seizures contributes to the occurrence of seizures with other causes although the size of the list and the common nature of many of the agents listed suggests that contribution is a large one. It is also perhaps revealing to note that in those cases with strictly drug-induced seizures, about 50% have multiple fits.

DIFFERENTIATING BETWEEN PRIMARY GENERALIZED AND PARTIAL SEIZURES

Once a diagnosis of seizure has been made, several decisions must be reached. Principal among these is to identify what type of seizure has occurred. The major point of differentiation is between primary generalized and partial seizures, as the pharmacologic approach to each is different. It is at this point that understanding of the current classification of the seizures is useful.

Primary generalized seizures always begin without an aura and usually start in childhood and adolescence. For example, quite often confused with complex partial seizures, the absence attack can be clearly differentiated by recognizing its abrupt onset and the prompt return of consciousness at the end of an attack, whereas the complex partial seizure is almost always followed by a period of postictal diminution of awareness. More particularly, the electroencephalogram (EEG) is specifically abnormal in over 95% of patients with absence, demonstrating the classical three-per-second

spike and wave. Although complex partial seizures are fairly easily differentiated from absence they are often quite difficult to diagnose in and of themselves as their symptomatology is quite often complex and can be bizarre (7). Unfortunately, these seizures are also the most common type that occur in adults, and the EEG is a less useful diagnostic procedure than in absence attacks.

A similar difficulty arises in distinguishing *primary generalized tonic clonic seizures* from those arriving from spread of an epileptic focus. This fact is particularly true in cases in which there is no preceding aura or it is too brief to be recognized or remembered. In general, those generalized tonic-clonic seizures that have their onset in adulthood are more likely to be secondarily generalized, whereas a juvenile onset points to a primary generalized disorder. There are, however, no clear distinguishing features that allow precise differentiation, and often the true situation becomes clear only after treatment either blocks the tonic clonic seizures and partial seizures become evident or treatment for secondarily generalized seizures fails. Another feature that may help differentiation is the presence of an initial clonic phase to the seizure, which is a feature seen in primary generalized seizures.

Agents particularly suitable for treatment of partial seizures, including partial seizures that secondarily generalize, are carbamazepine and, currently as a secondary agent, Dilantin. Within the last several years carbamazepine has become recognized as the agent of first choice for treatment of partial seizures, eclipsing Dilantin and phenobarbital and its congeners in this regard. Presently there is controversy regarding the role of carbamazepine in treatment of primary generalized seizures. Several studies have indicated its efficacy in this regard is no different than that of Dilantin; however, another school of thought recommends valproate for this seizure type. A resolution of this debate awaits further experience. Carbamazepine has a half-life of 6–12 hours and must be administered in divided dosages daily. Adverse effects include drowsiness, vertigo, and nausea. Much has been made in the past of the hematologic toxicity of this agent, which apparently was initially overestimated and is now felt to be rare. Nevertheless, serious bone marrow depression can occur and surveillance for this problem is warranted, especially when the drug is first begun. Drug interactions of this and other agents are given in Table 11.4. Carbamazepine (and other anticonvulsants) may accelerate the metabolism of a number of other drugs, for example oral contraceptives; however, a detailed analysis of these effects is beyond the scope of this discussion. Carbamazepine is available only as an oral agent.

Dilantin, previously a drug of choice for partial seizures, has been relegated to a secondary role as it is associated with an excessive number of side effects and may be associated with a depression of cognitive function with long-term use. It nevertheless retains usefulness, especially in cases in which carbamazepine cannot be employed, and, as discussed below, it is an initial drug of choice for treatment of status. It should be noted that different preparations of phenytoin have varying bioavailability, resulting in different absorption times and thus apparently different half-lives. Thus, caution should be exercised when using generic sources. Also, phenytoin is available in both oral and parenteral forms; the latter may be used only intravenously, as intramuscular administration produces precipitation in the muscle with consequent grossly reduced bioavailability and a sterile muscle abscess. Dilantin, as mentioned, has several side effects ranging from gum hypertrophy to production of a pseudolymphoma. The drug interactions of this agent are also especially complex and often difficult to predict. There are several congeners of phenytoin, for example mephenytoin, which have a very limited usefulness because of increased toxicity and no advantages over phenytoin.

Phenobarbital was the first modern anticonvulsant to be introduced and has enjoyed a long history of use. Today it is beginning to lose favor as a primary anticonvulsant for any kind of seizure, primarily because of the severe, undiminishing sedation associated with this agent. However, as it is the only anticonvulsant, besides phenytoin, available in parenteral form in the United States, it continues to play a central role in the treatment of status epilepticus, for which it is quite effective. Phenobarbital has a very long half-life (up to 96 hours), which may be still further prolonged by agents such as valproate, further exacerbating its sedating effects. As it is the archetypical hepatic enzyme inducer, it is associated with a number of drug interactions (Table 11.4). A closely related agent, primidone, was popular for many years as an agent for partial seizures, although it too has decreased in use, as much of the anticonvulsant activity of this drug can be attributed to its metabolism to phenobarbital. Thus, its properties are essentially those

of phenobarbital, save that there is a more prolonged time to onset of action because of the metabolic processing required.

Agents for primary generalized seizures include valproate and ethosuximide. The former is the most recent anticonvulsant to have been introduced into the United States and is experiencing a gradual increase in use as the spectrum of seizure types for which it has been found effective expands. Presently it is the agent of choice for mixed primary generalized absence and tonic clonic seizures and for tonic clonic seizures. As mentioned above, it is recommended by many as the agent of choice for all tonic clonic seizures as it controls many such disorders where the traditional agents fail. There are several studies that show it to be at least as effective as ethosuximide in the treatment of absence seizures. Unfortunately, valproate is available only in oral form. The half-life of this agent is from 6 to 15 hours; the longer values are associated with the enteric-coated form, which delays absorption somewhat. The most common adverse effect of this agent is gastric irritation and the most serious is idiosyncratic hepatotoxicity, which is seen particularly in children under 12 years of age who are also receiving other anticonvulsants and which is felt to be the consequence of the hepatic production of metabolites of valproate toxic to the liver. The effect on valproate of adding other anticonvulsants is given in Table 11.4. The other drug currently employed for primary generalized seizures is ethosuximide, an agent effective only for absence. If other seizure types are present this agent should not be used and valproate should be employed, as any of the other anticonvulsants available will aggravate absence. Ethosuximide is also available only in oral form and in adults has a half-life of up to 50–60 hours. The most common side effects of this drug are nausea, vomiting, and, in higher dosages, headaches. The most serious side effect is an increased risk of a psychotic reaction, which is more common than generally realized. A listing of the pharmacokinetic properties of the various anticonvulsants is found in Table 11.5.

Although the distinction between seizure types may be difficult, the patient appearing in the emergency room must be treated and several strategies may be of assistance. If the suspected seizure is the first one, two considerations are paramount. The first is that of diagnosis of seizure disorder—not a minor consideration as the societal consequences are often very profound for the patient and the

Table 11.5
Pharmacokinetic Data on Antiepileptic Drugs

Drug	Half-life (hr)	Time to Reach Steady State (days)	Therapeutic Range (μg/ml)	Protein Binding (%)
Phenytoin	10–34	7–28	10–20	69–96
Carbamazepine	14–27	3–4	4–12	66–89
Phenobarbital	46–136	14–21	15–40	40–60
Valproate	6–15	1–2	50–125	80–95
Ethosuximide	20–60	7–10	40–100	0

Adapted from Penry JK: *Diagnosis and Management of Epilepsy: Monotherapy of Primary Generalized Seizures.* New York, Biomedical Information Corporation, 1986.

family. The second is that if a seizure has taken place in an adult, even though no focality can be found, it strongly suggests a focal origin and therefore raises the question of an underlying disease process; for example a structural lesion, a cerebral ischemic process, or a metabolic abnormality. Attention must be directed as much to that issue as to the seizure itself, and an immediate diagnostic evaluation is indicated. There is justification then to consider withholding anticonvulsants until that evaluation is completed.

The patient most commonly presenting to the ER will be one who has an established seizure disorder and who has had either a single recurrent seizure or a flurry of these. It is critical to distinguish the circumstances of the individual situation. Clearly, the patient who has an established seizure disorder and has well-documented infrequent isolated seizures requires only a careful examination to assure that no injury has resulted from the seizure and to eliminate the unlikely possibility that an intercurrent process triggered the seizure. The most common cause of such recurrent seizures is medication noncompliance, and the most common mistake to make under such circumstances is to change the patient's medication even though it may actually be the correct medication and in the correct dosage. Thus, it is most important to diligently question a patient about possible omission of doses, recalling that the patient may be reluctant at first to admit that noncompliance has occurred. Once these considerations have been made and it has been established that no significant underlying problem is present, it is usually best to simply maintain the patient on the present regimen of anticonvulsants, obtain a blood level of the anticonvulsant(s) being given (even if those levels are not immediately available), and arrange for follow-up on a routine basis. If there is indication for a change of

anticonvulsants, this task can then be done in an orderly fashion.

On the other hand, the patient who has had a sudden flurry of seizures and then is brought to the ER represents a more significant problem and requires intervention as there is a risk that further seizures, and possibly even status epilepticus, may supervene. Of course, once again the common problems of medication noncompliance and underlying illness must be considered, as must the less common potential for drug interaction, in which concurrently administered medications (even anticonvulsants) can alter each other's metabolism and cause lowered serum levels of each other. This is especially a problem as these interactions occur on a somewhat unpredictable basis. Also, there is the possibility that the patient's seizure type has been incorrectly diagnosed and an ineffective anticonvulsant prescribed; this is a possibility more likely in the patient whose seizures are of recent onset or who has had a recent change in drug regimen. Thus, it is important to clearly review the basis for the patient's diagnosis. When that is accomplished, a decision can be made regarding anticonvulsant therapy. In the majority of cases requiring adjustment, it will be made in dosage rather than in the kind of anticonvulsant. If no explanation is found for the recurrences, the anticonvulsant appears appropriate for the seizures involved and there is no evidence, historical or otherwise of anticonvulsant toxicity, an increase of anticonvulsant (or, if the patient is on multiple anticonvulsants, the most appropriate one for the seizures involved) is indicated. This is simply a linear increase for almost all the agents currently used, with the sole exception of Dilantin. This agent exhibits nonlinear kinetics, such that in the therapeutic range small increases in dosage can produce dramatically large increases in blood levels. The situation is particularly confused in cases involving multiple anticonvulsants, and here it can be quite difficult to predict blood levels for a particular increase of medication. (This last factor is one of several that can be given in favor of monotherapy for epilepsy, i.e., the use of a single agent to control seizures.) A variety of schemes have been given for the rapid increase of anticonvulsant levels. Simply adding twice the difference between the old and new dosage to the old dosage of the anticonvulsant for one time and then continuing with the new dosage schedule is the method most often recommended to achieve that rapid increase. It should be recalled however that many of the currently employed anticonvulsants (particularly carbamazepine and valproate) when given in suddenly increased dosages produce transient symptoms of toxicity, particularly nausea and vomiting; as these medications must be given orally, those side effects will hardly promote compliance. In addition, following dosage changes, oral absorption of several of the anticonvulsants (e.g., carbamazepine) can be quite uncertain, which adds still further unpredictability. These potential pitfalls must be kept in mind when increasing anticonvulsants, especially in the outpatient setting. A compromise approach can be tried; when circumstances seem less urgent, one might simply increase the anticonvulsant employed to its new dosage level, with perhaps fewer toxic side effects. The relatively short half-lives of most of the agents currently used will result in increased blood levels in a short time. If this is too long a period, it may be advisable to consider that the patient is in status in a broad sense and begin parenteral agents. If the anticonvulsant in question is Dilantin, its relatively long half-life mandates that a parenteral approach be employed in any case, and the same applies to the other parenterally available agent, phenobarbital. Regardless, especially if outpatient treatment is elected, the patient must be carefully instructed about the possible complications mentioned above and the need to seek immediate follow-up should they occur.

STATUS EPILEPTICUS

Status epilepticus has been recognized for at least the last century and constitutes one of the true medical emergencies. There is a significant element of misunderstanding that surrounds the concept of status, and this problem is not helped by the existence of various definitions for the problem (2). For example, the World Health Organization (WHO) defines status epilepticus as any epileptic condition persisting long enough to constitute a permanent condition. Others have defined it as any seizure lasting longer than 30 minutes continually, or recurrent seizures without an intervening period of consciousness between events. It should be noted that none of these specify the kind of seizure involved, and indeed as several authors have pointed out, status epilepticus is a state not an illness in and of itself. Thus, any type of seizure can become continuous (elementary, complex partial, and generalized including tonic clonic, myoclonic, and absence). Perhaps as Leppik (10) has suggested, the most useful definition is to simply consider the appearance of three seizures in 24 hours as evidence of status, for the consequences of recurrent seizures are greater than the risks of treatment. This fact is specifically true of the most dangerous of the various forms of status, generalized tonic clonic. Other seizures that at least infrequently become continuous in adults include complex partial, elementary partial (Koshevnikov syndrome), and absence (see later sections in this chapter). Although generalized tonic clonic (GTC) status is easily recognized in the majority of cases, at times the seizures can become somewhat disorganized clinically, and thus may be difficult to diagnose if the seizures have been taking place for an extended period.

As in the case of isolated seizures, at times a variety of seizure-like entities can be mistaken for status. These may include a number of movement disorders, such as choreoathetosis and some forms of segmental myoclonus. Also, decorticate and decerebrate posturing, and a variety of rigors can be seen in obtunded patients, in whom the greatest difficulty arises in reaching the correct diagnosis. The key point regarding these seizure-like disorders is that none of these respond to anticonvulsants, which may lead ultimately to the use of greater and greater amounts of anticonvulsants to suppress them, resulting in patient toxicity. The key to recognizing seizure-like entities is often an awareness of the possibility of the diagnosis and the realization that the patient is not responding to treatment with anticonvulsant drugs. Still less frequently, the patient can present with psychogenic seizures, i.e., seizures without an organic basis. The EEG can also be of use in confirming that an epileptic condition does or does not exist; however, it is critical to realize that the usefulness of this diagnostic test depends on reliable interpretation of the data.

Precipitating Factors

Although it is surprising to many, the incidence of status is probably greater today than before the widespread use of anticonvulsants, probably because the inappropriate use of such drugs has been a major factor in precipitating status. The causes of status must be considered from a dual perspective: There must be both an underlying neurophysiologic cause for the seizure disorder and a precipitating factor that engendered the status. Several studies have considered this point; the most common causes have included underlying structural lesions such as metastatic and primary tumors. The latter most often involve low-grade gliomas such as astrocytomas, and these are more often found in the frontal area (9). Other processes predisposing to status include anoxic encephalopathy; Wernike's encephalopathy; drug abuse, including alcoholism; and various metabolic disorders influencing water and electrolytes, including calcium and magnesium. Vasculitis and other cerebrovascular disorders and particularly head injury are also numbered among the common underlying causes of status, as are meningeal and parenchymal infections of bacterial, fungal, and viral origin. In addition to these underlying etiologies, precipitating factors are usually present as well; for example, withdrawal from alcohol, withdrawal of anticonvulsants in a patient with a brain tumor and seizures, and so forth. These immediate causes vary from community to community, but a prevalent pattern of triggering factors can be characteristic of a given community, and thus, as Leppic has recommended, it is wise for the physician to be familiar with the mechanisms particularly common in the locality.

Failure to consider the aforementioned etiologic problems can severely impair the effectiveness of the therapeutic effort. For example, many metabolically induced seizures are quite resistant to anticonvulsants, and failure to correct that discrepancy can greatly prolong an episode of status. The consequences of status are evident both in the central nervous system and systemically. Despite full support for the metabolic stresses induced by status, including correction of hypoxia, etc., after a period of about 60 minutes, irreversible neuronal damage progressively appears, indicating that prolonged epileptic activity is capable of inducing damage to the brain directly and must be controlled (1). Clinical examples include the prolonged memory deficits seen in cases of complex partial status and permanent paralysis of the involved area following elementary partial status. Leppik (10) has also reviewed the systemic consequences of generalized tonic-clonic seizures, and they are detailed below. If these problems are sought and recognized, and current methods of treatment applied, survival of the patient will depend on the nature of the underlying pathology rather than the severity of the seizures themselves. This point even extends to patients with primary generalized seizures in status who may be expected to do well with prompt treatment.

Therapeutic Intervention for Control of Status

Although most authors agree that status epilepticus, particularly of the generalized tonic-clonic variety, requires prompt intervention, there is some considerable variation in the particulars of achieving that end. Porter has pointed out that status may be considered to exist in a bipolar form, consisting on the one hand of repetitive seizures continuing as the ER physician watches, and the more common history of a flurry of seizures in which the most recent seizure occurred shortly before the patient presented at the ER. Both require immediate intervention. In the case of repetitive seizures, there is often little or no time for casual contemplation of a plan, and a well-thought-out course of action must be developed ahead of time. This approach may even be extended to the point of having a specific team designated for response to a patient in status. Rothner and Morris (6) have described the following series of steps, which should be carried out in the sequence described next, but as close to simultaneously as possible.

It is essential that the airway be assured, and this goal takes absolute precedence. Early intubation should be considered to avoid aspiration and assure an adequate airway throughout the resuscitation. This point is important not only because of the usual concerns regarding mechanical obstruction but also because of the respiratory supressant effect of many anticonvulsants employed. Vital signs must be quickly monitored, and the patient protected from inadvertent injury, particularly head injuries. A brief history and physical examination should be obtained; this examination should emphasize a search for occurrence of prior seizures, a history of head injury, current major medical problems, alcoholism and drug abuse, and most especially the patient's anticonvulsant history if available. As well, the examination should be highly focused to include a determination of the vital signs and to seek evidence of head injury. Because of the side effects of status described below, continued observation of vital signs must be maintained, just as with a cardiac arrest. While the above is being done, blood studies are drawn, to include anticonvulsant levels even if there is no history of use of such agents, for the obvious reason that the history may simply not be available. Even if rapid anticonvulsant level determinations are not available, baseline studies for later comparison are of value. Also, blood for glucose, electrolytes (to include calcium), hepatic and renal functions should be monitored. Occasionally overlooked, a toxicological screen is important especially in cases where drug abuse is strongly suspected, not only because of concern regarding etiology for the status but also for possible interactions with the medications used to treat the status. An arterial blood gas should be drawn as well. Urinary catheterization should be performed for urinalysis and to monitor urinary output as significant fluid loads may accompany treatment. A secure intravenous access should be established; obviously, a large-bore catheter is appropriate. Fluid therapy should begin with a bolus of 50 ml of 50% glucose. As a history of alcohol abuse and therefore Wernike's encephalopathy is frequently found in patients in status, and as glucose infusion places such individuals at great risk of a worsening of their encephalopathy, infusion of 50 mg of thiamine is also indicated. At this point anticonvulsant therapy is begun.

ANTICONVULSIVE THERAPY

Benzodiazepines

Porter (5) has given useful guidance regarding the most effective approach to anticonvulsant administration at this stage. For those with continuous generalized tonic-clonic seizures, there is general agreement that immediate infusion of a benzodiazepine is appropriate. On the other hand, in the case of patients with repetitive seizures manifesting in-between periods of stupor, one has the option of avoiding the use of benzodiazepines and pro-

ceeding directly to administration of diphenlhydantoin (Dilantin). There are advantages to this course of action. Benzodiazepines are effective depressants of respiration and blood pressure and synergize with at least phenobarbital to worsen those effects, further complicating patient care in the likely event that barbiturates are subsequently administered. Moreover, in the case of drug-induced status, further supression of vital functions may occur with addition of benzodiazepines. Finally, the anticonvulsant effect of benzodiazepines is long outlived by the sedating effect, which can impede recovery of alertness after termination of the status. Indeed, if the seizures are sufficiently separated in time, administration of benzodiazepines may actually interfere with the primary therapeutic goal, long-term control of seizures with long-acting anticonvulsants. Thus use of benzodiazepines can be supported in the instance of a patient with seizures requiring immediate, urgent control but should not be used simply as an automatic reaction to every situation in which seizure control is sought.

Should it be necessary to resort to benzodiazepines, there are currently two choices available: diazepam and lorazepam. Traditionally, diazepam (Valium) has been used for this purpose, but in the last few years, a new agent, lorazepam, has come into vogue. Valium found favor initially because it distributes rapidly and quickly achieves therapeutic levels in the brain. That rapid distribution, along with other factors, unfortunately limits the usefulness of diazepam as its period of anticonvulsant action is only 30 minutes. This fact means that breakthrough seizures are likely, and thus, this medication must be followed up with a long-acting agent even if seizures stop with diazepam. A constant infusion with diazepam is no longer considered effective. The alternate agent, lorazepam, has a longer duration of central nervous system (CNS) action, and in a large study, it was found that 4 mg of lorazepam was as effective as 10 mg of diazepam. Lorazepam is available in parenteral form and is administered intravenously as a 4 to 8 mg bolus. However, as with diazepam, the anticonvulsant effect of lorazepam manifests tachyphylaxis; that is, repeated doses become progressively less effective in supressing seizures. Also, because of ethical considerations, it has not been possible to determine the duration of action of this agent, although early reports suggested a considerably longer effective period than diazepam. Regardless of that, however, as with diazepam, administration of a long-acting anticonvulsant on the heels of the benzodiazepine is mandatory for long-term seizure control.

Phenytoin

The anticonvulsant most often employed initially is phenytoin (10). The choice is based on its efficacy in controlling seizures, a nearly 50-year experience with the drug, ready penetration of the nervous system on parenteral administration, and a relative lack of CNS suppression, which allows quick recovery of consciousness in patients in whom it stops seizures. In animal preparations, significant anticonvulsant levels are achieved in the brain in a matter of minutes, and it is primarily for this reason that many authorities recommend that this agent be employed as the first-line anticonvulsant in the treatment of status. This fact is especially true in those cases in which seizures are interspersed by periods of quiescence or in circumstances that do not otherwise demand immediate intervention with benzodiazepines.

Phenytoin has the disadvantage of producing unwanted cardiovascular effects, such as hypotension and arrhythmias, especially with rapid administration. The rate of administration must be carefully regulated, and this problem limits the usefulness of this agent in circumstances requiring very rapid achievement of seizure control. (Of course, this agent must be given intravenously as it is quite alkaline and precipitates in muscle if given by that route.) Porter (5) also gives useful recommendations regarding administration of phenytoin:

1. An infusion rate of 50 mg/minute avoids the risks of cardiac arrhythmia and hypotension mentioned above, although young individuals otherwise in good health may be able to accept 100 mg/minute dosage without difficulty.
2. A cardiac monitor is useful, especially when more rapid infusion rates are used.
3. Frequent blood pressure determinations are indicated as a monitor for hypotension. If hypotension occurs, it is an obvious indication to decrease the rate of phenytoin administration.
4. Parenteral phenytoin, because of the necessity to bring it into solution with a highly alkaline vehicle, precipitates in neutral and acidic solutions, for example 5% dextrose. Prompt precipitation occurs under these circumstances and may occur even in saline preparations, particularly after 30 minutes. (Precipitation in the bloodstream presumably does not occur because of the avid adsorption of phenytoin by albumin.) Added advantages of direct administration are that it overcomes the uncertainty of administration of medication by non-physician personnel and obtains prompt achievement of therapeutic blood levels; also, significant fluid loading is avoided at a time when cerebral and pulmonary edema are real concerns.
5. Achievement of adequate blood levels is critical to the efficacy of phenytoin. The blood level sought by most authorities is $25\mu g/ml$, and in most cases this is achieved by administering 18 mg/kg. Toxicity from overdosage is less of a concern than cardiotoxicity from too rapid administration, as the former is primarily ataxia and unlikely to represent a problem in a patient who is most likely to be bedridden.

If seizure control is obtained, it is important to recall that blood levels of medication will be maintained for about 12–24 hours, and daily maintenance will have to begin about 12–18 hours after the initial administration of phenytoin. This therapy should be monitored with blood level determinations, and further parenteral dosages are not infrequently required, particularly in those patients with underlying pathology producing depression of consciousness.

Phenobarbital

About 40–50% of patients with convulsive status will not respond to intravenous phenytoin, and one must resort to phenobarbital, the other effective anticonvulsant available for parenteral use. As with phenytoin, phenobarbital quickly (in minutes) achieves peak brain levels. This medication inevitably produces sedation and possibly respiratory depression in the dosages required for supression of seizures, and the rate of administration does not significantly alter this. Thus most authorities recommend that a large loading dose (6–8 mg/kg) be administered, or if divided dosages are employed, that 10–20 mg/kg be given over 60–90 minutes. This dose should be administered even if it is more than the amount necessary to interrupt the status. Daily maintenance will need to begin about 12–24 hours later, and serum drug levels should be measured to assure therapeutic levels are achieved. This fact is especially true if drug-drug interactions or altered elimination of this medication is possible, e.g., in liver or renal disease. It is also important to realize that phenobarbital is a sedating drug and inevitably results in depression of a patient's level of consciousness in the dosages given above, and can significantly depress respiration and blood pressure, especially when a benzodiazepine has been used. Should seizures persist after the recommended dosages of phenobarbital have been administered, larger amounts can be used sufficient to achieve barbiturate coma with a burst-suppression pattern. This therapy should be performed under EEG control. Obviously under these circumstances, careful control of the airway must be emphasized again, as well as careful monitoring of blood pressure. An objection can be raised that phenobarbital, as it is a potent depressant, could worsen an already dangerous situation; however, if DPH fails, there are really few effective, efficient alternatives available beyond phenobarbital.

Paraldehyde, Lidocaine, and Valproate

Other medications have been used occasionally for control of seizures, including paraldehyde, lidocaine, and valproate. Paraldehyde is an agent with a long tradition of use in status epilepticus and about which little is actually known with confidence. It is a potentially quite toxic substance that when aged or exposed to light and heat is converted to acetic acid, an obviously dangerous property for any parenteral form. Intravenous administration is accompanied by serious risk of hypotension and pulmonary edema; for this reason it is given rectally at times. The latter route has variable rates of absorption and is therefore unreliable especially in cases of severe status. If the intravenous route is chosen, a solution of 4% paraldehyde in saline is used with dosages of 0.1–0.3 mg/kg given over about 30 minutes, with follow-up slow infusion of similar concentrations of the medication to control further seizures. Although it is possible to maintain a patient on paraldehyde for several days, long-acting anticonvulsants must be used eventually, and there is an urgency to this move, as dependence on this agent may appear. Paraldehyde is also incompatible with many of the plastics used in intravenous tubing, etc. and this problem also places obvious restrictions on its use. The drawbacks resulting from the above problems have led to its recent

withdrawal from general availability, still further diminishing its applicability for treatment of status. There is evidence to suggest that in the case of seizures due entirely to alcohol withdrawal, paraldehyde may be a drug of choice since it appears to suppress the appearance of delirium tremens beside being an effective anticonvulsant. Dilantin has been shown to be ineffective for such seizures. Paraldehyde may also be useful in cases in which the patient is allergic to more traditional agents.

Lidocaine is an agent that also has not been thoroughly studied in status, and the drug is somewhat paradoxical for use in this problem as it is known to be a convulsant agent in large doses. There is, nonetheless, evidence that it is effective for both generalized status and elementary partial status although it has variable brain distribution. Dosages of this agent are not well defined, however, the largest study recommends a single dose of 2–3 mg/kg, with an infusion of 3–10 mg/kg/hour if seizures persist. It should not be injected at rates greater than 25–50 mg/minute. It is considered nonsedating.

Valproate in general has been considered an adjunctive medication for status. It is as yet not available as a parenteral drug. Enemas of valproate were used originally to overcome this problem, although this practice has been subsequently replaced by the employment of suppositories, containing crushed 200-mg tablets. Rectal absorption is rapid and complete; following doses of 400 mg of valproate peak values are reached in 3–4 hours. On a 6 hourly dosage schedule, therapeutic plasma levels are reached in 24–48 hours and are well maintained. In most studies, valproate has not been used alone, and withdrawal of the other anticonvulsant, usually phenytoin, has precipitated a worsening or recurrence of seizures. There is also reason to believe that simultaneous administration of benzodiazepines with valproate may, through determined mechanisms, worsen seizures. Thus, the current role of valproate appears to be as an adjunct to phenytoin, to potentiate its effect and to "cover" a patient until therapeutic phenytoin levels are reached; it is possible that valproate may directly potentiate the effect of phenytoin.

EEG MONITORING

Although the termination of status may often appear clinically easy to recognize, this finding may be deceiving and at times EEG seizures may persist, presumably with the progressing neuronal damage that can follow prolonged seizures. For this reason EEG monitoring is always indicated when available. This test may be begun at any time during the course of treatment and should not take precedence over other life-saving interventions. A detailed discussion of the changes seen on the EEG is beyond the scope of this discussion; nevertheless it is worth recognizing that there is increasing awareness that somewhat specific EEG changes take place during most episodes of generalized tonic-clonic status and that these, when recognized, can give useful information about the progress toward control. There is increasing agreement that control of an episode of status cannot be considered achieved until EEG evidence of seizure activity is stopped as well. More prolonged monitoring, when available, is useful after the bout of status is over to further assure that there is no recurrence of the problem, a particularly significant point in obtunded patients in whom unrecognized recurrent seizures are a potential problem.

Medical Complications

Although the primary interest to this point has been pharmacologic treatment of status, it is important to realize that there are a number of medical complications of generalized tonic-clonic status that must be recognized. Simon has enumerated a number of these (11). Hyperthermia occurs frequently in status and is felt to be the result primarily of increased motor activity. Temperatures of 107°F have been reported, and this finding tends to parallel the duration and severity of the status. These temperature elevations may occur independent of infection, although infection must be ruled out. Thus, heat stress must be considered a risk of status. Hypothermia has also been reported in status, and in the majority it has been the result of drug effects and metabolic derangements such as hypoglycemia and hypothyroidism.

Another frequently encountered problem is leukocytosis, which can range above 25,000 cells/mm³ in the absence of any sign of infection. Up to 50% of patients demonstrate this effect, and it may manifest with either a polymorphonuclear or lymphocytic predominance. As Simon points out, there is rarely a shift toward immature forms, and that is a potential means of differentiating this phenomenon from a true infection. There may also be a mild cerebrospinal fluid pleocytosis; this finding has been reported in 2–6% of patients and consists of cell counts not exceeding 80 cells/mm³ with an initial polymorphonuclear predominance, although in days this count may tend to lymphocytosis. There may also be a slight elevation of CSF protein. Obviously, the critical point here is to rule out infection before the decision is made that the above mechanisms are in operation.

A significant acidosis as a result of lactate production also occurs, and up to one-half of patients have pH values less than 7.0 during status. The acidosis probably results from the vigorous muscle activity occasioned by the seizures, as it can be suppressed by motor paralysis. Although this acidosis would appear to increase the risk of development of a hyperkalemia and resultant cardiac arrhythmia, fortunately that does not seem to occur. There is also little evidence that the degree of acidosis correlates with the neurological outcome, and it rapidly resolves with cessation of seizures, and thus does not represent one of the potentially more serious effects of status.

Pulmonary edema can also occur with generalized tonic-clonic status: in one series over one-third of patients with status had this problem. It probably results at least in part from elevated pulmonary pressures that have been recorded in status. There, however, remains considerable uncertainty about the precise mechanism of this pulmonary edema. Pneumonia is also an unfortunately common accompaniment of status and can result from aspiration. The pulmonary vascular changes that accompany status may also contribute to this problem. Cardiac arrhythmias are common during status, and again extreme care must be used when administering anticonvulsants such as Dilantin.

The anoxia that can accompany status may also exacerbate underlying neurological dysfunction, and the medial temporal lobe and cerebellum are particularly susceptible. Recent work suggests that this problem may not be evident for as long as 24 hours or more following status, and reinforces the need for vigorous efforts to prevent anoxia during status.

Renal failure can also occur with resultant oliguria and uremia and may be associated with renal tubular necrosis and lower nephron nephrosis. The resultant hyperkalemia and azotemia obviously have the potential for increasing the likelihood of further seizures. Rhabdomyolysis is probably a significant factor in this issue, both from the vigorous muscle effort, and from pressure on dependent muscles after prolonged recumbency as in coma. The hyperpyrexia mentioned above may also contribute, with release of large amounts of myoglobin and resultant lower nephron nephrosis possibly leading to acute renal failure. The above factors associated with the profound sweating seen in status can lead to dehydration and marked electrolyte and osmolarity problems. This problem can be further worsened by alterations in blood glucose levels. Initially hyperglycemia may occur during an episode of status probably as the result of the profound sympathetic discharge that accompanies the event. The subsequent hypoglycemia that may follow is probably related to consumption of glucose by muscle and brain and by increased plasma insulin levels. Such a hypoglycemia might be harmful if sufficiently prolonged and could actually be a factor contributing to the precipitation of further seizures. As such it should be guarded against. Yet, hyperglycemia can also be harmful to the cerebrum under certain circumstances, for example during the course of a stroke; thus, the best advice that can be given is to maintain the blood glucose levels as close to the normal range as possible.

It is perhaps needless to say that primary causes of the deviations listed above must also be ruled out. It is also obvious that there are significant complexities in the treatment of tonic clonic status, and in general these require admission to an intensive care facility, at least until the status is controlled. There are certain exceptions to this rule, particularly patients who are otherwise known to be well but who are in status secondary to drug overdosage or other limited process; however, these are in the minority and the safest course is to admit the patient to an intensive care setting.

Postintervention Treatment

Also, the period following control of the status is critical. There is a natural tendency to consider the problem resolved when seizures have been controlled. This is a major error, and indeed, can be considered a fundamental point in the care of a patient with status. Aside from treatment of any underlying illnesses involved in the status, the major goal at this point is to establish a regimen that will both maintain control of the patient's seizure disorder and not result in toxicity. This approach will frequently require adjustments not only in dosage, but also in the kind of anticonvulsant administered. The major principles regarding anticonvulsant choice are the desirability of monotherapy and the recognition that nonsedating anticonvulsants are preferable. Both of the major anticonvulsants recommended in preceding sections (Dilantin and particularly phenobarbital) are sedating, and as a result it will almost certainly be preferrable to convert the patient to an oral monotherapy with the currently preferred agent for generalized tonic-clonic status, carbamazepine. This change must be done in a fashion that will not leave the patient uncovered by anticonvulsant therapy. Thus, one should begin with a carbamazepine dosage of about 200 mg four times a day, with the expectation that stable blood levels will be reached in 3–4 days. After that has been accomplished, an effort should be made to withdraw the most sedating agent, usually phenobarbital. This change can be done abruptly, as long as therapeutic levels of carbamazepine are maintained, for the long half-life of phenobarbital results in a gradual reduction of its blood level. Following this, withdrawal of Dilantin can be attempted as well.

An alternative anticonvulsant that can be employed for those patients with generalized tonic-clonic seizures is valproate, which is considered by some as a primary therapeutic agent for generalized seizures. Use of this agent in patients who are receiving phenobarbital must be approached with caution as valproate can significantly prolong the half-life of barbiturates, causing deep sedation and, potentially, coma. Also, many if not most tonic-clonic seizures in adulthood are secondarily generalized and valproate may not be effective in suppressing the underlying focal seizures. Thus, the circumstances surrounding the individual case require a tailored approach, and for that reason more specific recommendations cannot be made regarding long-term therapy. Since the treatment of seizure disorder is a long-term problem in which a strong patient-physician relationship must be developed, the involvement of the patient's primary-care giver should be sought if at all possible to allow coordinated long-term planning. Certainly the patient will require, even in the best of circumstances, observation in the hospital to recover from the effects of the status (which may produce significant depression for several days independent of medication effects and the underlying disease); during this time the careful monitoring of anticonvulsant levels should be undertaken and oral administration of anticonvulsants should be begun as soon as possible to achieve the basic goal of a course of therapy, the establishment of a therapeutically effective steady state of anticonvulsant medication. Oral loading dosages can be employed for this purpose, and, except for Dilantin, an initial dosage of twice the maintenance dosage can be tried, with the expectation that a therapeutic blood level will be established in 24 hours. This approach is more complicated than might be appreciated at first glance because of drug-drug interactions, making this an effort that must be guided by careful monitoring of blood levels. Also, it is frequently the case that initiation of large dosages can produce unwanted side effects, including gastrointestinal discomfort, particularly in the case of carbamazepine. Particular caution is warranted in the case of Dilantin, because the zero-order kinetics of this agent with drug levels in the therapeutic range make it particularly easy to overshoot into the toxic range. When circumstances permit, and this is a matter of judgement, consideration can be given to starting therapy at the maintenance dosage level, which may avoid many of the problems just stated.

NONCONVULSIVE STATUS AND ELEMENTARY PARTIAL STATUS

In addition to the most common form of status, generalized tonic-clonic status, several other forms of status are encountered, including nonconvulsive status and elementary partial status. Although these forms are not immediately life-threatening as is generalized tonic-clonic status, they are nevertheless associated with sufficiently significant complications that they also warrant immediate intervention. The first category is nonconvulsive status, and as the name implies, consists of seizures without a tonic-clonic component. The name was often taken to be synonymous with complex partial seizures, however, presently is considered to consist of two seizure types, complex partial seizures and adult onset absence status, sometimes called "petit mal". The latter is poorly named as the relation to the classic absence of childhood is problematical at best. The second category is elementary partial status.

Complex partial status is an entity that until recently was considered rare because few cases

had been reported (7, 12). Yet, at least one to two cases yearly can be expected in large referral centers, and recognition is important. Recognition of the various types of complex status that may occur usually requires specialized closed-circuit monitoring techniques. It is sufficient to say that complex partial status may be suspected when a patient manifests repeated episodes, usually with distinctive onset, of alterations of consciousness possibly associated with automatisms followed by a gradual progression toward recovery of full consciousness, if another episode does not intervene. There are clear-cut episodes, distinguishing this from the other likely diagnosis, adult onset absence status. In the case of the latter, there will more likely be a continued fluctuation of consciousness, with intervals of apparent relatively normal responsiveness grading into marked confusion, rather than a few distinct bouts of loss of consciousness.

The EEG can be of real value in differentiating complex partial status from absence status. It is again beyond the scope of this discussion to detail these, and the interested reader is referred to any of the several monographs listed among the references, that describe these in detail. The pertinence in differentiating these is based on the differences in anticonvulsants appropriate for each, and the recognition that improperly treated complex partial status have as a dire consequence the risk of prolonged memory deficit particularly. For this form of nonconvulsive status, initial treatment with lorazapam and then phenytoin as in generalized tonic-clonic status is appropriate; phenobarbital can be added if necessary, as in generalized status. This approach is appropriate as these seizures may easily secondarily generalize if not controlled. Determining that the seizures have stopped may be difficult, and, if available, the EEG may be of assistance. Adult onset absence status also responds to benzodiazepines, especially diazepam. That agent is used in dosages similar to the treatment of generalized tonic-clonic status, although the efficacy of lorazepam has not been established for this purpose. Following that, a maintenance anticonvulsant appropriate for absence seizures should be begun, for example, valproate. If that cannot be tolerated, and if the patient does not have generalized tonic-clonic seizures, ethosuximide can be used in the dosages given previously. If both of these are unsatisfactory, the third choice of anticonvulsant is Tegretol. For patients in whom a benzodiazepine fails to control the seizures, rectal valproate can be considered although the efficacy of this therapy has not been established. Dosages are as described previously for that agent.

The final entity to be considered is elementary partial status, sometimes called "epilepsia partialis continua." This condition usually consists of progressively spreading seizures that focally involve the motor cortex on one side, very often recruiting body parts in the order represented by the motor cortical homunculus (Jacksonian march), and that recur repeatedly. These seizures are often intermixed with myoclonias that may involve other parts of the body. The EEG often shows diffuse slowing and epileptiform rhythms may appear from a variety of foci, at times distant from the rolandic area, which is consistent with the observation that these focal seizures are associated with multifocal brain pathology. Treatment is aimed at preventing further spread of these seizures and discovering the underlying cause. Anticonvulsant therapy is similar to that for generalized tonic-clonic seizures, save that the urgency of administration is not so great, and if therapeutic levels of phenytoin do not control the seizures, most authorities agree that administration of phenobarbital should not produce blood levels exceeding the upper limits of the therapeutic range. Control of these seizures is often quite difficult and the toxicity of the agents used may exceed the risks from the focal seizures themselves.

References

1. Celesia G: Prognosis in convulsive status epilepticus. In Delgado-Escueta AV et al (eds): *Advances in Neurology Vol 34: Status Epilepticus*. New York, Raven Press, 1983, chap 5, pp 55–59.
2. Gastaut H. Classification of status epilepticus. In Delgado-Escueta AV et al (eds): *Advances in Neurology Vol 34: Status Epilepticus*. New York, Raven Press, 1983, chap 2, pp 15–35.
3. Klawans HL, Carvey PM, Tanner CM, Goetz, CG: Drug-induced myoclonus. In Fahn S et al (eds): *Myoclonus*. New York, Raven Press, 1986, pp 251–264.
4. Messing RO, Closson RG, Simon RP: Drug-induced seizures: a 10 year experience. *Neurology* 34:1582–1586, 1984.
5. Porter RJ: *Epilepsy: 100 Elementary Principles*. Philadelphia, WB Saunders, 1984.
6. Rothner AD, Morris HH: Generalized status epilepticus. In Luders H et al (eds): *Epilepsy: Electroclinical Syndromes*. New York, Springer Verlag, 1987, chap 10, pp 207–222.
7. Sharbrough FW: Complex partial seizures. In Luders H et al (eds): *Epilepsy: Electroclinical Syndromes*. New York, Springer Verlag, 1987, chap 12, pp 279–302.
8. Simon RP, Aminoff MJ: Electroencephalographic status epilepticus in fatal anoxic coma. *Ann Neurol* 20:351–355, 1986.
9. Hauser WA: Status epilepticus: frequency, etiology, and neurologic sequelae. In Delgaso-Esqueta AV (eds): *Advances in Neurology. Vol 34: Status Epilepticus*. New York, Raven Press, 1984, chap 1, 1984, pp 3–14.
10. Leppik IE, Patrick BK, Cranford RE: Treatment of acute seizures and status epilepticus with intravenous phenytoin. In Delgado-Esqueta AV et al (eds): *Advances in Neurology. Vol 34: Status Epilepticus*. New York, Raven Press, 1984, chap 45, pp 447–451.
11. Simon RP: Physiologic consequences of status epilepticus. *Epilepsia* 26 (Suppl 1):S58–S66, 1985.
12. Treiman DM, Delgado-Esqueta AV: Complex partial status epilepticus. In *Advances in Neurology. Vol 34: Status Epilepticus*. New York, Raven Press, 1984, chap 7, pp 69–81.

12

Catecholamines and Other Inotropes

Arno L. Zaritsky, M.D.
Bart Chernow, M.D., F.A.C.P., F.C.C.P.

Management of the critically ill patient often necessitates the use of one or more inotropic agents to maintain adequate tissue perfusion. Catecholamines and other sympathomimetics are the most important group of inotropic agents currently available; however, a number of new, noncatecholamine agents are being used in critically ill patients. This chapter reviews the pharmacology of both catecholamines and the new inotropes, arminone and milrinone. Adrenergic receptor physiology and endogenous catecholamine responses in the critically ill patient are highlighted, and the cardiovascular actions and clinical indications for these agents are reviewed.

Clinical use of inotropes requires an understanding of several important pharmacologic principles. These have been discussed in detail in chapter 1 but are reviewed briefly here. Whenever a drug is administered to a patient, its clinical actions are due to a complex interaction between the concentration of drug in the plasma, elimination from the body, diffusion to its site of action, and the response of the target tissue to the drug. Plasma drug concentration is modified by changes in the drug dose and pharmacokinetics, whereas the tissue response is influenced by changes in receptor and tissue responsiveness.

Pharmacokinetics is the mathematical expression of the time course of all processes leading to drug distribution and elimination. This time course is typically determined by quantifying drug concentration in the plasma compartment, although this approach may not be ideal since inotropic drug action occurs in the tissue. In the critical care setting, most inotropic agents are administered by continuous intravenous infusion, making the kinetics relatively simple. Pharmacodynamics is the relationship between drug concentration (again, usually measured in plasma samples) and drug effect. In the case of inotropic agents, measur-

able drug-induced physiologic action may be a change in cardiac output, blood pressure, and heart rate. When used clinically, the pharmacodynamic effects of inotropes are not related to the drug plasma concentration in a simple manner, since the patient's illness may influence the net hemodynamic effect observed.

In patients with circulatory shock, for example, drug within the plasma compartment may not be distributed to the active site because of poor perfusion. As the patient's clinical condition changes, the pharmacokinetics and pharmacodynamics of administered inotropes may also change, necessitating frequent reassessment of the patient and adjustment of the infusion rate. In the discussion of individual inotropes that follows, statements regarding hemodynamic effects observed with specific infusion doses should be recognized as being relative and that individual adjustment is needed for each patient.

ADRENERGIC RECEPTORS

The actions of catecholamines are determined by their binding at three major classes of receptors: α-adrenergic, β-adrenergic, and dopaminergic (DA) receptors. There are two subtypes of each of these receptors, termed α_1 and α_2, β_1 and β_2, and DA_1 and DA_2 (103, 138). Three of the four types of α- and β-adrenergic receptors mediate their cellular effects through stimulation (β-receptors) or inhibition (α_2-receptors) of adenylate cyclase activity. The α_1-receptor transduces the signal from receptor-agonist binding by increasing transcellular calcium flux through a recently described mechanism that results from phosphoinositol turnover at the cell membrane (117, 118).

Adrenergic receptor density on the cell surface is dynamic; the density of receptors can

Table 12.1
Disease and Conditions Altering Receptor Density on Effector Cells[a]

Disease or Condition	Receptor Altered	Change
Congestive heart failure	β (heart)	Increased[b]
Sepsis	α (liver, vasculature)	Decreased
Myocardial ischemia	β (heart)	Decreased
Myocardial ischemia	α (heart)	Increased
Asthma[c]	β (lung, leukocytes)	Decreased
Cystic fibrosis	β (leukocytes)	Decreased
Fetal and neonatal life	α, β (heart, platelets, leukocytes)	Decreased
Agonist administration	α, β (heart, platelets, leukocytes)	Decreased
Antagonist administration	α, β (heart, platelets, leukocytes)	Increased
Hyperthyroidism	β (heart)	Increased
Hypothyroidism	β (heart)	Decreased
Glucocorticoids	β (heart, leukocytes)	Increased

[a] From Zaritsky A, Eisenberg, MG: Ontogenetic considerations in the pharmaco-therapy of shock. In Chernow B, Shoemaker WC (eds): *Critical Care: State of the Art,* vol 7. Society of Critical Care Medicine, Fullerton, CA, 1986, pp 485–534.
[b] β-Adrenergic receptors are decreased in severe heart failure.
[c] If on β-agonist therapy for asthma.

be modulated by a number of disease states or conditions (Table 12.1). Changes in receptor density can have important implications in the pharmacotherapy of the patient with circulatory shock. Down-regulation (a decrease in the number of receptors on the cell surface) of β-adrenergic receptors in the myocardium of patients with chronic congestive heart failure results in decreased catecholamine sensitivity (21). In endotoxic shock, β-adrenergic receptors are down regulated in the liver, which may partially mediate the glucose dyshomeostasis seen in sepsis (149), and α_1-adrenergic receptor density and responsiveness is diminished in the peripheral vasculature (98), accounting for a portion of sepsis-mediated adrenergic vascular unresponsiveness (28). Similarly, adrenergic receptor density may be altered by ontogenetic influences (158). Infants have diminished catecholamine responsiveness; a portion of this phenomenon is probably due to diminished numbers and/or responsiveness of adrenergic receptors. (158).

Even when adrenergic receptor density is normal or increased, altered catecholamine-induced inotropic, chronotropic, or peripheral vascular effects may be noted because of postreceptor influences. This circumstance is observed, for example, in neonatal and young dogs (123), and following either chronic exposure to catecholamines or chronic blockade of α- or β-adrenergic receptors (115). β-Adrenergic receptors have two agonist-affinity states; changes being regulated by guanine nucleotides (115), and those affinity changes being modulated by small changes in plasma cate-

cholamine concentration (49). Differences in receptor affinity produce variations in adrenergic responsiveness, although our understanding of the β-adrenergic receptor coupling mechanism is currently limited. It is likely that changes in receptor affinity have important implications in the actions of exogenous or endogenous catecholamines. For example, repeated or prolonged exposure of the β-adrenergic receptor to an agonist results in an attenuated response that is partly mediated by altering the coupling state of the receptor (140).

ENDOGENOUS CATECHOLAMINE RESPONSE

The neurohumoral response to critical illness has important effects on the pharmacodynamics of inotropes. Besides altering adrenergic receptor affinity state and cell density as outlined above, endogenous catecholamines exert vasoactive effects: stimulating heart rate and cardiac contractility, modulating peripheral vascular tone, and partly mediating the metabolic changes characteristic of critical illness (27). When an inotrope is administered to a critically ill patient, the net hemodynamic effect reflects the pharmacodynamic action of the drug and the modifying influence of the patient's endogenous catecholamine response.

The majority of plasma norepinephrine is derived from synaptic nerve clefts. Norepinephrine is the neurotransmitter of the sympathetic nervous system; it is released from sympathetic nerves and acts locally. The concentration of norepinephrine in the plasma is used as a marker of sympathetic nerve activity (59), although it is influenced by the rate of norepinephrine release, the rate of norepinephrine reuptake by the sympathetic nerve, the rate of metabolic degradation at the effector site, and the rate of metabolic clearance from the plasma. Esler (48) has shown that a normal plasma norepinephrine concentration may be associated with an increased rate of norepinephrine release balanced by an increased rate of metabolic clearance. Plasma norepinephrine (and epinephrine) concentrations are also influenced by the site of sampling; epinephrine is increased and norepinephrine decreased in forearm arterial versus venous blood. (14). Therefore, caution should be used in the interpretation of plasma norepinephrine concentrations as a reflection of sympathetic nervous system activity. Finally, elevations in plasma norepinephrine concentration reflect neuronal activity and are *not* equivalent to norepinephrine infusions since circulating norepinephrine concentrations must exceed 1800 pg/ml to produce a clinically measurable hemodynamic effect (130), and these endogenous plasma concentrations are unusual in most stress states.

The release of norepinephrine from sympathetic nerves is controlled by a complex interplay between presynaptic receptors (for catecholamines, acetylcholine, angiotensin and other mediators) (129) and modulation by such other factors as pH, adenosine concentration, and prostaglandin E_2 (PGE$_2$) that can either increase or decrease norepinephrine release (129, 137). Many of these hormonal or metabolic systems are abnormal in critical illness and may modulate the local release and action of catecholamines.

Circulating epinephrine is largely derived from the adrenal gland and a small contribution is derived from other chromaffin tissue. Unlike norepinephrine, epinephrine functions as a circulating hormone; small changes in concentration can produce significant alterations in hemodynamic effects (31). Normal plasma epinephrine concentrations are in the range of 24–74 pg/ml; concentrations of 75–125 pg/ml produce increases in heart rate and systolic blood pressure (31).

Despite the limitations in the interpretation of plasma catecholamine concentrations noted above, it is apparent that the sympathetic nervous system functions as an important homeostatic mechanism to maintain blood pressure and cardiac output in response to shock and other stresses, and that this response can be approximately quantitated by measurement of plasma catecholamine concentrations.

Myocardial infarction (12) hemorrhagic hypotension (26), trauma (35, 70), and cardiopulmonary arrest (155), to name a few, are all associated with substantial increases in circulating norepinephrine and/or epinephrine concentrations. The extent of plasma catecholamine elevation has been correlated with the severity of congestive heart failure (32) and with the severity of injury early after trauma (35). This type of assessment may prove to be a useful means of assessing the severity of illness in critically ill patients. The increase in plasma catecholamines in critical illness may function in concert with other counterregulatory hormones to mediate some of the hemodynamic and metabolic alterations characteristic of stress (53), although the degree of correlation between plasma catecholamine concentrations and cardiac effects is unclear (156). Thus, endogenous catecholamine responses to critical illness influence the net hemodynamic response (pharmacodynamics) of exogenously administered catecholamines.

SPECIFIC INOTROPIC AGENTS

Epinephrine

PHARMACOLOGY

As noted previously, epinephrine is an important endogenous hormone (Fig. 12.1) that is largely produced and released from the adrenal gland in response to stress. The direct cardiac effects of epinephrine are mediated through β_1-adrenergic receptors. Epinephrine shortens systole more than diastole, in part by increasing conduction through the atrioventricular (AV) node and Purkinje system. It accelerates transmission through the SA node directly, and accelerates ectopic foci. Although epinephrine therapy may increase coronary blood flow, particularly in patients with coronary artery disease, epinephrine often increases myocardial oxygen demand more than oxygen delivery so that a mismatch occurs (127). In addition, it decreases the refractory period of ventricular muscle, predisposing the myocardium to arrhythmias.

When epinephrine is infused, its hemodynamic actions are determined by the infusion rate: at low rates (0.005–0.02 μg/kg/minute in adults) epinephrine principally stimulates β-

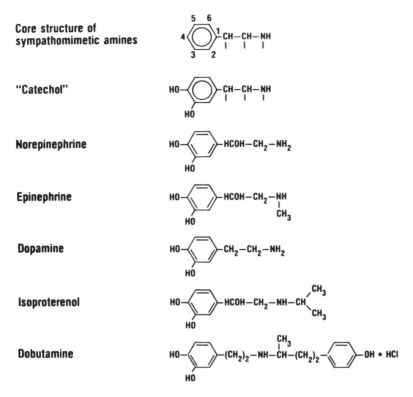

Figure 12.1. Chemical structure of the catecholamines. (From Chernow B, Rainey TG, Lake CR: Endogenous and exogenous catecholamines in critical care medicine. *Crit Care Med* 10:409–416, 1982.)

adrenergic receptors, resulting in peripheral vasodilation and increased heart rate and contractility. The net hemodynamic effects are to widen the pulse pressure, decrease systemic and pulmonary vascular resistance, and increase stroke volume, left ventricular stroke work, and cardiac output, provided that the patient's circulating blood volume is adequate. As the infusion rate is increased, more α-adrenergic mediated effects are seen, resulting in increased systemic vascular resistance, elevation of blood pressure, and variable effects on cardiac output (the latter action is dependent on the myocardium's ability to maintain stroke volume as afterload is increased).

Similar epinephrine-induced actions are seen in pediatric patients, although the dosage ranges are substantially different (based on infusion rate/weight). Thus, infusions up to 0.3 μg/kg/minute in infants and children often produce a predominant β-adrenergic effect with little evidence of increased systemic vascular resistance.

Epinephrine has important effects on the respiratory system. Activation of β_2-adrenergic receptors in bronchial smooth muscle results in bronchodilation, which combined with an inhibition of mast cell degranulation (mediated through β-2-adrenergic stimulation) has beneficial effects in asthma (7). Epinephrine is particularly important in the asthmatic patient since sympathetic nervous innervation of bronchial smooth muscle is scant (83), and, therefore, β-adrenergic mediated bronchodilation is largely determined by the amount of circulating epinephrine (148).

Epinephrine is a potent renal artery vasoconstrictor that limits its usefulness in patients with shock. Infusions as low as 0.035 μg/kg/minute induce a 10% fall in renal plasma flow in humans (60). A portion of epinephrine's vasoconstrictive effect is also probably mediated by increased renin activity following direct stimulation of β-adrenergic receptors of the juxtaglomerular apparatus (69). The net effect is to reduce renal blood flow and urine output. Despite these limitations, in patients with low cardiac output, epinephrine may increase urine output by increasing cardiac output and therefore renal blood flow (33).

Infusion of epinephrine to achieve plasma concentrations seen with exercise or stress causes plasma glucose, lactate, β-hydroxybutyrate, and free fatty acid concentrations to rise (31, 131), and serum potassium (22, 141) and phosphorus (18) concentrations to fall. The former are mediated by increased gluconeogenesis from the liver (131), skeletal muscle insulin resistance (13), and inhibition of insulin release (31). Epinephrine concentrations up to 1000 pg/ml do not alter plasma alanine, glucagon, growth hormone, or cortisol levels (31). Epinephrine-induced hypokalemia occurs through a β_2-adrenergic mechanism; mean plasma potassium falls 0.8 mEq/liter in response to epinephrine concentrations achieved during myocardial infarction (22, 141). Coincident with the decline in potassium, T-wave flattening and QT$_c$ prolongation were observed (141). These electrophysiologic effects in combination with epinephrine-induced hypokalemia may predispose the critically ill patient to serious dysrhythmias. Similar decreases in plasma potassium are seen with the use of other β_2-agonists, such as agents used in asthma or to inhibit labor (80).

INDICATIONS AND DOSE

Epinephrine infusions are most frequently used in pediatric patients; in adults, their potential toxicity in patients with coronary artery disease limits their utility. The recommended infusion rate in adults to produce principally a β-adrenergic effect is 0.005–0.02 μg/kg/minute (27). In pediatric patients, infusion rates of 0.05–0.3 μg/kg/minute are recommended in the treatment of cardiogenic or septic shock (160). Epinephrine may be particularly useful when combined with afterload reduction in cardiogenic shock, (10) and is preferable to dopamine in pediatric patients in whom catecholamine stores may be depleted (see "Dopamine", Table 12.2).

In the treatment of acute asthma, epinephrine may be administered subcutaneously in a dose of 0.01 mg/kg, up to 0.3 mg every 15–20 minutes. It is also administered subcutaneously in the treatment of acute allergic, local reactions (e.g., to bee stings), and may be administered intravenously (5–10 ml of the 1:10,000 solution) in the treatment of anaphylaxis. In cardiac arrest, epinephrine is the most effective pharmacologic agent (see Chapter 10) and may be administered intravenously (0.01 mg/kg) or endotracheally.

ADMINISTRATION AND TOXICITY

Epinephrine (adrenaline) is available in several forms: prediluted in syringes (1:10,000 concentration; 0.1 mg/ml) for use in cardiac arrest and anaphylaxis and in vials for subcutaneous administration (1-ml vials) and the preparation of intravenous infusions (30-ml vials) Tables 12.3 and 12.4).

The pharmacokinetics of epinephrine have been examined in a number of studies but always in normal adult volunteers (14, 31). Epinephrine is rapidly cleared from the plasma at mean rates of 35–89 ml/kg/minute, depending on the site of sampling and the rate of epinephrine infusion (14, 31). Clearance is largely by the liver and kidney, which contain

Table 12.2
Suggested Uses of Catecholamines by Age[a]

Condition	Infant	Child	Adult
Cardiogenic shock	EPI or Dobut DA[a]	Dobut DA or EPI	Dobut or DA EPI NE
Septic shock	EPI or Dobut DA	Dobut EPI or DA	Dobut or DA NE or EPI
Hypovolemic shock	Not Indicated	Not Indicated	Not Indicated
Shock from bradycardia	EPI or ISO	EPI or ISO	ISO or EPI
Anaphylactic shock	EPI	EPI	EPI
Decreased renal blood flow or urine output	DA	DA	DA

DA, dopamine; EPI, epinephrine; Dobut, dobutamine; NE, norepinephrine; ISO, isoproterenol.
[a] Listed in order of preference.
[b] DA at low infusion rates (1 to 2 μg/kg/minutes) may be used in combination with other catecholamines in shock to help maintain renal blood flow. DA is relatively contraindicated in patients with pulmonary artery hypertension.
From Zaritsky A, Eisenberg MG: Ontogenetic considerations in the pharmacotherapy of shock. In Chernow B, Shoemaker WC (eds): *Critical Care: State of the Art*, vol. 7. Fullerton, CA, Society of Critical Care Medicine, 1986, pp 485–534.

Table 12.3
Prescribing Infusions of Synthetic Catecholamines: Deriving Concentrations

Catecholamine	How Supplied	Diluent	Concentration
Epinephrine (Adrenalin chloride)	1 mg (1 ml) dosette ampules of 1:1000 epi; also in 30-ml vial of 1 mg/ml[a]	250 ml of either D$_5$W or 0.9% NaCl	4 μg/ml
Norepinephrine (Noradrenaline)	4-mg ampule of NE bitartrate; each ampule has 4 ml of fluid with 1 mg NE/ml[a]	250 ml of either D$_5$W, 0.9% NaCl or 0.45% NaCl	16 μg/ml
Dopamine	200-mg ampules (5 ml) of dopamine HCl (40 mg/ml); also available in 400-mg (10 ml) prefilled syringe.[a,b]	250 ml of D$_5$W or 0.9% NaCl	800 μg/ml
Dobutamine	250-mg lyophilized vials of dobutamine HCl which also contain 250 mg of mannitol; reconstitute with 10–20 ml of sterile water or D$_5$W; also in premixed solution– 400 mg/5 ml.[a,b]	250 ml of either D$_5$W or 0.9% NaCl	1000 μg/ml
Isoproterenol	1-mg ampule of 1:5000 isoproterenol HCL; each ampule has 1 mg/5 ml of fluid[a]	250 ml of either D$_5$W or 0.9% NaCl	4 μg/ml

[a] Protect ampules from light.
[b] Avoid use with alkaline solutions.

substantial concentrations of the enzymes catechol-O-methyl transferase and monoamine oxidase (78). This clearance results in a short half-life (about 2 minutes), which requires a continuous infusion to maintain hemodynamic effects. Perhaps more important is the degree of interindividual variation in epinephrine clearance reported in normal adults. In critical illness, greater variation in clearance would be expected, emphasizing the importance of individual titration of the infusion rate.

Epinephrine is also well absorbed from the tracheobronchial tree, although the plasma concentration and hemodynamic effects are about 1/10 those seen with a similar dose given intravenously (25). Endotracheal administration is reserved for patients in cardiac arrest or severe anaphylaxis in whom vascular access is not readily available. To improve absorption by this route, it is important to deliver the drug deeply into the airway, which may be accomplished by administration through a small feeding tube or other suitable catheter followed by flushing with air and manual hyperventilation (62, 116).

Epinephrine should preferably be administered through a central venous line, or at least a secure peripheral catheter, since infiltration from peripheral venous administration can result in local ulceration. If infiltration occurs and is recognized early, local injection of the site with 5–10 ml of phentolamine in 10–15 ml of saline may be effective. The epinephrine infusion rate should be controlled by a constant infusion pump to avoid inadvertent boluses. Epinephrine is compatible with a number of intravenous solutions (Table 12.3);

Table 12.4
Preparation of Catecholamine Infusions in Children

Catecholamine	Preparation	Dose
Isoproterenol Epinephrine Norepinephrine	0.6 mg × body weight (kg), added to diluent to make 100 ml	Then 1 ml/hr delivers 0.1 μg/kg/min
Dopamine Dobutamine	6 mg × body weight (kg), added to diluent to make 100 ml	Then 1 ml/hr delivers 1 μg/kg/minute

From Zaritsky A, Chernow B: Use of catecholamines in pediatrics. *J Pediatr* 105:341–350, 1984.

alkaline solutions should be avoided as diluents for epinephrine and other catecholamines that are inactivated at the higher pH.

Epinephrine-induced toxicities include restlessness, fear, throbbing headache, tachycardia, tachydysrhythmias (PVCs, ventricular tachycardia, and ventricular fibrillation), severe hypertension with secondary cerebral hemorrhage, and anginal pain resulting from an increase in myocardial oxygen demand relative to myocardial oxygen delivery.

Norepinephrine

PHARMACOLOGY

Norepinephrine is the neurotransmitter of the sympathetic nervous system and is the biosynthetic precursor of epinephrine, differing only by a methyl group on its amino terminus (Fig. 12.1). It possesses both α- and β-adrenergic receptor activity; low-infusion doses produce mainly β-adrenergic effects: cardiac contractility, conduction velocity, and chronotropy increase with little change in peripheral vascular resistance. More commonly, in the doses used during hypotensive shock, mixed α- and β-adrenergic effects occur. Peripheral vascular resistance is increased by α_1-adrenergic mediated vasoconstriction. Cardiac contractility, cardiac work and stroke volume all increase if the augmentation in afterload is tolerated by the ventricle. Chronotropy is generally blunted by baroreceptor-mediated vagal effects to slow the heart rate in response to norepinephrine-induced increase in blood pressure.

As with epinephrine, norepinephrine is a potent renal and splanchnic vasoconstrictor, which limits its clinical usefulness (63). It vasoconstricts the pulmonary as well as the systemic vascular bed and should be used with caution in patients with pulmonary artery hypertension. Norepinephrine infusion at 5.0 μg/minute in normal adults elevates blood glucose, glycerol, β-hydroxybutyrate, and acetoacetate (130); the metabolic effects of infusions in critical illness have not been reported.

INDICATIONS AND DOSE

Norepinephrine has limited usefulness in critically ill patients; its major indication is to elevate blood pressure in hypotensive patients who have failed to respond to adequate volume resuscitation and other, less potent, inotropes. The most frequent clinical condition generating this state is septic shock, and norepinephrine can help maintain perfusion pressure in this setting (29).

Norepinephrine may also be useful in myocardial infarction shock, since the major determinant of myocardial oxygen delivery is the diastolic blood pressure–left ventricular end diastolic pressure gradient (105). The goal should be to increase mean arterial pressure to 70–80 torr, at which time coronary blood flow improves (105). Use of a potent vasoconstrictor must be balanced against the increase in ventricular afterload, which heightens myocardial oxygen demand; therefore, norepinephrine should only be considered a temporizing measure. Intraaortic balloon counterpulsation is one of therapeutic approaches that is supplanting norepinephrine in hypotensive, cardiogenic shock patients since it has the advantage of both increasing diastolic coronary perfusion and decreasing ventricular afterload.

An additional concern with norepinephrine is renal vasoconstriction compromising renal function. Low-dose dopamine ameliorates the vasoconstrictive action of norepinephrine in dogs. (126). The clinical combination of dopamine and norepinephrine may therefore provide both the desired increase in coronary perfusion pressure and the maintenance of adequate renal function.

Initial norepinephrine infusion rate of 2 μg/minute is typical and is subsequently increased until the desired change in blood pressure is achieved. In pediatric patients, norepinephrine infusions may be prepared as seen in Table 12.4; initial infusion rates are 0.05–0.1 μg/kg/minute and are subsequently titrated up to 1.0 μg;/kg/minute.

ADMINISTRATION AND TOXICITY

Norepinephrine bitartrate (Levophed bitartrate) is available in 4-ml ampules of 1 mg/ml (Table 12.3). Intravenous infusions are constituted by adding 4 mg of norepinephrine to 250 or 500 ml of 5% dextrose in water or normal saline, which produces final concentrations of 16 or 8 μg/ml, respectfully. Norepinephrine is rapidly cleared from the plasma following intravenous administration; its average half-life is 2–2.5 minutes, although substantial interindividual variation has been noted (50). Norepinephrine is cleared by enzymatic degradation in the liver and kidney and by uptake and degradation in neuronal and nonneuronal effecter organ sites.

Norepinephrine infusions should preferably be given through a central vein. Careful monitoring of arterial pressure, perfusion, and renal function is necessary during norepinephrine infusions to prevent organ ischemia and excessive increases in ventricular afterload. Inadvertent boluses may precipitate profound hypertension, which may result in myocardial infarction or cerebral hemorrhage (150). Infiltrated infusions may produce local skin necrosis and ulceration, and if recognized early should be treated with phentolamine injuction (see "toxicity" under "Epinephrine"). Anxiety, respiratory difficulty, palpitations, angina, and transient headaches also occur.

Norepinephrine may also be added to gastric lavage solutions used in the treatment of acute gastrointestinal bleeding, with 16 mg of norepinephrine added to 200 ml of iced saline (40).

Isoproterenol

PHARMACOLOGY

Isoproterenol is a synthetic, N-alkylated catecholamine similar in structure to epinephrine (Fig. 12.1). It is a potent β-adrenergic agonist and therefore has potent effects on the heart; it stimulates an increase in cardiac contractility, heart rate, and conduction velocity. It also shortens arteriovenous nodal conduction and may incite either ventricular or atrial dysrhythmias. Stimulation of peripheral β_2-adrenergic receptors results in vascular smooth muscle relaxation, while systemic vascular resistance and diastolic blood pressure fall. Since β_2-adrenergic vascular receptors are most prevalent in the skeletal muscle vascular bed, cardiac output may be redirected from the splanchnic bed to the skeletal muscle bed producing a "splanchnic steal" (65).

The net hemodynamic effect produced by isoproterenol infusion is an increase in cardiac output, provided circulating blood volume is adequate. When circulating blood volume is low, vasodilation may impair venous return and cardiac output may fall. Pulse pressure increases because of a rise in systolic pressure generated by enhanced cardiac contractility and the fall in diastolic blood pressure mediated by peripheral vasodilation. Much of the increase in cardiac output is often related to the change in heart rate, rather than an increase in stroke volume, particularly in pediatric patients (43, 65).

Isoproterenol also relaxes pulmonary vascular and bronchial airway smooth muscle; pulmonary vascular resistance falls and bronchospasm may be reversed. By overcoming hypoxic pulmonary vasoconstriction, isoproterenol can increase intrapulmonary shunt and may result in a fall in arterial oxygen tension when used in patients with parenchymal lung disease.

Since heart rate and contractility are increased, myocardial oxygen demand is enhanced. At the same time, isoproterenol-induced decreases in diastolic filling time and diastolic coronary perfusion pressure may impair myocardial oxygen supply, which results in myocardial ischemia (104).

Isoproterenol does not produce the same degree of hyperglycemia as epinephrine, probably because β-adrenergic stimulation enhances insulin release, whereas α_2-adrenergic stimulation seen with epinephrine inhibits insulin release (114).

INDICATIONS AND DOSE

Once a popular inotrope, isoproterenol has fallen out of favor because of its propensity to produce myocardial ischemia and excessive tachycardia and because more selective inotropes are available. Isoproterenol may be used to treat hemodynamically significant bradycardia, particularly in the setting of heart block but should only be considered a temporizing measure until more definitive therapy, such as cardiac pacing, is obtained (135). In bradycardic pediatric patients, low-dose epinephrine infusion may be useful and has the advantage of maintaining diastolic coronary perfusion pressure better than isoproterenol.

Isoproterenol has been effective in pediatric patients with status asthmaticus (41) and those with pulmonary artery hypertension (100). Indeed, isoproterenol has been used to help assess the reversibility of pulmonary hypertension in pediatric patients prior to surgery in certain forms of congenital heart disease, as well as to reduce pulmonary artery pressure in the postoperative period (92, 100). Finally, isoproterenol may be used as an inotrope, although other agents that have fewer side effects are available. In adults with coronary artery disease, isoproterenol should be avoided since myocardial ischemia is likely (104).

Infusions are usually begun at 0.01 μg/kg/minute and are adjusted to produce the desired hemodynamic effect. In pediatric patients, infusions may be conveniently prepared as seen in Table 12.4. Initial infusion rates are 0.05–0.1 μg/kg/minute. As with other catecholamines, infusions should be administered through a secure intravenous line using a calibrated infusion pump, and the patient's heart rate and blood pressure should be carefully monitored.

ADMINISTRATION AND TOXICITY

The parenteral form of isoproterenol (Isuprel HCl) is available in 5-ml vials containing 1 mg (1:5,000 solution; Table 12.3). For adults, one vial (1 mg) is added to 250 ml of saline or D_5W giving a concentration of 4μgml.

After intravenous administration, isoproterenol is rapidly cleared from the plasma; it has a half-life of about 2 minutes (57). It is largely cleared in the liver and to a lesser extent it is taken up by effecter organs throughout the body. It is also well absorbed from the tracheobronchial tree and is thus available in an aerosol form for treatment of asthma, although more selective β-2-adrenergic agonists, such as metaproterenol and albuterol, have largely replaced aerosolized isoproterenol.

The major side effects of isoproterenol are tachycardia and tachydysrhythmias, particularly ventricular tachycardia. As noted previously, angina and myocardial infarction may result from the unfavorable action of isoproterenol on myocardial oxygen demand relative to oxygen delivery (104, 105), and has been reported in pediatric patients treated for status asthmaticus (81). Palpitation, headache, and flushing of the skin are common; whereas nausea, tremor, dizziness, and weakness are less common side effects.

Dopamine

PHARMACOLOGY

Dopamine is the immediate precursor of norepinephrine in the endogenous catecholamine biosynthetic pathway and differs from norepinephrine by the absence of a β-hydroxyl group (Fig. 12.1). Dopamine also serves as a neurotransmitter in both the central and peripheral nervous systems (82). In the latter, it appears to modulate autonomic activity at sympathetic ganglia, alter gastrointestinal activity, decrease aldosterone synthesis, and release (134) and increase renal blood flow (38, 82). When infused in pharmacologic concentrations, dopamine has complex actions because of its mixed direct and indirect sympathomimetic actions.

Unlike the other catecholamines, dopamine's hemodynamic effects are attributed to dopamine-stimulated release of norepinephrine from sympathetic nerves, as well as direct stimulation of α-, β- and DA receptors (42, 55). Pretreatment of dogs with reserpine to deplete endogenous norepinephrine stores suggests that as much as 50% of dopamine's hemodynamic action may be produced by norepinephrine release (42). In clinical studies, dopamine infusions increase plasma norepinephrine in a dose-dependent manner (77), and dopamine's hemodynamic effect is less pronounced than that observed with a direct-acting catecholamine, such as dobutamine, in clinical conditions characterized by myocardial norepinephrine depletion (30, 90).

When infused at 2–5 μg/kg/minute in normal subjects, dopamine increases cardiac contractility and cardiac output with little change in heart rate, blood pressure, or systemic vascular resistance (54, 55). Doses up to 10 μg/kg/minute in normal subjects further increase cardiac output, with small increases in heart rate and blood pressure (54). Renal blood flow and urine output increase at doses of 0.5–2.0 μg/kg/minute secondary to selective action at dopaminergic receptors (85); sodium excretion is enhanced by the increase in renal flow and dopamine-mediated inhibition of proximal tubular sodium reabsorption (112). Further improvement in renal function may occur at higher infusions rate related to improved global cardiac output. At infusion rates in excess of 10 μg/kg/minute an increasing α-adrenergic effect may be seen with increases in systemic vascular resistance and subsequently mean arterial pressure (122). The salutary effect of dopamine on renal blood flow may be lost at higher doses due to predominant α-adrenergic effects. (55).

In patients with pulmonary hypertension, dopamine infusions may lead to further increases in mean pulmonary artery pressure (67, 136), and dopamine enhances hypoxic pulmonary vasoconstriction (100). In the absence of pulmonary hypertension, dopamine increases pulmonary blood flow with little change in mean pulmonary artery pressure or pulmonary capillary wedge pressure (55). Dopamine constricts capacitance veins that may raise pulmonary capillary wedge pressure (84, 96); serious consequences may then result by increasing myocardial wall tension, and therefore myocardial oxygen demand, and by worsening hydrostatic pulmonary edema. (90).

Dopamine has several metabolic effects that may be important in the critically ill patient. Dopamine receptors located in the zona glomerulosa of the adrenal cortex decrease aldosterone secretion (151). Conversely, dopamine receptor blockade (for example, following the administration of metoclopramide) increases plasma aldosterone concentration (24). Dopamine inhibits thyroid-stimulating hormone (TSH) and prolactin release (157); the former blunts the response to thyroxine-releasing hormone (TRH), making discrimination between the patient with hypothyrodism and the one with the euthyroid-sick syndrome more difficult. Insulin secretion is also inhibited by a direct action of dopamine on pancreatic islet cells (161), although the clinical importance of this effect during dopamine infusion is unclear.

INDICATIONS AND DOSE

In cardiogenic shock due to myocardial infarction, a mean dopamine infusion rate of 17.2 μg/kg/minute was required to raise mean arterial pressure to 65–70 torr (106). In this study, dopamine infusion also increased heart rate, mean arterial pressure and cardiac index, and decreased pulmonary capillary wedge pressure (PCWP), central venous pressure (CVP), and systemic vascular resistance (SVR). Myocardial oxygen extraction significantly increased along with lactate production, indicating that the improvement in cardiac performance was at the expense of an increase in myocardial oxygen demand. Holzer et al. (68) also studied dopamine administration in cardiogenic shock. Survivors had improved cardiac output, urinary flow, PCWP, and heart rate at mean infusions of 9.1 μg/kg/minute, whereas nonsurvivors failed to show beneficial effects at mean infusion rates of 17.1 μg/kg/minute. Nonresponse to dopamine may have been because these patients were more acidotic.

Combined administration of dopamine and dobutamine may have advantages over the administration of either agent alone in cardiogenic shock (121). Dopamine alone (15 μg/kg/minute) consistently increased mean arterial pressure but also increased PCWP, had variable effects on stroke index, and reduced PaO_2. Dobutamine alone (15 μg/kg/minute) failed to increase mean arterial pressure, but

more consistently improved stroke volume. The combination of dopamine and dobutamine (7.5 μg/kg/minute each) had the most beneficial effects: mean arterial pressure, cardiac index, and stroke volume index all increased with no change in PCWP, mean pulmonary artery pressure, or PaO_2 (121). All three infusion combinations increased intrapulmonary shunt. This effect is common to inotropes that increase cardiac output, and is due to improved perfusion of poorly ventilated lung segments (72). Dopamine, however, caused hypoxemia, probably due to an increase in PCWP (90).

As in cardiogenic shock, dobutamine is superior to dopamine in chronic heart failure (90). Based on animal studies, dopamine's inotropic response is attenuated because myocardial norepinephrine stores are depleted in chronic cardiac failure (30). In addition, dopamine loses its inotropic effect after 24 hours of infusion in experimental myocardial infarction, presumably because of depletion of myocardial norepinephrine stores, and dopamine accentuates myocardial norepinephrine release, which may more rapidly deplete stores (93). Dopamine does not influence infarct size (6, 93), whereas dobutamine decreases the area of ischemic infarction (93).

After coronary artery bypass grafting, dopamine has frequently been used to support the circulation. Dopamine had increasing inotropic action during a 24-hour observation period after bypass graft (143), unlike the response seen in experimental myocardial infarction (93). Despite this beneficial effect, when compared with dobutamine, dopamine produces a relatively smaller enhancement of left ventricular contractility and it increases myocardial oxygen demand (142). Differences in the hemodynamic response to dopamine and dobutamine in the postoperative period may be related to the state of the ventricle (39). In normal ventricles, dobutamine had a greater chronotropic response; in volume-loaded ventricles, both drugs had similar effects on heart rate and cardiac output, but dobutamine caused a greater reduction in systemic vascular resistance and pulmonary vascular resistance (39). Neither agent (at 5 μg/kg/minutes) produces a hemodynamic effect in the pressure-loaded ventricle. Dobutamine appears to be superior to dopamine in the postoperative period.

In septic shock, dopamine is effective in improving cardiac output, although intrapulmonary shunting may increase as well (119). The latter can be prevented by the application of positive end-expiratory pressure (PEEP) (119). Since many septic patients are hypotensive, dopamine has the advantage of increasing systemic vascular resistance, and therefore blood pressure, and may be preferable over dobutamine in this clinical setting (153). An additional advantage of dopamine is its beneficial effect on urine output (37). Despite these advantages, dopamine has the disadvantage of increasing PCWP and pulmonary artery pressure in septic patients (37, 119).

Dopamine's major clinical benefit is that it causes a selective increase in renal and splanchnic blood flow. A low-dose infusion (1–4 μg/kg/minute) augments urine output following cardiopulmonary bypass (36), and in patients with oliguria and critical illness (111). Dopamine may also antagonize the vasoconstrictive action of norepinephrine and other adrenergic vasoconstrictors (126). In experimental studies, it improves blood flow and protein synthesis in the postischemic liver (66).

In pediatric patients, the pharmacodynamic effects of dopamine are further complicated by ontogenetic changes in response (158). In experimental animal studies, the more immature the animal, the smaller the relative hemodynamic response compared with adults (23, 42). Clinical studies reveal more consistent salutary effects of dopamine in premature neonates: infusions of 0.5–2 μg/kg/minute improve urine output, sodium excretion, and creatinine clearance (144), and dose-dependent improvement in blood pressure and cardiac output is seen at infusion rates between 2–8 μg/kg/minute (110). Recommendations for the use of dopamine and other catecholamines in pediatric patients are seen in Table 12.2.

Infusion rates of 0.5–2 μg/kg/minute result in selective dopaminergic actions on the renal and splanchnic vasculature. With infusion rates between 5–10 μg/kg/minute β-adrenergic effects usually dominate: infusions between 10–20 μg/kg/minute have mixed α- and β-adrenergic effects, whereas infusions in excess of 20 μg/kg/minute have predominant α-adrenergic effects.

ADMINISTRATION AND TOXICITY

Dopamine is available in a number of commercial formulations (Table 12.3). In adults, 200 mg may be diluted in 250 ml of diluent (e.g., D_5W), producing a final dopamine concentration of 800 μg/ml. In pediatric patients, infusions are prepared as seen in Table 12.4.

As with other catecholamines, dopamine should not be mixed in an alkaline solution.

After intravenous administration, dopamine is rapidly cleared from the plasma by a biphasic process and has a terminal elimination half-life of 9 minutes. Steady state plasma clearance of dopamine (50–70 ml/kg/minute) is similar in both adults and infants (73, 110).

Nausea, emesis, and tachyarrhythmias are the most frequent side effects (64). Anginal pain, myocardial ischemia (93), serious hypertension, and profound vasoconstriction may occur (56, 93). In patients dependent on hypoxic ventilatory drive, dopamine may depress ventilation and worsen hypoxemia (108).

Dobutamine

PHARMACOLOGY

Dobutamine was developed after the catecholamine molecule was systematically modified in the search for an agent that would have selective inotropic activity with little peripheral vascular effect (145). Dobutamine has a large substitution on the amino terminus of the catecholamine molecule (Fig. 31.1), and it is the only catecholamine administered as a racemic mixture of the (+)- and (−)- isomers. This racemic mixture provides dobutamine with its characteristic β_1-adrenergic selectivity: the (−)-isomer is an α-adrenergic agonist and the (+)-isomer acts as a competitive α-adrenergic receptor antagonist (125). The (+)-isomer is also the more potent form at the β-adrenergic receptor, although both isomers produce inotropic and chronotropic actions (125).

Dobutamine's hemodynamic effect is dependent on drug dose. At the usual infusion rates (5–15 μg/kg/minute) dobutamine's predominant effect is on the heart with an increase in contractility and a relatively smaller increase in heart rate. Dobutamine's comparatively selective inotropic action is probably multifactorial and attributed partly to the presence of both β_1- and β_2-adrenergic receptors in the sinoatrial node, which produce chronotropic effects, and dobutamine's higher affinity for the β_1-adrenergic receptor (152). Attenuated α-adrenergic effects in the peripheral vasculature are further balanced by a modest β_2-adrenergic effect so that peripheral vascular resistance is little changed (88). Dobutamine generally lowers central venous and pulmonary wedge pressure and has little effect on pulmonary vascular resistance. Like other inotropes, dobutamine can increase intrapulmonary shunt by augmenting cardiac output and thus perfusion of poorly ventilated lung regions (71).

Dobutamine does not have a selective vascular action, and significant metabolic side effects have not been reported. Although it lacks a selective renal vascular effect, dobutamine often enhances urine output by improving cardiac output and thus renal perfusion (87).

Unlike dopamine, dobutamine's pharmacologic action does not depend upon releasable stores of norepinephrine (125). Dobutamine loses its hemodynamic effect during prolonged infusion (146), presumably because of downregulation of receptors, but dobutamine maintains its hemodynamic effect much better than dopamine during continuous infusion since the latter depletes myocardial norepinephrine stores (97).

INDICATIONS AND DOSE

Dobutamine is indicated in clinical conditions where increased contractility with little effect on peripheral vascular resistance is desired. This setting most often occurs in normotensive patients with congestive heart failure (88). In patients with congestive heart failure, dobutamine increases stroke volume and cardiac output, while reducing the elevated filling pressure accompanying this clinical state (5, 87). When used in lower dosages (2–10 μg/kg/minute), little change in heart rate is seen (88). In patients with very poor myocardial function and higher baseline plasma norepinephrine concentrations, however, dobutamine's effect on cardiac index is attenuated (34).

In patients with myocardial failure and nonobstructed coronary arteries, dobutamine improves coronary blood flow and myocardial oxygen supply equal to, or in excess of, the increase in myocardial oxygen demand elicited by its positive inotropic action (94). Supplementation of myocardial perfusion may partly explain dobutamine's ability to produce sustained improvement of cardiac function in patients with congestive heart failure following short-term infusions (89). In one study, a 72-hour dobutamine infusion improved endomyocardial ATP/creatinine ratio and the ultrastructural appearance of mitochondria (147).

Dobutamine generally improves the balance between myocardial oxygen supply and demand in patients with myocardial failure resulting from coronary artery disease (88). Patients with myocardial infarction also benefit from dobutamine infusion, even those having hypotension prior to therapy (76, 120). Patients with hypotensive cardiogenic shock, however, may not be improved by dobutamine since it has relatively less peripheral vascular action, and dopamine may be superior in this setting (52, 88).

In postoperative cardiovascular surgical patients, dobutamine improves stroke volume and decreases ventricular filling pressures with less positive chronotropy than observed with dopamine (61). In addition, dobutamine has a more beneficial effect on myocardial blood flow than dopamine (51). In patients following a heart transplant, myocardial sympathetic innervation is destroyed. Since dobutamine's inotropic action does not depend on myocardial stores of norepinephrine, it should be a better inotrope than dopamine, and indeed this finding has been observed (46).

Because dobutamine lacks clinically important vasoconstrictive effects, it may be disadvantageous in the patient with septic shock and hypotension. Dobutamine should ideally be reserved for septic patients with combined ventricular dysfunction and elevated filling pressures (71, 88).

Dobutamine is also a useful inotropic agent in pediatric patients with a variety of clinical conditions: cardiovascular failure (128), postoperative cardiovascular surgery (11), and septic shock (113). Clinical studies suggest that dobutamine is most useful in children >12 months of age since the cardiac index in younger patients failed to increase and PCWP rose in response to 10 μg/kg/minute of dobutamine (113). Depending on the clinical state, dobutamine-induced increases in cardiac index may be entirely due to increases in heart rate with little change in stroke volume (11, 19).

Initial infusion rates of dobutamine are the same in adult and pediatric patients: 2–5 μg/kg/minute. Maximal beneficial effects are generally observed with 10–15 μg/kg/minute; higher infusion rates increase the risk of drug-induced toxicity (88).

ADMINISTRATION AND TOXICITY

Dobutamine (Dobutrex) is supplied in 250-mg vials (Table 12.3). One vial is usually diluted into 250 ml of an appropriate diluent, achieving a final drug concentration of 1000 μg/ml. A good correlation exists between dobutamine dose, plasma concentration, and hemodynamic effects (88). Dobutamine is rapidly cleared and has a plasma half-life of 2.37 ± 0.7 minutes in patients with congestive heart failure (75). The drug is cleared by catechol-O-methyl transferase and rapid redistribution from the plasma compartment.

With drug infusion, steady state plasma concentration is achieved in about five half-lives, thus like the other catecholamines, maximal effect is seen approximately 10 minutes after starting or changing the infusion rate. As with the other catecholamines, dobutamine should preferably be administered into a central venous site using a continuous infusion pump.

Dysrhythmias are the most frequent toxic side effect, although they are less frequent than with dopamine or isoproterenol (132). Other side effects include excessive tachycardia, headaches, anxiety, tremors, and excessive increases or decreases in blood pressure (88).

Amrinone and Milrinone

PHARMACOLOGY

The bipyridine, amrinone, was discovered in the search for positive inotropic drugs with a better therapeutic/toxic ratio than digoxin. Amrinone possesses positive inotropic and, to a lesser extent, chronotropic actions on the heart and has potent vasodilator properties (3, 47). Amrinone has recently been approved by the Food and Drug Administration (FDA) for intravenous administration but is not useful orally. Milrinone is a methyl carbonitrile derivative of amrinone that is orally effective and produces few side effects. The addition of a methyl group to the carbon-3 atom (Fig. 12.2) greatly increases the efficacy of the compound. Based on studies in isolated animal hearts, milrinone is 10–30 times more potent than amrinone (4).

Pharmacologically, these compounds differ from the catecholamines and the cardiac glycosides. They possess a unique structure, unlike any of the other inotropic agents (Fig. 12.2). Although their mechanism of action is still not completely understood, they do not stimulate either α- or β-adrenergic receptors nor provoke the release of either histamine or prostaglandins (1, 2). Unlike cardiac glycosides, the bipyridines do not inhibit cell membrane sodium-potassium ATPase (1, 2) but do share a similar pharmacologic action with methylxanthines (3); both inhibit phosphodiesterase resulting in an increase in intracellu-

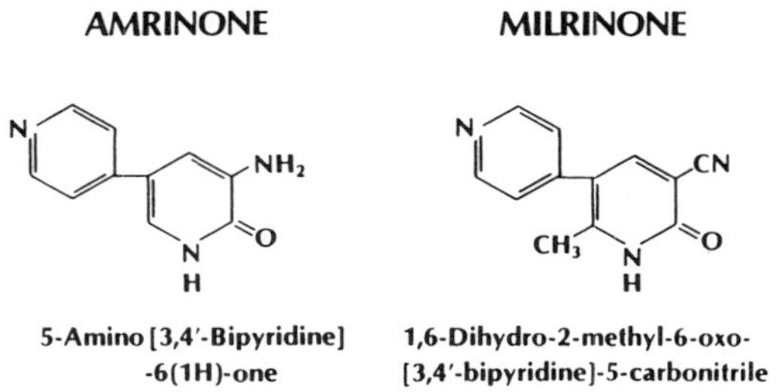

Figure 31.2. Chemical structure of amrinone and milrinone.

lar cyclic AMP (cAMP), although it is unlikely that the inotropic action of the bipyridines is simply due to phosphodiesterase inhibition (3). Finally, like most other inotropic agents, the bipyridine's inotropic action is characterized by an increase in intracellular calcium concentration (102), which can be attenuated by pretreatment with calcium channel blockers (3). Unlike catecholamines and other drugs whose inotropic effect is mediated only by increasing cAMP concentration, amrinone also appears to prolong the release and/or delay the reuptake of calcium by the sarcoplasmic reticulum (102).

Amrinone increases cAMP concentrations in vascular smooth muscle, relaxing tone (99) and thus decreasing peripheral and pulmonary vascular resistance, and dilating coronary vessels (157). Based on studies in isolated tissue, the potency of these drugs in vascular tissue is 10–100 times greater than their inotropic action (102).

In intact animals and humans, the bipyridines increase cardiac contractility, stroke volume, heart rate, and cardiac output. Although the bipyridines decrease systemic vascular resistance, systemic blood pressure is unchanged with low doses because the drug-induced increase in stroke volume compensates for the fall in resistance (3, 9). In the pulmonary vascular bed, pulmonary systolic and diastolic blood pressures usually decline (3, 9). The bipyridines are particularly beneficial in cardiac failure since they reduce afterload by peripheral vasodilation and increase cardiac contractility, often without an increase in myocardial oxygen consumption (8). The net hemodynamic effect is dose related: increasing doses produce greater afterload reduction and increased contractility, although with little further increase in cardiac output in intact dogs (3).

Complicating the pharmacology of amrinone

and milrinone is the observation of species-dependent and age-dependent differences in their inotropic effects (17). In newborn puppies, amrinone administration induces a significant *decrease* in both peak myocardial tension developed and the rate of myocardial tension development, which changed to a positive inotropic effect by 3 days of age and increased in magnitude thereafter (16). These effects are not a result of developmental changes in the effects of amrinone on phosphodiesterase (17). It is speculated that the observed ontogenetic differences are related to inadequate development of the T-tubule-sarcoplasmic reticulum system in the newborn (3, 86). Supporting this theory is the observation that amrinone has negative inotropic effects in adult Purkinje fibers, another tissue that lacks a T-tubular system (124).

Both amrinone and milrinone are largely eliminated by renal excretion (79); milrinone's half-life in normal volunteers is approximately 50 minutes (139) compared with 2 hours in patients with congestive heart failure (45). Even with drug-induced improvement in cardiac function, however, milrinone kinetics remain constant for up to 30 days with oral administration (45). Studies with amrinone reveal a mean half-life of 3.6 hours, with somewhat slower elimination seen in patients with congestive heart failure (5–8 hours) (44, 45). The relatively slow elimination observed in sicker patients has potential therapeutic implications since a continuous infusion (as currently recommended) of amrinone or milrinone may result in progressive increase in drug plasma concentrations over several hours.

INDICATIONS AND DOSE

Most of the clinical data on these drugs are derived from studies in either normal populations or patients with chronic congestive heart failure, and little data are available in patients with acute, critical illness.

When compared with dobutamine, milrinone has similar beneficial effects on stroke volume and cardiac output in normal subjects; a greater portion of the improved stroke volume observed with milrinone results from afterload reduction (20). In addition, milrinone decreases myocardial oxygen demand while enhancing cardiac output. Monrad and co-workers (101) compared milrinone to dobutamine and nitroprusside in patients with advanced congestive heart failure. All three drugs consistently improved cardiac output, but do-

butamine increased myocardial oxygen consumption and heart rate, whereas nitroprusside produced a much greater fall in blood pressure. Milrinone had little effect on heart rate or blood pressure; myocardial oxygen consumption was unchanged and pulmonary capillary wedge pressure was lowered (101). Sonnenblick et al. (133) demonstrated in patients with severe heart failure (left ventricular ejection fraction of 9–37%) that milrinone exhibited a moderate positive inotropic and potent vasodilating action; mean cardiac index increased from 1.75 to 2.36 liter/minute/m². Similar findings have been described with amrinone (8).

In patients with heart failure, amrinone augments dP/dt without significant changes in heart rate or blood pressure (58). Both amrinone and milrinone reduce left ventricular filling pressure, mean pulmonary artery pressure, right atrial pressure, and pulmonary and systemic vascular resistances (58, 74). The magnitude of these changes is variable depending on the underlying clinical state of the patient and the dosage regimen employed. Thus, milrinone and amrinone appear to have ideal hemodynamic properties in patients with severe heart failure: cardiac index is enhanced and filling pressure is reduced with minimal effect on myocardial oxygen demand.

Individual variation in the peripheral vascular and myocardial response makes it difficult to select the correct dose of either drug in critically ill patients. Since the half-life of amrinone and milrinone is substantially longer than that with either catecholamines or intravenous vasodilators used in cardiogenic shock, it is probably preferable to individually titrate an inotrope and vasodilator rather than use an agent, such as milrinone, that possesses both activities. By virtue of their vasodilator action, both amrinone and milrinone may also result in clinically important hypotension (74), which could compromise diastolic coronary filling in the patient with cardiogenic shock.

With the above considerations in mind, the recommended dosage for amrinone is an initial intravenous loading dose of 0.75 mg/kg over 3–5 minutes, followed by a second equal bolus 30 minutes later if required. The bolus should be followed by a continuous intravenous infusion of 5–10 μg/kg/minute with the total daily dose not exceeding 10 mg/kg (58). After an intravenous bolus, peak effects are seen in several minutes; with an intravenous infusion alone, peak effects occur at about 7 hours (58). Milrinone is not currently approved for intravenous infusion, and dosage recommendations are therefore not available.

ADMINISTRATION AND TOXICITY

Amrinone lactate (Inocor) is available as a solution of 100 mg in 20-ml vials. The drug is generally diluted in normal or half-normal saline to a concentration of 1–3 mg/ml. Glucose-containing solutions should not be used since a slow chemical interaction occurs when amrinone is mixed in dextrose. This interaction does not preclude the coinfusion of amrinone with dextrose-containing solutions using a Y-connector.

Neither drug is approved for use in infants or children, and caution against the use of amrinone in newborns is raised because of observed negative inotropic effects in neonatal puppies (15), although positive inotropic effects have been reported in lambs (95).

The relatively long half-life, and thus slow attainment of a new steady state with changes in continuous infusion rate of amrinone, make it less attractive in the critical care setting. There is no information about drug excretion in patients with renal failure, and amrinone should be used cautiously, if at all, in this population.

Several studies in adults with chronic congestive heart failure report small, statistically insignificant, increases in ventricular ectopy during long-term therapy with either amrinone or milrinone (91, 107). Thus, these agents may be safer than currently used inotropes that have much greater arrhythmogenic potential.

Intravenous amrinone produces reversible thrombocytopenia in approximately 4% of patients (79); the frequency increases with total daily doses in excess of 24 mg/kg. Elevation of liver enzymes has been reported with long-term but not short-term use (79). In addition, oral long-term therapy has produced numerous side effects, especially gastrointestinal disturbances and thrombocytopenia, which preclude its clinical use (109).

SUMMARY

The pharmacology of catecholamines and bipyridines have been reviewed in this chapter. These compounds possess potent myocardial and peripheral vascular actions that may be used in critically ill patients to maintain cardiac function and manipulate peripheral and pulmonary vascular tone. Optimal use of these potent and useful drugs requires an understanding of their pharmacology, and the influence of critical illness on the hemodynamic actions resulting from their administration. In pediatric applications, age-related changes in drug kinetics or dynamics may occur, further complicating their administration to infants and children and emphasizing the need to individually titrate the infusion rate to observed hemodynamic changes.

References

1. Alousi AA, Canter JM, Montenaro MJ, et al: Cardiotonic activity of milrinone, a new and potent cardiac bipyridine, on the normal and failing heart of experimental animals. *J Cardiovasc Pharmacol* 5:792, 1983.
2. Alousi AA, Farah AE, Lesher GY, et al: Cardiotonic activity of amrinone-Win 4080 [5-amino- 3.4'-bipyridin-6(1H)-one]. *Circ Res* 45:666, 1979.
3. Alousi AA, Johnson DC: Pharmacology of the bipyridines: amrinone and milrinone. *Circulation* 73(Suppl 3):3–10, 1986.
4. Alousi AA, Stankus GP, Stuart JC, et al: Characterization of the cardiotonic effects of milrinone, a new and potent cardiac bipyridine on isolated tissue from several animal species. *J Cardiovasc Pharmacol* 5:804, 1983.
5. Andy JJ, Curry CL, Ali N, et al: Cardiovascular effects of dobutamine in severe congestive heart failure. *Am Heart J* 94:175, 1977.
6. Arnold JMO, Braunwald E, Sandor T, et al: Inotropic stimulation of reperfused myocardium with dopamine: Effects on infarct size and myocardial function. *J Am Coll Cardiol* 6:1026, 1985.
7. Assem ESK, Schild HO: Inhibition by sympathomimetic amines of histamine release induced by antigen in passively sensitized human lung. *Nature* 224:1028, 1969.
8. Benotti JR, Grossman W, Braunwald E, et al: Effects of amrinone on myocardial energy metabolism and hemodynamics in patients with severe congestive heart failure due to coronary disease. *Circulation* 62:23, 1980.
9. Benotti JR, Grossman W, Braunwald E, et al: Hemodynamic assessment of amrinone. A new inotropic agent. *N Engl J Med* 299:1373, 1978.
10. Benzing G III, Helmsworth JA, Schreiber JT, et al: Nitroprusside and epinephrine for treatment of low output in children after open-heart surgery. *Ann Thorac Surg* 27:523, 1979.
11. Berner M, Rouge JC, Friedli B: The hemodynamic effect of phentolamine and dobutamine after open-heart operations in children: influence of the underlying heart defect. *Ann Thorac Surg* 35:644, 1983.
12. Bertel O, Buhler FR, Baitsch G, et al: Plasma adrenaline and noradrenaline in patients with acute myocardial infarction. *Chest* 82:64, 1982.
13. Bessey PQ, Brooks DC, Black PR, et al: Epinephrine acutely mediates skeletal muscle insulin resistance. *Surgery* 94:172, 1983.
14. Best JD, Halter JB: Release and clearance rates of epinephrine in man: Importance of arterial measurements. *J Clin Endocrinol Metab* 55:263, 1982.
15. Binah O, Banilo P, Rosen MR: Development changes in the effects of amrinone on cardiac contraction. *Am J Cardiol* 49:993, 1982.
16. Binah O, Legato MJ, Danilo P Jr, et al: Developmental changes in the cardiac effects of amrinone in the dog. *Circ Res* 52:747, 1983.

17. Binah O, Sodowick B, Vulliemoz Y: The inotropic effects of amrinone and milrinone on neonatal and young canine cardiac muscle. *Circulation* 73(Suppl 3):3–46, 1986.

18. Body J-J, Cryer PE, Offord KP, et al: Epinephrine is a hypophosphatemic hormone in man. *J Clin Invest* 71:572, 1983.

19. Bohn DJ, Poirier CS, Edmonds JF, et al: Hemodynamic effects of dobutamine after cardiopulmonary bypass in children. *Crit Care Med* 8:367, 1980.

20. Borow KM, Neumann A, Lang RM: Milrinone versus dobutamine: contribution of altered myocardial mechanics and augmented inotropic state to improved left ventricular performance. *Circulation* 73(Suppl 3):3–153, 1986.

21. Bristow MR, Ginsburg R, Minobe W, et al: Decreased catecholamine sensitivity and β-adrenergic receptor density in failing human hearts. *N Engl J Med* 307:205, 1982.

22. Brown MJ, Brown DC, Murphy MB: Hypokalemia from beta$_2$-receptor stimulation by circulating epinephrine. *N Engl J Med* 309:1414, 1983.

23. Buckley NM, Brazeau P, Frasier ID: Cardiovascular effects of dopamine in developing swine. *Biol Neonate* 43:50, 1983.

24. Carey RM, Thorner MO, Ortt EM: Dopaminergic inhibition of metoclopramide-induced aldosterone secretion in man. *J Clin Invest* 66:10, 1980.

25. Chernow B, Holbrook P, D'Angona DS Jr, et al: Epinephrine absorption after intratracheal administration. *Anesth Analg* 63:829, 1984.

26. Chernow B, Lake CR, Barton M, et al: Sympathetic nervous system sensitivity to hemorrhagic hypotension in the subhuman primate. *J Trauma* 24:229, 1984.

27. Chernow B, Rainey TG, Lake CR: Endogenous and exogenous catecholamines in critical care medicine. *Crit Care Med* 10:409, 1982.

28. Chernow B, Roth BL: Pharmacologic manipulation of the peripheral vasculature in shock: Clinical and experimental approaches. *Circ Shock* 18:141, 1986.

29. Chernow B, Roth BL: Pharmacologic support of the cardiovasculature in septic shock. In Sibbald WJ, Sprung CL (eds): *Perspectives on Sepsis and Septic Shock.* Fullerton, CA, Society of Critical Care Medicine, 1986, pp 173.

30. Chidsey CA, Braunwald E, Morrow AG, et al: Myocardial norepinephrine concentration in man: effects of reserpine and of congestive heart failure. *N Engl J Med* 269:653, 1963.

31. Clutter WE, Bier DM, Shah SD, et al: Epinephrine plasma metabolic clearance rates and physiologic thresholds for metabolic and hemodynamic actions in man. *J Clin Invest* 66:94, 1980.

32. Cohn JN, Levine TB, Olivari MT, et al: Plasma norepinephrine as a guide to prognosis in patients with chronic congestive heart failure. *N Engl J Med* 311:819, 1984.

33. Coffin LH Jr, Ankeney JL, Beheler EM: Experimental study and clinical use of epinephrine for treatment of low cardiac output syndrome. *Circulation* 33(Suppl 1):78, 1965.

34. Colucci WS, Wright RF, Jaski BE, et al: Milrinone and dobutamine in severe heart failure: differing hemodynamic effects and individual patient responsiveness. *Circulation* 73(Suppl 3):175, 1986.

35. Davies CL, Newman RJ, Molyneux SG, et al: The relationship between plasma catecholamines and severity of injury in man. *J Trauma* 24:99, 1984.

36. Davis RF, Lappas DG, Kirklin JK, et al: Acute oliguria after cardiopulmonary bypass: renal functional improvement with low-dose dopamine infusion. *Crit Care Med* 10:852, 1982.

37. DeLaCal MA, Miravalles E, Pascual T, et al: Dose-related hemodynamic and renal effects of dopamine in septic shock. *Crit Care Med* 12:22, 1984.

38. Dinerstein RJ, Jones RT, Goldberg LI: Evidence for dopamine-containing renal nerves. *Federation Proc* 42:3005, 1983.

39. DiSesa VJ, Brown E, Mudge GH Jr, et al: Hemodynamic comparison of dopamine and dobutamine in the postoperative volume-loaded, pressure-loaded, and normal ventricle. *J Thorac Cardiovasc Surg* 83:256, 1982.

40. Douglas HD Jr: Levarterenol irrigation: control of massive gastrointestinal bleeding in poor risk patients. *JAMA* 230:1653, 1974.

41. Downes JJ, Wood DW, Harwood I, et al: Intravenous isoproterenol infusion in children with severe hypercapnia due to status asthmaticus. *Crit Care Med* 1:63, 1973.

42. Driscoll DJ, Gillette PC, Ezrailson EG, et al: Inotropic responses of the neonatal canine myocardium to dopamine. *Pediatr Res* 12:42, 1978.

43. Driscoll DJ, Gillette PC, Fukushige J, et al: Comparison of the cardiovascular action of isoproterenol, dopamine and dobutamine in the neonatal and mature dog. *Pediatr Cardiol* 1:307, 1980.

44. Edelson J, LeJemtel TH, Alousi AA, et al: Relationship between amrinone plasma concentration and cardiac index. *Clin Pharmacol Ther* 29:723, 1981.

45. Edelson J, Stroshane R, Benziger DP, et al: Pharmacokinetics of the bipyridines amrinone and milrinone. *Circulation* 73(Suppl 3):145, 1986.

46. Edwards H, Olafsson O, Hyman AI, et al: Dobutamine in the rejecting transplanted heart. *Crit Care Med* 9:498, 1981.

47. Einzig S, Rao GH, Pierpont ME, et al: Acute effects of amrinone on regional myocardial and systemic blood flow distributions in the dog. *Can J Physiol Pharmacol* 60:811, 1982.

48. Esler M, Leonard P, O'Dea K, et al: Biochemical quantification of sympathetic nervous activity in humans using radiotracer methodology: fallibility of plasma noradrenaline measurements. *J Cardiovasc Pharmacol* 4:S152, 1982.

49. Feldman RD, Limbird LE, Nadeau J, et al: Dynamic regulation of leukocyte β-adrenergic receptor-agonist interactions by physiological changes in circulating catecholamines. *J Clin Invest* 72:164, 1983.

50. FitzGerald GA, Hossman V, Hamilton CA, et al: Interindividual variation in kinetics of infused norepinephrine. *Clin Pharmacol Ther* 26:669, 1979.

51. Fowler MB, Alderman EL, Oesterle SN, et al: Dobutamine and dopamine after cardiac surgery: greater augmentation of myocardial blood flow with dobutamine. *Circulation* 70(Suppl 1):103, 1984.

52. Francis GS, Sharma B, Hodges M: Comparative hemodynamic effects of dopamine and dobutamine in patients with acute cardiogenic circulatory collapse. *Am Heart J* 103:995, 1982.

53. Gelfand RA, Matthews DE, Bier DM, et al: Role of counterregulatory hormones in the catabolic response to stress. *J Clin Invest* 74:2238, 1984.

54. Goldberg LI: Dopamine-clinical uses of an endogenous catecholamine. *N Engl J Med* 291:707, 1974.

55. Goldberg LI, Hsuh Y, Resnekov L: Newer catecholamines for treatment of heart failure and shock: an update on dopamine and a first look at dobutamine. *Prog Cardiovasc Dis* 19:327, 1977.

56. Goldbrauson F, Lurie L, Vance RM, et al: Multiple extremity amputations in hypotensive patients with dopamine. *JAMA* 243:1145, 1980.

57. Goldstein DS, Zimlichman R, Stull R, et al: Plasma catecholamine and hemodynamic response during isoproterenol infusions in humans. *Clin Pharmacol Ther* 40:233, 1986.

58. Goldstein RA: Clinical effects of intravenous amrinone in patients with congestive heart failure. *Circulation* 73(Suppl 3):191, 1986.

59. Goldstein DS: Plasma norepinephrine as an indicator

of sympathetic neural activity in clinical cardiology. *Am J Cardiol* 48:1147, 1981.

60. Gombos EA, Hulet WH, Bopp P, et al: Reactivity of renal and systemic circulations to vasoconstrictor agents in normotensive and hypertensive subjects. *J Clin Invest* 41:203, 1962.

61. Gray R, Shah PK, Singh B, et al: Low cardiac output states after open heart surgery: comparative hemodynamic effects of dobutamine, dopamine and norepinephrine plus phentolamine. *Chest* 80:16, 1981.

62. Greenberg MI, Spivey WH: Comparison of deep and shallow endotracheal administration of dionosil in dogs and effect of manual hyperventilation. *Ann Emerg Med* 14:209, 1985.

63. Greenway CV, Stark RD: Hepatic vascular bed. *Physiol Rev* 51:23, 1971.

64. Guller B, Fields AI, Coleman MG, et al: Changes in cardiac rhythm in children treated with dopamine. *Crit Care Med* 6:151, 1978.

65. Halloway EL, Stinson EB, Derby GC, et al: Action of drugs in patients early after cardiac surgery. I. Comparison of isoproterenol and dopamine. *Am J Cardiol* 35:656, 1975.

66. Hasselgren P-O, Biber B, Fornander J: Improved blood flow and protein synthesis in the postischemic liver following infusion of dopamine. *J Surg Res* 34:44, 1983.

67. Holloway El, Palumbo RA, Harrison DC: Acute circulatory effects of dopamine in patients with pulmonary hypertension. *Br Heart J* 37:482, 1975.

68. Holzer J, Karliner JS, O'Rourke RA, et al: Effectiveness of dopamine in patients with cardiogenic shock. *Am J Cardiol* 32:79, 1973.

69. Insel PA, Snavely MD: Catecholamines and the kidney: Receptors and renal function. *Ann Rev Physiol* 43:625, 1981.

70. Jaattela A, Alho A, Avikainen V, et al: Plasma catecholamines in severely injured patients: a prospective study on 45 patients with multiple injuries. *Br J Surg* 62:177, 1975.

71. Jardin F, Sportiche M, Bazil M, et al: Dobutamine: a hemodynamic evaluation in septic shock. *Crit Care Med* 9:329, 1981.

72. Jardin F, Eveleigh MC, Gurdjian F, Margairaz A: Venous admixture in human septic shock. *Circulation* 60:155, 1978.

73. Jarnberg P-O, Bengtsson L, Ekstrand J, et al: Dopamine infusion in man. Plasma catecholamine levels and pharmacokinetics. *Acta Anaesth Scand* 25:328, 1981.

74. Jaski BE, Fifer MA, Wright RF, et al: Positive inotropic and vasodilator actions on milrinone in patients with severe congestive heart failure: dose-response relationship and comparison to nitroprusside. *J Clin Invest* 75:643, 1985.

75. Kates RF, Leier CV: Dobutamine pharmacokinetics in severe heart failure. *Clin Pharmacol Ther* 24:537, 1978.

76. Keung ECH, Siskind SJ, Sonnenblick EH, et al: Dobutamine therapy in acute myocardial infarction. *JAMA* 245:144, 1981.

77. Kho TL, Henquet JW, Punt R, et al: Influence of dobutamine and dopamine on hemodynamics and plasma concentrations of noradrenaline and renin in patients with low cardiac output following acute myocardial infarction. *Eur J Clin Pharmacol* 18:213, 1980.

78. Kopin IJ: Catecholamine metabolism (and the biochemical assessment of sympathetic activity). *Clin Endocrinol Metab* 3:525, 1977.

79. Kullberg MP, Freeman GB, Biddlecome C, et al: Amrinone metabolism. *Clin Pharmacol Ther* 29:394, 1981.

80. Kung M, White JR, Burki NK: The effect of subcutaneously administered terbutaline on serum potassium in asymptomatic adult asthmatics. *Am Rev Respir Dis* 129:329, 1984.

81. Kurland G, Williams J, Lewiston NJ: Fatal myocardial toxicity during continuous intravenous isoproterenol therapy of asthma. *J Allergy Clin Immunol* 63:407, 1979.

82. Lackovic Z, Relja M: Evidence for a widely distributed peripheral dopaminergic system. *Federation Proc* 42:3000, 1983.

83. Laitinen A, Partanen M, Hervonen N, et al: Electron microscopic study on the innervation of the human lower respiratory tract: evidence of adrenergic nerves. *Eur J Respir Dis* 67:209, 1985.

84. Lang P, Williams RG, Norwood WI, et al: The hemodynamic effects of dopamine in infants after corrective cardiac surgery. *J Pediatr* 96:630, 1980.

85. Lee MR: Dopamine and the kidney. *Clin Sci* 62:539, 1982.

86. Legato MJ: Cellular mechanisms of normal growth in the mammalian heart. II. A quantitative and qualitative comparison between the right and left ventricular myocytes in the dog from birth to five months of life. *Circ Res* 44:263, 1979.

87. Leier CV, Hebran PT, Huss P, et al: Comparative systemic and regional hemodynamic effects of dopamine and dobutamine in patients with cardiomyopathic heart failure. *Circulation* 58:466, 1978.

88. Leier CV, Unverferth DV: Dobutamine. *Ann Intern Med* 99:490, 1983.

89. Liang C-S, Sherman LG, Doherty JU, et al: Sustained improvement in patients with congestive heart failure after short-term infusion of dobutamine. *Circulation* 69:113, 1984.

90. Loeb HS, Bredakis J, Gunnar RM: Superiority of dobutamine over dopamine for augmentation of cardiac output in patients with chronic low output cardiac failure. *Circulation* 55:375, 1977.

91. Ludmer PL, Baim DS, Gauthier DF, et al: Effect of milrinone on complex ventricular arrhythmias in congestive heart failure. *Circulation* 72(Suppl 3):405, 1985.

92. Lupi-Herrera E, Sandoval J, Seoñane M, et al: The role of isoproterenol in the preoperative evaluation of high blood pressure high resistance ventricular septal defect. *Chest* 81:42, 1982.

93. Maekawa K, Liang C-S, Hood WB Jr: Comparison of dobutamine and dopamine in acute myocardial infarction. *Circulation* 67:750, 1983.

94. Magorien RD, Unverferth DV, Brown GP, et al: Dobutamine and hydralazine: comparative influences on positive inotropy and vasodilation on coronary blood flow and myocardial energetics in nonischemic congestive heart failure. *J Am Coll Cardiol* 1:499, 1983.

95. Mammel MC, Einzig S, Kulik TJ, et al: Pulmonary vascular effects of amrinone in conscious lambs. *Pediatr Res* 17:720, 1983.

96. Marino RJ, Romagnoli A, Keats AS: Selective venoconstriction by dopamine in comparison with isoproterenol and phenylephrine. *Anesthesiology* 43:570, 1975.

97. MacCannel KL, Giraud GD, Hamilton PL, et al: Haemodynamic response to dopamine and dobutamine infusions as a function of duration of infusion. *Pharmacology* 26:29, 1983.

98. McMillan M, Chernow B, Roth BL: Hepatic alpha$_1$-adrenergic receptor alteration in a rat model of chronic sepsis. *Circ Shock* 19:185, 1986.

99. Meisheri KD, Plamer RF, van Breemen C: The effects of amrinone on contractility, Ca^{2+} uptake and cAMP in smooth muscle. *Eur J Pharmacol* 61:159, 1980.

100. Mentzer RM Jr, Alegre CA, Nolan SP: The effects of dopamine and isoproterenol on the pulmonary circulation. *J Thorac Cardiovasc Surg* 71:807, 1976.

101. Monrad ES, Baim DS, Smith HS, et al: Milrinone, dobutamine and nitroprusside: comparative effects on hemodynamics and myocardial energetics in patients with severe congestive heart failure. *Circulation* 73(Suppl 3):3–168, 1986.

102. Morgan JP, Gwathmey JK, DeFeo TT, et al: The effects of amrinone and related drugs on intracellular calcium

in isolated mammalian cardiac and vascular smooth muscle. *Circulation* 73(Suppl 3):65, 1986.

103. Motulsky HJ, Insel PA: Adrenergic receptors in man. *N Engl J Med* 307:18, 1982.

104. Mueller HS, Ayres SM, Gregorry JJ, et al: Hemodynamics, coronary blood flow and myocardial metabolism in coronary shock: response to L-norepinephrine and isoproterenol. *J Clin Invest* 49:1885, 1970.

105. Mueller HS: Treatment of acute MI. In Shoemaker WC, Thompson WL (eds): *Critical Care Medicine: State of the Art*, vol. 3. Fullerton, CA, Society of Critical Care Medicine, 1982, pp G1.

106. Mueller HS, Evans D, Ayres SM: Effect of dopamine on hemodynamics and myocardial metabolism in shock following acute myocardial infarction in man. *Circulation* 57:361, 1978.

107. Naccarelli GV, Gray EL, Dougherty AH, et al: Amrinone: electrophysiologic and hemodynamic effects in patients with congestive heart failure. *Am J Cardiol* 54:600, 1984.

108. Olson LG, Hensley MJ, Saunders NA: Ventilatory responsiveness to hypercapnic hypoxia during dopamine infusion in humans. *Am Rev Respir Dis* 126:783, 1982.

109. Packer M, Medina N, Yushak M: Hemodynamic and clinical limitations of long-term inotropic therapy with amrinone in patients with severe chronic heart failure. *Circulation* 70:1038, 1984.

110. Padbury JF, Agata Y, Baylen BG, et al: Dopamine pharmacokinetics in critically ill newborn infants. *J Pediatr* 110:293, 1987.

111. Parker S, Carlon GC, Isaacs M, et al: Dopamine administration in oliguria and oliguric renal failure. *Crit Care Med* 9:630, 1981.

112. Pelayo JC, Fildes RD, Eisner GM, et al: Effects of dopamine blockade on renal sodium excretion. *Am J Physiol* 245:F247, 1983.

113. Perkin RM, Levin DL, Webb R, et al: Dobutamine: a hemodynamic evaluation in children with shock. *J Pediatr* 100:977, 1982.

114. Porte D Jr: Sympathetic regulation of insulin secretion. *Arch Intern Med* 123:252, 1969.

115. Post G: New insights into receptor regulation. *J Appl Physiol* 57:1297, 1984.

116. Ralston SH, Voorhees WD, Babbs CF: Intrapulmonary epinephrine during prolonged cardiopulmonary resuscitation: Improved regional blood flow and resuscitation in dogs. *Ann Emerg Med* 13:79, 1984.

117. Rasmussen H: The calcium messenger system (Part I). *N Engl J Med* 314:1094, 1986.

118. Rasmussen H: The calcium messenger system (Part II). *N Engl J Med* 314:;1164, 1986.

119. Regnier B, Kapin M, Gory G, et al: Hemodynamic effects of dopamine in septic shock. *Intensive Care Med* 3:47, 1977.

120. Renard M, Bernard R: Clinical and hemodynamic effects of dobutamine in acute myocardial infarction with left heart failure. *J Cardiovasc Pharmacol* 2:543, 1980.

121. Richard C, Ricome JL, Rimailho A, et al: Combined hemodynamic effects of dopamine and dobutamine in cardiogenic shock. *Circulation* 67:620, 1983.

122. Robie NW, Goldgerg LI: Comparative systemic and regional hemodynamic effects of dopamine and dobutamine. *Am Heart J* 90:340, 1975.

123. Rockson SG, Homcy CJ, Quinn P: Cellular mechanisms of impaired adrenergic responsiveness in neonatal dogs. *J Clin Invest* 67:319, 1981.

124. Rosenthal J, Ferrier G: Inotropic and electrophysiologic effects of amrinone on untreated and digitalized ventricular tissues. *J Pharmacol Exp Ther* 221:188, 1982.

125. Ruffolo RR Jr, Spradlin TA, Pollock GD, et al: Alpha- and beta-adrenergic effects of the stereoisomers of dobutamine. *J Pharmacol Exp Ther* 219:447, 1981.

126. Schaer GL, Fink MP, Parrillo JE: Norepinephrine alone vs. norepinephrine plus low-dose dopamine: enhanced renal blood flow with combination pressor therapy. *Crit Care Med* 13:492, 1985.

127. Schechter E, Wilson MF, Kong Y-S: Physiologic responses to epinephrine infusion: The basis for a new stress test for coronary artery disease. *Am Heart J* 105:554, 1983.

128. Schranz D, Stopfkuchen H, Jungst B-K, et al: Hemodynamic effects of dobutamine in children with cardiovascular failure. *Eur J Pediatr* 139:4–7, 1982.

129. Shepherd JT, Vanhoutte PM: Local modulation of adrenergic neurotransmission. *Circulation* 64:655, 1981.

130. Silverberg AB, Shag SD, Haymond MW, et al: Norepinephrine: hormone and neurotransmitter in man. *Am J Physiol* 234:E252, 1978.

131. Soman VR, Shamoon H, Sherwin RS: Effects of physiologic infusion of epinephrine in normal humans: relationship between the metabolic response and β-adrenergic binding. *J Clin Endocrinol Metab* 50:294, 1980.

132. Sonnenblick EH, Frishman WH, LeJental TH: Dobutamine. A new synthetic cardioactive sympathetic amine. *N Engl J Med* 300:17, 1979.

133. Sonnenblick EH, Grose R, Strain J, et al: Effects of milrinone on left ventricular performance and myocardial contractility in patients with severe heart failure. *Circulation* 73(Suppl 3):162, 1986.

134. Sowers JR, Brickman AS, Sowers DK, et al: Dopaminergic modulation of aldosterone secretion in man is unaffected by glucocorticoids and angiotensin blockage. *J Clin Endocrinol Metab* 52:1078, 1981.

135. Standards and Guidelines for Cardiopulmonary Resuscitation and Emergency Cardiac Care. *JAMA* 255:2841, 1986.

136. Stephenson LW, Edmunds LH, Raphaely R, et al: Effects of nitroprusside and dopamine on pulmonary arterial vasculature in children after cardiac surgery. *Circulation* 60(Suppl 1):106, 1979.

137. Stjarne L, Brundin J: Frequency dependence of ^{3}H-noradrenaline secretion from human vasoconstrictor nerves: modification by factors intering with alpha- or beta-adrenoceptor or prostaglandin E_2 mediated control. *Acta Physiol Scand* 101:199, 1977.

138. Stoof JC, Kebabian JW: Two dopamine receptors: biochemistry, physiology, and pharmacology. *Life Sci* 35:2281, 1984.

139. Stroshane RM, Koss RF, Biddlecome CE, et al: Oral and intravenous pharmacokinetics of milrinone in human volunteers. *J Pharm Sci* 73:1438, 1984.

140. Strulovici B, Cerione RA, Kilpatrick BF, et al: Direct demonstration of impaired functionality of a purified desensitized β-adrenergic receptor in a reconstituted system. *Science* 225:837, 1984.

141. Struthers AD, Whitesmith R, Reid JL: Metabolic and haemodynamic effects of increased circulating adrenaline in man. *Br Heart J* 50:277, 1983.

142. Trigt PV, Spray TL, Pasque MK, et al: The comparative effects of dopamine and dobutamine on ventricular mechanics after coronary artery bypass grafting: a pressure dimension analysis. *Circulation* 70(Suppl I):I–112, 1984.

143. Trigt PV, Spray TL, Pasque MK, et al: The influence of time on the response to dopamine after coronary artery bypass grafting: assessment of left ventricular performance and contractility using pressure/dimension analyses. *Ann Thorac Surg* 35:3, 1983.

144. Tulassay T, Seri I, Machay T, et al: Effects of dopamine on renal functions in premature neonates with respiratory distress syndrome. *Int J Pediatr Nephrol* 4:19, 1983.

145. Tuttle RR, Mills J: Dobutamine. Development of a new catecholamine to selectively increase cardiac contractility. *Circ Res* 36:185, 1975.

146. Unverferth DV, Blanford M, Kates RE, et al: Tolerance

to dobutamine after a 72-hour continuous infusion. *Am J Med* 69:262, 1980.

147. Unverferth DV, Magorien RD, Altschuld R, et al: The hemodynamic and metabolic advantages gained by a three-day infusion of dobutamine in patients with congestive cardiomyopathy. *Am Heart J* 106:29, 1983.

148. Warren JB, Dalton N: A comparison of the bronchodilator and vasopressor effects of exercise levels of adrenaline in man. *Clin Sci* 64:475, 1983.

149. Watters JM, Wilmore DW: Metabolic responses to sepsis and septic shock. In Sibbald WJ, Sprung CL, (eds): *Perspectives on Sepsis and Septic Shock*. Fullerton, CA, Society of Critical Care Medicine, 1986, p 97.

150. Weiner N: Norepinephrine, epinephrine, and the sympathomimetic amines. In Gilman AG, Goodman LS, Rall TW, Murad F (eds): *The Pharmacologic Basis of Therapeutics*. New York, Macmillan, 1985, pp 145.

151. Whitfield L, Sowers JR, Tuck ML, et al: Dopaminergic control of plasma catecholamine and aldosterone response to acute stimuli in normal man. *J Clin Endocrinol Metab* 51:724, 1980.

152. Williams RS, Bishop T: Selectivity of dobutamine for adrenergic receptor subtypes. *J Clin Invest* 67:1703, 1981.

153. Wilson RF, Sibbald WJ, Jaanimagi JL: Hemodynamic effects of dopamine in critically ill septic patients. *J Surg Res* 20:163, 1976.

154. Wortsman J, Frank S, Cryer PE: Adrenomedullary response to maximal stress in humans. *Am J Med* 77:779, 1984.

155. Young MA, Hintze TH, Vatner SF: Correlation between cardiac performance and plasma catecholamine levels in conscious dogs. *Am J Physiol* 248:H82, 1985.

156. Zaloga GP, Smallridge RC: Thyroidal alterations in acute illness. *Semin Resp Med* 7:95, 1985.

157. Zannad F, Juillere Y, Royer RJ: The effects of amrinone on cardiac function, oxygen consumption and lactate production of an isolated, perfused working guinea pig heart. *Arch Int Pharmacodyn Ther* 263:264, 1984.

158. Zaritsky AL, Eisenberg MG: Ontogenetic considerations in the pharmacotherapy of shock. In Chernow B, Shoemaker WC (eds): *Critical Care: State of the Art*, vol 7. Fullerton, CA, Society of Critical Care Medicine, 1986, pp 485.

159. Zaritsky A, Chernow B: Use of catecholamines in pediatrics. *J Pediatr* 105:341, 1984.

160. Zern RT, Foster LB, Blalock JA, et al: Characteristics of the dopaminergic and noradrenergic systems of the pancreatic islets. *Diabetes* 28:185, 1979.

13

Antimicrobials

Henry Masur, M.D.

Infection is frequently suspected or documented in critically ill patients either as the primary process that brings the patient to an intensive care unit (ICU) or as a complication of diagnostic procedures, surgical intervention, drug therapy, or nosocomial exposure in patients who originally entered the ICU for other indications. Therapy of suspected infections in critically ill patients must often be more empirical than in other hospitalized patients, because the critically ill patient may be too sick to tolerate diagnostic procedures. Treatment must also be more encompassing since the critically ill patient may not survive if a causative organism is not immediately treated, whereas a less ill patient may be able to tolerate inadequately treated infection for a few days until the specific pathogens are identified.

Another major consideration for treating critically ill patients is the route of drug administration and the dose and interval that are required. Oral and intramuscular routes usually must be avoided because of uncertainty of absorption. Hepatic and renal dysfunction must be carefully monitored and the fluid and colloid status assessed so that drug levels are maintained in therapeutic but nontoxic ranges.

The focus of this chapter is on the antimicrobial agents commonly employed for critically ill patients in the United States. In the late 1980s a plethora of antimicrobial agents has become available, and a major issue is which of these agents really represent an advance in terms of improved efficacy, lower cost, or reduced toxicity (2, 3, 15, 51, 59, 60). These newer drugs vary greatly in their antimicrobial spectrum, toxicity, doses, distribution, half-lives, and routes of elimination. It is probably preferable for intensivists to be very familiar with a limited number of antimicrobial drugs so that these drugs are used correctly rather than attempting the use of numerous costly agents, many of which are quite similar to each other.

SPECIFIC ANTIMICROBIAL AGENTS

Antibacterial Agents

PENICILLINS

The penicillins are a group of natural and semisynthetic compounds that share a basic structure that consists of a thiazolidine ring connected to a β-lactam ring with an attached side chain. The biologic activity of the penicillins is determined by the integrity of the thiazolidine and β-lactam structures. The antibacterial and pharmacologic properties of penicillin are modified by altering the side chain, resulting in a wide variety of available penicillin compounds (Table 13.1). These penicillins are most usefully classified according to their antibacterial spectrum. They all have similar, though not necessarily identical, mechanisms of action, the details of which are currently being elucidated. Penicillins kill bacteria by interfering with synthesis of the peptidoglycan component of the bacterial cell wall (28). Without effective cell walls the bacteria either fail to divide or swell and rupture.

Penicillins do not kill or inhibit all bacteria. Bacteria may be intrinsically resistant or may acquire resistance to the penicillins (72, 73). Differential permeability to penicillins and differential binding of a specific penicillin to receptor proteins account for different activity of various penicillin compounds against specific bacteria. Other bacteria contain enzymes that inactivate the drugs (72). In Gram-positive bacteria, for instance, the peptidoglycan polymer is near the cell surface and is thus readily acted upon. In Gram-negative bacteria, however, the cell wall is protected from the hydro-

Table 13.1
Antimicrobial Agents for Bacterial, Fungal, and Viral Infections in Critically Ill Patients

Drug	Usual Adult Daily Dose (Recommended Dose Interval)	Route of Administration	Peak Serum Concentration (μg/ml) (i.v. Dose)	Hepatic Metabolism/Excretion	Dose Alteration with Renal Dysfunction	Serum Concentration Altered by: Hemodialysis	Peritoneal Dialysis
Penicillins							
Aqueous crystalline penicillin G	0.6–20 million units/day (continuous-q4h)	i.v., i.m.	18 (1×10^6 U/hr)	No	Major	No	No
Ampicillin	4–12 g/day (q4–6h)	i.v., i.m.	6 (0.5 g)	Yes	Major	Yes	No
Carbenicillin	0.5 g/kg/day (q4h)	i.v., i.m.	150 (2 g)	Yes	Major	Yes	Yes
Ticarcillin	0.25 g/kg/day (q4h)	i.v., i.m.	140 (3g)	Yes	Major	Yes	Yes
Timentin	18.6 g/day (q4–6h)	i.v., i.m.		Yes	Major	Yes	Yes
Piperacillin	0.2–0.5 g/kg/day (q4h)	i.v., i.m.	320 (4 g)	Yes	Minor	Yes	Yes
Oxacillin	4–8 g/day (q4–6h)	i.v., i.m.	50 (0.5 g)	No	Minor	No	No
Nafcillin	4–8 g/day (q4h)	i.v., i.m.	11 (0.5 g)	Yes	Minor	No	No
Methicillin	6–12 g/day (q4–6h)	i.v., i.m.	72 (2.0 g)	No	Minor	No	No
Cephalosporins and Cephamycins							
Cephalothin	4–12 g/day (q4–6h)	i.v., i.m.	100 (2 g)	Yes	Minor	Yes	Yes
Cefazolin	2–6 g/day (q6–8h)	i.v., i.m.	188 (1 g)	Yes	Major	Yes	No
Cefoxitin	4–12 g/day (q4–6h)	i.v., i.m.	110 (1 g)	Yes	Major	Yes	
Cefamandole	4–12 g/day (q4–6h)	i.v., i.m.	80 (1 g)	Yes	Major	No	No
Cefotaxime	4–12 g/day (q6–8h)	i.v., i.m.	214 (2 g)	Yes	Minor	No	No
Ceftazidime	4–6 g/day (q6–8h)	i.v., i.m.	130 (2 g)	No	Major	Yes	Yes
Ceftriaxone	2–4 g/day (q12h)	i.v., i.m.	250 (2 g)	Yes	Minor	No	No
Other β-Lactams							
Imipenem/Cilastatin	3 g/day (q6–8h)	i.v., i.m.	70 (1 g)	No	Major	Yes	
Aztreonam	8 g/day (q8–12h)	i.v., i.m.	125 (1 g)	Yes	Major	Yes	Yes
Aminoglycosides							
Gentamicin	3–6 mg/kg/day (q6–8h)	i.v., i.m.	3–6 (1 mg/kg)	No	Major	Yes	Yes
Tobramycin	3–6 mg/kg/day (q6–8h)	i.v., i.m.	4–10 (1 mg/kg)	No	Major	Yes	Yes
Amikacin	15 mg/kg/day (q12h)	i.v., i.m.	20 (1.0 g)	No	Major	Yes	Yes

	Dose	Route	Level (serum)				
Antimycobacterial Agents							
Isoniazid	300 mg/day (q24h)	p.o.	1.0 (10 mg/kg)	Yes	Minor	Yes	No
Rifampin	600 mg/day (q24h)	p.o.	7 (600 mg)	Yes	Minor	No	No
Ethambutol	15 mg/kg/day (q24h)	p.o.		No	Major	Yes	Yes
Other Antibacterial Agents							
Trimethoprim/sulfamethoxazole	320–960 mg trimethoprim/day	i.v.	100–150 S (25 mg/kg)	Yes	Major	Yes	Yes
Vancomycin	2 g/day (q6h or q12h)	i.v.	20–40 (0.5 g)	No	Major	Yes	No
Erythromycin lactobionate	2 g/day (q6h)	i.v.	9.9 (0.50g)	Yes	No	No	No
Clindamycin	2.4 g/day (q6h)	i.v.	14 (0.6 g)	Yes	Minor	No	No
Chloramphenicol	2–6 g/day (q6h)	i.v.	11 (1.0 g)	Yes	Minor	No	No
Metronidazole	2.25 g/day (q6–8h)	i.v.	26 (0.5 g)	Yes	Major	Yes	No
Tetracycline	2 g/day (q6h)	i.v.	8.5 (0.5 g)	Yes	Avoid	Yes	No
Antiprotozoal Agents							
Pentamidine	4 mg/kg/day (q24h)	i.v.	0.612 (4 mg/kg)	?	No	No	No
Trimethoprim/sulfamethoxazole	20 mg/kg/day (T) and 100 mg/kg/day (S) (q6h)	i.v., p.o.	100–150 S (25 mg/kg)	Yes	Major	Yes	Yes
Sulfadiazine	4–8 g/day (q6h)	i.v.		Yes	Yes	Yes	Yes
Pyrimethamine	25 mg/day (q24h)	p.o.		No	No	No	
Antifungal Agents							
Amphotericin B	0.6 mg/kg/day (q24h)	i.v.		No	Minor	No	Yes
Flucytosine	150 mg/kg/day (q6h)	p.o.	75 (2.0 g)	No	Yes	Yes	No
Ketoconazole	400 mg/day	p.o.	3.5 (200 mg)	No	No	No	
Antiviral Agents							
Acyclovir	15–30 mg/kg/day (q8h)	i.v.	20 (10 mg/kg)	No	Yes	Yes	
Amantadine	100–200 mg/day (q24h)	p.o.	0.3 (100 mg)	No	Yes	Yes	
Azidothymidine	1000 mg/day (q4h)	p.o.		Yes			
Ribavirin	aerosol	aerosol			Yes		
DHPG	10 mg/kg/day (q12h)	i.v.		No	Yes		

philic penicillins by a complex surface structure. While some microorganisms are inherently resistant to the penicillins, other microorganisms produce enzymes that can inactivate various β-lactam drugs. Gram-positive organisms generally secrete extracellular enzymes, whereas Gram-negative organisms produce small quantities of enzymes that remain in the periplasmic space between the inner and outer cell membranes. Each bacterial species produces a somewhat different β-lactamase, and each specific penicillin, or cephalosporin, varies in its susceptibility to the particular enzyme produced. The information for penicillinase is encoded on a plasmid that can be transferred by phages to other organisms. Ability to produce the enzyme is often inducible by exposure to the appropriate substrate. Some of the β-lactamases secreted by Gram-negative bacteria are inducible while others are constitutive.

Penicillins are most readily classified for clinical purposes on the basis of their antimicrobial spectrum. Table 13.1 lists the most commonly used penicillins, and their major routes of excretion. Table 13.2 indicates organisms for which penicillin drugs are effective therapy.

Distribution and Elimination

Most penicillins are widely distributed throughout the body though local concentrations may vary substantially. In CSF, levels are generally well below serum concentrations, though the presence of fever or meningeal inflammation usually augments penetration such that subarachnoid concentrations are therapeutic for the most common community acquired organisms that cause meningitis. Concentrations in obstructed bile and in prostatic tissue are often subtherapeutic for the most likely pathogens.

Adverse Reactions

The most common adverse reactions to the penicillins are hypersensitivity reactions. All of the penicillin compounds have potential to cause allergic phenomena (66). In order of decreasing frequency, these reactions are maculopapular rash, urticaria, fever, bronchospasm, vasculitis, serum sickness, exfoliative dermatitis, and anaphylaxis. The true incidence of such reactions is probably between 0.5% and 10%, although some hypersensitivity

reactions may occur particularly frequently with one penicillin compound. A hypersensitivity response after one administration of a drug does not guarantee a similar response for each of its subsequent administrations. It is not safe clinical practice to give a patient a penicillin compound if the patient has a reliable history of immediate hypersensitivity response to any drug in the penicillin group (41, 66). Whether or not desensitization of the patient to the penicillin compound decreases the likelihood of a subsequent allergic response is uncertain, but desensitization in a controlled medical setting, such as an ICU, is a standard practice for patients who have no therapeutic alternative to penicillin. Skin testing with both major and minor determinants of penicillin is useful for predicting which patients are most likely to have a hypersensitivity response. Reliable preparations of antigens should be used for skin testing. Both major and minor determinants must be employed.

Serious toxic reactions to the penicillins are unusual events. The drugs provoke an inflammatory response that appears to be concentration dependent; inflammation at injection sites and thrombophlebitis occasionally occur. Very high serum concentrations are associated with confusion, lethargy, and seizures, especially in those patients with pre-existing cerebral disorders. Intrathecal administration of penicillins can cause arachnoiditis, but such administration is almost never warranted. Other toxic reactions reported include nephritis (especially with methicillin) (34), bone marrow depression (especially with methicilin or nafcillin) (35), hepatitis (especially with oxacillin) (54), and impaired platelet aggregation (especially with carbenicillin and ticarcillin) (12, 67).

Because of their proven clinical efficacy and their safety, penicillins are commonly used in critically ill patients. Table 13.1 indicates the recommended doses for the commonly used penicillin drugs.

Numerous new penicillin compounds have appeared in recent years. The acylamino penicillins, for example (azlocillin, mezlocillin, piperacillin) are broad-spectrum penicillins with activity against many enterobacteriaceae and *Pseudomonas aeruginosa* (22). Piperacillin is widely used because of its excellent in vitro activity against *P. aeruginosa*, but the major determinant of the drug of choice among these acylamino penicillins is probably cost rather than efficacy or safety, because the efficacy and safety profiles of these drugs are so similar. Ticarcillin has been marketed as a combination with potassium clavulanate, a noncompetitive inhibitor of many β-lactamases. The combination is available as Timentin, and has increased in vitro activity against a variety of organisms (55, 77). This drug combination may be useful against certain aerobic Gram-negative bacilli, anerobes, and *Staphylococcus aureus* that produce β-lactamase, but it has no clear advantage over older drugs or drug combinations.

CEPHALOSPORINS

Cephalosporins are a group of natural and semisynthetic compounds with broad antibacterial activity. They are structurally similar to penicillins and inhibit bacterial cell wall synthesis in much the same manner as the penicillins. Cephamycins are structurally similar to cephalosporins and act in a similar manner, and thus are also considered in this section.

A large and expanding number of cephalosporin and cephamycin compounds are avail-

Table 13.2
Antimicrobial Drugs of Choice for the Treatment of Specific Infectious Agents in Critically Ill Patients

Organism	Antimicrobial Agent of Choice	Alternative Agents
BACTERIA		
Gram-positive cocci (aerobic)		
Staphylococcus aureus		
Non-penicillinase-producing	Penicillin	Vancomycin, cephalosporin
Penicillinase producing	Nafcillin, oxacillin	Vancomycin, cephalosporin
α-Streptococci (viridans streptococcus	Penicillin	Erythromycin, clindamycin, cephalosporin
β-Streptococci (A,B,C,G)	Penicillin	Cephalosporin, erythromycin
Streptococcus fecalis		
Serious infection	Ampicillin + aminoglycoside	Vancomycin + aminoglycoside
Uncomplicated urinary infection	Ampicillin	Vancomycin
Streptococcus bovis	Penicillin	Cephalosporin, vancomycin
Streptococcus pneumoniae	Penicillin	Erythromycin, vancomycin, cephalosporin
Gram-negative cocci (aerobic)		
Neisseria meningitidis	Penicillin	Cefotaxime, chloramphenicol
Neisseria gonorrheae	Penicillin	Spectinomycin, ceftriaxone
Gram-positive bacilli (aerobic)		
Corynebacterium JK	Vancomycin	
Gram-negative bacilli (aerobic)		
Acinetobacter sp.	Aminoglycoside + carbenicillin	Trimethoprim-sulfamethoxazole
Campylobacter sp.	Erythromycin	Tetracycline
Enterobacter sp.	Aminoglycoside	Third generation cephalosporin
Escherichia coli	Ampicillin	Cephalosporin, aminoglycoside
Haemophilus influenza	Second- or third-generation cephalosporin	Trimethoprim-sulfamethoxazole
Klebsiella pneumoniae	Aminoglycoside	Cephalosporin, aztreonam
Legionella sp.	Erythromycin + rifampin	Rifampin, quinolones
Proteus mirabilis	Ampicillin	Aminoglycoside, cephalosporin
Other proteus species	Aminoglycoside	Cephalosporin, aztreonam
Providencia sp.	Aminoglycoside (amikacin)	Cephalosporin, aztreonam
Pseudomonas aeruginosa	Aminoglycoside + carbenicillin	Third-generation cephalosporin, aztreonam
Salmonella sp.	Trimethoprim-sulfamethoxazole	Ampicillin, chloramphenicol, third-generation cephalosporins
Serratia marcescens	Aminoglycoside	Third generation cephalosporin
Shigella sp.	Ampicillin	Chloramphenicol
Anaerobes		
Anaerobic streptococci	Penicillin	Clindamycin, metronidazole
Bacteroides sp.		
Oropharyngeal strains	Penicillin	Clindamycin
Gastrointestinal strains	Clindamycin	Metronidazole, cefoxitin
Clostridium sp. (except *C. difficile*)	Penicillin	Clindamycin, metronidazole

Organism	Antimicrobial Agent of Choice	Alternative Agents
Clostridium difficile	Vancomycin	Metronidazole
Other Bacteria		
Actinomyces and *Arachnia*	Penicillin G	Tetracycline
Nocardia sp.	Trimethoprim-sulfamethoxazole	Minocycline
Mycobacterium tuberculosis	INH + rifampin	Ethambutol, streptomycin
FUNGI		
Aspergillus sp.	Amphotericin B	
Elastomyces dermatitidis	Amphotericin B	
Candida sp.	Amphotericin B	Ketoconazole
Coccidioides immitis	Amphotericin B	
Cryptococcus neoformans	Amphotericin B + flucytosine	
Histoplasma capsulatum	Amphotericin B	Ketoconazole
Mucor-Absidia-Rhizopus	Amphotericin	
PROTOZOA		
Pneumocystis carinii	Trimethoprim-sulfamethoxazole	Pentamidine
Toxoplasma gondii	Sulfadiazine + pyrimethamine	
VIRUSES		
Herpes simplex	Acyclovir	
Influenza A	Amantadine	
Herpes zoster	Acyclovir	
OTHER ORGANISMS		
Mycoplasma pneumoniae	Erythromycin	Tectracycline
Chlamydia psittaci	Tetracycline	Chloramphenicol
Chlamydia trachomatis	Erythromycin	Tetracycline
Leptospira sp.	Penicillin G	Tetracycline
Rickettsia sp.	Tetracycline	Chloramphenicol

able, which vary considerably in antibacterial spectrum, pharmacokinetics, and cost (3, 50). For most clinicians it is necessary to be knowledgeable about only a few of these many compounds but to be aware that if the cephalosporin they are accustomed to using does not have the desired antimicrobial spectrum or tissue penetration, other cephalosporin compounds should be considered. The availability of new, extended-spectrum cephalosporins often makes it possible now to use a relatively nontoxic cephalosporin drug as a single agent rather than a multiple-drug regimen that includes an aminoglycoside. The relative role of newer cephalosporins compared with imipenem, timentin, aztreonam, or the quinolones is currently a matter of great debate (2, 3, 15, 51, 59).

Cephalothin and cefazolin are the prototype compounds against which subsequent cephalosporins should be judged. They have wide activity against almost all aerobic cocci including *Staphylococcus aureus* (but not *Streptococcus faecalis*) and against many enteric Gram-negative bacilli (but not against *P. aeruginosa*). Cefazolin is less phlebogenic than cephalothin, and can be given either intramuscularly or intravenously as opposed to cephalothin, which should not be given intramuscularly.

Cefoxitin offers the advantage, compared with cephalothin or cefazolin, of outstanding activity against almost all anaerobic organisms including *Bacteroides fragilis*, and more activity for indole positive proteus and serratia. Thus it can be of particular use for purulent pulmonary infections such as empyemas and abscesses and for mixed abdominal infections. Cefamandole has excellent activity against *Haemophilus influenzae* as well as aerobic Gram-positive cocci and an extended spectrum of enteric bacilli. Cefuroxime, however, probably has more activity than cefamandole and is preferred over cefamandole by some experts. Its usefulness is primarily for mixed upper and lower respiratory infections that are likely to involve Gram-positive cocci and *H. influenzae*.

The extended-spectrum cephalosporins (the so called third generation) offer improved in vitro activity compared with second-generation cephalosporins for aerobic Gram-negative bacilli (3, 23, 49, 50, 51, 52, 58, 59). As a group these drugs are active against most aerobic Gram-positive cocci (but not *S. faecalis*, methicillin resistant *S. aureus,* or many *Staphylococcus epidermidis*), *Neisseria meningitidis,* and *Neisseria gonorrheae,* many anaerobic organisms (but not *B. fragilis*), and aerobic Gram-negative bacilli including, for a few cephalosporins, *P. aeruginosa.* Cefotaxime, ceftizoxime, and ceftriaxone are the most commonly used third-generation cephalosporins that have broad spectrum activity which does not include *P. aeruginosa.* Ceftriaxone has the advantage of a longer half-life (49). Ceftazidime has a similar (but not identical) spectrum of activity to these latter drugs but is also active against *P. aeruginosa* (58, 59). All the third-generation cephalosporins mentioned above cross inflamed meninges (17, 40). The emergence of resistance during therapy has been reported for third-generation cephalosporins (62). The major advantage of this group of cephalosporins is their low toxicity compared with aminoglycosides, activity against certain unusual multiple-drug-resistant bacilli, and the opportunity in many situations to administer a single drug rather than multiple agents. These drugs are clearly effective clinically, but their relative efficacy compared with older antibiotic combinations has not been clearly established, particularly when these agents are used as monotherapy for immunologically abnormal patients (e.g., the efficacy of ceftazidime compared with combination regimens for therapy of fever and neutropenia or sepsis and neutropenia has not been unequivocally established) (58, 59, 77).

Distribution and Elimination

Therapeutic cephalosporin levels can be found in most body sites including bile, synovial fluid, and pericardial fluid. Cephalothin, cefazolin, cefoxitin, and cefamandole penetrate the subarachnoid space poorly, but several of the third-generation cephalosporins appear to penetrate sufficiently to have therapeutic potential (17). These include cefotaxime, ceftriaxone, ceftizoxime, and ceftazidime. The elimination of cephalosporins varies with the specific agent (Table 13.1).

Adverse Effects

Hypersensitivity reactions are the most common adverse effects for the cephalosporins and cephamycins (66). No one cephalosporin or cephamycin seems to cause dramatically more hypersensitivity responses than the others. Clinical manifestations of hypersensitivity are similar to those described with the penicillins. Clinically, about 5–10% of patients with a penicillin allergy demonstrate an allergic response when challenged with a cephalosporin (57). Skin test antigen is not available to assess cephalosporin hypersensitivity. It is imprudent to administer a cephalosporin to any patient with a history of immediate hypersensitivity reactions to a penicillin drug.

Other serious adverse effects are uncommon. They include positive Coombs test, hemolytic anemia, nephrotoxicity (especially when cephalosporins are used in combination with aminoglycosides), thrombocytopenia, and granulocytopenia.

OTHER β-LACTAM DRUGS

Imipenem is a β-lactam antibiotic that is sold in a fixed combination with cilastatin (Primaxin) (15, 53). Cilastatin inhibits the renal metabolism of imipenem and is included to decrease the production of potentially nephrotoxic compounds. Imipenem has the broadest activity of any β-lactam drug including extended-spectrum cephalosporins: its spectrum includes Gram-positive cocci (except some *Streptococcus fecium,* *S. epidermis,* and some methicillin-resistant staphylococci), most aerobic Gram-negative bacilli including *P. aeruginosa,* (but excluding *Pseudomonas capacia* and *Pseudomonas maltophilia*), and many anaerobic bacteria including *B. fragilis;* it does not cover *Corynebacterium JK.* Emergence of resistance during therapy, particularly for *P. aeruginosa,* is a concern, as is superinfection and the induction of β-lactamases, which would make Gram-negative bacilli more resistant to other β-lactam drugs. The role for imipenem is similar to that for extended-spectrum cephalosporins, but imipenem should not be used as a single agent for *P. aeruginosa* infections because of the possible emergence of resistance (61, 64). Patients allergic to other β-lactam drugs are likely to be allergic to imipenem. Imipenem should be avoided in patients with seizures.

Aztreonam is a synthetic β-lactam antibiotic that is structurally different from cephalosporins and penicillins (2). It is the first monobactam approved for clinical use. Aztreonam has broad activity against aerobic Gram-negative organisms including *N. gonorrheae,* most enteric Gram-negative rods, and *P. aeruginosa.* It has no activity against Gram-positive organisms or anerobes. Aztreonam is clinically effective against a broad range of Gram-negative organisms, although its efficacy for meningitis has not been established. Adverse effects are similar to other β-lactam drugs. There appears to be little cross allergenicity with penicillins and cephalosporins. The major advantage of aztreonam is that it has potent activity against Gram-negative bacilli without the toxicity of aminoglycosides. It remains to be determined whether for therapy of Gram-negative bacillus infections there is any advantage of aztreonam over imipenem or cephalosporins for patients who are not allergic to these β-lactam drugs.

AMINOGLYCOSIDES

The aminoglycosides are a group of natural and semisynthetic compounds that have broad activity against Gram-negative bacilli. The clinically useful drugs are gentamicin, tobramycin, amikacin, and netilmicin (5, 60). The group also includes streptomycin, neomycin, and kanamycin, which are infrequently used in the 1980s. Because aminoglycosides have broad activity against Gram-negative bacilli and because they are proven to be clinically efficacious, they are a major component of the antimicrobial armamentarium for the critically ill. They are widely used as part of multiple-drug empiric therapy and as specific therapy for infections caused by organisms not susceptible to less toxic drugs.

Gentamicin, tobramycin, netilmicin, and amikacin have excellent activity against aerobic Gram-negative bacilli including most *Pseudomonas* species. These drugs have no activity against anaerobic organisms and limited activity against aerobic Gram-positive cocci. S. *faecalis* are susceptible to aminoglycosides in the presence of penicillins. Aminoglycosides have excellent activity against most *P. aeruginosa*: they act synergistically against these organisms and against some enterobacteriaceae when used in combination with carbenicillin or ticarcillin or piperacillin (22, 39). Aminoglycosides are active in vitro against most *S. aureus* and *S. epidermidis*, but clinical efficacy against staphylococci has never been proved, and staphylococci rapidly become resistant when treated with aminoglycosides alone. The aminoglycosides act at the 30S bacterial ribosomal unit, where they inhibit protein synthesis and interfere with the translation of mRNA. These mechanisms do not, however, explain the bactericidal effects of these drugs. Bacterial resistance to aminoglycosides is usually caused by elaboration of enzymes that inactivate the drugs, though failure to penetrate into the bacteria

and low affinity of the drug for ribosomes are also factors (21, 46). These enzymes are located in the bacterial membrane. They adenylate, acetylate, and phosphorylate the aminoglycosides at numerous sites. Aminoglycosides that are poor substrates for these enzymes are active against more organisms. Thus amikacin, a compound that is a substrate for only one of the common enzymes, an acetylase, is active against more Gram-negative bacilli than the other aminoglycosides. However, it is not clear whether clinicians should use this semisynthetic compound in preference to the other aminoglycosides since resistance to amikacin could spread if this drug were used more commonly. Many consultants prefer to withhold amikacin for the treatment of microorganisms that are suspected or documented to be resistant to other aminoglycosides.

Distribution and Elimination

Aminoglycoside concentrations are high in the renal cortex. Levels are low in other tissues, and aminoglycosides do not reliably penetrate into the subarachnoid space. Concentrations in bile are about 30% of serum levels unless the biliary system is obstructed, in which case levels are even lower. Aminoglycosides are eliminated by glomerular filtration. Some tubular reabsorption of these agents probably occurs.

Adverse Effects

Aminoglycosides are toxic to renal, auditory, and cochlear function (4, 5, 48). Toxicity is concentration dependent and the predilection for site of toxicity varies with each specific drug. Ototoxicity occurs due to progressive destruction of vestibular or cochlear sensory cells when the aminoglycoside is concentrated in the perilymph of the inner ear. Ototoxicity can occur abruptly or gradually. Gentamicin and streptomycin primarily affect auditory function, and tobramycin affects both equally. All the aminoglycosides are nephrotoxic (4). The frequency of clinical nephrotoxicity is influenced by the frequency and severity of concurrent nephrotoxic insults and by pre-existing renal pathology. Nephrotoxicity characteristically occurs after 5–7 days of therapy: proteinuria and tubular casts initially occur, followed by a reduction in glomerular filtration. The process is usually reversible. Tobramycin is slightly less nephrotoxic than gentamicin; the difference is probably not clinically important. In patients who are seriously ill it is important to measure serum levels of aminoglycosides in order to avoid drug accumulation and toxicity, and conversely to avoid inappropriately low levels and ineffectiveness. Peak serum levels of 2–3 μg/ml are usually needed to produce concentrations greater than the minimum inhibitory concentration of most *Pseudomonas* and many *Enterobacteriaceae* (47). Gentamicin or tobramycin levels greater than 12 mg/ml are associated with toxicity. There is controversy concerning the optimal peak and trough levels to maximize efficacy but avoid toxicity. It seems reasonable to try to maintain peak gentamicin or tobramycin levels of 6–12 μg/ml, and trough levels of 1–2 μg/ml. Peak amikacin levels should be maintained at 25–30 μg/ml. Serum aminoglycoside levels (peak and trough) should be measured at least two or three times weekly in seriously ill patients regardless of renal function. Many factors affect serum level, including the underlying disease and fever. Although nomograms and formulas are available, measurement of serum levels is the only accurate method of assuring the desired range. Either the total daily dose or the interval between doses can be altered. A useful method of estimating the appropriate interval between 1-mg/kg doses of gentamicin or tobramycin while awaiting laboratory results is to estimate the interval in hours to be equal to the product of eight times the serum creatinine. Thus, if the serum creatinine is 3 mg/dl, 1 mg/kg of gentamicin should be given every 24 hours (8×3). Peak and trough levels should then be measured, and the dose readjusted as indicated by the levels.

MACROLIDE ANTIBIOTICS

The macrolide antibiotics are a group of compounds that contain a lactone ring to which are attached one or more deoxy sugars. Because of their excellent gastrointestinal absorption, erythromycin and clindamycin are widely used antibiotics in ambulatory medicine. In critically ill patients, their use as intravenous preparations relates primarily to their excellent activity against agents causing atypical pneumonia and anaerobic infections, respectively.

Erythromycin

Erythromycin is either bacteriostatic or bacteriocidal depending on the microorganism and the serum concentration. The drug is effective in vitro for almost all *Streptococcus pyogenes*, *Streptococcus pneumoniae*, and *Viridans streptococcus*, though a few strains of these organisms may be resistant, particularly if the patient has recently been exposed to a macrolide antibiotic. The antibiotic is also useful against all *Mycoplasma pneumoniae*, *Legionella pneumophila*, and *N. gonorrheae*. Erythromycin is active against only some *S. aureus* and *H. influenzae*, and thus is not recommended as first-line therapy for infections involving these organisms. Erythromycin has little activity against most Gram-negative bacilli with the exception of *Campylobacter* species. In critically ill patients the major role for erythromycin is to treat suspected *legionella* or *mycoplasma* pneumonias.

Erythromycin binds to the 50S subunit of bacterial ribosomes and thus interferes with protein synthesis.

Distribution and Elimination. Erythromycin diffuses into intracellular fluids and adequate concentration is attained in almost all tissues except the brain and CSF. It penetrates the prostate well, though its antimicrobial spectrum renders it of little utility in prostatic infections.

Erythromycin is concentrated in the liver and excreted in the bile. About 15% of the intravenous form is excreted in the urine.

Adverse Effects. Serious adverse effects due to erythromycin are rare. The drug is irritating in its intravenous form and frequently causes phlebitis. Fever, eosinophilia, and rashes occasionally occur. Cholestatic hepatitis rarely occurs with the intravenous preparations. This complication is more often observed with the oral estalate.

Clindamycin

Clindamycin is a macrolide antibiotic that, like erythromycin, has excellent activity against *S. pyogenes*, *S. pneumoniae*, and *V. streptococcus*. It is active against many but not all *S. aureus*. Because clindamycin is only bacteriostatic against *S. aureus*, and because resistance develops during experimental infection, clindamycin is not first-line antistaphylococcal therapy. Clindamycin differs from erythromycin in that it has excellent activity against almost all anaerobic bacteria except for a few peptococci, a few *Clostridium perfringens*, a few *B. fragilis*, and many nonperfringens clostridia. The major role for clindamycin in the treatment of critically ill patients is to provide therapy for anaerobic infections (6).

Clindamycin inhibits protein synthesis by binding to the 50S subunit of bacterial ribosome.

Distribution and Elimination. Clindamycin penetrates most body sites well, particularly bone. It does not reliably enter the CSF. Only about 10% of clindamycin is excreted unchanged in the urine. The rest of the drug is metabolized in the liver and excreted in the bile and urine.

Adverse Effects. The most prominently described adverse effect of clindamycin is pseudomembranous colitis, which is a serious inflammatory process caused by the toxin of *Clostridium difficile*, a normal bowel organism (7, 8). This syndrome presents as persistent copious watery stool or sudden bloody stool associated with fever and abdominal pain. The frequency of its occurrence differs sharply in various series from 0.2% to 20% of patients. It must be recognized, however, that pseudomembranous colitis has been reported with almost every currently used antibiotic, not just clindamycin, and concern about this potential complication should not be an important factor in deciding whether or not to include clindamycin in an antibiotic regimen.

Skin rashes, transaminasemia, and bone marrow suppression have occasionally been associated with clindamycin administration. Diarrhea without pseudomembrane formations is quite common. This form of diarrhea is probably due to alteration of bowel flora. It usually resolves when antimicrobial therapy is stopped.

CHLORAMPHENICOL

Chloramphenicol is a natural compound with a unique structure unrelated to other antimicrobials. Like the macrolide antibiotics, chloramphenicol binds to the 50S ribosomal subunit, preventing formation of peptide bonds. Chloramphenicol also inhibits mitrochondrial protein synthesis in mammalian cells, especially those in the erythropoietic system. This drug can be useful in critically ill patients because of its antibacterial spectrum and distribution; its marrow toxicity, however, is a major drawback that results in this drug being used with decreasing frequency, now that clindamycin, metronidazole, and extended spectrum β-lactam drugs are available as less toxic alternatives.

Chloramphenicol is bacteriostatic for a wide variety of Gram-positive and Gram-negative organisms including almost all nonenterococcal streptococci, *Neisseria meningitidis*, *N. gonorrhoae*, *Salmonella* species, most anaerobes, *H. influenzae* and many enteric Gram-negative bacilli. *P. aeruginosa* is not inhibited. High concentrations inhibit many *S. aureus*. Resistance of Gram-negative bacilli is spread by a R factor.

Distribution and Elimination

Chloramphenicol penetrates all body tissue including the brain and CSF. Only about 5–10% of biologically active chloramphenicol is excreted in the urine. The rest of the drug is metabolized in the liver. The half-life of the drug correlates with the plasma bilirubin concentration. The dosage must therefore be reduced for patients with hepatic insufficiency but not for patients with renal insufficiency.

Adverse Effects

There are two separate and distinct types of bone marrow toxicity that are the major toxicities. The idiopathic type of marrow aplasia is usually irreversible especially if the onset occurs more than 2 months after the last dose. Aplastic anemia is the most common manifestation. This form occurs only once per 25,000 treated patients, and almost exclusively in young women receiving oral therapy who had previous exposure to the drug.

A dose-related hematologic toxicity also occurs, producing increased serum iron levels, cytoplasmic vacuolization of granulocyte and erythroid precursors, and anemia, often with leukopenia and thrombocytopenia. This syndrome regularly occurs when the serum level is greater than $25\mu g/ml$. It should be watched for by monitoring the serum iron level and the percent saturation of the total iron binding capacity and the platelet count. This type of marrow toxicity is reversible when the drug is stopped. Blurred vision, digital paresthesias, and allergic phenomena are observed rarely.

VANCOMYCIN

Vancomycin is a natural compound that is structurally unlike the other antimicrobial compounds (19, 24). It is bactericidal against essentially all staphylococci (both *S. aureus* and *S. epidermidis*), all *S. pneumoniae*, *S. pyogenes*, and *V. streptococci*. It is bacteriostatic against all *S. faecalis* and most *Corynebacterium* species. A few anaerobes are susceptible, but virtually no Gram-negative organisms are susceptible to vancomycin. Vancomycin has a prominent role in therapy of critically ill patients (19, 24). To an increasing extent critically ill patients have temporary or permanent foreign bodies implanted as pacemakers, vascular access, valves, or shunts. These devices are especially predisposed to infection by staphylococci including S. aureus, and S. epidermidis, an increasing fraction of which are methecillin resistant. In addition, the importance of S. epidermidis and diphtheroid species in patients with prosthetic valves or malignant tumors and the emergence of drug-resistant S. pneumoniae has made vancomycin a particularly useful bactericidal antibiotic. Vancomycin is also useful for patients with Gram-positive infection and a history of serious penicillin allergy (24).

Distribution and Elimination

Vancomycin penetrates most body tissues well, including the brain and inflamed meninges. It is excreted almost unchanged by the kidneys.

Adverse Effects

Nephrotoxicity and ototoxicity are uncommon with the modern drug preparation if peak serum levels are maintained below 50 μg/ml. Phlebitis is common with intravenous vancomycin. Flushing, tingling, and erythema ("red neck syndrome") are usually associated with rapid infusion, especially if 1-g doses are used. Leukopenia occasionally occurs.

SULFONAMIDES, TRIMETHOPRIM, AND PYRIMETHAMINE

Sulfonamides are a large group of compounds that were the first chemotherapeutic agents employed systematically for the prevention and treatment of bacterial infection in humans. They have a wide antibacterial spectrum that includes Gram-positive cocci, Gram-negative rods, chlamydia, nocardia, neisseria, and protozoa (toxoplasma, pneumocystis, malaria). More effective drugs have taken the place of sulfonamides for the treatment of most bacterial processes. They have an important role for treating uncomplicated urinary tract infections. They are also first-line therapy for nocardia, pneumocystis, and toxoplasma infections, particularly when combined with trimethoprim and pyrimethamine (33, 71).

The sulfonamides are structural analogs and competitive antagonists of para-aminobenzoic acid, and thus interfere with the production of folic acid. Sulfonamides exert a synergistic effect when they are combined with agents such as trimethoprim or pyrimethamine that act at sequential steps in folic acid synthesis. For this reason a fixed combination preparation of two of these sequential blockers, trimethoprim-sulfamethoxazole (in a ratio of 1:5), has proven to be an effective and widely used therapeutic product (71). It is the drug of choice for pneumocystosis. Sulfadiazine or sulfasoxazole are still preferred for nocardiosis. Pyrimethamine is the preferred choice in combination with sulfadiazine for toxoplasmosis.

Distribution and Elimination

Sulfonamides are widely distributed throughout the body including the CSF. They are metabolized in the liver to varying degrees depending on the compound involved. The parent drug and the metabolites are excreted in the urine.

Adverse Effects

For most patient groups, about 5% of recipients have adverse reactions to sulfonamides. Hypersensitivity reactions, especially skin, mucous membrane, and vasculitic lesions can be life threatening. Acute hemolytic anemia, often associated with glucose-6-phosphate dehydrogenase deficiency, and agranulocytosis, thrombocytopenia, aplastic anemia, crystalluria, and hepatic necrosis are also seen. For AIDS patients, up to 70% can have fever, leukopenia, hepatitis, nephritis, or rash when treated with trimethoprim-sulfamethoxazole: these reactions appear to be related to the sulfamethoxazole rather than the trimethoprim, and often necessitate cessation of therapy.

METRONIDAZOLE

Metronidazole is a synthetic nitroimidazole that has an increasingly important role in the treatment of serious anaerobic infections as well as in the treatment of certain protozoal infections (27). Metronidazole is active against almost all anaerobes; some cocci and a few non-spore-forming Gram-positive bacilli are resistant. Ameba, giardia, and trichomonas are generally susceptible. Because metronidazole is the only bactericidal drug available for most anaerobic organisms, it has a potentially important role for critically ill patients with anaerobic infections. Its role compared to clindamycin or chloramphenicol is currently being defined. With regard to mechanism of action, the nitro group of metronidazole is reduced by electron transport proteins with low redox potentials. The cell is thus deprived of reducing equivalents, and the reduced form of metronidazole is able to alter the helical structure of DNA.

Although metronidazole is well absorbed after oral administration, it should be given intravenously to seriously ill patients.

Distribution and Elimination

Good drug levels are attained in most tissues; particularly high levels are found in the CSF. Both metabolized and unmetabolized metronidazole are excreted in the urine.

Adverse Effects

Metronidazole causes considerable headache and gastrointestinal symptoms including anorexia, nausea, vomiting, diarrhea, epigastric pain, and cramps. Neurotoxic effects such as dizziness, vertigo, and ataxia and peripheral neuropathy may occur. Reversible neutropenia may be noted during therapy.

PENTAMIDINE

Pentamidine is a diamidine compound that is effective for the therapy of pneumocystis pneumonia (33, 56). Formerly available only from the Centers for Disease Control, this drug is now available commercially. For protozoa the mechanism of action of pentamidine is unclear; it may inhibit replication of protozoan kinetoplast DNA.

Pentamidine isethionate should be reconstituted in sterile water and administered by slow intravenous infusion (30–60 minutes). Clinically important hypotension is not frequently associated with slow intravenous infusion despite older reports to the contrary (42). Intramuscular administration often causes painful sterile abscesses and is no longer recommended. Aerosolized pentamidine appears to be well tolerated and effective as either therapy or prophylaxis for pneumocystis pneumonia in preliminary studies, but further studies concerning dose, delivery devices, schedules, efficacy, and safety are needed.

Distribution and Elimination

Concentrations of drug are detectable for at least 24 hours after a 4 mg/kg dose. The half-life after intravenous administration is about 6.5 hours (18). The routes of metabolism and elimination are not well worked out.

Adverse Effects

Parenteral pentamidine is associated with renal failure in a high percent of patients, as well as dysglycemia (hypoglycemia followed by hyperglycemia, both of which can be clinically severe) and pancreatitis. AIDS patients appear to be particularly predisposed to leukopenia, which is usually quickly reversed when drug is discontinued.

ANTIMYCOBACTERIAL THERAPY

Although many antituberculous drugs are available, the most important drugs for therapy of critically ill patients are isoniazid, rifampin, streptomycin, and ethambutol (69). The first three of these drugs are available for intramuscular administration.

Isoniazid (INH) is the hydrazide of isonicotinic acid. It is bactericidal against dividing typical mycobacteria (*Mycobacterium tuberculosis*) and some atypical mycobacteria. It appears to work by inhibiting synthesis of the cell wall. About one in 10^6 *M. tuberculosis* are genetically impermeable to INH.

Isoniazid is readily absorbed orally. The drug penetrates all body tissues including the CSF. The drug is acetylated and hydrolyzed, and then excreted in the urine. The rate of acetylation is racially dependent. The serum INH concentration of rapid acetylators is 50–80% less than that of slow acetylators.

About 5% of patients develop INH-induced untoward reactions including rash, jaundice, peripheral neuritis, fever, seizures, bone marrow depression, hypersensitivity reactions and arthritis. The peripheral neuritis is quite common if pyridoxine is not given concurrently (30). The most common concern with isoniazid therapy is hepatic injury. Mild transaminasemia (SGOT and SGPT two to three times normal) is a common occurrence that does not predict more serious injury. Bridging necrosis can be caused by isoniazid. The drug should immediately be stopped in patients with symptoms of hepatitis (anorexia, nausea, malaise, and jaundice) and transaminases that are more than three times normal. Older patients are more likely to have substantial hepatic damage than are younger patients.

Rifampin is a zwitterion that inhibits many

Gram-positive and Gram-negative organisms by inhibiting DNA-dependent RNA polymerase, leading to suppression of the initiation of RNA chain synthesis. *In vitro* and *in vivo* resistance develops rapidly.

The drug is well absorbed orally; the parenteral form is available only as an investigational drug. Rifampin is metabolized in the liver via an active deacetylation and ultimately excreted via bile in the gastrointestinal tract. Rifampin is widely distributed in body tissue, including the CSF.

Less than 4% of patients suffer fever, rash, jaundice, various gastrointestinal complaints, and hypersensitivity reactions.

Ethambutol is an oral compound with excellent tuberculostatic activity. The drug is widely distributed. About 50% is excreted unchanged in the urine. Optic retinitis occurs only rarely in patients who are receiving 15 mg/kg or less of the drug. Other adverse effects are rare.

Streptomycin is tuberculocidal. Vestibular toxicity, auditory toxicity, and nephrotoxicity are not uncommon.

A variety of other antimycobacterial drugs are available for the therapy of *M. tuberculosis* or atypical mycobacteria such as *M. avium intracellulare*. Clofzimine and ansamycin are investigational agents that have been used in AIDS patients to treat *M. avium intracellulare*, but their efficacy or the efficacy of any other agents for the treatment of this organism has not been shown yet.

Antifungal Agents

AMPHOTERICIN B

Amphotericin B is a polyene antibiotic that is fungistatic or fungicidal for a wide variety of fungi but has no activity against bacteria or viruses (11, 14, 44). Amphotericin B is active against most *Candida* species, *Cryptococcus neoformans*, and *Torulopsis glabrata* as well as some *Aspergillus* and *Rhizopus* species, and most *Histoplasma capsulatum*, *Coccidioides immitis*, *Blastomyces dermatiditis*, and *Sporotichum schenkii*. Amphotericin B binds to the sterol component of fungal membranes, creating channels that increase the permeability of the membrane. Amphotericin B does not bind to the membranes of resistant organisms. Fungi do not become resistant to amphotericin B *in vivo*.

Amphotericin B must be administered by slow intravenous infusion after the amphotericin B has been dissolved in 5% dextrose in water. The drug precipitates in solutions containing acids, preservatives, or electrolytes. Because of the serious adverse effects, a 1-mg test dose is usually given in 20 ml of 5% dextrose solution over 1 hour. The next dose can be given immediately if there are no adverse effects. Although some experts suggest a gradual increase in dosage by 5-mg steps, it is prudent in critically ill patients to proceed directly to 0.6 mg/kg/day, administered in 500 ml of 5% dextrose solution over 2–6 hours. Few patients tolerate higher daily doses. Alternate-day therapy may be useful for some critically ill patients, especially after their fungal disease is clearly controlled. Hypersensitivity effects can be diminished by premedication with meperidine (50 mg intravenously administered) and diphenhydramine HCL (50 mg intravenously administered), and heparin (1000 units) added to the infusion. Premedication with hydrocortisone (10–100 mg intravenously administered) may be necessary to reduce the adverse effects, but this immunosuppressive agent should not be automatically given unless the other premedications are not effective. Amphotericin B can be administered intrathecally though there are few cases where this is warranted. Coccidioidomycosis meningitis may be one such indication.

Amphotericin B is a highly tissue bound drug that penetrates most body compartments, though concentrations in CSF and vitreous humor are low. Its metabolic pathways are incompletely understood. Very little of the drug is excreted in the urine, though the drug can be detected in the urine for 6–8 weeks after the last dose is given. Altered renal function or hemodialysis do not necessitate changes in drug dosage.

Adverse Effects

Amphotericin B is associated with a substantial number of adverse reactions such as flushing, chills, fever, anorexia, and headache. When severe, these untoward effects can be associated with tachypnea, hypoxemia, and hypotension. Slowing the infusion and premedicating the patient can diminish or eliminate these untoward effects.

Renal function is impaired by long courses of amphotericin B in over half of patients (13). Renal dysfunction can be reduced in severity and frequency by maintaining good hydration for the patient. Often the patient's serum creatinine, initially normal, will plateau in the 2–3 mg/dl range. In most cases, the renal dysfunction is largely but not completely reversible. If the serum creatinine rises about 3.0 mg/dl, the amphotericin B should be discontinued or the dose should be reduced if the danger of uremia outweighs the acute danger of the fungal process. Renal tubular function is often impaired by amphotericin B, resulting in hypokalemia, hypomagnesemia, and renal tubular acidosis that may be permanent. Anemia is also reported as a consequence of amphotericin B therapy, but leukopenia and thrombocytopenia are rare.

FLUCYTOSINE

Flucytosine, or 5-fluorocytosine, is a fluorinated pyrimidine that has activity against *C. neoformans*, some *Candida* species, and occasional isolates of other fungal species. Because 30% of cryptococci develop resistance during therapy, and resistance has also been observed to develop during therapy of *Candida* infection, flucytosine has no role as a single agent except perhaps in the treatment of chronic blastomyeosis. Its primary use is in combination with amphotericin B for cryptococcal infections and some candida infections (10).

Flucytosine is converted to fluorouracil by fungal cells, but not by host cells. The fluorouracil ultimately inhibits hymidylate synthetase.

Flucytosine is well absorbed orally and is widely distributed in body tissues, penetrating CSF and aqueous humor quite well. About 80% of the drug is excreted unchanged in the urine.

Adverse Effects

Bone marrow depression is a common occurrence in patients receiving flucytosine, especially those whose marrows have been previously compromised by malignancy, radiation, or myelosuppressive drugs. Bone marrow suppression can be minimized by maintaining peak serum levels below 100–125 μg/ml. Hepatomegaly, transaminasemia, nausea, rash, emesis, diarrhea, and enterocolitis are also seen occasionally.

KETOCONAZOLE

Ketoconazole is an oral agent that is effective against mucosal candidiasis as well as less common fungal diseases such as histoplas-mosis, coccidiomycosis, and blastomycosis. For patients with life-threatening fungal disease, ketoconazole has no role as a single agent. Nausea is the major adverse effect; numerous endocrinologic effects have also been described although their clinical importance when conventional doses are used is unclear. Ketoconazole is not absorbed unless there is gastric acidity.

MICONAZOLE

The indications to use miconazole in an intensive care setting are extremely rare although this imidazole does have activity against yeasts and filamentous fungi (70).

Antiviral Agents

RIBAVIRIN

Aerosolized ribavirin is effective therapy for severe respiratory syncytial virus (RSV) infections in children. Precipitation of the aerosolized drug on the valves and tubing of mechanical ventilators can lead to potentially hazardous malfunctions, especially if prefilters are not used. Other adverse effects associated with its use include anemia. There is no clear role for ribavirin in adults.

ACYCLOVIR

Acyclovir is a purine nucleoside analogue that has excellent activity against herpes simplex and herpes zoster but not against cytomegalovirus or Epstein-Barr virus (32, 37). The drug acts by inhibiting viral DNA synthesis. Some herpesviruses are resistant by virtue of thymidine kinase deficiency as well as by other mechanisms. Resistance developing during therapy has been described (20). Intravenous acyclovir is the drug of choice for life-threatening herpes simplex or herpes zoster infections such as disseminated disease or Herpes simplex encephalitis. Because herpes zoster is less sensitive to acyclovir than is herpes simplex, serious herpes zoster disease requires higher doses of acyclovir than serious herpes simplex. Acyclovir is excreted largely unchanged by the kidney, so dose adjustments must be made in the presence of renal dysfunction.

Adverse Effects

Intravenous acyclovir is well tolerated: phlebitis, rash, hypotension, nausea, headache, and encephalopathic changes can occur, as can reversible renal dysfunction.

9-1,3 DIHYDROXY-2-PROPOXYMETHYL-GUANINE

9-1,3 Dihydroxy-2-propoxymethyl-guanine (DHPG) inhibits the replication of all herpes viruses *in* vitro including cytomegalovirus, herpes zoster, and herpes simplex (16, 43, 68). DHPG is highly bone marrow suppressive in the doses employed clinically, so it is less desirable than acyclovir for therapy of Herpes simplex and herpes zoster infections. Its major clinical role is for therapy of cytomegalovirus disease. In AIDS patients it has been used to successfully treat cases of cytomegalovirus retinitis, pneumonia, esophagitis, and colitis. As of 1987 the specific indications for its use and the optimal treatment regimens are being delineated.

AZIDOTHYMIDINE

Azidothymidine (AZT, zidovudine) is a synthetic thymidine analog that has activity against human immunodeficiency virus (HIV). It is the first drug that has been shown to clearly prolong the life of patients with acquired immunodeficiency syndrome (AIDS). It is currently available commercially only in oral form. There is no evidence that therapy during life-threatening illness improves short-term survival. Major adverse effects including neutropenia, anemia, and headache. Little data are available about its interactions with other marrow suppressive drugs.

VIDARABINE

Vidarabine (adenosine arabinoside) is a derivative of adenosine. It is effective for herpes simplex encephalitis and keratoconjunctivitis, but there is almost no occasion to use it since intravenous acyclovir has become available (32, 75, 76). Acyclovir is at least as effective and considerably less toxic. The vidarabine must be administered intravenously in large volumes of fluid (15 mg/kg dissolved in 2.5 liters) given over 12–24 hours. This fluid bolus presents a management problem for patients with increased intracranial pressure, or with renal failure.

Adverse Effects

Thrombophlebitis occasionally occurs at the site of administration. Nausea, emesis, diarrhea, and malaise can also occur. Ataxia, tremor, seizures, and psychiatric disturbances can occur, particularly when serum levels are high.

CLINICAL USE OF ANTIMICROBIAL AGENTS IN CRITICALLY ILL PATIENTS

General Considerations

The successful use of antimicrobial therapy in the critically ill depends on an understanding of the pharmacology of the agents employed. For optimal therapy of an infectious process the drug must have good activity against the suspected or documented pathogen, it must be administered in such a way that active forms of the drug reach the site of infection at concentrations greater than the minimum inhibitory concentration (MIC) of the organism, and adverse effects must be avoided (9, 25). The activity of the drug against the presumed pathogens must be based on both *in* vitro susceptibility testing and clinical trials. Certain antibiotics have excellent *in* vitro activity but poor clinical efficacy. For example, polymixins may be quite active against Gram-negative bacilli, yet clinical response is unimpressive. *Salmonella* species may be susceptible to cephalothin, and S. *aureus* may be susceptible to chloramphenicol, yet patients do not have dramatic clinical response to these drugs compared with ampicillin and methicillin, respectively. Similarly, drugs may fail because organisms quickly develop resistance such as rifampin and S. *aureus* or carbenicillin and P. *aeruginosa*.

The mechanism of antimicrobial action is frequently considered in the choice of an antimicrobial agent. Common sense deems it preferable to use an agent that is bactericidal rather than bacteriostatic, especially if the patient's immune function is abnormal. In bacterial endocarditis, bactericidal agents are much more efficacious than bacteriostatic compounds (36, 45, 65, 74). For the treatment of other infections the importance of microbicidal as opposed to microbistatic drugs is unconvincing (38). Thus, the optimal antibiotic is probably best chosen on the basis of activity against the pathogen, distribution, and toxicity rather than mechanism of action.

Additive or synergistic drug combinations are popular approaches to the treatment of infectious processes (1, 36, 45, 63, 65). For bacterial endocarditis the addition of an aminoglycoside to a penicillin enhances serum bactericidal activity and the likelihood of clinical cure. These observations have been applied to other clinical situations where *in vitro* testing shows synergy for the offending microbe. In fact, there are little data, except for endocarditis, that document the clinical usefulness of these drug combinations, and in many situations, toxicity of the second drug can outweigh its usefulness (36, 45, 63). In some situations, however, the addition of a second drug may provide sufficient synergy that the dose of the first drug can be reduced, thus decreasing the toxicity. This is the case when flucytosine is added to amphotericin B for the treatment of cryptococcal meningitis (10).

Antagonism between bactericidal and bacteriostatic drugs is another in vitro phenomenon that is frequently applied to clinical situations (1, 63). With the exception of a trial of penicillin plus tetracycline for the treatment of pneumococcal meningitis, however, there is little documentation that antibiotic antagonism should be an important consideration in the choice of antibiotics. To ascertain that adequate antibiotic concentration reaches the site of infection is an essential consideration. An antibiotic must be present at a concentration equal to or greater than the MIC of the organism. Measuring antibiotic levels or measuring bacteriostatic activity in joint fluid, CSF, or bone may help determine the adequacy of drug dose (38). For anesthetic agents or for pressors, augmented clinical responses can be obtained by augmenting drug concentrations. With antibiotics, however, increased drug concentrations over the MIC for the pathogen do not correlate with enhanced clinical response in any predictable manner. The clinician often takes solace in attaining serum or body fluid drug levels that are much higher than the MIC of the causative organism. Attaining very high serum levels at peak and trough periods may in fact be useful: They ensure the clinician that sufficient antibiotic will be available if renal or hepatic drug excretion suddenly increases or if the infection occurs at a site where drug diffusion is poor. Only in bacterial endocarditis, however, does a specific measurement of serum killing activity correlate with clinical efficacy.

* Measuring serum levels of antibiotics is important for ensuring adequate dosing and for preventing toxicity. In critically ill patients, renal and hepatic function may be difficult to assess and may fluctuate rapidly. Formulas and nomograms may help to estimate proper drug dose. Drug levels should be measured on a regular basis, particularly if the drug is potentially toxic, such as an aminoglycoside or vancomycin. Measuring drug levels several times weekly may be expensive on an absolute basis, yet such measurements represent a small fraction of total patient cost and prevent distressing and expensive complications.

Empirical Therapy

When patients are critically ill their survival is often dependent on the prompt initiation of appropriate antimicrobial therapy. If the identity of the etiologic microorganism(s) is uncertain, empirical therapy that covers the full range of likely pathogens pending the outcome of diagnostic procedures must be initiated. For many critically ill patients, however, the optimal diagnostic procedure cannot be performed because the patient is too hypoxic for a bronchoscopy, too thrombocytopenic for a biopsy, or too hemodynamically unstable to be transported to radiology or the operating suite. This scenario is especially common when dealing with immunosuppressed patients.

Traditionally, empirical antimicrobial regimens were likely to include multiple drugs, since no one agent has broad coverage that included aerobic and anaerobic organisms, Gram-positive and Gram-negative bacteria, rods, and cocci. The past few years have been characterized by the appearance of third-generation cephalosporins, thienamycin, quinolones, and β-lactam/β-lactamase inhibitor combinations that can provide broad coverage. Single agents have the advantage of being less time consuming to administer. Moreover, several of these drugs are considerably less toxic than the aminoglycosides that were previously included in most multiple-drug empirical regimens, particularly those used for neutropenic patients. In the middle 1980s a major unresolved issue was whether single agents such as ceftazidine, or imipenem, or timentin would be as effective as multiple-drug regimens, thus allowing clinicians the ease of monotherapy and the diminution in direct toxicity (15, 51, 53, 58, 59). Whether these benefits will outweigh the high absolute cost of many of these newer drugs remains to be determined.

Epidemiological and Other Factors

The epidemiology of highly pathogenic or multiple antibiotic resistant organisms is an important consideration in the choice of antimicrobial agents in critically ill patients. Many patients who are critically ill have been exposed to hospital flora during previous hospitalization. Many critically ill patients are hospitalized in an ICU where they can acquire resistant organisms and become superinfected. Substantial antibiotic pressure on these patients can also select out endogenous flora that are multiply antibiotic resistant (26). These organisms can cause serious disease in the infected patient and they can be transmitted to other patients. A physician caring for a critically ill patient is obligated to use the most efficacious antimicrobial therapy available. The physician must also, however, introduce antibiotics appropriately so that resistance to newer antibiotics is delayed, thus saving these drugs for unusual situations where they are uniquely useful. For instance, amikacin has decided advantages over gentamicin and tobramycin because it is often more active against more Gram-negative bacilli. Gram-negative bacilli that are resistant to gentamicin and tobramycin will sometimes be susceptible to amikacin, yet the more frequently this latter drug is used, the more amikacin resistant organisms will likely appear. Thus, amikacin should probably be used only if the organism is known to be resistant to other therapeutic agents, or if there is some reason to strongly suspect such resistance. Similarly, some third-generation cephalosporins appear to be useful, nontoxic agents for the treatment of organisms that previously required toxic agents such as the aminoglycosides. If they are used indiscriminately to treat organisms susceptible to more conventional agents, however, resistance may rapidly develop, thus decreasing their usefulness and the usefulness of other β-lactam drugs.

The cost of newer antibiotics should also influence the drug selected. Newer drugs are often much more expensive than older, generically available agents, and their routine use can dramatically increase a hospital's pharmacy expenditure.

Finally, the choice of antimicrobial agent must be influenced by a physician's familiarity with the drug. The rapid explosion of penicillin, cephalosporin and quinolone agents makes it impossible for physicians to be familiar with the doses, pharmacokinetics, and adverse effects of all agents. Errors in selection and administration are more frequent if the physician attempts to use too large an armamentarium of drugs, especially when dealing with critically ill patients with changing hepatic and renal function and when considering the interaction of the drug with other medications. It seems preferable for the physician to be very familiar with the pharmacology of a limited antibiotic armamentarium and to select other agents or newer agents only when clearly indicated.

References

1. Acar JF, Sabath JP, Ruch PA: Antagonism of the antibacterial action of some penicillins by other penicillins and cephalosporins. *J Clin Invest* 55:446–453, 1975.
2. Acar JF, Neu HC (eds): Gram-negative aerobic bacterial infections: a focus on directed therapy, with special reference to aztreonam. *Rev Infect Dis* 7(Suppl 4):5537–5840, 1985.
3. Allan JD, Eliopoulos GN, Moellering RC: The expanding spectrum of beta-lactam antibiotics. *Adv Intern Med* 00:119–146, 1986.
4. Appel GB, Neu HC: The nephrotoxicity of antimicrobial agents. *N Engl J Med* 296:663, 676, 1977.
5. Appel GB, Neu HC: Gentamicin in 1978. *Ann Intern Med* 89:528, 538, 1978.
6. Bartlett JG, Gorbach SL: Penicillin or clindamycin for primary lung abscess? An Editorial. *Ann Intern Med* 98:546, 1983.
7. Bartlett JG, Chang TW, Gurwith M, et al: Antibiotic associated psuedomembranous colitis due to toxic producing clostridia. *N Engl J Med* 298:531, 534, 1978.
8. Bartlett JG, Onderdonk AB, Cisneros RL: Clindamycin. Associated colitis due to a toxin producing species of clostridia in hamsters. *J Infect Dis* 136:701–707, 1977.
9. Bauer AW, Kirby WMM, Sherris JC, et al: Antibiotic susceptibility testing by a standardized single disc method. *Am J Clin Pathol* 45:493–496, 1966.
10. Bennett JE, Dismukes NE, Duma RJ, et al: A comparison of amphotericin B alone and combined with flucytosine in the treatment of cryptococcal meningitis. *N Engl J Med* 301:126–131, 1979.
11. Bennett JE: Antifungal agents. In Mandell GL et al: *Principles and Practices of Infectious Diseases.* New York, John Wiley & Sons, 1985, pp 263–269.
12. Brown CH, Natelson EA, Bradshaw E, et al: The hemostatic defect produced by carbenicillin. *N Engl J Med* 291:265–270, 1974.
13. Burgess JL, Birchall R: Nephrotoxicity of amphotericin B with emphasis on changes in tubular function. *Am J Med* 53:77–84, 1972.
14. Carrizosa J, Kaye D: Antibiotic concentrations in serum, serum bactericidal activity and results of therapy of streptococcal endocarditis in rabbits. *Antimicrob Agents Chemother* 12:479–483, 1977.
15. Clissold SP, Todd PA, Campoli-Richards DM: Imipenem/Cilastin—A review of its antibacterial activity, pharmacokinetic properties, and therapeutic efficacy. *Drugs* 33:183–241, 1987.
16. Collaborative DHPG Treatment Study Group. Treatment of serious cytomegalovirus infections with 9-(1,3-dihydroxy-2-propoxymethyl) guanine in patients with AIDS and other immunodeficiencies. *N Engl J Med* 314:801–805, 1986.
17. Congeni BL: Comparison of ceftriaxone and traditional therapy of bacterial meningitis. *Antimicrob Agents Chemother* 25:40–44, 1984.
18. Conte JE, Upton RA, Phelps RT, et al: Use of a specific and sensitive assay to determine pentamidine pharma-

cokinetics in patients with AIDS. *J Infect Dis* 154:923–929, 1986.

19. Cook RV, Farrar WE Jr: Vancomycin revisited. *Ann Intern Med* 88:318–321, 1978.
20. Crupacker CS, Schnipper LE, Marlowe SI, et al: Resistance to antiviral drugs of Herpes simplex virus isolated from patients treated with acyclovir. *N Engl J Med* 306:343, 1982.
21. Davies J, Courvalin P: Mechanisms of resistance to aminoglycosides. *Am J Med* 62:868–877, 1977.
22. Elipoulos GM, Moellering RC: Azlocillin, mezlocillin, piperacillin: new broad spectrum penicillins. *Ann Intern Med* 97:755–760, 1982.
23. Farrar WE Jr, O'Dell NM: Comparative beta-lactamase resistance and antistaphylococcal activities of parenterally and orally administered cephalosporins. *J Infect Dis* 137:490–493, 1978.
24. Geraci JE, Hermans PE: Vancomycin. *Mayo Clin Proc* 58:88–91, 1983.
25. Fekety FR Jr, Norman PS, Cluff LE: Treatment of Gram-negative bacillary infections with colistin. *Ann Intern Med* 57:214–227, 1962.
26. Finland M: Emergence of antibiotic resistance in hospitals, 1935–1975. *Rev Infect Dis* 1:4, 1979.
27. Galgiani JN, Busch DF, Brass C, et al: *Bacteriodes fragilis* endocarditis bacteremia and other infections treated with oral or intravenous metronidazoles. *Am J Med* 65:284–289, 1978.
28. Ghysen JM: Penicillin-sensitive enzymes of peptidoglycon metabolism. In Schlessinger D: *Microbiology-1977*. Washington, DC, American Society for Microbiology, 1977, p 195.
29. Gilman AG, Goodman LS, Gilson: *The Pharmacologic Basis of Therapeutics*, ed 8. New York, Macmillian, 1980.
30. Gronhagen-Riska C, Hellstrom PE, Froseth B: Predisposing factors in hepatitis induced by isoniazide-rifampin treatment of tuberculosis. *Am Rev Respir Dis* 105:292–295, 1978.
31. Handbook on antimicrobial therapy: *Med Lett Drugs Ther* 1986.
32. Hirsch MS, Schwartz ML: Antiviral agents. *N Engl J Med* 302:903–907, 949–953, 1980.
33. Hughes WT, Feldman S, Chaudhary SC, et al: Comparison of pentamidine isethionate and trimethoprim-sulfamethoxazole in the treatment of *Pneumocystis carinii* pneumonia. *J Pediatr* 92:285–291, 1978.
34. Kancir LM, Tuazon CU, Cardella TA, et al: Adverse reactions to methicillin and Naficillin during treatment of serious *Staphylococcus aureus* infections. *Arch Intern Med* 138:909–911, 1978.
35. Kaufman C, Frame PT: Bone marrow toxicity associated with 5-fluorocytosine therapy. *Antimicrob Agents Chemother* 11:244–247, 1977.
36. Kaye D: *Infective Endocarditis*. Baltimore, University Park Press, 1976.
37. King DHJ, Galasso G (ed): Proceedings of a symposium on acyclovir. *Am J Med* July 20, 1982.
38. Klastersky J, Daneau D, Weerts D: Antibacterial activity in serum and urine as a therapy guide to bacterial infection. *J Infect Dis* 129:187–193, 1974.
39. Kluge RM, et al: Carbenicillin-gentamicin combination against *Pseudomonas aeruginosa*. *Ann Intern Med* 81:584, 1974.
40. Landesman SH, Corrado ML, Shah PM, et al: Past and current roles for cephalosporin antibiotics in treatment of meningitis. Emphasis on use in gram-negative bacillary meningitis. *Am J Med* 71:693, 1981.
41. Levine BB: Skin rashes with penicillin therapy: current management. *N Engl J Med* 286:42–43, 1972.
42. Mallory DL, Parrillo JE, Lane HC, et al: The hemodynamic effects and safety of intravenous pentamidine. *Critical Care Med* 15:503–505, 1987.
43. Masur H, Lane HC, Palestine A, et al: Effect of 9-(1,3-dihydroxy-2-propoxymethyl) guanine on serious cytomegalovirus disease in eight immunosuppressed homosexual men. *Ann Intern Med* 104:41–44, 1986.
44. Medoff G, Kobayashi GS: Strategies in the treatment of systemic fungal infections. *N Engl J Med* 302:145–148, 1980.
45. Moellering RC Jr, Wennersten C, Weinberg AN: Synergy of penicillin and gentamicin against enterococci. *J Infect Dis* 124:5207, 1971.
46. Moellering RC Jr, Wennersten C, Kung LJ, et al: Resistance to gentamicin, tobramycin, and amikacin among clinical isolates of bacteria. *Am J Med* 62:873–877, 1977.
47. Moore RD, Smith CR, Lietman PS: The association of aminoglycoside plasma levels with mortality in patients with gram-negative bacteremia. *J Infect Dis* 149:443, 1984.
48. Moore RD, Smith CR, Lipsky JJ, et al: Risk factors for renal dysfunction in patients treated with aminoglycosides. *Ann Intern Med* 100:352, 1984.
49. Nahata MC, Barson WJ: Ceftriaxone: A third generation cephalosporin. *Drug Intell Clin Pharm* 19:900–906, 1985.
50. Neu HC: The new β-lactamase stable cephalosporins. *Ann Intern Med* 97:408–413, 1982.
51. Neu HC: Antibiotics in the second half of the 1980's—Areas of future development and the effect of new agents on aminoglycoside use. *Am J Med* 80(Suppl 6B):195–203, 1986.
52. Neu HC, Turck M, Phillips I: Ceftizoxime: A broad spectrum beta-lactamase stable cephalosporin. *J Antimicrob Agents Chemother* 10(Suppl C):1, 1982.
53. Neu HC: Beta-lactamase inhibitors. In Mandel GL, Douglas RG, Bennett JE (eds): *Principles and Practice of Infectious Diseases*, ed 2, New York, John Wiley & Sons, 1985, pp 190–192.
54. Onorato IM, Axelrod JL: Hepatitis from intravenous high dose oxacillin therapy. Findings in an adult inpatient population. *Ann Intern Med* 89:497–500, 1978.
55. Parter RH, Eggleston M: Beta-lactamase inhibitors: Another approach to overcoming antimicrobial resistance. *Inf Control* 8:36–40, 1987.
56. Pearson RD, Hewlett EL: Pentamidine for the treatment of pneumocystis pneumonia and other protozoal disease. *Ann Intern Med* 103:783–786, 1985.
57. Petz LD: Immunologic cross reactivity between penicillins and cephalosporins: a review. *J Infect Dis* 137:574–579, 1978.
58. Pizzo PA, Hathorn JW, Hiemenz J, et al: A randomized trial comparing ceftazidime alone with combination antibiotic therapy in cancer patients with fever and neutropenia. *N Engl J Med* 315:552–558, 1986.
59. Pizzo PA, Thaler M, Hathorn JW, et al: New Beta-lactam antibiotics in granulocytopenic patients: new options and new questions. *Am J Med* 79(Suppl 2A):75–82, 1985.
60. Pratt WB, Fekety R: *The Antimicrobial Drugs*. New York, Oxford University Press, 1986.
61. Quinn JP, Dudek EG, Divincenzo CA, et al: Emergence of resistance to imipenem during therapy for *Pseudomonas aeruginosa* infections. *J Infect Dis* 154:289, 1986.
62. Quinn JP, Divincenzo CA, Foster J: Emergence of resistance to ceftazidime during therapy for Enterobacter-cloacal infections. *J Infect Dis* 155:942–947, 1987.
63. Rahall JJ Jr: Antibiotic combinations: clinical relevance of synergy and antagonisms. *Medicine* 570:179–183, 1978.
64. Rouveix E, Bure AM, Regnier B, et al: Experience with imipenem/cilastatin in the intensive care unit. *J Antimicrob Agents Chemother* 18(Suppl):153–180, 1986.
65. Sande MA, Courtney KB: Nafcillin-gentamicin synergism in experimental staphylococcal endocarditis. *J Lab Clin Med* 88:118, 1976.
66. Saxon A: Immediate hypersensitivity reactions to Beta-lactam antibiotics. *Rev Infect Dis* 5(Suppl 2):5368, 1983.

67. Shattil JS, Bennett JS, McDonough M, et al: Carbenicillin and penicillin inhibit platelet functions in vitro by impairing the interactions of agonists with the platelet surface. *J Clin Invest* 65:329–337, 1980.

68. Shepp DH, Dandliker PS, Myers JD: Treatment of *Varicella* zoster virus infection in severely immunocompromised patients: a randomized comparison of acyclovir and vidarabine. *N Engl J Med* 314:208–212, 1986.

69. Snider DE, Cohn CL, Davidson PT, et al: Standard therapy for tuberculosis. *Chest* 1985 87(supp):1175–1245, 1985.

70. Stevens DA: Miconazole in the treatment of systemic fungal infection. *Am Reve Respir Dis* 116:801–806, 1977.

71. Symposium. Trimethoprim-sulfamethoxazole. *J Infect Dis* 128(Suppl):425–816, 1973.

72. Tomasz A: The mechanism of the irreversible effects of penicillins. How the β-lactam antibiotics kill and lyse bacteria. *Ann Rev Microbiol* 33:113, 1979.

73. Weinstein L, Dalton AC: Host determinants of response to antimicrobial agents. *N Engl J Med* 279:467, 1968.

74. Weinstein L: Experimental staphylococcal endocarditis. *J Lab Clin Med* 88:118, 1976.

75. Whitley RJ, Alford CA, Hirsch MS, et al: Vidarabine versus acyclovir therapy in Herpes simplex encephalitis. *N Engl J Med* 314:144–149, 1986.

76. Whiteley RJ, Ch'ien LT, Dolin R, et al: Adenosine arabinoside therapy of Herpes zoster in the immunosuppressed. *N Engl J Med* 297:289–294, 1977.

77. Williams ME, Harman C, Scheld M, et al: A controlled study: Ticarcillin plus clavulanic acid versus piperacillin as empiric therapy for fever in the immunosuppressed host. *Am J Med* 79(Suppl 5B):67, 1985.

14

Poisoning

Glenn C. Freas, M.D., F.A.C.E.P.

Mortality from poisoning ranges from 5,000 to 12,000 deaths per year (20, 67). Accidents are the leading cause of death in Americans up to age 40. In this category, poisoning is outranked only by motor vehicle fatalities. Suicide from poisoning is the second leading cause of death among adolescents and young adults (46). Current estimates attribute 1% to 10% of all emergency room visits to poisoning (46). Roughly 15% of all ICU admissions are for acute poisoning (8). Only a minority of poisoned patients presenting to a hospital are cared for in a critical care setting since less than 15% of self-poisonings result in changes in level of consciousness (21). The overall mortality rate from poisoning in hospitalized patients is low, less than 1% of admitted patients (28). Preschoolers (children less than 5 years of age) tend to be victims of accidental, nontoxic ingestions or exposures. Ingestion in older patients is more likely to be purposeful and toxic. Data from the National Clearinghouse for Poison Control Centers in 1978 revealed that only 2% of poisoned preschoolers required hospitalization, and preschoolers were involved in only 9% of fatal poisonings. The 1978 NCPCC data show that the mode of poisoning was accidental in only 36% of cases involving the older population, as opposed to essentially 100% of cases in preschoolers (46).

Carbon monoxide, alcohols, acetaminophen, opioids, salicylates, sedative-hypnotics, psychotherapeutic agents, cardiac glycosides, β-blockers, and anticonvulsants account for the large majority of poisoning deaths and ICU admissions in this country (20, 90). Carbon monoxide is the most common cause of death by poisoning.

PHARMACOLOGY

Poisons may be inhaled, injected, absorbed through the skin and mucous membranes, and ingested. Many drugs can be used and abused via all four routes. The pharmacokinetics of drugs or toxins taken in toxic doses may be much different than when taken in therapeutic dosages. Absorption, distribution, metabolism, and excretion may all be altered by an overdose (137).

Many poisons can alter absorption rates by delaying gastric emptying; this is especially true of drugs that possess anticholinergic properties. Delayed absorption may have some indirect benefit in the poisoned patient because most drugs are not absorbed in the stomach but in the small intestine. Many authors advocate inducing emesis or gastric lavage even several hours after ingestion because of this delay in gastric emptying (19).

This concept of gastric emptying as one of the determinants of intestinal absorption rates is important when considering the use of dilutents, with or without syrup of ipecac. When copious fluids are given in an effort to dilute a poison or to follow a dose of ipecac, gastric emptying may be increased because of gastric distention. Animal studies demonstrate that the oral lethal dose of a variety of drugs is decreased as the volume of diluent is increased (48). These considerations make judicious use of fluids (limited to 8–10 oz in adults or 5 ml/kg of body weight in children) imperative when used as a diluent or "chaser" for ipecac.

Enterohepatic circulation plays a major role in drug overdoses. Recent reports indicate that repeated doses of orally administered activated charcoal increase clearance of certain agents from the systemic circulation. The proposed mechanism is adsorption of drug that has passively diffused or has been actively secreted from the systemic circulation into the gastrointestinal tract. This mode of therapy is called "gastrointestinal dialysis" (95).

Many drugs are eliminated by first-order kinetics in which the amount of drug eliminated is directly proportional to the concentration of that drug. Zero-order kinetics (e.g., the amount of drug eliminated is constant and independent of drug concentration) may result if enzyme systems are saturated. Methanol, ethanol, salicylates, and phenytoin exhibit zero order or saturation kinetics at all clinically important blood concentrations (4).

The reader is referred to other sources for a more indepth discussion of the pharmacology of poisoning (6). Concepts such as solubility, volume of distribution, protein binding, and active metabolites have important implications for the clinician. The choice of interventional means such as hemodialysis or hemoperfusion is based on these concepts. Later in this chapter, in the discussion of specific poisons, significant pharmacologic characteristics will be addressed as they relate to management of each toxin.

RESUSCITATION AND STABILIZATION

In most cases the intensivist assumes care for the poisoned patient when the patient is transferred from the emergency room to the intensive care setting. It is imperative that all prior therapy, intervention, and perhaps aborted attempts at intervention be carefully reviewed once the patient is admitted to the ICU. In the vast majority of poisoned patients nonspecific supportive therapy is all that is necessary to assure complete recovery. Some basic points about resuscitation bear re-emphasizing.

Airway

Poisoned patients may lose their ability to protect their airway rather rapidly. Obtundation, hypoventilation, a weak or absent gag reflex, signs of airway obstruction, or associated maxillofacial injuries all warrant immediate management with nasotracheal or orotracheal intubation. Aspiration of gastric contents is the most frequent complication of poisoning (127). Nasotracheal intubation, if possible, is preferable because it is better tolerated by the semiconscious patient and it allows easier access for eventual placement of a large-bore orogastric tube.

A question often arises regarding airway protection for the patient who is not a candidate for ipecac (and who consequently requires gastric lavage), yet who is responsive enough to fight insertion of a nasotracheal tube.

Although some might consider paralysis with succinylcholine prior to intubation and lavage, this approach may be hazardous. Succinylcholine may affect the ingested toxin; for example, succinylcholine may produce cardiac arrhythmias and obscure the clinical picture in tricyclic antidepressant overdose (69). A safer approach would be to attempt nasotracheal intubation without the use of succinylcholine. Should patients be so combative as to inflict harm on themselves or the staff, one can cease attempts at intubation and observe the patient carefully during insertion of the orogastric tube and subsequent lavage.

Breathing

Proper oxygenation is required to meet metabolic needs (often increased by seizures, hyperpyrexia, etc.) and is specifically therapeutic in the treatment of toxins such as carbon monoxide, which interferes with the transport of oxygen. In paraquat poisoning tissue damage is mediated by superoxide ions. In this type of poisoning, supplemental oxygen should be avoided (47). Supplementing a hypoventilating patient's respirations with a bag-valve-mask for prolonged periods is to be discouraged because it may overdistend the stomach and result in vomiting and aspiration. Respiratory rate, effort, and breath sounds must be constantly reassessed. Noncardiogenic pulmonary edema or direct gaseous toxins may complicate pulmonary function.

Circulation

Maintenance of adequate end organ perfusion requires that intravascular volume, cardiac function, and systemic vascular resistance be controlled. Hypotension on admission is the most important prognostic factor for mortality in severe poisoning (3). Even if normotensive initially, at least one large-bore intravenous line should be inserted to provide venous access should hypotension later develop. Direct arterial monitoring and measurements of pulmonary capillary wedge pressures may need to be initiated in the patient whose fluid management is complex. Use of pressor agents should be reserved until failure of fluid resuscitation is clearly demonstrated; toxins that cause hypotension by venous pooling far outnumber the agents, such as propranolol, that might cause myocardial depression (46).

Other Stabilizing Measures

All patients with a depressed sensorium or in coma should receive naloxone hydrochloride in an initial intravenously administered dosage of at least 0.8 mg (two ampules). This specific narcotic antagonist will reverse the central nervous system depression associated with the overdose of opiates as well as other drugs. Larger doses and repeated doses may be necessary to achieve or maintain the desired response. All patients with a depressed sensorium should also receive 50 g of dextrose intravenously if indicated by a spot, bedside glucose determination. Thiamine 100 mg, intravenous or intramuscular, should be given prior to or concomitant with dextrose to prevent the development of Wernicke-Korsakoff syndrome in the patient who may be severely thiamine depleted (67).

DIAGNOSIS

The history may be unreliable in the poisoned patient as a result of drug induced confusion, amnesia, misinformation (particularly important in recreational drug overdoses), and deliberate attempts at deception (68). Despite these handicaps the physician must elicit as much information from as many sources as possible. Family, friends, emergency department personnel, pre-hospital-care providers, pharmacists, bystanders, and police can be contacted and significant historical clues can emerge, even when the patient is comatose. It is incumbent upon the physician to determine what toxin (or toxins) is involved, the mode of exposure, the amount ingested, the time since ingestion, and the circumstances surrounding the overdose. One should also attempt to determine coexisting medical, surgical, or psychiatric conditions, current medications, and any drug allergies. If applicable, an occupational and vocational history should be obtained.

The aim of the physical examination is to detect signs that may lead to a determination of the type and severity of poisoning, as well as evidence of underlying systemic disease or trauma. Additionally, the intensivist must look for complications of therapy that may have occurred in the pre-hospital-care setting or the emergency room.

Particular attention should be paid to vital signs, the integument, the cardiopulmonary system, the abdomen, the neurologic examination, and products of secretion and excretion. Patients may be profoundly hypothermic due to prolonged periods of exposure and inactivity as well as prolonged resuscitation and stabilization. Temperature elevation may be due to specific poisons (salicylates or anticholinergics) or related to coexistent medical problems producing a fever.

Many severely poisoned patients will have alterations in blood pressure, heart rate, and respiratory rate. These must be followed closely and appropriate therapy initiated when indicated by the clinical picture.

Along with a general description of the patient and vital signs, the examiner should note any characteristic odors on the patient's breath. The breath may smell like alcohol (e.g., ethanol, methanol, ethylene glycol), gasoline (hydrocarbons), or fruit (diabetic ketoacidosis or alcoholic ketoacidosis).

Fresh or old, scarred needle puncture or "tracks" suggest intravenous drug abuse. Cutaneous bullae may be seen in barbiturate, glutethamide, and carbon monoxide poisoning (69). Diaphoresis may be due to salicylates or organophosphates. Hot, dry skin may be characteristic of anticholinergic poisoning, as well as severe heat stroke. Cyanosis may be due to oxidizing agents that cause methemaglobinemia.

A whole host of poisons may cause noncardiogenic pulmonary edema and a wide variety of toxins can cause alterations in cardiac function. In the intravenous drug abuser with a cardiac murmur, the examiner should think of endocarditis with embolic phenomenon as a source for persistent neurologic signs. In hydrocarbon ingestion, the onset of wheezing or rales may precede the development of chest x-ray findings.

The abdominal examination should focus on the presence or absence of bowel sounds, presence of involuntary guarding, evidence of urinary retention, and the presence of signs such as hepatomegaly and/or splenomegaly that may signify chronic alcohol abuse or other medical conditions. In the poisoned trauma victim with changes in mental status the abdominal examination can be unreliable as an indicator of a potential surgical problem. In most cases further investigation by peritoneal lavage or abdominal imaging techniques will be necessary.

A careful neurological examination is mandatory. Serial determinations of level of consciousness by a standardized evaluation system or by the same examiner is invaluable. Changes in level of consciousness not consistent with the suspected ingestion should lead the examiner to further investigate other possible etiologies. Pinpoint pupils suggest either a pontine lesion or use of opiates, organophosphates, phenothiazines, or chloral hydrate. Midpoint or dilated pupils are less specific. Extraocular movements and the presence of nystagmus should be examined and noted. Ingestion of PCP may cause nystagmus. Testing the cranial nerves and checking the gag reflex are mandatory. The presence of focal neurological findings is highly suggestive of a structural lesion and further investigation is warranted, it is re-emphasized that repeated neurological examinations may detect expanding masses (e.g., hemorrhage) or evolving metabolic abnormalities.

Finally, attention to secretory and excretory products may yield characteristic findings. Salivation, lacrimation, urination, and defecation (SLUD) are characteristic of muscarinic signs of anticholinesterase poisoning (63). On the other hand, anticholinergic agents can cause dry mouth, urinary retention, and decreased gastrointestinal motility.

Careful and selective use of laboratory tests can be extremely valuable. An indiscriminate "shotgun" approach or delaying therapy while awaiting results can be disastrous. In general, any severely poisoned patient should have blood collected for hemoglobin, hematocrit, blood counts, serum electrolytes, blood urea nitrogen, creatinine, glucose, prothrombin time, and arterial blood gases. A urine analysis should also be obtained. Depending on the clinical scenario, other commonly needed studies include a carboxyhemaglobin, serum ketones, serum osmolality, and liver function studies. Specific laboratory abnormalities will be discussed in the sections dealing with individual poisons.

Judicious use of the toxicology lab can help confirm a suspected diagnosis. In most cases a qualitative urine screen is sufficient for the poisoned patient. If positive, it confirms the suspected diagnosis and may add additional unsuspected information. If negative, it suggests the presence of another etiology.

Quantitative drug concentrations are essential in the management of some toxins. These include acetaminophen, digoxin, ethanol, methanol, ethylene glycol, carbon monoxide, salicylates, iron, lead, and lithium. If a toxic blood level is reported by the laboratory but is not supported by the clinical picture, the level

should be repeated before instituting specific treatment based on that result.

Tablets that are radiopaque on x-ray flat plate of the abdomen include chloral-hydrate, heavy metals (arsenic, lead, iron), iodides, psychotropics (phenothiazines and tricyclics), and enteric-coated tablets. ECGs, while nonspecific, can have some important therapeutic considerations in certain overdoses such as tricyclic antidepressants. Since many poisons can complicate pulmonary function (e.g., cause pulmonary edema or aspiration pneumonitis) a chest x-ray is a valuable adjunct as well.

DRUG REMOVAL

Once the patient is stabilized and diagnostic measures have been undertaken the focus of therapy shifts to removal of the offending agent(s). This goal can be accomplished by decreasing absorption of the poison and hastening its elimination.

While the vast majority of poisons are ingested and absorbed via the gastrointestinal tract, it bears emphasizing that some toxins are absorbed in other ways and it is necessary to decontaminate any portal of entry. When the portal of entry is dermal, it is imperative that all clothing be removed and the skin washed so as to prevent continued absorption.

Measures to Decrease Absorption

Spontaneous emesis often occurs with such substances as theophylline, iron, and salicylates. This is probably not an efficacious way of decontaminating the gastrointestinal tract, and the clinician should not let an episode of spontaneous emesis deter further attempts to empty the upper part of the gastrointestinal tract (44). Mechanically induced emesis (e.g., tongue blade, finger) is likewise ineffective in emptying the stomach (35).

Induced emesis is most frequently accomplished with either ipecac syrup or apomorphine. Ipecac is the agent of choice for most clinicians. The best candidate for induced emesis is the awake, alert, cooperative patient who demonstrates an intact gag reflex. Contraindications to induced emesis include coma, manifest or incipient seizures, loss of a gag reflex, ingestion of a caustic agent, or ingestion of a hydrocarbon where the risk of aspiration outweighs the risk of systemic toxicity if intestinal absorption is permitted (46).

Syrup of ipecac is derived from the dried root of *Cephaelis ipecacuanha*. The principle alkaloids producing emesis are emetine and cephaline. Both agents exert central effects on the medulla's chemoreceptor trigger zone, as well as a local irritant effect on the gastric mucosa. Fluid extract of ipecac is no longer used. It is 14 times more concentrated than syrup of ipecac, and it caused a variety of cardiovascular complications.

Recommended doses of ipecac are 10 ml for children under 1 year of age, 15 ml for children 1–12 years of age, and 30 ml for those over 12 years of age. This dose should be followed by 8–12 oz of water in adults or 5 ml of water per kilogram of body weight in children (165). In more than 90% of cases, emesis will ensue within 30 minutes (98). If emesis has not occurred within 30 minutes the dose of ipecac may be repeated. A recent prospective study showed that the use of syrup of ipecac in the 9- to 12-month-old child appears to be safe and effective (57).

Most authorities caution against the simultaneous use of ipecac and activated charcoal. The proposed reasoning is that activated charcoal significantly absorbs the ipecac and thus decreases its efficacy. In a recent, small prospective study, administration of activated charcoal 10 minutes after ipecac (and prior to emesis) found no significant decrease in the ability of ipecac to produce emesis. After emesis subsided, a repeat dose of charcoal was given (53). These results take on significant implications when one considers the recent recommendations that activated charcoal be given as rapidly as possible (discussed below). Ipecac is effective when administered to patients who have ingested an overdose of antiemetics (161).

Apomorphine is a morphine congener that acts by stimulating the medullary chemoreceptor trigger zone. It is unstable in solution and only effective when used parenterally. Thus, a tablet must be crushed and dissolved to create a fresh, stable solution. Apomorphine causes respiratory depression and CNS sedation, which can be reversed with naloxone (39). Because of the inconvenience in preparation and its CNS sedation and respiratory depression, apormorphine is not used extensively.

Gastric lavage is an alternate method for preventing absorption of toxin from the gastrointestinal tract. It is commonly employed when the need to empty the stomach is present but the patient does not meet the criteria for induced emesis or in the rare case where ipecac (two doses) has not produced emesis. Contraindications to gastric lavage include caustic ingestions, hydrocarbon poisoning, and lack of ability to protect the airway (46).

A large-bore gastric tube of at least 36-F diameter should be used and the stomach lavaged with 4 ml/kg/cycle to a maximum of 200 ml/cycle of fluid. The patient should be on the left side to pool gastric contents in the fundus, tilted head down to deter aspiration, and turned slightly on the stomach. Lavage should be continued until the gastric return is "clear" but this approach does not guarantee removal of dissolved toxin (138). Protection of the airway is important during lavage. Repeated assessments of the level of consciousness and the presence of a gag reflex are mandatory.

The use of tap water is advocated by many. It is just as efficacious as saline solutions, can be warmed easily, causes no demonstrable electrolyte imbalances in adults, and is much less expensive (138). Use of saline when lavaging children is advocated by some because it is less likely than tap water to produce electrolyte imbalances. In selected cases it may be advantageous to modify the lavage fluid. In cases of oxalate poisoning it is useful to add calcium to the lavage fluid to precipitate these ions. In poisoning with enteric-coated tablets or with iron it is useful to use a bicarbonate solution (152). In glutethamide overdose it is recommended that a lavage solution of castor oil and water be used.

An age-old debate in clinical toxicology is the question of the comparative efficacy of gastric lavage and induced emesis in gastrointestinal decontamination. This question is still unresolved. The clinician must tailor his approach to the clinical setting. Effective results from induced emesis or gastric lavage might take anywhere from 30 minutes to 2 hours. One prospective study showed that gastric-emptying procedures in the emergency room were not of benefit unless gastric lavage was performed within 1 hour of ingestion in obtunded patients (90).

Large pill concretions, which are resistant to easy removal via traditional gastric emptying methods, can form in the stomach. Successful removal of tablets of meprobamate, ferrous sulfate, and aspirin has been accomplished by endoscopy or removal of the mass via gastrotomy (100). These techniques should be reserved for the patient in whom ongoing absorption of the poison from the concretion is deleterious and cannot be prevented by repeated doses of activated charcoal.

Activated charcoal is formed by burning such substances as wood, bone, starch, and other organic substances. The residue is "activated" by treatment with superheated steam or with other chemicals to remove any adsorbed substances and to increase the surface area available for adsorption. When charcoal is used in poisoning, the quantity of drug adsorbed at equilibrium is proportional to the amount of internal surface area. There is a wide variety of commercially available activated charcoal preparations, and they vary in their adsorption capacity. Activated Charcoal Merck, Norit A, and Nuchar C are the most efficient commercial preparations (89).

Activated charcoal is administered orally as a suspension, or alternately the suspension can be instilled via an orogastric tube (after lavage) or via a nasogastric tube (after induced emesis). The desired ratio of activated charcoal to ingested toxin is 10:1. However, the amount of poison is frequently unknown. For most adults, 50–100 g in 8 oz of water creates the desired slurry. For children, 20–50 g is recommended, depending on age and habitus. Activated charcoal is nontoxic and completely inert if aspirated. The sooner charcoal is administered, the more efficacious it is for preventing absorption of toxin (96). Activated charcoal is poorly tolerated orally, and it may be necessary to insert a small-bore nasogastric tube (which is left in place when repeated doses are necessary) for installation of the slurry. This method saves precious time and nursing efforts.

Activated charcoal should be withheld when N-acetylcysteine is going to be administered for the treatment of acetaminophen overdose. This approach is based on the assumption that activated charcoal will adsorb this antidote. Although a recent study has challenged this assumption, the recommendation to withhold charcoal in this situation should stand until further in vivo studies are completed (138).

Repeated doses of activated charcoal are advised for those toxins that undergo enterogastric or enterohepatic recirculation. This method of enhancing gastrointestinal clearance by activated charcoal has been termed "gastrointestinal dialysis" (95). Drugs amenable to this form of treatment include phenobarbital and cyclic antidepressants and related compounds, phenylbutazone, digitoxin, theophylline, glutethamide, and meprobamate (32, 50, 73). Recommended doses for this purpose are 50 g every 2–6 hours for four doses. Charcoal is not efficacius in treatment of poisoning with cyanide, lithium, iron, alkalies, or mineral acids.

Measures to Enhance Elimination

The administration of cathartics to hasten elimination of both adsorbed toxin and free toxin has traditionally been advocated. Commonly used agents are sodium sulfate, magnesium sulfate, or magnesium citrate. However, there have been no clinical studies confirming that catharsis decreases the total adsorption of an ingested toxin (44). On the other hand, there are many reports of complications related to cathartic therapy, including a case report of profound cathartic-induced magnesium toxicity (86).

Clinical studies on cathartics have examined only immediate-release dosage forms of potential poisons. Studies need to be done which evaluate the effect of rapid catharsis on the bioavailability of sustained-release preparations such as theophylline or delayed-release, enteric-coated products. Recommended doses of cathartics in these situations is 15–30 g of magnesium citrate in adults and 250 mg/kg in pediatric patients. Cathartics should not be used in the very young, the patient who may have an ileus, the patient in renal failure, or the patient in whom fluid and electrolyte balance is problematic.

Fluid loading and forced diuresis may help eliminate toxic agents from the body but may also lead to complications that include electrolyte disturbance, acid-base disorders, cerebral edema, and pulmonary edema.

The following general criteria should be considered before instituting forced diuresis: (a) renal excretion of the unchanged drug is the major route of elimination, (b) the drug is extensively reabsorbed in the renal tubules, and (c) the drug is distributed mainly in the extracellular fluid compartment and is minimally protein bound.

Cell membranes are relatively impermeable to ionized (polar) molecules, whereas nonionized (nonpolar) molecules can easily cross cell membranes. By increasing the ratio of ionized to nonionized drug by altering urine pH, less drug is available for absorption through cell membranes.

Alkalinization of urine is achieved with sodium bicarbonate, 1 to 2 mEg/kg intravenously every 3–4 hours. Maintenance of a urinary pH of 7.5–8.5 is desired and the amount of bicarbonate administered is guided by this endpoint. A urine flow of 5 ml/kg/hour is desired. Toxins amenable to alkaline diuresis are salicylates and barbiturates (156, 97). Cyclic antidepressant poisoning is treated with systemic alkalinization (but not forced diuresis).

Acid diuresis is usually accomplished with ammonium chloride (either orally or intravenously). Hydration is maintained with 5% dextrose in saline. Ammonium chloride, 4 g every 2 hours orally or a 1–2% solution in normal saline intravenously, should be given to maintain a urinary pH of 5.5–6 (171). Forced acid diuresis can increase the excretion of phencyclidine, amphetamines, quinine, fenfluramine, and quinidine (171, 128).

Hemoperfusion or hemodialysis is indicated (171, 128) when (a) progressive deterioration of the patient occurs despite careful and intensive supportive care, (b) severe clinical intoxication occurs with abnormal vital signs signifying depression of midbrain functioning, (c) the compound ingested has been absorbed or ingested in a potentially lethal dose, (d) a blood or plasma concentration of the compound is in the lethal range, (e) there is impairment of the patient's normal excretory capacity for eliminating the ingested poison, or (f) the drug ingested can be removed at a rate that exceeds the endogenous elimination by the liver or kidneys.

Drugs that can effectively be removed by hemodialysis include ethylene glycol (124), methanol (102), lithium (171), salicylates (77), and ethanol (171). Drugs in which hemoperfusion plays a role in active removal include quinine (109); isopropyl alcohol (9); diquat (171); barbiturates (195); digitalis glycosides; tricyclic antidepressants (188); other lipid soluble drugs (171); and nonbarbiturate hypnotics, sedatives, and tranquilizers (171).

SPECIFIC TOXINS

Acetaminophen

Acetaminophen is currently available in more than 250 pharmaceutical products in the United States (25). Cases of acute hepatocellular necrosis in association with paracetamol (acetaminophen) overdoses were reported in 1966 (38). Two-hundred patients die every year from acetaminophen overdose in the United Kingdom, where the drug is the leading cause of acute hepatic necrosis (75). In the United States

the incidence of poisoning from acetaminophen overdose is rising, and in some areas may constitute 10–12% of patients who are admitted for poisoning (141).

Acetaminophen is primarily metabolized to glucuronide and sulfate conjugates, which are nontoxic. A small proportion of the parent compound (about 4%) is metabolized by the cytochrome P-450 dependent, mixed function oxidase enzymes to a poorly described reactive intermediate (105). With therapeutic doses of acetaminophen this intermediate is detoxified by conjugation with glutathione and excreted by the kidney as cysteine and mercapture metabolites of acetaminophen (79). However, when acetaminophen is given in toxic doses, glutathione becomes depleted and the hepatotoxic metabolite cannot be adequately detoxified. The metabolite binds to sulfhydryl groups in hepatic intracellular proteins and causes acute, widespread hepatocyte death (19). Acetylcysteine can prevent this process. N-acetylcysteine is metabolized to cysteine, a glutathione precursor, thereby providing additional glutathione for use in the detoxification of acetaminophen metabolite (139).

Toxic ingestion of acetaminophen is characterized by four clinical stages (139). Stage 1 occurs 12–24 hours after ingestion and is typified by nausea, vomiting, diaphoresis, and anorexia. There may be some patients with few symptoms in this stage, even after ingesting large amounts. Stage 2 occurs 1–2 days after ingestion. Typically the previous stage's symptoms abate, however, liver enzymes and prothrombin time begin to rise. Some right upper quadrant pain and tenderness may develop at the end of this stage. Stage 3 develops 3 days postingestion and correlates with peak hepatotoxicity. This phase is characterized by jaundice, coagulopathy, hypoglycemia, encephalophathy, and occasionally renal failure and cardiomyopathy. The SGOT may reach 20,000 IU or more, and in one case the SGOT reached 321,900 IU (145). Stage 4 occurs 7–8 days after ingestion and is the recovery stage for patients who survive.

Treatment of acetaminophen overdose is centered around N-acetylcysteine. Treatment is most effective with N-acetylcysteine when it is administered within 16 hours after acetaminophen ingestion. Current recommendations are to institute treatment if the ingestion occurred within 24 hours. Use of a nomogram (Fig. 14.1) to guide therapy requires that plasma levels be drawn at least 4 hours after ingestion. It is important to note that nonspecific colori-

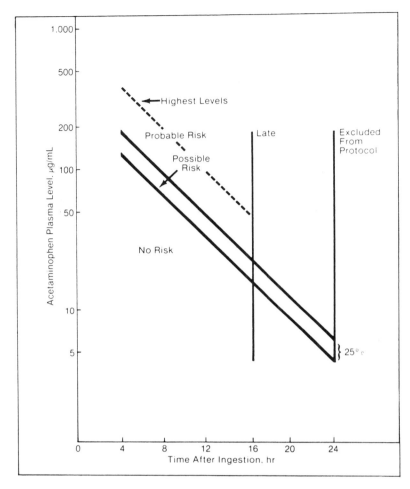

Figure 14.1. Revised nomogram for estimating toxicity from acetaminophen overdose. (From Rumack BH, Peterson RG, Koch GG, Amara IA: Acetaminophen overdose: 662 cases with evaluation of oral acetylcysteine treatment. *Arch Intern Med* 141:380, 1981. Copyright 1981, American Medical Association.)

metric assays may underestimate acetaminophen levels by as much as 700% (123). If levels are not readily available, starting treatment with N-acetylcysteine is advised until a plasma level can be obtained. If a pretreatment plasma level is in the nontoxic range then treatment can be stopped. If a previously toxic plasma level becomes nontoxic during therapy, treatment should continue for the full course of therapy. Most authorities agree that 7.5 g of acetaminophen represents a toxic dose in adults and 150 mg/kg represents a toxic dose in children. Because of inaccuracies in some patient's histories, it is best to draw a level (at least 4 hours postingestion), start therapy, and continue or stop treatment based on the pretreatment serum acetaminophen level.

N-acetylcysteine should be given after appropriate stabilizing measures have been accomplished. If activated charcoal has been instilled, it is recommended that the stomach be lavaged clear of charcoal prior to the first dose of N-acetylcysteine. An initial loading dose of 140 mg/kg is given orally. The solution is prepared by mixing one part (20%) N-acetylcysteine with three parts soda, or water, or grapefruit juice. This yields a 5% solution. Maintenance doses are 70 mg/kg administered every 4 hours for a total of 68 hours (17 doses). Intravenous N-acetylcysteine is used in the United Kingdom with good success. Currently, this is not available in the United States. Palatability of N-acetylcysteine is its major drawback. If the patient vomits less than 1 hour after ingestion of any dose of N-acetylcysteine, it should be repeated. An occasional patient will require placement of a duodenal tube for administration of the antidote.

Salicylates

Children make up the largest group of patients who present with salicylate poisoning (20, 156, 159). The most commonly encountered salicylates are acetylsalicylic acid (aspirin), sodium salicylate, and salicylic acid. A less common yet very concentrated form of salicylate is methyl salicylate (oil of wintergreen), which is a component of Ben-Gay. Oral ingestion of a little as 5 ml of oil of wintergreen is equivalent to 21 325-mg tablets of aspirin, a lethal dose in young children (22).

Salicylates follow zero-order kinetics; thus an increase in dose does not result in a linear increase in serum level. Rather, at saturation an increase in dose causes a higher than expected serum level. In addition, children's metabolic pathways are more rapidly saturated than adults (156).

The two major modes of presentation of severe salicylism are metabolic alterations and CNS manifestations. The biochemical actions responsible for the metabolic derangements include direct stimulation of the medullary respiratory center (respiratory alkalosis), uncoupling of oxidative phosphorylation, inhibition of amino acid metabolism, inhibition of Krebs Cycle enzymes, stimulation of gluconeogenesis, and inhibition of glycolysis (149). Metabolis acidosis predominates in young children (less than 4 yours of age) while respiratory alkalosis is more common in older children and in adults (130).

Neurologic disturbances such as confusion, delirium, and coma are the best clinical indications of severe intoxication (129). CNS toxicity is most frequently demonstrated in those patients in whom a picture of metabolic acidosis dominates (130). The acidosis is thought to favor a shift of salicylates from extracellular fluid into cells, particularly the brain (78). Additionally it is postulated that some CNS effects may be caused or exacerbated by a relatively hypoglycemic environment in the brain despite normal serum glucose levels.

Patients with mild toxicity typically show nausea and vomiting, tinnitus and other hearing disturbances, hyperpnea, respiratory alkalosis, and slight restlessness or lethargy. Those with moderate toxicity have more pronounced

hyperpnea, fever, varying degrees of dehydration, metabolic acidosis, and marked lethargy and/or excitability. Severe toxicity can manifest as stupor, coma, seizures, severe metabolic acidosis, noncardiogenic pulmonary edema, renal failure, and hepatic failure (156, 159).

Severity of salicylate poisoning can be determined from a serum salicylate level (Fig. 14.2). The Done nomogram is only useful in estimating severity of acute poisoning. The serum level should be drawn at least 6 hours postingestion. Peak levels correlate best with toxicity (41). With ingestion of large amounts, or with ingestion of enteric-coated preparations, there may be prolonged absorption and levels may continue to rise for 24 hours after

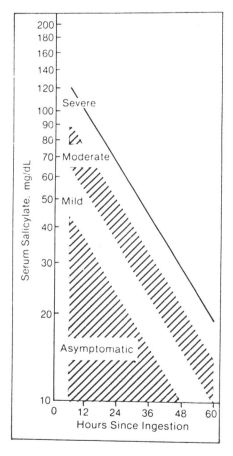

Figure 14.2. Nomogram for estimating the severity of poisoning from the serum salicylate level at varying intervals after ingestion of a single dose. (From Done AK: Salicylate intoxication. Significance of measurements of salicylate in blood in cases of acute ingestion. *Pediatrics* 26:800, 1960. Reproduced with permission of the publisher.)

ingestion. Salicylate ingestion is also suggested by positive results on several qualitative screening tests. These include an increased anion gap, a positive urine Clinitest with a negative glucose oxidase strip test, and a positive ferric chloride test on a boiled sample of urine. Prior to return of the serum salicylate level, the severity of toxicity can be estimated as follows: (a) no toxic reaction if ingested dose is 150 mg/kg, (b) mild to moderate toxicity if ingested dose is 150 –300 mg/kg, (c) serious toxicity if ingested dose is 300–500 mg/kg, and (d) potentially lethal reaction if ingested dose is 500 mg/kg.

The diagnosis of chronic salicylism may be very difficult since typically symptoms are minimal and nonspecific. Many elderly patients undergo a neurologic workup for altered mental status before the diagnosis of chronic salicylism is entertained. Delayed diagnosis is associated with a higher morbidity and mortality (5).

Treatment of salicylate poisoning is aimed at correcting fluid, electrolyte, and acid-base disturbances and enhancing elimination of the salicylate. Initial measures include hydration, administration of dextrose for hypoglycemia, correction of acidemia with sodium bicarbonate, and administration of vitamin K (2–5 mg/ kg administered intravenously) if the patient manifests any evidence of a bleeding disorder secondary to hypoprothrombinemia. Gastrointestinal decontamination with lavage and activated charcoal is important, particularly when large amounts or enteric-coated preparations are ingested. Elimination of salicylates is enhanced by alkaline diuresis (107), as previously described.

Hemodialysis can be used in the severely poisoned patient. It is usually reserved for the patient who is likely to develop fluid overload and pulmonary edema with forced diuresis (as in cardiac or renal failure). Other indications for hemodialysis are a plasma salicylate level of greater than 100 mg/dl and acidemia with neurotoxicity, refractory to bicarbonate administration.

Cyclic Antidepressants

Tricyclic antidepressants are used by over 25 million people annually (99) and are the fourth most common cause of drug overdose in the United States (26). There is an associated 3% mortality (26). The narrow and sometimes overlapping margin of safety between therapeutic and toxic effects mandates close follow-up of all patients taking these medications.

The active agents responsible for both therapeutic and toxic effects are the parent tertiary amine compound (e.g., imipramine, amitriptyline, doxepin) and their metabolites (desipramine, nortriptyline, desmethyldoxepin). It should be noted that cyclobenzaprine (Flexeril) and carbamazepine (Tegretol) are similar to the cyclic antidepressants in their presentation and management of overdose.

Cyclic antidepressants undergo rapid absorption from the gastrointestinal tract. Metabolism takes place mainly via N-demethylation, N-oxidation, and hydroxylation reactions in the liver. They all possess a large volume of distribution, signifying extensive tissue binding (81). Because of the extensive protein binding of these compounds and the large volume of distribution, forced diuresis, hemoperfusion, and hemodialysis have no role in the management of these overdoses (33).

Additionally, because of their wide volume of distribution, serum levels of these compounds are not reflective of potential toxicity. Tissue levels may be 10 times serum levels (51). Cyclic antidepressant medications also undergo an enterohepatic circulation that makes repeated doses of activated charcoal advisable in treatment of overdoses (33).

Cyclic antidepressants and related compounds exert four pharmacological actions that can result in both therapeutic and toxic effects. They sedate, exert both central and peripheral anticholinergic effects, block presynaptic uptake of amine neurotransmitters (norepinephrine, serotonin, and dopamine), and exert a quinidine-like effect on the cardiac conduction system.

As a result of these pharmacological effects there are three major manifestations of toxicity: CNS signs, anticholinergic signs, and cardiopulmonary signs. CNS effects may occur with both toxic and therapeutic doses. In a typical overdose, an initial phase of excitement and restlessness is followed by sedation, which may progress to coma, seizures, and autonomic changes (132). Amoxapine and maprotiline are associated with a higher incidence of seizures compared with older tricyclic antidepressants and trazodone (167). Typical anticholinergic signs include fever, fixed dilated pupils, dry mouth, flushed hot skin, excitement, hallucinations, and coma. Cardiopulmonary toxicity is manifested by supraventricular and ventricular dysrhythmias, conduction disturbances, hypotension, and pulmonary edema.

Cardiac toxicity is the major concern in tricyclic overdose. There have been various attempts to establish criteria for predicting the likelihood of cardiac toxicity from an overdose. In the absence of an atrioventricular conduction disturbance it is reasonable to assume that the absence of a tachycardia means there is a low probability of significant cardiac toxicity (80). A QRS duration greater than 100 ms signifies cardiac toxicity and is usually associated with serum levels of greater than 1000 mg/dl (18). Others have found that a prolonged corrected QT interval and a terminal QRS vector of 130° to 270° indicate significant cardiac toxicity. It was also found that a QRS duration of 100 ms or more was associated with a higher incidence of seizures, whereas a QRS duration of greater than 160 ms was associated with a higher incidence of ventricular dysrhythmias (18). Despite these guidelines, there is still a paucity of data predicting the likelihood of cardiac disturbances from cyclic antidepressant overdose, as well as predicting when a patient is "out of the woods" and can be transferred to an unmonitored setting.

Treatment for the patient with a cyclic antidepressant overdose is based on general supportive measures and liberal criteria for admitting the patient to the intensive care setting. Early airway control cannot be overemphasized. Patients with a significant overdose may initially present awake, alert, and with an intact gag reflex. Within minutes they can become obtunded and lose their gag reflex. Because of the delayed gastric emptying associated with these medications, measures to empty the upper gastrointestinal tract (lavage or induced emesis) should be attempted within 4–6 hours of ingestion. Repeated doses of activated charcoal may help remove the drug because of its enterohepatic circulation. Because of the possibility of pulmonary edema, intravenous fluids should be kept at maintenance infusion rates unless hypotension is present.

The use of physostigmine salicylate in the management of cyclic antidepressant overdose remains controversial. In this setting, physostigmine can arouse a comatose patient, stop seizures, and terminate tachydysrhythmias. However, arousal after physostigmine administration is not diagnostic of poisoning with anticholinergics because it can arouse victims of other poisonings (117). Physostigmine can aggravate conduction abnormalities and produce asystole in patients with severe tricyclic poisoning (125). Physostigmine may also precipitate seizures (115). Thus, physostigmine should be used only when other measures have failed. The usual dose in adults is 0.2 mg/minute intravenously over 10 minutes.

Diazepam is the agent of choice for treating seizures (82). Intractable seizures can be treated with phenytoin or other anticonvulsants. Sodium bicarbonate administration to achieve a pH of 7.5 has been shown to suppress dysrhythmias, narrow the QRS complex, and significantly improve hypotension (24). When bicarbonate is unsuccessful in terminating ventricular dysrhythmias in adults, phenytoin is recommended (59, 103). In children, propranolol is recommended for dysrhythmias unresponsive to bicarbonate (134). In the patient with hypotension resistant to bicarbonate therapy, fluid and pressor therapy is indicated. Logical pressors to choose are norepinephrine or dopamine since they are two of the amine neurotransmitters that cyclic antidepressants affect.

Several patients have died from dysrhythmias as late as 6 days postingestion despite apparent hemodynamic stability (54). However, absence of tachycardia, absence of QRS, PR, and QT prolongation, absence of ventricular dysrhythmias, and absence of anticholinergic and CNS signs for at least 24 hours suggest that the patient can be safely discharged from a monitored bed.

Carbon Monoxide

Carbon monoxide (CO) poisoning accounts for one-half of all poisoning deaths in the United States (120) and may contribute to many others (116). CO is a tasteless, odorless, and colorless gas that is the product of incomplete combustion of carbon-containing substances. Some common sources include combustion engine exhaust fumes, defective heating systems, smoke, fires, faulty gas and kerosene space heaters, and improperly ventilated charcoal briquette or Sterno fires. Methylene chloride is a volatile solvent used in many home and industrial preparations. Accidental exposure or purposeful inhalation of this solvent may result in CO poisoning (155). The resting carboxyhemoglobin level in normal nonsmokers is about 0.8–1.0% while the level in normal smokers is about 4–6.8% (30, 112).

The effects of acute CO poisoning vary depending on the inspired concentration of

CO, the activity level of the victim, and the duration of the exposure. The nonspecific nature of the initial presentation forces the clinician to have a high index of suspicion, if the condition is to be correctly and promptly diagnosed. Over-reliance on carboxyhemoglobin levels and inadequate attention to clinical signs and symptoms may lead to incomplete treatment with subsequent permanent neurological sequelae.

CO has two major actions as a poison. It crosses the alveolar-capillary membrane and binds to hemoglobin with an affinity 200–250 times greater than that of oxygen. CO also causes the oxyhemoglobin dissociation curve to shift to the left. These effects dramatically reduce the blood's oxygen carrying capacity. In addition, CO is a direct cellular toxin for the cytochrome A3 oxidase system, preventing aerobic cellular metabolism (29).

These toxic effects primarily impact on the tissues with the highest oxygen consumption, such as the myocardium and the brain. The principal initial clinical manifestations of CO poisoning are neurological. The symptoms are nonspecific and are easily confused with those caused by ingestion of other substances, particularly alcohol. The diagnosis may further be confused by the fact that up to 60% of CO poisoning victims also ingest alcohol in varying amounts (173). Some of the presenting symptoms and signs include headache, nausea, confusion, poor judgment, visual disturbances, shortness of breath, fatigability, memory deficits, somnolence, coma, and seizures. Dermatologic manifestations include erythema, bullae, and edema. Cherry red discoloration of the lips or skin is usually a postmortem finding and rarely seen as a presenting sign in the alive patient. Rhabdomyolysis may occur from pressure necrosis of muscle or as a direct toxic effect (166). Fever and leukocytosis may also be present. An ECG should be obtained to rule out evidence of myocardial ischemia from hypoxia.

The intensivist is cautioned against over-reliance on carboxyhemoglobin levels. Past attempts to correlate these blood levels with severity of symptoms have been unsuccessful. Carboxyhemoglobin levels obtained in the ICU do not reflect peak levels that may have been partially treated by EMS personnel or emergency room physicians. A normal carboxyhemoglobin level does not rule out CO poisoning (113). Levels between 10 and 70% may be associated with the entire spectrum of clinical CO poisoning. In general, brief exposures to high levels of CO will have much less clinical toxicity than prolonged exposures to lower levels (166).

The mainstay of treatment for victims of CO poisoning is oxygen. The half-life of CO in a patient breathing room air is about 5 hours. With 100% oxygen administration, the half-life is reduced to about 1½ hours. Hyperbaric oxygen at 3 atm reduces the half-life to 23 minutes (113). The mode of oxygen therapy depends on the clinical condition, the carboxyhemoglobin level, and the availability and proximity of a hyperbaric chamber. In suspected cases of CO poisoning, immediate applications of 100% oxygen should precede any other therapy while awaiting a laboratory report on carboxyhemoglobin levels. Since CO is eliminated by adequate ventilation, patients demonstrating inadequate ventilation should be intubated and mechanically ventilated. Treatment of other medical or surgical conditions should be instituted simultaneously. Arterial pH should be monitored and corrected as necessary.

Current recommendations for the use of hyperbaric oxygen therapy following CO exposure include (120) (a) any patient with a carboxyhemoglobin level of 25% or more; (b) any patient exhibiting neurological symptoms other than a mild headache and nausea, regardless of carboxyhemoglobin level; (c) a patient with a history of unconsciousness; and (d) a patient with new cardiac abnormalities such as arrhythmias or ischemic changes.

Oxygen therapy should continue until the patient clinically improves. Clinical recovery usually lags hours to days behind normalization of carboxyhemoglobin levels.

Cyanide

Cyanide poisoning, although relatively rare, represents one of the most severe poisonings a clinician can encounter. More importantly, cyanide is one of the few poisons that can be successfully treated with a specific antidote. The intensivist must be able to rapidly recognize a victim of cyanide poisoning, initiate resuscitative efforts promptly, and administer the antidote in the proper sequences and dosages.

Cyanide can exist in several forms. Hydrocyanic acid is the highly volatile acid that liberates the deadly gas hydrogen cyanide. The gas has the distinctive smell of bitter almonds.

Cyanide also exists as the sodium and potassium salts of hydrocyanic acid. Derivations of hydrogen cyanide include acrylonitrile, cyanamide, cyanogen chloride, and nitroprusside (31). Industrial sources for cyanide compounds include fumigation, ore extraction, electroplating, synthetic ruber production, fertilizers, silver polishes, and rodenticides. Natural sources of cyanide include amygdalin, which is found in the seeds of many fruits such as cherries, plums, peaches, pears, and apricots. Amygdalin is harmless unless the seed that contains it is crushed and moistened, which allows the enzyme emulsin to drive the chemical reaction that produces cyanide. Laetrile is a synthetic agent, allegedly antineoplastic, that contains amygdalin usually from apricot or peach pits. There have been several cases of cyanide poisoning from Laetrile, at least one resulting in death (43). Recently, there have been several tragic deaths from apparently purposeful contamination of over-the-counter medications with cyanide salts.

Cyanide causes hypoxia by binding to the ferric $(Fe+3)$ iron of mitochondrial cytochrome oxidase. This results in an almost total inhibition of cytochrome oxidase activity and thus inhibition of cellular respiration. This leads to anaerobic metabolism and an accumulation of lactic acid (71).

The clinical presentation depends on the amount inhaled or absorbed and the duration of exposure. Symptoms begin within minutes to an hour after oral ingestion; skin absorption usually produces symptoms in minutes; and inhalation may produce symptoms and even death within seconds. The symptoms occur in rapid succession and include giddiness, palpitations, headache, dyspnea, and unconsciousness. Usually, gastrointestinal symptoms from ingestion of the salts do not occur because of the rapidity of the onset of CNS depression. Seizures and dysrhythmias result from profound hypoxia. Lactic acidosis occurs because of anaerobic metabolism and hypoxia.

Diagnosis rests on a history of potential exposure and rapidly progressive clinical signs, as described above. Lactic acidosis is helpful but nonspecific. Other clinical clues include equally red arteries and veins on funduscopic examination and signs and symptoms of severe hypoxia in patients who do not appear cyanotic (71). Cyanide levels are not usually available in the acute setting. Plasma thiocyanate (an indication of the amount of endogenous detoxification of cyanide by the naturally occurring enzyme rhodanase) may be measured and followed to detect cyanide poisoning in patients on nitroprusside therapy.

Successful treatment involves simultaneous resuscitation and stabilization efforts, and administration of the appropriately sequenced and dosed antidotes. All emergency rooms and intensive care units should have the Lilly Cyanide Antidote kit. This contains instructions, pediatric dose tables, and prepackaged forms of amyl nitrite "perles," 10% sodium nitrite, and 25% sodium thiosulfate.

Inhalation of amyl nitrite and intravenous injection of sodium nitrite causes a methemoglobinemia $(Fe+3)$ which has a greater affinity for cyanide than does the ferric iron $(Fe+3)$ of cytochrome oxidase. Methemoglobin remove cyanide from the respiratory enzyme, allowing normal cellular respiration to resume. Sodium thiosulfate is given intravenously to enhance the metabolism of cyanide to thiocyanate, a relatively nontoxic substance that is excreted by the kidneys. In adults, amyl nitrite "perles" should be broken in a gauze pad and inhaled by the patient while the sodium nitrite solution is being prepared. Usually 10 ml of the sodium nitrite (330 mg) is given intravenously (slowly to prevent hypotension). Subsequently 50 ml (12.5 g) of sodium thiosulfate is given intravenously. Repeat doses may be necessary as clinically indicated.

Theophylline

The incidence of theophylline poisoning is on the rise (45). Some cases are a result of intentional overdoses, but many others are the result of physician-prescribing errors (110). The availability of slow-release preparations has also contributed to the increased incidence of theophylline poisonings. Available forms of theophylline include aminophylline, oxtriphylline, dyphylline, slow-release theophylline, and slow-release aminophylline. Theophylline is a methylxanthine similar in structure to caffeine. Short-acting preparations are rapidly absorbed from the gastrointestinal tract, and peak blood levels occur within 2 hours. Slow-release preparations have delayed absorption and peak serum levels may not occur for 8–12 hours depending on the preparation. Once absorbed, approximately 60% of theophylline is protein bound. Only free theophylline is pharmacologically active. Serum levels measure both bound and unbound theophylline.

Theophylline is metabolized in the liver, and diseases or drugs affecting the liver's ability to metabolize theophylline may result in higher blood levels.

At therapeutic levels, theophylline is metabolized by first-order kinetics. However, at blood levels of 10 μg/ml or above, metabolizing enzymes become saturated and zero-order kinetics ensues. Thus, patients with therapeutic blood levels of theophylline, may become toxic if doses are increased or liver function is decreased. Medical conditions that may predispose patients to theophylline toxicity include age over 60 years, liver disease (cirrhosis, hepatitis, cholestasis), COPD, cor pulmonale, congestive heart failure, viral illnesses, febrile illnesses, and influenza vaccine. Medications that can predispose to toxicity include cimetidine, erythromycin, and noncardioselective β-blockers (103).

Serum theophylline levels are best determined by high-pressure liquid chromotography. Both symptoms of toxicity and clinical response to therapy correlate well with peak serum levels. Therapeutic serum concentrations range from 10 to 20 μg/ml. Acute single ingestions (in a patient not on maintenance therapy) of less than 10 mg/kg are unlikely to produce symptoms of toxicity. Acutely toxic patients can tolerate much higher theophylline levels than patients on chronic therapy who become toxic (121).

Mild manifestations of toxicity usually occur with serum levels between 20 and 35 μg/ml. These signs and symptoms include nausea and vomiting, tremors, irritability, polyuria, tachycardia, tachypnea, and headaches. Severe toxic manifestations occur above serum levels of 80 μg/ml in acute toxicity and above 50 μg/ml in chronic toxicity. Severe toxicity includes supraventricular arrhythmias, ventricular arrhythmias, hypotension, seizures, coma, and cardiopulmonary arrest. Metabolic abnormalities of toxicity include hypokalemia, hyperglycemia, leukocytosis, respiratory alkalosis, metabolic acidosis, hypomagnesemia, and hypophosphatemia (72). The presence of seizures carries up to a 50% mortality in some series (179).

The hypotension seen in severe toxicity is usually mediated by a decrease in systemic vascular resistance. It is proposed that this decrease in systemic vascular resistance is secondary to an increase in β-adrenergic activity causing vasodilation in skeletal muscle (36). This has led some authorities to advocate the use of β-blockers or pure α-agonists (methoxamine) for the treatment of hypotension. In one limited series, β-blockers did indeed raise blood pressure (17). Many of the metabolic abnormalities may also result from a hyperadrenergic state (17).

Treatment includes general supportive measures, institution of gastrointestinal dialysis with repeated doses of activated charcoal, and careful selection of patients for charcoal or resin hemoperfusion. Theophylline levels should be drawn every 2 hours until a trend is established and efficacy of therapeutic measures is proven. Once theophylline toxicity is established, anticipation of life-threatening dysrhythmias or seizures is paramount.

Early and repeated doses of activated charcoal can decrease ongoing absorption of theophylline and increase elimination, because of theophylline's enterohepatic circulation (144, 96). Initial doses of activated charcoal range from 50–100 g and are followed by 30–50 g every 2–4 hours until levels are below the toxic range. Sorbitol (100 ml of 70% solution) may be given as a cathartic along with the charcoal (160).

Treatment of arrhythmias from theophylline toxicity follows conventional guidelines. Seizures associated with theophylline overdose may be prolonged and intractable. They carry a high mortality and survivors may show permanent neurologic sequelae. Diazepam should be used as a first-line drug. If diazepam (or one of its benzodiazepine analogues) is given to a total dose of 20–30 mg and the seizures persist beyond 15–20 minutes, phenobarbital should be added. Phenobarbital can be given at a dose of 10 mg/kg intravenously. A repeat dose of 10 mg/kg may be given in 15 minutes. If seizure activity persists beyond 45 minutes, thiopental general anesthesia is recommended (103).

Hemoperfusion may be useful in removing theophylline and minimizing life-threatening complications of toxicity. Criteria for selecting patients for hemoperfusion are poorly defined. Some recommend hemoperfusion in the setting of a rising serum concentration greater than 60 μg/ml (17). Others recommend it when levels exceed 80 μg/ml (61). In chronic toxicity, hemoperfusion may be instituted when levels exceed 50 μg/ml in a patient who is over 60 years of age and has heart or liver failure. Hemoperfusion may also be useful in the elderly patient who is unable to tolerate oral activated charcoal. While decisions are being made about hemoperfusion, all patients should have oral charcoal therapy started.

Alcohols

An osmolal gap of greater than 10 suggests the presence of osmotically active substances such as the alcohols, mannitol, or glycerol. The most commonly ingested alcohols are ethanol, methanol, ethylene glycol, and isopropyl alcohol.

ETHANOL

Ethyl alcohol is the most common drug consumed (49). It is oxidized in the liver to carbon dioxide and water by the alcohol dehydrogenase system. This is a nicotinamide adenine dinucleotide (NAD) dependent enzyme. Other enzyme systems may play a role in ethanol metabolism, but alcohol dehydrogenase is the major route by which ethanol is detoxified. Hepatic ethanol metabolism follows zero-order kinetics, with 7–10 g of ethanol metabolized each hour in the adult. Chronic alcoholics and children metabolize alcohol more rapidly than the average adult (131).

Whisky and wine are involved in most reported serious ethanol poisonings in children. Mouthwashes and colognes may also be involved. In the very small child, a potentially lethal dose is provided by just 5–10 oz of mouthwash or 1–2 ounces of cologne (170). Ethanol serum concentrations of 338–575 mg/dl have been associated with coma and subsequent survival without sequelae in toddlers (131). The occurrence of concomitant hypoglycemia in children is of major concern.

Although serum ethanol levels may be helpful in establishing a diagnosis, they frequently do not correlate well with the level of intoxication because of tolerance. For the novice drinker, or the person never exposed to alcohol, death from medullary failure may occur at serum ethanol levels of 500 mg/dl. However, there is one anecdotal report of a patient with an ethanol level of 999 mg/dl, who was treated and discharged from an emergency room (162).

The clinical features of ethanol intoxication range from mild mental impairment to coma and death. The degree of intoxification depends upon the rapidity of the rise of the blood ethanol level, the level reached, and the length of time high levels are maintained. With severe toxicity, hypotension, hypoventilation, hypothermia, and coma may develop. Tachycardia is commonly seen, even without hypotension. Patients must be examined for evidence of complications of the acute intoxication (such as aspiration, gastrointestinal bleeding, or core hypothermia) as well as coexistent medical or surgical conditions (such as multiple trauma, diabetes, or other ingestions).

Treatment of the acutely poisoned patient is supportive. Early airway protection is paramount. Alcohol is a gastric irritant and carries high risk of aspiration in the obtunded patient. Lavage and instillation of charcoal are indicated if the ingestion is acute (e.g., within 2 hours of presentation). After blood is drawn for a glucose determination, administer 50 g of dextrose intravenously and 100 mg of thiamine intravenously or intramuscularly. Hypotension usually responds to fluid therapy. The Wernicke-Korsakoff Syndrome (ataxia, dysarthria, and sixth-nerve palsy or oculomotor paralysis) requires the administration of 500–1000 mg of thiamine intravenously.

Some have tried the administration of naloxone in order to reverse the CNS and respiratory depression associated with ethanol poisoning. There are some data to indicate that naloxone reverses the ethanol-induced depression of the hypercapnic drive. There are also anecdotal reports of boluses of naloxone dramatically improving the mental status of the acutely intoxicated patient. However, this same effect reportedly is not operative in the acutely intoxicated chronic alcoholic (104). Further studies are needed to determine its place, if any, in the treatment of acute ethanol intoxication. Hemodialysis can be employed when ethanol levels are high and the patient exhibits profound midbrain and medullary dysfunction despite supportive measures.

The intensivist must also be aware of the potential for alcohol withdrawal syndromes in their poisoned patients. Alcohol withdrawal seizures ("rum fits") are major motor seizures that may manifest before the onset of other withdrawal symptoms. They occur typically in burst of two to three seizures and begin 8–12 hours after cessation of drinking. Prior to the onset of full-blown delirium tremens, the patient may show tremors, tachycardia, insomnia, and irritability. These symptoms may occur even in the presence of elevated blood ethanol levels. The full spectrum of delirium tremens usually manifests 36–96 hours after cessation of drinking. Symptoms and signs include marked tachycardia, diaphoresis, hypertension, visual hallucinations, psychosis, and uncontrollable tremors. Intravenous diazepam or easily titratable short-acting benzodiazepines are effective in controlling delirium tremens. Huge doses may be necessary, mandating careful monitoring of the patient's airway and respiratory status. Withdrawal seizures rarely require treatment because status epilepticus is unusual. Use of phenothiazines is contraindicated because they decrease the seizure threshold. Those patients with underlying seizure disorders should receive phenytoin intravenously both therapeutically and prophylactically.

METHANOL

Methyl alcohol (methanol) in its distilled form is a nearly odorless and palatable alcohol. Crude wood alcohol (methanol) has many impurities that give it a very disagreeable odor and taste. Methanol is obtained from the destructive distillation of wood and is found in antifreeze fluid, windshield de-icers, varnishes, and shellacs. "Bootleg" whiskey may contain significant amounts of methanol. Methanol is not taxed, and because of its low cost has led the occasional unwary alcoholic to imbibe it in lieu of more expensive ethanol.

Methanol is rapidly absorbed from the gastrointestinal tract, with peak levels occurring 30–60 minutes after ingestion. Toxicity can also result from inhalation and skin absorption. Methanol, being water soluble, distributes in total body water.

The primary route of elimination of methanol is oxidation to formaldehyde, formic acid, and carbon dioxide. The rate limiting step in methanol metabolism is its conversion by alcohol dehydrogenase to formaldehyde. Formaldehyde is then rapidly converted to formic acid. Formic acid, in turn, is metabolized by a folate-dependent enzyme to carbon dioxide and water. Formaldehyde and formic acid are much more toxic than methanol, and it is now believed that formic acid is the major toxin. Formic acid levels correlate with the degree of acidosis and magnitude of the anion gap (143). Clinically, mortality rates and severity of visual symptoms also correlate with the degree of acidosis (12). There is an enormous variability in the reported doses necessary to cause acidosis, blindness, or death. This variability is partially due to the total amount of methanol ingested, the extent of concomitant ethanol ingestion, and the folate levels present at the time of ingestion. The generally accepted lethal dose of methanol is 30 ml.

Typically there is a lag time of 8–72 hours from ingestion to onset of symptoms. The onset of symptoms correlates with the appearance of metabolic acidosis (162). The most important initial symptom is altered visual perception, which may be described as blurred vision or photophobia. Permanent and complete blindness may eventually develop. Initially, optic disc hyperemia and papillary edema are evident. With permanent visual sequelae, optic atrophy and attenuation of blood vessels occur. No patient with normally reactive pupils has suffered permanent visual loss (14). Conversely, decreased pupillary function may occur in patients who recover completely. Other signs and symptoms of methanol poisoning are abdominal pain, vomiting, dyspnea with Kussmaul respirations, headache, nuchal rigidity, weakness, confusion, seizures, and coma. The most striking laboratory finding is a high anion gap metabolic acidosis. Serum bicarbonate levels may reach zero. Other characteristic laboratory values include increased osmolal gap, increased amylase, increased serum glucose, and lactic acidemia. The finding of a profound metabolic acidosis in a patient with visual disturbances should lead the clinician to consider methanol poisoning.

After initial resuscitation and gastric decontamination, treatment of suspected methanol poisoning centers on (a) prompt correction of metabolic acidosis, (b) prompt initiation of ethanol therapy, (c) administration of folate, and (d) selection of patients for hemodialysis. Large doses of sodium bicarbonate may be necessary to correct the metabolic acidosis. Arterial blood gases and serum bicarbonate determinations should be used to guide therapy.

Ethanol competitively inhibits alcohol dehydrogenase from converting methanol to formaldehyde because ethanol has a ninefold higher affinity for this enzyme. Ethanol therapy should be instituted in all cases of suspected or confirmed methanol poisoning. Therapy should precede the return of blood methanol determinations. Ethanol therapy is given to maintain a serum ethanol concentration of 100 mg/dl. McCoy (102) suggests the following regimen: (a) a loading dose of 0.6 g/kg, (b) a maintenance dose for nondrinkers of 66 mg/kg/hr, and (c) a maintenance dose for drinkers of 153 mg/kg/hour. If hemodialysis is instituted, the ethanol infusion will need to be increased because ethanol is removed by dialysis. McCoy suggests increasing the infusion rate in adults to 7.2 g/hour (102). Folate doses of 1 mg/kg (up to 50 mg/dose) intravenously every 4 hours for a total of six doses is given to replete folate stores.

Patients with a serum methanol level of 50 mg/dl should undergo hemodialysis. Ethanol therapy increases methanol's half-life from 8 hours to 30 or more hours. Hemodialysis will decrease the half-life to about 2.5 hours and thus shorten the length of time intensive care management is necessary (67). Hemodialysis will remove both methanol and formic acid. Other indications for hemodialysis include a history of ingestion of more than 30 ml of methanol, intractable acidosis, and deterioration of vision or CNS function (64). Hemodialysis should be continued until the serum methanol level is reduced to 20 mg/dl or below.

ETHYLENE GLYCOL

Ethylene glycol is a colorless, and sweet-tasting liquid. It is a common component of antifreeze, lacquer, polish, and de-icers. Approximately 1.4–1.6 ml/kg constitutes a minimum lethal dose, about 100 ml in adults (23).

Unmetabolized ethylene glycol has about the same CNS toxicity as ethanol. Once ingested it is rapidly absorbed and peak serum levels occur in 1–4 hours. Like methanol, it is distributed evenly throughout the body tissues. Although the parent compound is relatively nontoxic, the metabolic by-products are extremely toxic. Metabolism takes place mainly in the liver and, like methanol, the major converting enzyme is alcohol dehydrogenase. Toxic by-products are aldehydes, glycolate, oxalate, and lactate. Ethanol, with its higher enzyme affinity, prevents the metabolism of ethylene glycol into its more toxic by-products.

Toxic manifestations are due primarily to the development of metabolic acidosis and tissue destruction due to the deposition of oxalate crystals. Hypocalcemia may result from calcium chelation with oxalate. The onset of symptoms may be delayed up to 12 hours or more depending on the amount of ethylene glycol ingested and the extent of coingestion of ethanol. Berman (15) described three stages of intoxication: stage 1 (occurring 20 minutes to 12 hours after ingestion) consists of symptoms of intoxication such as nausea, vomiting, seizures, and coma; stage 2 (12–24 hours post-ingestion) is manifest by tachypnea, tachycardia, congestive heart failure, or pulmonary edema; and stage 3 (24–72 hours after ingestion) is characterized by renal failure secondary to acute tubular necrosis. In reality, the distinction between the phases is not clear cut, particularly between the CNS manifestations (stage 1) and the cardiovascular manifestations (stage 2). Other prominent CNS signs include nystagmus, myoclonus, and ophthalmoplegia. Pulmonary edema may result from both congestive heart failure and the adult respiratory distress syndrome (ARDS) (27). Laboratory findings include a high anion gap metabolic acidosis, hypocalcemia, and calcium oxalate crystals in the urine. With the onset of renal failure, there will be an elevation in BUN and creatinine. Hematuria and proteinuria may also be seen.

Ethylene glycol intoxication is suggested by the presentation of a patient who appears markedly intoxicated but does not have the smell of ethanol on the breath, the presence of coma with a large anion gap acidosis and an osmolal gap, and the presence of calcium oxalate crystals in the urine.

After initial resuscitation measures and gastrointestinal decontamination, therapy consists of maintenance of a high urine flow, administration of ethanol, administration of thiamine and pyridoxine supplements, correction of acidosis, correction of hypocalcemia, and hemodialysis. Some authorities advocate maintaining a high urine output until crystalluria disappears (164). Urine output may need to be augmented by furosemide or mannitol. If congestive heart failure or ARDS ensues, fluid therapy should be appropriately altered.

Ethanol should be administered to maintain a blood level of 100 mg/dl. Peterson suggests a loading dose of 0.6 to 0.8 g/kg, followed by a maintenance dose of 110–130 mg/kg/hour. If dialysis is performed the maintenance dose must be increased to 250–350 mg/kg/hour (126).

Correction of acidemia may require large amounts of sodium bicarbonate. To correct hypocalcemia the intensivist may use calcium chloride or calcium gluconate. Thiamine and pyridoxine are administered to prevent depletion of these cofactors, which are necessary for ethylene glycol detoxification. Thiamine (100 mg) and pyridoxine (100 mg) are given intramuscularly or intravenously every 6 hours for the first 24 hours (62).

Hemodialysis is recommended in ethylene glycol poisoning when ethylene glycol levels are above 50 mg/dl or if severe toxicity occurs. With ethanol blocking therapy, the half-life of ethylene glycol increases from 3 hours to 17 hours or more (126). In a small series, patients who had hemodialysis instituted prior to the onset of renal failure did better clinically than those in whom it was instituted after renal failure developed (9). Both ethylene glycol and intermediate toxic aldehydes are dialyzable. For these reasons, early and aggressive use of hemodialysis is recommended, rather than waiting for symptoms and signs of severe toxicity to develop. An exception to early hemodialysis would be rapid clinical improvement and/or rapidly falling ethylene glycol levels associated with ethanol therapy. All treatment should continue until ethylene glycol is undetectable in serum.

ISOPROPANOL

Isopropanol (isopropyl alcohol) is a clear, colorless, volatile liquid with a characteristic odor and a slightly bitter taste. Ingestion is common in young children and in suicidal or derelict adults. It is commonly found in the home as rubbing alcohol. It is also found in disinfectants, solvents, cleaning agents, and cosmetics.

Absorption from the stomach is rapid, occurring within 30 minutes, and peak blood levels are achieved within 1–1½ hours. It is more toxic than ethanol; its clinical effects last two to four times longer; and CNS depression is more pronounced. Dermal absorption is insignificant yet inhalation can be a significant route of exposure, particularly in children who are being sponged down with isopropanol for treatment of fever. Serious toxicity has been reported with this type of exposure (56).

Approximately 80% of isopropyl alcohol is metabolized by the liver to acetone, which is excreted by the kidneys (primarily) and the lungs. A small amount of unchanged isopropanol is resecreted into the stomach and saliva. Isopropanol appears to follow first-order kinetics, with a half-life of 2.5–3 hours (37). Acetone elimination occurs much more slowly. A lethal dose of isopropanol in adults is about 3 ml/kg.

Symptoms of acute intoxication, including abdominal pain, vomiting, and CNS effects usually occur within 30 minutes of ingestion. The CNS manifestations are similar to those of ethanol except they are more pronounced and they last longer. The acetone probably contributes to the more prolonged symptoms. Deep coma may develop rapidly and respiratory arrest may ensue. Gastrointestinal symptoms are more severe than with ethanol, and hemorrhagic gastritis has been reported (94). With severe toxicity (serum concentrations above 300–400 mg/dl) myocardial depression and severe hypotension can result. Less common effects include renal tubular necrosis, hypothermia, acute myopathy, and hemolytic anemia (91). The most characteristic and specific laboratory findings are an elevated anion gap, elevated osmolal gap, acetonemia, and acetonuria. Acidosis is less common, and when present, it is not as severe as that associated with methanol or ethylene glycol. Acidosis with isopropanol poisoning is likely due to lactic acidosis associated with hypotension and hypoxia. Hypotension is a poor prognostic indicator. In one series, the presence of hypotension carried a 45% mortality, while those patients in grade III or IV coma without hypotension had a 25% mortality (92).

Treatment involves gastric emptying, lavage, and activated charcoal if the ingestion was within 2 hours, and continuous nasogastric suction to remove re-secreted isopropanol. The clinician should be alert to the possibility of significant gastrointestinal bleeding and intervene appropriately.

Hemodialysis is effective in removing both isopropanol and acetone. Some investigators have reported beneficial clinical outcomes with the early institution of hemodialysis (171). No widely accepted guidelines are available for the use of dialysis. In view of the mortality figures associated with deep coma and hypotension, hemodialysis is appropriate in these settings as well as with blood levels in excess of 400 mg/dl. As is the trend with treatment of other alcohol poisonings, early institution of dialysis before severe complications set in may decrease mortality. Controlled studies comparing this approach with supportive treatment alone are not yet available.

Opiates

The term *opiates* generally refers to all drugs with pharmacological effects similar to the parent drug opium. For the purpose of this chapter opiates include medications derived from opium (morphine and codeine), drugs that are semisynthetic derivatives of opium (heroin, oxycodone, hydromorphone, etc.), and drugs that are synthetic compounds with opiate-like properties (meperidine, methadone, propoxyphene, and newer generation synthetics). The intensivist will most frequently face opiate overdoses in the setting of intravenous drug abuse (e.g., heroin, methadone), childhood ingestions of diphenoxylate or propoxyphene, or adolescent or adult oral overdoses of prescribed pain medications or antitussives.

Opiates are readily absorbed from the gastrointestinal tract, nasal mucosa, pulmonary mucosa, and parenterally (subcutaneous, intravenous, and intramuscular). When orally ingested, a significant percentage of the dose undergoes first-pass hepatic metabolism. Thus, there is less effect from an oral dose than an intravenous dose. Opiates are well distributed throughout the body. Blood levels may not correlate with the clinical picture nor reflect the ingested dose. Hemodialysis does not remove significant amounts of opiates from the body (2). Hepatic metabolism is relatively rapid, and major metabolic pathways differ with each opiate. Metabolism and toxic effects can be prolonged in hepatic disease and with delayed gastric emptying (2). About 90% of an ingested or injected drug is excreted in the urine, making this the fluid of choice for toxicology screening.

Opiates have their most pronounced effects on the central nervous system and the respiratory system. CNS effects include analgesia, euphoria, sedation, suppression of the cough reflex, dysphoria, nausea and vomiting, respiratory depression, fixed miotic pupils, and seizures. Seizures are due to a brief excitatory effect early after ingestion. The respiratory depression is secondary to a blunted medullary response to hypercarbia. In addition, patients may develop noncardiogenic pulmonary edema (13, 154). Other clinical effects include peripheral vasodilation with orthostatic hypotension, flushed skin, pruritis, diminished peristalsis, delayed gastric emptying, and urinary retention. A clue to diagnosis may be the presence of fresh or sclerotic needle puncture marks overlying blood vessels. Laboratory tests are not helpful in making the diagnosis of opiate overdose, with the exception of qualitative urine toxicology screens. A significant percentage of the time, other drugs or toxins are coingested with opiates. Opiates may mask manifestations of other drugs and vice versa.

Supportive measures are the mainstay of therapy. Once the airway is secured and respirations controlled or supplemented, the remainder of the resuscitation can take place in a controlled orderly fashion. Intravenous access should be established, blood and urine collected for routine laboratory tests, and toxicology screens and glucose and thiamine should be given. Naloxone is then administered. Once aroused with naloxone, the patients may be quite agitated and uncooperative with further procedures. Some clinicians favor

application of therapeutic restraints prior to reversing the CNS depression of opiates.

Naloxone is a superior antidote. It has no agonist properties and there are no contraindications to its use. Naloxone is a competitive antagonist at all three proposed opiate receptor subtypes (87). Naloxone restores pulmonary ventilation, reverses postural hypotension, and improves the patient's level of consciousness. It can also reverse the delay in gastric emptying caused by opiates. An initial dose of 0.8–2.0 mg may be given intravenously. If no response is elicited, repeat doses may be given every 3–5 minutes to a total of 4 mg. If no improvement is noted, the clinician should suspect another cause for the patient's clinical status. With a child, initial doses can be given in the range of 0.01–0.02 mg/kg. Repeated doses up to 0.05 mg/kg should produce the desired response (85). Subsequent administration is titrated to the desired clinical response. Naloxone has a half-life of 12–20 minutes (a fraction of the half-life of the ingested opiate), and frequent repeat doses or initiation of a naloxone drip (0.4–0.8 mg/hr) may be necessary. Naloxone has also been successfully administered via the endotracheal tube (158).

Delayed gastric emptying occurs following oral ingestion and may be a reason to institute a gastric lavage. As mentioned above, administration of naloxone can speed gastrointestinal transit. Naloxone should not be administered to awaken a comatose patient so that ipecac syrup can be administered.

Organophosphates

Insecticides come under two general classes, organophosphates and carbamates. The organophosphate compounds are the type of insecticide most commonly associated with serious toxicity, accounting for more than 80% of pesticide-related hospitalizations (157). The popularity of these agents for commercial use has been growing because after application, they are rapidly hydrolyzed in the environment and little long-term accumulation occurs. Poisoning usually occurs in children who accidentally ingest the substance, in farmworkers who are accidentally exposed, and in victims of suicide attempts. Organophosphates sold for household use are usually made of more dilute formulations, about 1–2%, in contrast to the 40–50% concentrations in agricultural compounds (65). Just a few drops of the agricultural compounds can be fatal in children (42). Organophosphate poisoning can be rapidly fatal. One study (157) revealed that in hospitalized patients the fatality rate was 50% in children and 10% in adults.

Organophosphate poisoning can be successfully treated with chemical and physiological antidotes. However, recognizing a victim or organophosphate poisoning can be difficult. Organophosphate toxicity results from the disruption of normal cholinergic neurotransmission at multiple sites in the body (11). The organophosphates gain entrance to the body via gastrointestinal absorption, dermal absorption, and absorption through the ocular and respiratory mucosa. Acetylcholine is the neurotransmitter at the affected synaptic junctions. Normally acetylcholine is broken down into acetic acid and choline by the enzyme acetylcholinesterase. Acetylcholinesterase (true cholinesterase) is found primarily in erythrocytes and nervous tissue. Another cholinesterase, pseudocholinesterase, is found in the serum and in the liver. Organophosphates are powerful inhibitors of both cholinesterases, irreversibly binding to them within 24–48 hours (147).

The clinical effects depend on the site and type of acetylcholine synapse affected. The anatomic sites are muscarinic synapses (autonomic effector cells), nicotinic synapses (autonomic ganglia and the adrenal medulla), and central nervous system synapses. Excessive amounts of acetylcholine initially excite and subsequently paralyze normal function of these synapses producing the characteristic effects (11).

The onset of muscarinic effects depends on the route of exposure. In a case of inhalation of fumes or vapors, the ocular and respiratory effects may appear first. These include miosis, eye pain, blurred vision, excessive lacrimation and salivation, wheezing and tightness in the chest (bronchoconstriction and increased tracheobronchial secretions), and dyspnea. Following ingestion, gastrointestinal symptoms may predominate or appear earliest. These include diarrhea, abdominal cramps, nausea, vomiting, and fecal incontinence. Other muscarinic signs and symptoms are bradycardia, diaphoresis, and urinary incontinence.

Nicotinic effects of organophosphates manifest in striated muscle and sympathetic ganglia. These effects include muscle fasciculations, fatigability, weakness, cramps, paralysis (with apnea), tachycardia, hypertension, and, rarely, mydriasis. Central nervous system effects manifest as confusion, slurred speech, ataxia, anxiety, fatigue, psychosis, seizures, coma, and central respiratory paralysis.

A history, if available, should attempt to determine what was taken, how much, and when. The physical examination should search for the muscarinic, nicotinic, and CNS signs just described. Laboratory tests are of limited usefulness. A red cell cholinesterase level is most specific but not readily available in most institutions (115). The serum cholinesterase level is usually more readily available. This is more sensitive but less specific than a red cell cholinesterase. Other conditions that may depress serum cholinesterase levels include hepatitis, cirrhosis, hepatic congestion, metastatic carcinoma, malnutrition, acute infections, anemia, myocardial infarction, and dermatomyositis.

A trial with atropine may be useful in aiding the diagnosis. In organophosphate poisoning, intravenous administration of atropine in doses of 1–2 mg does not result in flushing, dry mouth, tachycardia, or mydriasis. In fact, the ability to administer large doses of atropine without observable adverse effects is virtually diagnostic of organophosphate poisoning.

Treatment of organophosphate poisoning must be individualized. Administration of the antidote atropine prior to stabilization and oxygenation can be catastrophic. Seriously poisoned patients must have their airway controlled. Seizures, aspiration, increased tracheobronchial secretions, and bronchospasm can be managed more easily with adequate airway protection and control. Once the airway is controlled, maximum oxygenation should be accomplished. Suctioning and administration of atropine can lessen the effects of increased secretions. Diazepam can be used to control seizures.

Decontamination of the portal of entry is imperative. Continuous absorption from the clothing and/or skin must be prevented by completely stripping all clothes off and thoroughly washing skin, hair, and under nails. Copious irrigation of eyes should take places in cases of ocular exposure. Even when the vehicle for an ingested organophosphate is a hydrocarbon, gastric lavage or induced emesis should take place. Initial and repeated doses of charcoal are indicated.

Once the patient is stabilized and properly oxygenated, pharmacological treatment can ensue. The use of morphine, aminophylline, phenothiazines, and reserpine are contraindicated (108). Hypoxia and a direct toxic effect of organophosphates often results in a hyper-irritable myocardium, and epinephrine may cause irreversible ventricular fibrillation in such cases (135). Pharmacological treatment is based on the use of atropine and the cholinesterase "activator" pralidoxime. Atropine counters the muscarinic and CNS manifestations of organophosphate poisoning, whereas pralidoxime reverses both the muscarinic and the nicotinic effects.

Atropine may need to be given in large and repeated doses. The most common cause of treatment failure is inadequate atropinization (108). The therapeutic endpoint is evidence of atropinization as manifested by mydriasis, tachycardia, flushing, xerostomia, or anhydrosis. Two milligrams of atropine should be administered intravenously every 15 minutes until atropinization is apparent. The pediatric dose is 0.05 mg/kg every 15 minutes. The severely poisoned patient may require a continuous atropine infusion. Atropine should be tapered slowly during its discontinuation.

Pralidoxime (2-PAM chloride) has three major biochemical effects that are beneficial to the patient poisoned with organophosphates (11). It cleaves the organophosphate bond from cholinesterases, which reactivates the cholinesterase enzyme. It directly reacts with and detoxifies the organophosphate molecule, and it has an anticholinergic atropine-like effect. Pralidoxime should be used in the presence of muscle fasciculations or muscle weakness. For optimum effects, pralidoxime must be administered immediately after poisoning. Early administration may lessen the need for large doses of atropine. Reactivation of cholinesterases may not occur in patients administered the drug more than 36 hours after exposure (11).

The dosage of pralidoxime for adults is 1 g administered intravenously, with a maximum infusion rate of 0.5 g/minute and 20–50 mg/kg with a maximum infusion of one-half the total dose per minute for children (108). Repeat doses depend upon the clinical response. Reversal of muscle weakness and fasciculations usually begins within 10–40 minutes of administration (115).

The major complications of organophosphate poisoning are pulmonary and include aspiration pneumonitis, pulmonary edema, ARDS, and respiratory paralysis. Untreated patients usually die within 24 hours of exposure. In all other cases, provided cerebral hypoxia has been successfully prevented or treated, clinicians can expect total symptomatic recovery within 7–10 days (115).

Digitalis

Digitalis preparations have been used in contemporary medicine for over 200 years and are among the top 10 drugs prescribed in the United States. Iatrogenic digitalis intoxication is one of the most common toxic reactions in clinical medicine and is the most common cause of unintentional poisoning deaths in the elderly (176). Digitalis intoxication causes a morbidity of 8–35% and a mortality of 3–21% (148). Single, massive overdoses of digitalis are a relatively uncommon but significant mode of suicide. Deliberate digoxin overdose is fatal in 50% of patients (122).

Digitalis exerts its action at the cellular level by altering the activity of the sodium-potassium-ATPase membrane transport system. Digitalis preparations come in the form of digoxin (half-life of about 33 hours) and digitoxin (half-life of 6–7 days). Drug action depends on tissue concentration, which is relatively constant in relation to serum levels. The major human depot is skeletal muscle (40). Digoxin is excreted primarily via the kidneys; digitoxin is eliminated after being metabolically inactivated in the body. Both substances undergo enterohepatic circulation. Children are believed to be less sensitive to digoxin and require higher doses (89). Digitalis preparations possess a relatively narrow therapeutic index, with 40–60 percent of the lethal dose being required to achieve maximal therapeutic effect.

Digitalis cardiotoxicity is caused by its effects on cardiac conduction and automaticity, coexistent cardiac disease (both myocardial and conduction system disease), and other noncardiac disease states or medications. Almost any rhythm or conduction disturbance can result from this complex interaction of factors. More characteristic disturbances associated with digitalis toxicity include profound bradycardias with or without associated atrioventricular conduction disturbances, atrial tachycardias with atrioventricular block, and ventricular ectopy and tachydysrhythmias. Ventricular dysrhythmias are associated with a higher mortality, up to 50% in some series (111).

Gastrointestinal manifestations of digitalis toxicity include nausea, vomiting, and anorexia. Hypokalemia appears to be a consistent finding with chronic toxicity (106), while hyperkalemia is a prominent finding in acute, massive overdose (40). Neurologic symptoms include blurred and altered color vision, headache, fatigue, depression, confusion, hallucinations, and delirium. These latter symptoms are not a consistent finding with acute ingestions (142).

Diagnosis of digitalis toxicity is based on a history of ingestion of a digitalis preparation, a history of nausea, vomiting, and anorexia, an ECG demonstrating "digitalis effects" (prolonged PR interval, AV block, ST depression), the presence of arrhythmias, and confirmation with serum levels. The magnitude of the serum level, and its correlation with the degree of toxicity, depend upon the presence or absence of other host disease states or medications. In one study, a significant increase in mortality was correlated with an increasing digoxin level, with a 50% mortality occurring with digoxin levels of above 6 ng/ml. Quinidine causes an increase in serum digoxin in up to 90% of patients. This finding is best explained by the displacement of digoxin from tissue binding sites (70).

Therapy of digitalis intoxication is aimed at intensive cardiovascular support and hastening digitalis removal from the body. Gastric emptying and administration of activated charcoal are indicated. Repeat doses of charcoal may be useful in view of the presence of an enterohepatic circulation. Conduction disturbances of arrhythmias require treatment only if hemodynamic compromise is manifest. Bradydysrhythmias can be treated with atropine and/or placement of a temporary pacemaker. Correction of hypoxia and hypokalemia is imperative for successful treatment of ventricular ectopy and arrhythmias. Lidocaine and phenytoin are the most efficacious agents. Phenytoin doses are similar to those used for anticonvulsant treatment (e.g., 50–100 mg can be given slowly every 5 minutes to a total dose of 600 mg). Direct-current countershock is to be withheld unless all other therapy fails.

Immunotherapy with Fab fragments from digoxin antibodies has recently been reported to dramatically reverse signs of profound digoxin poisoning. Use of these antibodies can terminate life-threatening arrhythmias, lower serum digoxin levels, terminate gastrointestinal side effects, and reverse life-threatening hyperkalemia, all within 1–2 hours of administration (153). Use of immunotherapy is limited mostly to tertiary care institutions.

Sporadic cases of the successful use of hemoperfusion for treating digitalis intoxication are reported in recent literature (93). It is said to cause a more rapid fall in plasma digoxin levels than supportive treatment alone. It is a good therapeutic alternative in digoxin poisoning when adverse factors, such as hyperkalemia, pre-existing heart disease, and chronic renal failure are present. Hemodialysis may be necessary for recalcitrant, life-threatening hyperkalemia; however, it will not eliminate digoxin because of high protein binding.

Benzodiazepines

The popularity of the benzodiazepines needs little re-emphasis here. They are among the most widely prescribed drugs every year. Between 1964 and 1973 the number of prescriptions nearly tripled. In the last 10 years, the number of available benzodiazepine compounds has increased. The popularity of these medications is based on their relative safety as compared with their predecessor sedative, hypnotic-type medications and barbiturates. Indeed, despite sometimes massive doses (2 g of diazepam in one ingestion), patients who ingest benzodiazepines alone seldom suffer any serious medical complications (66). It is their ingestion as part of a polydrug overdose that may result in death or serious consequences. The potentiating effect of alcohol on benzodiazepines is well known.

Benzodiazepines are all derived from a common nucleus. Alterations of this basic nucleus produce the variety of compounds available today. The pharmacokinetics of these compounds can vary widely. Although these pharmacokinetic differences may suggest therapeutic differences, currently there are no data clearly demonstrating the clinical superiority of one compound over another when based solely upon pharmacokinetic properties. In general, the benzodiazepines are rapidly and completely absorbed after oral ingestion. Once into the systemic circulation, all benzodiazepines bind to plasma albumin and are then distributed to tissues at rates dependent upon their lipid solubility. Essentially all benzodiazepines are hepatically biotransformed via oxidation and/or conjugation pathways. Oxidation frequently results in the production of multiple metabolites, some of which are pharmacologically active. Certain benzodiazepines, including diazepam, undergo enterohepatic circulation. These agents primarily affect the CNS. They potentiate the effects of the neurotransmitter GABA without themselves being GABA-mimetic compounds.

Benzodiazepine overdose is characterized by sedation without cardiovascular compromise.

Drowsiness, ataxia, dizziness, and weakness are usual symptoms. Severe CNS depression (deep coma) is unusual and should suggest other coingestants. Patients may take 2 g or more of diazepam and still be oriented and conversant (66). The diagnosis is made by history and qualitative toxicological examination. Since polysubstance ingestion is found in over 80% of hospitalized patients, the intensivist should search carefully for clues revealing other more dangerous toxins (16). In one study, almost 40% of patients who were hospitalized for polydrug ingestion involving benzodiazepines required ventilatory support (3).

Treatment is purely supportive. Ingestion of alcohol or other toxins may depress the patient's ability to protect their airway. In pure benzodiazepine overdoses, the efficacy of gastric emptying is minimal. Repeated doses of activated charcoal may be helpful; but again, given the excellent prognosis for even massive single ingestions of benzodiazepines alone, the indication for even this relatively benign form of therapy is questioned. Observation is usually all that is necessary. Specific therapy is directed at other more toxic agents that may have been ingested. Hemodialysis, hemoperfusion, forced diuresis, physostigmine, and naloxone are not of any proven clinical utility. Recovery from huge, single-dose ingestions is rapid and complete, usually within 24–48 hours.

Calcium Channel Blockers

As the use of calcium channel blockers increases, so has the incidence of both accidental and purposeful poisoning with these agents. Presently, therapeutic modalities are derived mainly from case reports of overdoses and the rational assumption that parenteral calcium administration should and does reverse some of the toxic effects in an overdose scenario. Three preparations of calcium channel blockers are currently in use: verapamil, nifedipine, and diltiazem. These agents are used for the treatment of dysrhythmias, coronary artery spasm, hypertensive emergencies, heart failure, and angina pectoris.

The mechanism of action of these compounds rests on their ability to inhibit the slow calcium channel current. These drugs may cause (106) myocardial depression (negative inotropism), bradycardia, decrease in atrioventricular conduction, inhibition of vascular tone with peripheral and coronary vasodilation, CNS depression, nausea and vomiting, and disordered glucose metabolism and mild acidosis.

Data regarding the pharmacokinetics and toxic effects of calcium channel blockers in a massive overdose scenario are lacking. Most comparisons are limited to side effects or therapeutic effects with therapeutic doses. Documented adverse cardiovascular manifestations with overdoses of diltiazem and verapamil include hypotension, bradycardia, sinus arrest, and cardiogenic shock (151). There are also documented case reports of verapamil causing terminal ventricular fibrillation after being administered to patients with Wolff-Parkinson-White syndrome and atrial tachyarrhythmias (83).

Treatment is aimed at reversing these life-threatening cardiovascular manifestations. Intravenous calcium administration should follow initial resuscitative measures if the patient is not responding to general supportive measures alone. Ten percent calcium chloride can be given in doses of 10 ml for adults and 0.1–0.2 ml/kg in pediatric patients (174). Repeat doses with careful monitoring of the serum calcium concentration may be necessary. Gastrointestinal decontamination should be accomplished. Dopamine or dobutamine can be used for persistent hypotension. For symptomatic persistent bradycardias or sinus arrest, glucagon (177), atropine, or isoproterenol can be tried. A temporary pacemaker may be necessary in some cases. There is one case report of a patient who ingested large quantities of diltiazem and metoprolol who responded well to charcoal hemoperfusion (7). No controlled data are available regarding the use of hemoperfusion in calcium channel blocker overdoses.

β-Blockers

Propranolol is the best known of the β-blocking drugs. Other drugs in this class include metoprolol, nadolol, timolol, atenolol, pindolol, and oxyprenolol. β-blockers are used widely in the treatment of hypertension, arrhythmias, glaucoma, angina, migraine disease, and prophylaxis against sudden death in the postmyocardial infarction period. The rise in β-blocker popularity for treatment of these various disorders has also been accompanied by a rise in the incidence of overdoses with these agents (168). Massive overdoses with β-blockers can pose a significant challenge for the intensivist because frequently, traditional pharmacologic management of decreased cardiac output with catecholamines has been unsuccessful.

β-blocking agents differ in their pharmacologic properties. Metoprolol and atenolol are "cardioselective" (β_1 only) in therapeutic doses. Propranolol exhibits the most pronounced membrane depression (168). Membrane-active drugs are more likely to cause CNS effects (e.g., sedation, coma, and convulsions). Pindolol and oxyprenolol possess partial adrenergic receptor agonist activity, leading to tachycardia and hypertension in overdose situations. The more lipophilic drugs tend to be extensively distributed in body tissues and rapidly metabolized by the liver. They are well absorbed but undergo extensive first-pass metabolism. Less lipophilic drugs are distributed less extensively to tissues and are excreted mostly unmetabolized by the kidneys. Half-lives of the metabolized drugs tend to be shorter than those of the drugs excreted by the kidney (34).

β-blockers function at the β-adrenergic receptors in the body. β-1 stimulation increases sinoatrial rate, myocardial contractility, and conduction velocity. β-2 stimulation dilates bronchial smooth muscle and arterioles in skeletal muscle, stimulates insulin secretion, and increases lactic acid production, lipolysis, and glycogenolysis. β-blockade reverses these adrenergic effects.

β-blocker overdose is manifested by bradycardia (72%), hypotension (76%), seizures (28%), peripheral cyanosis (23%), and coma (26%) (168). Heart failure and/or bronchoconstriction can appear in patients with pre-existing heart or lung disease. Hyperglycemia is uncommon but may be a more prominent problem in children and diabetics (76). Cardiogenic shock, intraventricular conduction delays, and asystole due to direct myocardial depression can occur in previously healthy people (146). As mentioned previously, β-blockers with partial adrenergic agonist activity can produce mild to moderate degrees of tachycardia and hypertension.

Diagnosis rests on the suspicion of β-blocker ingestion coupled with profound hypotension and bradycardia resistant to standard therapy. Patients may initially be ambulatory and conversant and within minutes deteriorate to seizures and severe hemodynamic compromise (169). Blood levels are not necessary to management, yet a qualitative toxicology screen may be helpful in the unknown ingestion. Close monitoring of blood glucose may be necessary, particularly during treatment with glucagon. Serum electrolytes, electrocardiograms, and chest x-rays may be helpful but are not diagnostic.

Management of patients with overdoses of β-blockers primarily focuses on reversal of life-threatening hypotension and bradycardia. Standard resuscitative and decontamination measures should be employed. In a patient with a history of a massive ingestion, anticipation of rapid clinical deterioration should include withholding ipecac, achieving early airway control, and keeping diazepam readily available to treat seizures. When treating ventricular arrhythmias, lidocaine is the agent of choice. Use of quinidine, procainamide, and disopyramide is contraindicated because of their myocardial depressant effects.

Although there are no prospective human studies comparing the efficacy of glucagon alone with β-agonists, atropine, and vasopressors, retrospective studies and case reports clearly point out the superiority of glucagon in reversing hypotension and bradycardia associated with massive β-blocker overdose in patients with low cardiac output and normal capillary wedge pressures (168, 169, 178). Glucagon is the agent of choice in this clinical situation. Glucagon produces a positive inotropic and chronotropic effect on the heart via stimulation of glucagon specific receptors in the myocardium that are not blocked by even massive doses of β-blockers (88). Glucagon can have salutary effects within 5–10 minutes after intravenous administration. The optimal dose is not precisely known, but an initial dose of 2–5 mg is advised. Repeat doses may be administered as necessary. Alternately a continuous intravenous infusion of about 1–5 mg/hour, titrated to desired response, can be employed.

While not proven to be more effective than glucagon, atropine, β-agonists, and fluid treatment in the treatment of bradycardia and hypotension have been recommended by most authors. This author favors maximizing treatment with glucagon (after establishing adequate hydration) prior to initiating other therapy. Glucagon can cause persistent vomiting and hyperglycemia. Airway protection and monitoring of the serum glucose are imperative. Bradydysrhythmias resistant to pharmacological management should be treated with a transvenous pacemaker.

Iron

The accidental ingestion of iron-containing compounds by children less than 5 years old continues to be a very common problem. Most iron preparations are over-the-counter vitamins or vitamin supplements that are available in large quantities. Some vitamins are brightly colored, which makes them appealing to children; many parents still do not recognize the potential danger of these compounds to their children. While the majority of iron ingestions can be managed easily without hospital admission, a small percentage of patients will present after significant and sometimes massive ingestion and present a complex management problem for the intensivist. Despite the widespread experience with iron poisoning over the years, several important aspects of treatment remain controversial, including the techniques of gastric lavage, the route of administration of the complexing agent deferoxamine, and the use of the clinical laboratory in management of iron overdose.

The common ferrous salts are sulfates, fumarates, and gluconates. Iron toxicity is related to the total amount of elemental iron ingested. In ferrous sulfate tables, iron content is 20%. Ferrous fumarate preparations contain 33% elemental iron. Ferrous gluconate tablets are 12% iron. A generally accepted lethal dose is 200–250 mg/kg, although fatal ingestions have been recorded with smaller quantities (136).

Iron content of the body is controlled by alterations in absorption. There is no specific mechanism for excretion. Iron is absorbed in the duodenum and jejunum. After oxidation to the ferric state, iron is complexed to a storage protein called ferritin. When iron is released to plasma from ferritin it is transported by binding to the protein transferrin. When transferrin's capacity to bind iron is exceeded, free iron circulates unbound and exerts its toxic effects by depositing into tissues, particularly cells in the liver.

Iron poisoning has classically been divided into stages. Perhaps the most useful approach is that of Lovejoy and Lecoutre (91), which looks at clinical changes in relation to time after ingestion. Early changes occur from 30 minutes to 6 hours after ingestion. Prominent amongst these early changes are gastrointestinal effects. Vomiting and diarrhea occur; frequently they are severe and complicated by gastrointestinal bleeding. Fever and leukocytosis may also be present. Shock may ensue from various mechanisms including gastrointestinal blood loss, venous pooling, and increased capillary permeability, all of which lead to a decrease in cardiac output. Acidosis and hyperglycemia may also occur. Intermediate changes occur between 6 and 48 hours postingestion. A brief period of quiescence is followed by profound shock and vascular collapse (84). Hepatic failure may occur with jaundice, elevated liver enzymes, and bleeding disorders. Hypoglycemia may manifest during this phase, secondary to hepatic damage (60). Late changes manifest from 3 days to 3 weeks after ingestion. Characteristic changes include strictures of the stomach, small bowel infarction, liver cirrhosis, and fatty degeneration of the liver.

Diagnosis and therapy in part depend upon timely and selective use of ancillary studies. Specifically, serum iron levels, total iron binding capacity (TIBC), and flat plate abdominal radiographs can be most helpful. Normal serum iron levels range from 100 to 125 ug/dl. Levels above 300 ug/dl should be treated with chelation therapy until the TIBC becomes available. Iron concentrations measured between 4 and 6 hours after ingestion are the most reliable. Iron levels above 1000 μg/dl carry a large increase in mortality (60). If the serum iron exceeds the TIBC, chelation therapy is recommended. Others caution against overreliance on the TIBC (10). The abdominal flat plate can be helpful in assessing the adequacy of gastric lavage since iron is radiopaque. A positive flat plate is usually associated with a serum iron level above 300 μg/dl (74).

Treatment of iron overdose centers on gastric decontamination and chelation therapy with deferoxamine. Deferoxamine is a highly specific chelator of ferric (Fe + 3) iron and has affinity for iron that is 10 times greater than any other known chelator of iron (136). Iron in the gut can be bound by orally administered deferoxamine. Parenterally administered deferoxamine enhances iron elimination through the formation of the water-soluble, renally excreted ferrioxamine.

Gastric emptying is extremely important because of the direct corrosive effect that iron has on the gastric mucosa. Iron preparations tend to form concretions in the stomach with large ingestions (52). Copious gastric lavage should be performed. Although some recommend addition of bicarbonate or deferoxamine to the lavage solution, this is not proven to be more efficacious than saline or tap water alone. In large ingestions, flat plate abdominal radiographs can demonstrate the efficacy of lavage attempts. Large pill concretions resistant to voluminous lavage may need to be removed endoscopically or surgically (52). After lavage is complete, instillation of 100 ml of a 1% sodium bicarbonate solution is recommended. Bicarbonate promotes formation of a ferrous carbonate salt that is less irritating and poorly absorbed. Others recommend instillation of deferoxamine (10 g in 50 ml of water) at the completion of lavage to chelate any iron remaining in the stomach (74). Activated charcoal is not indicated.

Any patient with a serum iron level greater than 300 ug/dl should undergo parenteral chelation therapy. However, a level below 300 ug/dl does not rule out serious toxicity. Because of this, patients exhibiting clinical signs or symptoms of toxicity should also undergo chelation therapy. Other indications for parenteral chelation are a positive deferoxamine challenge test (appearance of vin rosé urine after a single intramuscular dose of deferoxamine) and evidence of radiopaque densities after gastric lavage. Any patient with a history of significant iron ingestion should receive 2 g of deferoxamine intramuscularly (after serum studies are drawn) until further decisions can be made about indications for continuing chelation therapy.

For normotensive patients, deferoxamine can be given intramuscularly. Doses are 50–100 mg/kg, up to 2 g, every 6–8 hours to a maximum of 6 g/24 hours. For hypotensive patients, a continuous infusion of 15 mg/kg/hour is given (10). Chelation therapy should continue until the disappearance of the vin rosé color from the urine, signifying disappearance of the iron-deferoxamine complex. Others recommend continuing chelation therapy for an additional 24 hours after the urine has cleared in patients with initial serum iron levels above 500 μg/dl (58).

Because of the high incidence of shock and acidosis in severe poisoning aggressive supportive therapy is mandatory. Fluid and pressor therapy should be guided by hemodynamic monitoring and clinical response. Blood therapy for gastrointestinal bleeding should be anticipated. Administration of sodium bicarbonate for acidosis may be necessary on repeated occasions. Intensive supportive therapy, combined with aggressive decontamination and chelation therapy, can successfully treat even the most severe overdoses.

References

1. Abramowitz M (ed): Acute drug abuse reactions. *Med Letter* 696:77–80, 1985.
2. Achong MR: Clinical pharmacology of analgesic drugs. *Can Fam Physician* 25:179, 1979.
3. Afife AA, Sacks ST, Liu VY, et al: Accumulative prognostic index for patients with barbiturate glutethamide, and meprobamate intoxication. *N Engl J Med* 285:1497–1502, 1971.
4. Ambre J: Principles of pharmacology for the clinician. Winchester, Haddad (eds): *Clinical Management of Poisoning and Drug Overdose*, Philadelphia, WB Saunders, 1983.
5. Anderson RJ, Potts DE, et al: Unrecognized adult salicylate intoxication. *Ann Intern Med* 85:745, 1976.
6. Anonymous: Carbon monoxide, an old enemy forgot. *Lancet* 2:75–76, 1981.
7. Anthony T, Jastremski M, et al: Charcoal hemoperfusion for the treatment of combined diltiazem and metaprolol overdose. *Ann Emerg Med* 15:1344–1348, 1986.
8. Aquilonius SN, Hedstrand V: The use of physostgimine as an antidote in tricyclic antidepressant intoxication. *Acta Anaesthiol Scand* 22:40–45, 1978.
9. Baker MD: Theophylline toxicity in children. *J Pediatr* 109:538–542, 1986.
10. Banner W, Tong TG: Iron Poisoning. *Pediatr Clin North Am* 33:393–409, 1986.
11. Becker C, Sullivan JB: Prompt recognition and vigorous therapy for organophosphate poisoning. *Emerg Med Rep* 7:33–40, 1986.
12. Bennet IL, Cary FH, Mitchell GL: Acute methyl alcohol poisoning: review based on experiences in outreach of 323 cases. *Medicine* 32:431–463, 1953.
13. Benowitz NL, Rosenberg J, Becker CE: Cardiopulmonary catastrophes in drug overdose patients. *Med Clin North Am* 63:267, 1979.
14. Benton CD, Calhoun FP: The ocular effects of methyl alcohol poisoning: report of a catastrophe involving 320 persons. *Am J Ophthalmol* 36:1677–1685, 1952.
15. Berman LB, Schreiner GE, Feys J: The nephrotoxic lesion of ethylene glycol. *Ann Intern Med* 46:611–619, 1957.
16. Bertino JS, Reed MD: Barbiturate and nonbarbiturate sedative hypnotic intoxication in children. *Pediatr Clinics North Am* 33:703–720, 1986.
17. Biberstein MP, Ziegler MG, Ward DM: Use of beta-blockade and hemoperfusion for acute theophylline poisoning. *West J Med* 141:485–490, 1984.
18. Biggs JT, Spiker DG, et al: Tricyclic antidepressant overdose: incidence of symptoms. *JAMA* 238:135, 1977.
19. Black M: Acetaminophen hepatotoxicity. *Ann Rev Med* 35:377, 1984.
20. Brancato JC, Fow MI: Poisoning. Poisoning mortality in the United States, 1978. *Natl Clearingh Poison Control Cent Bull* 25:11–15, 1981.
21. Brandwin MA: Drug overdose emergency room admissions. *Am J Drug Alcohol Abuse* 3:605–619, 1976.
22. Brenner BE, Simon RR: Management of salicylate intoxication. *Drugs* 24:335, 1982.
23. Brown CG, Trumbull D, et al: Ethylene glycol poisoning. *Ann Emerg Med* 12:501–506, 1983.
24. Brown TC: Tricyclic antidepressant overdosage: experimental studies on the management of circulatory complications. *Clin Toxicol* 9:55, 1976.
25. Byers AJ, Traylor TR, Semmer JR: Acetaminophen overdose in the third trimester of pregnancy. *JAMA* 247:3114–3115, 1982.
26. Callaham M: Epidemiology of fatal tricyclics: antidepressant ingestion: management. *Ann Emerg Med* 14:1–9, 1985.
27. Catchings TT, Beane LC, et al: Adult respiratory distress syndrome secondary to ethylene glycol ingestion. *Ann Emerg Med* 14:594–596, 1985.

28. Clemmensen C, Nilsson E: Therapeutic trends in the treatment of barbiturate poisoning: The Scandanavian method. *Clin Pharmacol Ther* 2:220, 1961.
29. Coburn RF: Mechanisms of carbon monoxide poisoning toxicity. *Prev Med* 8:310–322, 1979.
30. Coburn RF, Danielson GK, et al: Carbon monoxide in blood: analytical method and sources of error. *J Appl Physiol* 19:510, 1964.
31. Cotrell JE, Casthel P, et al: Prevention of nitroprusside induced cyanide toxicity with hydroxycolbalamin. *N Engl J Med* 298:809–811, 1978.
32. Crome P, Dawling S, et al: Effect of activated charcoal on nortriptyline. *Lancet* 2:1203, 1977.
33. Crome P, Braithwaite G, et al: Hemoperfusion in clinical and experimental poisoning. Chang (ed): *Hemoperfusion: Kidney and Liver Support and Detoxification.* Washington, Hemisphere Pub, 1980.
34. Cruickshank JM: The clinical importance of cardioselectivity and lipophilicity in beta blockers. *Am Heart J* 100:160, 1980.
35. Cupit GC, Temple AR: Gastrointestinal decontamination in the management of the poisoned patient. *Emerg Med Clin North Am* 1:3–14, 1984.
36. Curry SC, Vance MV, et al: Cardiovascular effects of toxic concentrations of theophylline in the dog. *Ann Emerg Med* 14:547–553, 1985.
37. Daniel DR, McAnalley BH, Garriot JC: Isopropyl alcohol metabolism after acute intoxication in humans. *J Anal Toxicol* 5:110–112, 1981.
38. Davidson DGD: Acute liver necrosis following overdose of paracetamol. *Br Med J* 2:497–499, 1966.
39. deCastro FJ, Jaeger RW, et al: Apomorphine: clinical trial of a stable solution. *Clin Toxicol* 12:65–68, 1978.
40. Doherty JE, deSoyza N, et al: Clinical pharmacokinetics of digitalis glycosides. *Prog Cardiovas Dis* 21:141, 1978.
41. Done AK: Salicylate intoxication: significance of measurements of salicylate in blood in cases of acute ingestion. *Pediatrics* 26:800–807, 1960.
42. Done AK: The toxic emergency. The great equalizer? Anticholinesterases. *Emerg Med* 11:167, 1979.
43. Dorr RT, Paxinos J: The current status of laetrile. *Ann Intern Med* 89:387–389, 1978.
44. Easom JM, Lovejoy FH: Efficacy and safety of gastrointestinal decontamination in the treatment of oral poisoning. *Pediatr Clin North Am* 26:827, 1979.
45. Ellis EF: Theophylline toxicity. *J Allergy Clin Immunol* 76:297, 1985.
46. Epstein FB, Eilers MA: Rosen, et al (eds): Poisoning. Emergency Medicine. *Concepts and Clinical Practice* St. Louis, CV Mosby, 1983.
47. Fairshter RD, Wilson AF: Paraquat poisoning, manifestations and therapy. *Am J Med* 59:751–753, 1975.
48. Ferguson HC: Dilution of dose and acute oral toxicity. *Toxicol Appl Pharmacol* 4:759, 1962.
49. Fifth Special Report to the US Congress on Alcohol and Health. Washington, DC, US Govt Printing Office, 1983.
50. Fiser RH, Maetz HM, et al: Activated charcoal in barbiturate and glutethamide poisoning. *J Pediatrics* 78:1045, 1971.
51. Food and Drug Administration, Bureau of Drugs: Minutes of Ad Hoc Panel on *Toxicity of the Tricyclic Antidepressants* of the Psychopharmacological Agents Advisory Committee, Rockville, MD, September 10, 1975.
52. Foxford R, Goldfrank L: Gastrotomy—A surgical approach to iron overdose. *Ann Emerg Med* 14:1123–1126, 1985.
53. Freedman GE, et al: A clinical trial using syrup of ipecac and activated charcoal concurrently. *Ann Emerg Med* 2:164–166, 1987.
54. Freeman JW, Mundy GR, et al: Cardiac abnormalities in poisoning with tricyclic antidepressants. *Br Med J* 2:610, 1969.
55. Frejaville JP, Nicaise AM, et al: Etude statistique d'une seconde certaine d'intoxications aiques par les derive de l'iminobenzle. *Bul Soc Med Hop Paris* 117:1151, 1966.
56. Garrison RF: Acute poisoning from use of isopropyl alcohol in tepid sponging. *JAMA* 152:317–318, 1953.
57. Gaudreault P, McCormick MA, et al: Poisoning exposures and use of ipecac in children less than one year old. *Ann Emerg Med* 7:808–810, 1986.
58. Ghandi R, Roberts F: Hourglass stricture of the stomach and pyloric stenosis due to ferrous sulfate poisoning. *Br J Surg* 49:613–617, 1962.
59. Glassman AH: Cardiovascular effects of tricyclic antidepressants. *Annual Rev Med* 35:503–511, 1984.
60. Gleason WA, deMello, et al: Acute hepatic failure in severe iron poisoning. *J Pediatr* 95:138–140, 1979.
61. Goldberg MJ, Park GP, Berlinger WG: Treatment of theophylline intoxication. *J Allerg Clin Immunol* 78:811–817, 1986.
62. Goldfrank L, Flomenbaum N, et al: The liquid time bomb. *Hospital Physician* 18:38–60, 1982.
63. Goldfrank LR, Kirstein R: *Toxicologic Emergencies: A Comprehensive Handbook in Problem Solving.* New York, Appleton-Century-Crofts, 1984.
64. Gonda A, Gault H, et al: Hemodialysis for methanol intoxication. *Am J Med* 64:749–758, 1978.
65. Gosselin RE, Smith RP, Hodge HC: *Clinical Toxicology of Commercial Products,* ed 5. Baltimore, Williams & Wilkins, 1984.
66. Greenblatt DJ, Allen MD, et al: Acute overdosage with benzodiazepine derivatives. *Clin Pharmacol Ther* 21:497–514, 1977.
67. Gross PL, Schwartz HS: Toxicology emergencies. In Wilkens EW (ed): *MGH Textbook of Emergency Medicine.* Baltimore, Williams & Wilkins, 1982.
68. Guzzardi LJ: Role of the emergency physician in the management of the poisoned patient. *Emerg Med Clinics North Am* 1:3–14, 1984.
69. Haddad L: A general approach to the emergency management of poisoning. In Winchester, Haddad (eds): *Clinical Management of Poisoning and Drug Overdose.* Philadelphia, WB Saunders, 1983.
70. Hager WD, Fenster P, et al: Digoxin-quinidine interaction: Pharmacokinetics evaluation. *N Engl J Med* 300:1238, 1979.
71. Hall AH, Rumack BH: Clinical toxicity of cyanide. *Ann Emerg Med* 15:1067–1074, 1986.
72. Hall KW, Dobson KE, et al: Metabolic abnormalities associated with intentional theophylline overdose. *Arch Intern Med* 101:457–462, 1984.
73. Hassan E: Treatment of meprobamate overdose with repeated oral doses of activated charcoal. *Ann Emerg Med* 15:73–76, 1986.
74. Henretig FN, Karl SR, Weintraub WH: Severe iron poisoning treated with enteral and intravenous deferoxamine. *Ann Emerg Med* 12:306–309, 1983.
75. Henry J, Volans G: ABC of poisoning. Analgesics: II paracetamol. *Br Med J* 289:907, 1984.
76. Heese B, Pederson JT: Hypoglycemia after propanolol in children. *Acta Med Scand* 193:551, 1973.
77. Hill JB: Salicylate intoxication. *N Engl J Med* 292:250, 1975.
78. Hill JB: Experimental salicylate poisoning: Observations on the effects of altering blood pH on tissue and plasma salicylate concentrations. *Pediatrics* 47:658, 1971.
79. Hinson J, Pohl K, et al: Acetaminophen—induced hepatotoxicity. *Life Sci* 29:107, 1981.
80. Hornback KD: Overdoing the anticholinergics. *Emerg Med* 13:45–53, 1981.
81. Jackson JE, Bressler R: Prescribing tricyclic antidepressants, Part I. General considerations. *Drug Ther* 11:87–96, 1981.
82. Jackson JE, Bressler R: Prescribing tricyclic antide-

pressants. Part III. Management of overdose. *Drug Ther* 12:49–63, 1982.

83. Jacob AS, Nielsen DH, Gianelly RE: Fatal ventricular fibrillation following verapamil in Wolff-Parkinson-White syndrome with atrial fibrillation. *Ann Emerg Med* 14:159–160, 1985.

84. Jacobs J, Greens H, Gendel BR: Acute iron intoxication. *N Engl J Med* 273:1124, 1965.

85. Jaffe JH, Martin WR: Opioid analgesics and antagonists. In Goodman, Gilman (eds): *The Pharmacologic Basis of Therapeutics.* ed. 6. New York, MacMillian, 1980.

86. Jones J, Heiselman D, et al: Cathartic-induced magnesium toxicity during overdose management. *Ann Emerg Med* 15:1214–1218, 1986.

87. Kallos T, Smith TG: Naloxone reversal of pentazocine-induced respiratory depression. *JAMA* 204:932, 1968.

88. Kazmers A, Whitehouse W, et al: Dissociation of glucagon's central and peripheral hemodynamic effects: Mechanism of reduction and redistribution on canine hindlimb blood flow. *J Surg Res* 30:384–390, 1981.

89. Kearin M, Kelly JG, O'Malley K: Digoxin "receptors" in neonates an explanation of less sensitivity to digoxin than in adults. *Clin Pharmacol Ther* 28:346–349, 1980.

90. Kulig K, et al: Management of acutely poisoned patients without gastric emptying. *Ann Emerg Med* 14:562–567, 1985.

91. Lacouture PG, Lovejoy FH: Iron. Haddad, Winchester (eds): *Clinical Management of Poisoning and Drug Overdose.* Philadelphia, WB Saunders, 1983.

92. Lacouture PG, Wason S, et al: Acute isopropyl alcohol ingestion: diagnosis and management. *Am J Med* 75:680–686, 1983.

93. Lai KN, Swaminathan R, et al: Hemofiltration in digoxin overdose. *Arch Intern Med* 146:1219–1220, 1986.

94. Lehman AJ, Chase HF: The acute and chronic toxicity of isopropyl alcohol. *J Lab Clin Med* 29:561, 1944.

95. Levy G: Gastrointestinal clearance of drugs with activated charcoal. *N Engl J Med* 307:676–678, 1982.

96. Lim DT, Singh P: Absorption inhibition and enhancement of elimination of sustained-release theophylline tablets by oral activated charcoal. *Ann Emerg Med* 15:1303–1307, 1986.

97. Linton AL, Luke RG, Briggs JD: Methods of forced diuresis and its application in barbiturate poisoning. *Lancet* 2:7512, 1967.

98. Manno BR, Manno JE: Toxicology of ipecac: A review. *Clin Toxicol* 10:221, 1977.

99. Marshall JB, Forker AD: Cardiovascular effects of tricyclic antidepressant drugs: therapeutic usage, overdosage, and management of complications. *Am Heart J* 103:401–414, 1982.

100. Marstellar H, Gugler R: Endoscopic management of toxic masses in the stomach. *N Engl J Med* 196:1003, 1977.

101. McCarthy LG, Speth CP: Diquat intoxication. *Ann Emerg Med* 12:394–396, 1983.

102. McCoy HG, Cipolle RJ, et al: Severe methanol poisoning: application of a pharmacokinetic model for ethanol therapy and hemodialysis. *Am J Med* 67:804, 1979.

103. McGuigan MA: Planning an effective strategy for theophylline poisoning in adults. *Emerg Med Rep* 8:41–48, 1987.

104. Michiels TM, Light RW, Mahutte CK: Naloxone reverses ethanol-induced depression of hypercapnic drive. *Am Rev Respir Dis* 128:823–826, 1983.

105. Mitchell JR, Jollow DT, et al: Acetaminophen-induced hepatic necrosis, role of drug metabolism. *J Pharmacol Exp Ther* 187:184–194, 1973.

106. Mofenson HC, Caraccio TR, Schauber J: Poisoning by antidysrhythmic drugs. *Ped Clinics North Am* 33:723–738, 1986.

107. Morgan AG, Polak A: The excretion of salicylate in salicylate poisoning. *Clin Sci* 41:475–484, 1971.

108. Morgan DP: *Recognition and Management of Pesticide Poisonings,* 3rd ed. Wash DC, US Environmental Protection Agency, 1982.

109. Morgan MD, Pusey CD, et al: Treatment of quinine poisoning with charcoal hemoperfusion, *Post Med J* 59:365–367, 1983.

110. Mountain RD, Neff TA: Oral theophylline intoxication: a serious error of patient and physician understanding. *Arch Intern Med* 144:724–727, 1984.

111. Murphy DJ, Bremer WF, Haber E: Massive digoxin overdose treated with FAB: fragment of digoxin specific antibodies. *Pediatrics* 70:;472, 1982.

112. Myers RAM, Linberg SE, Crowley RA: Carbon monoxide poisoning, the injury and its treatment. *JACEP* 8:479–484, 1979.

113. Myers RAM, Synder SK, et al: Value of hyperbaric oxygen in suspected carbon monoxide poisoning. *JAMA* 246:2478–2480, 1981.

114. Namba T: Diagnosis and treatment of organophosphate insecticide poisoning. *Med Times* 100:100–126, 1972.

115. Namba T, Nolte C, et al: Poisoning due to organophosphate insecticides. *Am J Med* 50:475–492, 1975.

116. National Safety Council: Accident Facts. Chicago, National Safety Council, 1982.

117. Nattel S, Bayne L, Ruedy J: Physostigmine in coma due to drug overdose. *Clin Pharmacol Ther* 25:96–102, 1979.

118. Newton RW: Physostigmine in the treatment of tricyclic antidepressant overdose. *JAMA* 231:941–943, 1975.

119. Niemann JT, Besser HA, et al: Electrocardiographic criteria for tricyclic antidepressant cardiotoxicity. *Am J Cardiol* 57:1154–1159, 1986.

120. Norkool DM, Kirkpatrick JN: Treatment of acute carbon monoxide poisoning with hyperbaric oxygen: a review of 115 cases. *Ann Emerg Med* 14:1168–1171, 1985.

121. Olson KR, Benowitz NC, et al: Theophylline overdose: acute single ingestion versus chronic repeated overmedication. *Am J Emerg Med* 3:408, 1985.

122. Ordog GI, Benaron S, et al: Serum digoxin levels and motality in 5,100 patients. *Ann Emerg Med* 16:32–39, 1987.

123. Osterpoh J: Limitations of acetaminophen assays. *J Toxicol Clin Toxicol* 20:19, 1983.

124. Parry MF, Wallack R: Ethylene glycol poisoning. *Am J Med* 57:143, 1974.

125. Pentel P, Peterson CD: Asystole complicating physostigmine treatment of tricyclic antidepressant overdose. *Ann Emerg Med* 9:588–590, 1980.

126. Peterson C, Collins A, et al: Ethylene glycol poisoning: pharmacokinetics during therapy with ethanol and hemodialysis. *N Engl J Med* 304:21–23, 1981.

127. Piper KW, Griner PF: Suicide attempts with drug overdose. *Arch Intern Med* 134:703–706, 1974.

128. Pond SN: Diuresis, dialysis, and hemoperfusion. *Emerg Med Clin North Am* 2:29–45, 1984.

129. Proudfoot AT: Toxicity of salicylates. *Am J Med* 75:99–103, 1983.

130. Proudfoot AT, Brown SS: Acidemia and salicylate poisoning in adults. *Br Med J* 2:547–550, 1969.

131. Ragan FA, Samuels MS, Hite SA: Ethanol in children. *JAMA* 242:2787–2788, 1979.

132. Reed K: Tricyclic antidepressant blood levels—eight practical questions. *Postgrad Med* 70:81–88, 1981.

133. Renzi FP, Donovan JW, et al: Concomitant use of activated charcoal and N-acetylcysteine. *Ann Emerg Med* 4:568–572, 1985.

134. Roberts RJ, Mueller S, Lauer RM: Propanolol in the treatment of cardiac arrythmias associated with amitryptiline intoxication. *J Pediatr* 82:65, 1973.

135. Roberts RJ, Morgan DP: Organophosphate and N-methyl

carbamate insecticides. Edlick and Spyker (eds): *Current Emergency Therapy*. Rockville, Aspen Systems, 1985.

136. Robotham JL, Lietman PS: Acute iron poisoning. *Am J Dis Child* 134:875–878, 1980.

137. Rosenberg J, Benowitz NL, Pond S: Pharmacokinetics of drug overdose. *Clin Pharmacokinet* 6:161–192, 1981.

138. Rudolph JP: Automated gastric lavage and a comparison of 0.9% normal saline solution and tap water irrigant. *Ann Emerg Med* 14:1156–1159, 1985.

139. Rumack BH: Acetaminophen overdose. *Am J Med* 76:104–111, 1983.

140. Rumack BH, Matthew H: Acetaminophen poisoning and toxicity. *Pediatrics* 55:871–876, 1975.

141. Rumack BH, Peterson RG: Acetaminophen overdose: incidence, diagnosis, and management in 416 patients. *Pediatrics* 62:898–903, 1978.

142. Rumack BH, Wolfe RR, Gilfrick H: Phenytoin treatment of massive digoxin overdose. *Br Heart J* 36:405–408, 1974.

143. Sejersted OM, Jacobson D, et al: Formate concentrations in plasma in patients poisoned with methanol. *Acta Med Scand* 213:105–110, 1983.

144. Sessler CN, Glauser FL, Cooper KR: Treatment of theophylline toxicity with oral activated charcoal. *Chest* 87:325–329, 1985.

145. Severance H: Vomiting and abdominal pain. *Case Stud Emerg Med* 12:4–6, 1986.

146. Shore ET, Cepin D, Davidson MJ: Metoprolol overdose. *Ann Emerg Med* 10:524–526, 1981.

147. Smith PW: Bulletin: Medical problems in aerial applications. Office of Aviation Medicine, Federal Aviation Administration, Department of Transportation, Washington DC, 1977.

148. Smith TW, Haber E: Digitalis IV. *N Engl J Med* 289:1125, 1973.

149. Snodgras WR: Salicylate toxicity. *Ped Clin North Am* 33:381–391, 1986.

150. Snodgras WR, Rumack BH, et al: Salicylate toxicity following therapeutic doses in young children. *Clin Toxicol* 18:247–259, 1981.

151. Snover SW, Bocchino V: Massive diltiazem overdose. *Ann Emerg Med* 15:1221–1224, 1986.

152. Sogge MR, Griffith JL, et al: Lavage to remove enteric coated aspirin and gastric outlet obstruction. *Ann Int Med* 87:721, 1977.

153. Spiegel A, Marchlinski FE: Time course for reversal of digoxin toxicity with digoxin—specific antibody fragments. *Am Heart J* 109:1397, 1985.

154. Steinberg AD, Karliner JS: The clinical spectrum of heroin pulmonary edema. *Arch Intern Med* 122:122, 1968.

155. Sturman K, Mofenson H, Carracio T: Methylene chloride inhalation: an unusual form of drug abuse. *Ann Emerg Med* 14:903–905, 1985.

156. Sullivan JB, Lander DH: Planning an effective therapeutic strategy in salicylate poisoning. *Emerg Med Rep* 7:89–96, 1986.

157. Tafuri J, Roberts J: Organophosphate poisoning. *Ann Emerg Med* 16:193–202, 1987.

158. Tandberg D, Abercrombie R: Treatment of heroin overdose with endotracheal naloxone. *Ann Emerg Med* 11:443–445, 1982.

159. Temple AR: Acute and chronic effects of aspirin toxicity and their treatment. *Arch Intern Med* 141:364, 1981.

160. Tenenbein M: Multiple dose charcoal therapy. *Curr Probl Pediatr* 7:214, 1986.

161. Thompson ME, Verhulst HL: Ipecac syrup in antiemetic ingestion. *JAMA* 196:433, 1966.

162. Tintinalli JE: The alcohols. In Tintinalli, et al (eds): *Emergency Medicine: A Comprehensive Study Guide*. New York, McGraw-Hill, 1985.

163. Uhl JA: Phenytoin: The drug of choice in tricyclic overdose? *Ann Emerg Med* 10:270–274, 1984.

164. Underwood E, Bennet W: Ethylene glycol intoxication. *JAMA* 226:1453–1454, 1978.

165. Veltri JC, Temple AR: Telephone management of poisonings using syrup of ipecac. *Clin Toxicol* 9:407, 1976.

166. Walls RM, Sloan MB: Coma in a fire victim. *Case Stud Emerg Med* 11:10–12, 1985.

167. Weden GP, Oderda GM, et al: Relative toxicity of cyclic antidepressants. *Ann Emerg Med* 15:797–804, 1986.

168. Weinstein RS: Recognition and management of poisoning with beta-adrenergic blocking agents. *Ann Emerg Med* 13:1123–1131, 1984.

169. Weinstein RS, Cole S, et al: Beta blocker overdose with propanolol and atenolol. *Ann Emerg Med* 14:161–163, 1985.

170. Weller-Fahy ER, Berger LR, Troutman WG: Mouthwash: A source of acute ethanol intoxication. *Pediatrics* 66:302–304, 1980.

171. Winchester JF: Active methods for detoxification: oral sorbents, forced diuresi hemoperfusion, and hemodialysis. In Winchester, Haddad (eds): *Clinical Management of Poisoning and Drug Overdose*. Philadelphia, WB Saunders, 1983.

172. Winchester JF, Gelfand MC, et al: Dialysis and hemoperfusion of poisons and drugs. *Trans Am Soc Artif Organs* 23:762, 1977.

173. Winter PM, Miller JN: Carbon monoxide poisoning. *JAMA* 236:1502–1504, 1976.

174. Worthley LIG: Treating the adverse effects of verapamil. *JAMA* 252:1129, 1984.

175. Yatzides H, Voudiclari S, et al: Treatment of severe barbiturate poisoning. *Lancet* 2:216, 1965.

176. Yearly Report. Washington, DC, National Center for Health Statistics, 1977.

177. Zaloga GP, Malcolm D, Holaday J, Chernow B: Glucagon reverses the hypotension and bradycardia of verapamil overdose in rats. *Crit Care Med* 13:273, 1985.

178. Zaloga GP, Delacey W, Holmebae E, Chernow B: Glucagon reverses the hypotension of anaphylactic shock. *Ann Intern Med* 105:65–66, 1986.

179. Zwillich CW, Sutton FD, et al: Theophylline-induced seizures in adults: correlation with serum concentration. *Ann Intern Med* 82:784–787, 1975.

15

Electrolyte and Acid-Base Disorders

Man S. Oh, M.D.
Hugh J. Carroll, M.D.

Electrolyte and acid-base disorders are common problems in clinical medicine. This chapter reviews some of these disorders with particular reference to those problems that occur frequently in critically ill patients. Discussions stress pathophysiology, diagnosis, and pharmacological aspects of management.

HYPONATREMIA

Hyponatremia, which is defined as a reduced plasma sodium concentration, is the most common electrolyte disorder. The term *pseudohyponatremia* is applied to a spurious reduction in serum sodium concentrations due to a measurement error caused by hyperlipidemia, hyperproteinemia, or increased viscosity of the plasma. Although the sodium concentration in plasma water is normal in pseudohyponatremia, the dilution of the sample causes an error in measurement (33). When measurement is made with an ion-specific electrode without dilution of the sample (direct method), the concentration is normal. However, the error occurs when serum sodium is measured with a flame photometer, because the sample is always diluted before flame-photometric measurement. The error also occurs even when an ion-specific electrode is used, if an indirect method (dilution of the sample) is used (15, 23). In pseudohyponatremia, plasma osmolality, which is customarily measured without dilution, is normal (33). A low plasma sodium concentration with a normal plasma osmolality does not always indicate the presence of pseudohyponatremia; true hyponatremia may be accompanied by a normal plasma osmolality because of hyperglycemia, azotemia, mannitol, or alcohol (31).

Hyponatremia usually signifies a proportionate reduction in plasma osmolality, which causes cellular overhydration by the shift of water into the cells. Cell overhydration, especially when it occurs abruptly, can cause neuromuscular dysfunction, convulsions, and death. Cellular overhydration in hyponatremia is independent of extracellular volume, since the shift of water across the cell membrane depends solely on the osmotic gradient. Accumulation of a substance such as mannitol or glucose that is restricted to the extracellular fluid can cause hyponatremia by increasing extracellular (effective) osmolality and hence causing the shift of water from the intracellular space to the extracellular space. In such situations, despite hyponatremia, cells are dehydrated rather than swollen. Some authors extend the definition of pseudohyponatremia to those hyponatremic states accompanied by increased effective osmolality. However, since the sodium concentration in mannitol- or hyperglycemia-induced hyponatremia is truly low, such an extended definition of pseudohyponatremia is inappropriate and also confusing.

Glucose, sodium, and mannitol are effective osmols, whereas urea and alcohol are ineffective osmols because the former can effectively cause the shift of water across the cell membrane, whereas the latter diffuse freely into the cell and therefore do not cause the water shift (12). Thus, the clinical importance of hyponatremia must be judged in the context of the effective plasma osmolality, which may be determined in two ways. It can be measured by summation of all effective osmols in plasma:

Effective osmolality = Plasma Na (mEq/liter)

$$\times\, 2 + \frac{\text{glucose (mg/dl)}}{18} + \frac{\text{mannitol (mg/dl)}}{18} +$$

Alternatively, the total osmolality can be meaured and the osmolality due to ineffective osmols subtracted. Table 15.1 lists the cate-

Table 15.1
Hyponatremia According to Effective Osmolality

Normal effective osmolality-pseudohyponatremia:
hyperlipidemia, hyperproteinemia, increased
viscosity
Increased effective osmolality: hyperglycemia,
mannitol infusion
Low effective osmolality: usual hyponatremia

Table 15.2
Causes of Hyponatremia According to Mechanism of Maintenance

Increased water intake, e.g., primary polydipsia
Reduced water excretion
  Reduced delivery of fluid to the distal nephron
    because of low effective arterial volume (ADH
    is usually present as well)
  Heart failure
  Nephrotic syndrome
  Cirrhosis of the liver
  Gastrointestinal sodium loss
  Sweating
  Diuretic therapy or renal salt wasting
  Adrenal insufficiency
  Hypothyroidism
  Advanced renal failure
  Inappropriate secretion of ADH (SIADH)
  Tumors
  Pulmonary diseases
  Central nervous system disorders
  Drugs, e.g., chlorpropamide, barbiturates,
    morphine, indomethacin
  Physical and emotional stress, nausea
  Glucocorticoid deficiency
  Myxedema
  Idiopathic
  Reset osmostat

gories of hyponatremia associated with increased, normal, and low effective plasma osmolality.

Causes and Pathogenesis of True Hyponatremia

The initiating mechanism of hyponatremia will be one of the following: (a) shift of water from the cell caused by accumulation of extracellular solutes other than sodium salts; (b) retention of excess water in the body; (c) loss of sodium; and (d) shift of sodium into the cells.

The appropriate physiological response to hyponatremia is suppression of antidiuretic hormone (ADH) release, leading to rapid excretion of excess water and correction of hyponatremia. Persistence of hyponatremia indicates the failure of this compensatory mechanism. In most instances hyponatremia is maintained because the kidney fails to produce water diuresis, but sometimes excessive ingestion of water is responsible.

Among the reasons for the inability of the kidney to excrete water and therefore correct hyponatremia are renal failure, reduced delivery of glomerular filtrate to the distal nephron, and the presence of ADH. The mechanism for impaired water excretion in renal failure is obvious and needs no further explanation. Reduced distal delivery of filtrate results from the low glomerular filtration rate and enhanced proximal tubular reabsorption that characterize volume-depletion states. The normal dilution of urine requires delivery of adequate amounts of fluid to the diluting segment and the reabsorption of solute without water at that segment. ADH impairs urine dilution by reabsorption of water in the collecting duct. The presence of normal amounts of ADH despite hyponatremia would be considered inappropriate, but the release of ADH caused by reduced effective arterial volume is not considered inappropriate. The term "the syndrome of inappropriate ADH secretion" (SIADH) is therefore reserved for hyponatremia with a

normal or increased effective arterial volume. There are many causes of SIADH: tumors, pulmonary diseases including tuberculosis and pneumonias, central nervous system diseases, drugs, etc. (Table 15.2).

Hyponatremia in clinical states associated with reduced effective arterial volume such as congestive heart failure and cirrhosis of the liver is caused by a combination of reduced delivery of fluid to the distal nephron and elaboration of ADH (74). The same appears to be true of myxedema and glucocorticoid deficiency states (24, 34, 67).

Finally, mild hyponatremia may be caused by "resetting of the osmostat" at an osmolality lower than the usual level. In such cases urine dilution occurs normally when the plasma osmolality is brought down below the reset level. Resetting of the osmostat would be considered a form of SIADH, since ADH secretion occurs inappropriately at hyponatremic levels. Patients with chronic debilitating diseases such as pulmonary tuberculosis often manifest this phenomenon (17).

Diagnosis

The presence of a low plasma sodium and normal osmolality suggests pseudohyponatremia, but does not confirm it; hyponatremia accompanied by a high concentration of urea or alcohol might give a normal osmolality. More direct proof is the demonstration of a normal sodium concentration using a sodium-specific electrode or demonstration of reduced water content of plasma. Pseudohyponatremia due to hyperlipidemia is caused by accumulation of chylomicrons, which consist mostly of triglycerides (33), and is obvious from the milky appearance of serum or plasma. Substantial hyponatremia due to hyperlipidemia requires accumulation of more than 5–6 g/dl of lipids, and that degree of hyperlipidemia does not occur with hypercholesterolemia alone. Pseudohyponatremia due to hyperproteinemia can be confirmed by measurement of plasma proteins. Hyponatremia caused by mannitol or glucose is easily detected from the history and simultaneous measurements of plasma sodium, osmolality, and glucose.

In evaluating hyponatremia associated with hypoosmolality, the main concern is to distinguish between SIADH and hyponatremia due to other causes, for the most part volume-depletion states and edematous states. The major distinction between SIADH and other causes of hyponatremia lies in the status of effective arterial volume (EAV); EAV is normal or increased in the former, whereas the latter are associated with reduced EAV. However, there is no diagnostic test that measures effective arterial volume with certainty. A convenient and thus widely practiced technique for estimating EAV consists of measurement of urinary sodium and serum urea nitrogen (SUN), creatinine, and uric acid. Urinary sodium excretion > 20 mEq/liter, SUN < 10 mg/dl (16), serum creatinine < 1 mg/dl, and serum urate < 4.0 mg/dl (5) are suggestive of normal or increased effective arterial volume. In contrast, the measurement of urine osmolality has virtually no diagnostic value, and often misleads physicians. Contrary to common belief, SIADH may be associated with urine osmolality less than plasma osmolality (4). Similarly, other causes of hyponatremia can also be accompanied by urine osmolality higher than plasma osmolality, and a high urine osmolality in hyponatremia does not necessarily favor the diagnosis of SIADH.

The only situation in which urine osmolality may be appropriately low in the presence of hyponatremia is the hyponatremia caused by primary polydipsia, and this is usually apparent when a careful history reveals polyuria (53). In all other disorders that cause hyponatremia urine osmolality is inappropriately increased, i.e., greater than 100 mOsm/liter.

Management and Pharmacology

Hyponatremia is treated either by the addition of sodium or by removal of water. Salt is given to patients with hyponatremia due to salt depletion, and water is to be removed in hyponatremic states with normal or increased sodium content. The speed of correction of hyponatremia is very important and should depend on the speed of development of hyponatremia and the patient's symptoms. Clearly, severe symptomatic hyponatremia is a life-threatening condition (2), but there are considerable dangers associated with treatment of hyponatremia. In addition to the danger of volume overload that may occur with administration of a large quantity of salt-containing solution, the possibility of central pontine myelinolysis is now considered a major danger associated with rapid correction of hyponatremia (40, 73). This demyelinating disease of the central pons, which is characterized by motor nerve dysfunction including quadriplegia, may develop following rapid correction of hyponatremia. The complication tends to occur more with chronic hyponatremia in a malnourished and debilitated patient than with acute hyponatremia, and may be avoided by slow correction of hyponatremia (at a speed < 0.5 mEq/liter/hour). Since there is less danger of central pontine myelinolysis with acute hyponatremia than with chronic hyponatremia, and chronic hyponatremia is usually asymptomatic, rapid correction (at a rate of 1–2 mEq/liter/hour) should be restricted to those with acute symptomatic hyponatremia. Even then, there is no advantage in rapidly increasing serum sodium above levels of 125–130 mEq/liter. For patients admitted with hypotonic dehydration and chronic asymptomatic hyponatremia who suffer mainly from volume depletion, the traditional recommendation has been administration of isotonic saline. However, sometimes rapid excretion of water following isotonic saline administration in these patients may leave them particularly vulnerable to the development of central pontine myelinolysis. For those patients, the use of 0.45% sodium chloride solution may be safer (43).

RAPID TREATMENT

For hyponatremia with sodium depletion, intravenous administration of sodium as hypertonic saline will correct hyposmolality effectively. The amount of sodium necessary to increase the sodium to a desired level of serum sodium is calculated as follows:

$$\text{Sodium requirement (in mEq)} = \text{TBW} \times \text{(the desired serum sodium} - \text{actual serum sodium)}$$

Sodium may be administered as a 3% or 5% NaCl solution. If the main purpose of treatment is correction of volume depletion rather than of hyponatremia, normal saline may be administered instead. As the ADH release caused by low EAV is suppressed with the volume expansion, excess water is excreted in the urine, resulting in correction of hyponatremia. This approach is feasible, of course, only if there is sufficient renal function for water excretion.

When accumulation of excess water is primarily responsible for hyponatremia, as in SIADH, water may be rapidly removed by administration of intravenous osmotic diuretics such as mannitol. An easier technique to use is to administer a loop diuretic (e.g., furosemide, which causes sodium and water diuresis) and simultaneously to administer hypertonic saline; the net result is removal of water (27). The usual adult dose of furosemide for this purpose is 40 mg. The same dose can be repeated at 2 to 4-hour intervals while hypertonic saline is being given. The response to this regimen cannot be predicted with precision, and frequent follow-up measurements of serum sodium level must be made. There is no theoretical advantage of replacing exactly the amount of sodium lost in urine with hypertonic saline. Administration of hypertonic saline alone usually causes a salt and water diuresis, but addition of a loop diuretic makes the correction of hyponatremia easier by preventing excretion of concentrated urine. Another advantage of adding a diuretic is prevention of fluid overload that may result from the administration of hypertonic saline. Potassium supplements are usually needed with this therapy.

CHRONIC THERAPY

Chronic hyponatremia may be treated by a reduction of water intake or by an increase in renal water excretion. Reduction of water intake is preferable but is not always feasible. If water restriction is difficult or unsuccessful, the latter approach may be used. Increased renal water excretion can be achieved by the use of pharmacological agents that interfere

with urine concentration. Lithium and demeclocycline increase urine output by reducing the production of cyclic AMP and also by interfering with its action (18, 65, 66). Demeclocycline is more effective and has fewer side effects (19), but it may cause nephrotoxicity in patients with liver diseases (11). The usual dose of lithium for this purpose is 300 mg twice or three times a day, and the usual dose of demeclocycline is 300 mg twice to three times a day.

Administration of a loop diuretic such as furosemide in conjunction with increased salt and potassium intake is a safer method of treating chronic hyponatremia than the above methods. The mechanism of action of the diuretic is prevention of high medullary interstitial osmolality by limiting the reabsorption of salt in Henle's loop and hence prevention of urine concentration. The increased salt and potassium intake leads to increased delivery of solutes and hence to increased water output (61). There is evidence that ethacrynic acid may impair ADH-stimulated water movement across the collecting duct, and furosemide may have the same effect. The usual dose of furosemide is 40 mg twice to three times a day.

Finally, the recently discovered vasopressin antagonists, which are not yet commercially available, may become an important addition to the chronic as well as acute treatment of hyponatremia in the future (60). The vascular effect as well as the antidiuretic effect of vasopressin is antagonized by the vasopressin antagonists.

HYPERNATREMIA

Hypernatremia is defined as an increased sodium concentration in plasma water. Whereas hyponatremia may not be accompanied by hyposmolality, e.g., hyponatremia due to hyperglycemia, hypernatremia is always associated with an increased effective plasma osmolality and hence with a reduced cell volume. However, the extracellular volume may be normal, decreased, or increased, depending on the pathogenesis of the hypernatremia.

Pathogenesis

Hypernatremia is caused by either loss of water or gain of sodium (Table 15.3). Loss of water could be due to increased loss or reduced intake, and gain of sodium is due either

Table 15.3
Pathogentic Mechanism of Hypernatremia

Loss of Water
  Reduced water intake
    Defective thirst
    Unconsciousness
    Inability to drink water
    Lack of access to water
  Increased water loss
    Gastrointestinal loss; vomiting, osmotic diarrhea
    Cutaneous loss; sweating and fever
    Respiratory loss; hyperventilation
    Renal loss, diabetes insipidus, osmotic diuresis
Gain of Sodium
  Increased intake
    Hypertonic saline infusion
    Ingestion of sea water
    Hypertonic sodium bicarbonate
  Renal salt retention
    Usually in response to primary water deficit

to increased intake or to reduced renal excretion. Increased loss of water can occur through the kidney (e.g., in diabetes insipidus or osmotic diuresis), the gastrointestinal tract (e.g., gastric suction or osmotic diarrhea), or the skin. Reduced water intake occurs most commonly in comatose patients or in those with a defective thirst mechanism. Less frequent causes of reduced water intake include continuous vomiting, lack of access to water, and mechanical obstruction such as esophageal tumor. The excess gain of sodium leading to hypernatremia is usually iatrogenic, e.g., from hypertonic saline infusion, abortion with hypertonic saline, or administration of hypertonic sodium bicarbonate during cardiopulmonary resuscitation or treatment of lactic acidosis (35). Reduced renal sodium excretion leading to sodium gain and hypernatremia is most commonly observed in patients who are water depleted.

Water depletion due to diabetes insipidus, osmotic diuresis, or insufficient water intake commonly leads to secondary renal sodium retention in those who continue to ingest or are given sodium. Often, hypernatremia observed in such cases is due more to sodium retention than to water loss (Table 15.3). Whether hypernatremia is due to sodium retention or water loss can be determined by examination of the patient's volume status. For example, if a patient with a serum sodium of 170 mEq/liter is normotensive and does not have obvious evidence of dehydration, hypernatremia cannot be caused entirely by water loss. In order to increase a serum sodium to 170 mEq/liter by water deficit alone, one would have to lose more than 20% of total body water.

Whereas the most effective defense against hyponatremia is increased renal water excretion, the most effective defense against hypernatremia is increased water drinking in response to thirst. Because thirst is such an effective and sensitive defense mechanism against hypernatremia, it is virtually impossible to increase serum sodium by more than a few milliequivalents per liter if the water drinking mechanism is intact. Therefore, in a patient with hypernatremia, there will always be a reason for reduced water intake (Table 15.3).

Management

ACUTE TREATMENT

Hypernatremia is treated either by the addition of water or the removal of sodium. The choice depends on the status of the body sodium and water content. If water depletion is the cause of hypernatremia, water is added. If sodium excess is the cause, sodium needs to be removed. When the water deficit is substantial, circulatory disturbances may result from extracellular volume depletion. In this situation, isotonic (0.9%) NaCl or 0.45% NaCl may be given initially to stabilize circulatory dynamics, with subsequent administration of more hypotonic solutions to normalize the tonicity. Administration of 5% dextrose solution would also correct the extracellular volume depletion, but a larger volume than isotonic saline is needed to expand the extracellular volume by the same extent and too rapid reduction of the plasma osmolality may result in cerebral edema. In acute symptomatic hypernatremia, serum sodium may be reduced by 6–8 mEq/liter in the first 3–4 hours, but thereafter the rate of decline should not exceed 1 mEq/liter/hour. As with hyponatremia, chronic hypernatremia usually does not cause CNS symptoms, and therefore does not require rapid correction. The amount of water needed to correct hypernatremia can be estimated with the following equation:

$$\text{Water deficit (in liters)} = \text{TBW} \left(\frac{\text{Na2}}{\text{Na1}} - 1 \right)$$

where Na1 is the desired serum sodium level, Na2 the observed serum sodium, and TBW is total body water. Total body water (in liters) can be estimated using the following formula:

$$\text{TBW} = \text{body weight in lb}/4.$$

In hypernatremia with excess sodium, the restoration of a normal volume usually initiates natriuresis, but if natriuresis does not occur promptly, sodium may be removed with diuretics. Furosemide plus 5% dextrose solution might be an appropriate regimen to treat hypernatremia associated with excess sodium, but care must be taken not to allow serum sodium concentration to decline too rapidly. Furosemide can be given at 40–60 mg intravenously at 2–4 hour intervals while 5% dextrose solution is being infused. If the patient has renal failure, salt can be removed by dialysis.

CHRONIC TREATMENT

Hypernatremic disorders that require chronic preventive therapy include diabetes insipidus and primary hypodipsia. If diabetes insipidus is the primary cause of hypernatremia, the distinction should first be made between nephrogenic and neurogenic (pituitary) diabetes insipidus. Administration of pitressin or stimulation of endogenous ADH secretion is helpful only for pituitary diabetes insipidus. Exogenous pitressin is available in three forms: pitressin tannate in oil, which is administered intramuscularly; I, desmopressin (dDAVP), a synthetic analog of ADH, which is administered through a plastic nasal tube (56); and a synthetic lysine vasopressin (lypressin, Diapid), which is administered as a nasal spray. The usual dose of dDAVP is 0.2 ml twice a day, and the usual dose for Diapid is 1–2 sprays in each nostril four times a day.

Some patients may prefer oral agents, and the two that have been used extensively with relatively few side effects are chlorpropamide and thiazide diuretics. Chlorpropamide (100–250 mg/day) stimulates the secretion of endogenous ADH and may also enhance the effect of ADH. Thiazide diuretics produce vascular volume depletion and enhanced reabsorption of fluid in the proximal tubule. Thus, they increase urine concentration by reducing the delivery of fluid to the distal diluting segment of the nephron. Addition of a thiazide diuretic to chlorpropamide may prevent the hypoglycemia that may occur if the latter is used alone. Two other drugs that have been used for the treatment of neurogenic diabetes insipidus are clofibrate (the usual dose, 2 g/day) (38) and carbamazepine (600 mg/day) (52). Since both drugs are less effective than chlorpropamide and have serious side effects, they should be the last resources in the treatment of diabetes

insipidus. Nephrogenic diabetes insipidus cannot be treated with ADH preparations or an agent that stimulates ADH release, but measures to reduce the distal delivery of salt and water, i.e., low salt diet and thiazide diuretics, have been used successfully. Subjects with primary hyodipsia should be educated to drink on schedule. In some instances, stimulation of the thirst center with chlorpropamide has met with success (8).

POTASSIUM METABOLISM

Although most of the body potassium is intracellular, the plasma potassium concentrations usually reflect the total body store of potassium. However, in conditions such as periodic paralysis or acid-base disorders, where abnormal shifts in potassium take place across the cell membrane, the plasma potassium concentration may not accurately reflect body stores. In both hyperkalemic and hypokalemic types of periodic paralysis, abnormal plasma potassium concentrations are explained by transmembrane potassium shifts. Similarly, in acute acidosis hyperkalemia may occur because of the shift of potassium from the cell, while acute alkalosis leads to hypokalemia because of potassium shift into the cells. Catecholamines and respiratory alkalosis are often responsible for hypokalemia in critical care units.

HYPOKALEMIA

Hypokalemia refers to a reduction in the plasma potassium concentration. Except for the situations where hypokalemia is caused by intracellular shift, it usually represents depletion of cellular potassium.

Pathogenesis

There are three basic mechanisms for hypokalemia: (a) intracellular shift, (b) reduced intake, and (c) increased loss (Table 15.4). An intracellular shift of potassium occurs with an increase in blood pH (62). This shift may occur when a patient develops alkalosis or when acidosis is being corrected. Administration of glucose and insulin also causes an intracellular shift of potassium, in part by stimulation

Table 15.4
Causes and Mechanism of Hypokalemia

Shift into the cell
   Correction of acidosis
   Administration of insulin and glucose
   Alkalosis
   Hypokalemic periodic paralysis
   Barium poisoning
   Increased catecholamines due to acute stress
Reduced intake
Increased loss
   Renal loss
      Primary hyperaldosteronism
      Secondary hyperaldosteronism, e.g., diuretic
         therapy, malignant hypertension, Bartter's
         syndrome, renal artery stenosis
      Mineralocorticoids other than aldosterone, e.g.,
         licorice, fluoro-prednisolone ointment,
         carbenoxolone
      Miscellaneous, e.g., hypercalcemia, Liddle's
         syndrome, magnesium deficiency, L-DOPA,
         RTA, acute myelocytic and monocytic
         leukemia, poorly reabsorbable anions
   Gastrointestinal loss
      Vomiting or nasogastric suction
   Diarrhea or fistula drainage

of glucose metabolism, but also by a direct effect of insulin on the cellular uptake of potassium (32, 58). The mechanism of intracellular shift of potassium in familial periodic paralysis is not clearly known.

The ingestion of absorbable barium salts, e.g., carbonate or chloride, causes a prompt reduction in the plasma potassium concentration by an intracellular shift (57). The intracellular shift is due to a decrease in passive outward diffusion of potassium because of decreased conductance of potassium (69).

The major routes of potassium loss are the kidneys and the gastrointestinal tract. There are numerous causes for renal potassium loss, but the two most constant factors are increased sodium delivery to the distal nephron and increased mineralocorticoid activity. Increased sodium delivery with reduced mineralocorticoid activity (e.g., high salt diet), or increased mineralocorticoid activity with reduced renal sodium excretion (e.g., extrarenal salt loss) does not lead to increased renal potassium excretion. Conditions such as primary hyperaldosteronism or chronic diuretic therapy are associated with increased sodium delivery to the distal nephron, even though sodium intake and urinary excretion may be normal. In primary hyperaldosteronism the proximal tubular sodium reabsorption is reduced because of volume expansion, resulting in greater sodium delivery to the distal ne-

phron. Enhanced sodium reabsorption at the Na-K exchange site allows normal amounts of sodium to come out in the urine despite increased delivery of sodium to the distal nephron.

A similar mechanism is responsible for the maintenance of increased sodium delivery to the Na-K exchange site during chronic diuretic therapy even when sodium excretion equals the intake. Hypercalcemia causes hypokalemia through increased renal potassium loss, but the exact mechanism is unknown. Increased urinary sodium excretion, which occurs with calcium infusion, is suggested as a possible mechanism (3). The degree of hypokalemia appears to be positively correlated with the serum calcium concentration. Hypokalemia caused by magnesium deficiency is due to increased renal loss of potassium, perhaps caused by increased production of aldosterone (21). PRA in magnesium deficiency is normal, and the mechanism of increased aldosterone is not known. Although the causal relationship is not entirely clear, the prevalence of hypokalemia in familial hypomagnesemia suggests that they are related (68). L-Dopa also occasionally causes hypokalemia possibly through increased aldosterone secretion (25). Kaliuresis and hypokalemia in renal tubular acidosis are commonly attributed to secondary hyperaldosteronism caused by renal salt wasting. Although renal salt wasting occurs in chronic metabolic acidosis, there is little convincing evidence for secondary hyperaldosteronism. There may be a specific tubular defect causing increased potassium loss in renal tubular acidosis (63). The mechanism of hypokalemia in acute myelocytic and acute monocytic leukemias is increased renal loss of potassium, but the mechanism of this loss is controversial (36). Delivery to the distal nephron of poorly reabsorbable anions such as penicillin and carbenicillin, leads to increased urinary loss of potassium because increased luminal negativity enhances potassium secretion (29). Vomiting and nasogastric suction cause hypokalemia, in part, because of direct loss of potassium from the stomach, but to a larger extent because of renal loss attributable to the renal bicarbonate wasting that occurs with metabolic alkalosis. Excretion of large amounts of bicarbonate causes renal potassium loss because bicarbonate acts as a poorly reabsorbable anion. Secondary hyperaldosteronism due to volume depletion is an additional factor involved in the pathogenesis of hypokalemia in this setting.

Management

Hypokalemia is usually treated either by potassium administration or by prevention of the renal loss of potassium. Renal loss of potassium is prevented either by treating its cause (e.g., removal of aldosterone-producing adenoma or by discontinuation of diuretics) or by the administration of potassium-sparing diuretics. The potassium-sparing diuretics in current use are aldosterone antagonists (e.g., spironolactone), triamterene, and amiloride. Aldosterone antagonists are effective in preventing renal potassium loss only if an increased mineralocorticoid concentration is responsible for hypokalemia. In disorders such as Liddle's syndrome, spironolactone is ineffective because plasma aldosterone is reduced, whereas triamterene and amiloride are effective regardless of the plasma aldosterone concentration. The daily dose of spironolactone ranges from 25 to 400 mg. The usual doses of triamterene range from 50 to 150 mg twice a day, whereas amiloride is administered at 5 mg/day, and can be slowly increased up to 20 mg/day. Amiloride should be administered with food to avoid gastric irritation. Because reduced delivery of sodium to the distal nephron always reduces potassium secretion, a low salt diet may be effective in reducing renal potassium loss of any cause, independent of the plasma aldosterone concentration.

HYPERKALEMIA

Hyperkalemia may be caused by one of three mechanisms: (a) shift of potassium from the cells to the extracellular space, (b) increased potassium intake, and (c) reduced renal potassium excretion (Table 15.5). Hyperkalemic familial periodic paralysis, use of succinylcholine in paralyzed patients (14), use of cationic amino acids such as epsilon-aminocaproic acid, arginine or lysine (13, 28), rhabdomyolysis or hemolysis, and acute acidosis all cause hyperkalemia by extracellular potassium shift. Rhabdomyolysis and hemolysis cause hyperkalemia only in the presence of renal failure. Acute acidosis has long been regarded as a cause of extracellular potassium shift, irrespective of the type of acidosis, but recent evidence suggests that hyperkalemia is not as predictable with organic acidosis as with inorganic acidosis (46). Furthermore, there is little change in serum potassium concentration with either respiratory acidosis or alkalosis.

Table 15.5
Causes of Hyperkalemia

Pseudohyperkalemia
  Thrombocytosis, massive leucocytosis, use of tourniquet with fist exercise, in vitro hemolysis
True hyperkalemia
  Due to extracellular shift
    Severe acidosis (especially inorganic acidosis)
    Catabolic states
    Periodic paralysis
    Succinylcholine
    Cationic amino acids
  Due to excessive ingestion: rare if renal excretion is normal
  Decreased renal excretion
    Hypoaldosteronism; Addison's disease; selective hypoaldosteronism (hyporeninemic hypoaldosteronism, heparin, congenital adrenal enzyme deficiencies, angiotensin converting enzyme inhibitors)
    Tubular unresponsiveness to aldosterone: congenital, salt-losing nephropathy
    Potassium-sparing diuretics
    Severe dehydration

However, hyperkalemia is common in diabetic ketoacidosis and phenformin-induced lactic acidosis (1). The more frequent occurrence of hyperkalemia in clinical organic acidosis than in experimental organic acidosis may be explained by the longer duration of acidosis and the presence of other factors such as dehydration and renal failure in organic acidosis. Hyperkalemia can also occur in severe digitalis intoxication by extracellular shift of potassium as digitalis inhabits the Na^+-K^+ pump (6).

The kidney's ability to excrete potassium is so great that hyperkalemia rarely occurs solely on the basis of increased intake of potassium. However, increased intake can lead to hyperkalemia when renal excretion of potassium is reduced. There are three major mechanisms of diminished renal potassium excretion: reduced aldosterone or aldosterone responsiveness, renal failure, and reduced distal delivery of sodium.

Aldosterone deficiency may be part of a generalized deficiency of adrenal hormones (e.g., Addison's disease) or it may represent a selective process (e.g., hyporeninemic hypoaldosteronism). Hyporeninemic hypoaldosteronism is not only the most common cause of selective hypoaldosteronism, but also the most common cause of all aldosterone deficiency states (48). Selective hypoaldosteronism with normal glucocorticoid function can also occur with heparin therapy (49). Renal tubular unresponsiveness to aldosterone (pseudohypoaldosteronism) may be congenital, but it is more often an acquired defect. This defect may involve only potassium secretion (pseudohypoaldosteronism type II) (59) or sodium reabsorption as well as potassium secretion. Most cases of so-called salt-losing nephritis appear to represent the latter defect (76). Severe dehydration may cause hyperkalemia despite secondary hyperaldosteronism because delivery of sodium to the distal nephron is markedly reduced (41). Pseudohyperkalemia is defined as an increase in potassium concentration only in the local blood vessel or in vitro, and has no physiological consequences. Prolonged use of a tourniquet with fist exercises can increase the serum potassium level by as much as 1 mEq/liter (10). Thrombocytosis and severe leucocytosis cause pseudohyperkalemia through potassium release from the platelets and white blood cells respectively during blood clotting (9, 26).

Management

Hyperkalemia may be treated by removal of potassium from the body, relocation of extracellular potassium into the cells, and by antagonism of potassium action on the membrane of the cardiac conduction system. Removal of potassium may be accomplished by several routes: through the gastrointestinal tract with a potassium exchange resin given orally or by enema; through the kidney by diuretics, mineralocorticoids, and increased salt intake; or by hemodialysis or peritoneal dialysis. A potassium exchange resin, sodium polystyrene sulfonate (kayexalate), is more effective when it is given with agents that cause osmotic diarrhea such as sorbitol or mannitol. One tablespoon of Kayexalate mixed with 100 ml of 10% sorbitol or mannitol can be given by mouth two to four times a day. When it is given as an enema, a larger quantity is given more frequently. Shift of potassium into cells can be accomplished with glucose and insulin or by increasing the blood pH with sodium bicarbonate. Antagonism of the action of potassium on the heart with intravenous calcium salts or hypertonic sodium solution is the quickest method of treating hyperkalemia, and is used in cases of life-threatening hyperkalemia. Reduced intake is often important in the long-term management of hyperkalemia. Prolonged administration of diuretics and a high salt diet is an effective treatment for hyporeninemic hypoaldosteronism, the most common cause of chronic hyperkalemia. This regimen ensures

the delivery of an adequate amount of sodium to the distal nephron without causing further volume expansion. Mineralocorticoid may be required as an adjunct therapy for hyporeninemic hypoaldosteronism, and the agent most commonly used is a synthetic mineralocorticoid, fludrocortisone (Florinef), 0.1 mg once or twice daily. Since renal salt retention may be an important mechanism in the pathogenesis of hyporeninemic hypoaldosteronism (48), mineralocorticoid replacement may lead to salt retention and worsening hypertension.

METABOLIC ACIDOSIS

Metabolic acidosis is defined as a reduction in extracellular pH resulting from a primary decrease in the bicarbonate concentration. The kidney plays a major role in maintaining the extracellular bicarbonate concentration, and the failure of the kidney in this function results in metabolic acidosis referred to as renal acidosis (Table 15.6). The term "extrarenal acidosis" is used when factors other than defective renal acid-excretory function are responsible. Renal acidosis may occur because of specific defects of tubular function in acid excretion or bicarbonate reabsorption (renal tubular acidosis) (64) or because of reduced nephron mass due to renal parenchymal disease (uremic acidosis). Three types of metabolic acidosis occur most frequently in critically ill patients: lactic acidosis (Table 15.7), ketoacidosis, and uremic acidosis.

When lactic acidosis results from tissue hypoxia, it is called type A lactic acidosis (the most common type). The most common cause

Table 15.6
Causes of Metabolic Acidosis

Renal acidosis
  Uremic acidosis
  Renal tubular acidosis
    Distal renal tubular acidosis (type I)
    Proximal renal tubular acidosis (type II)
    Aldosterone deficiency (type IV)
Extrarenal acidosis
  Gastrointestinal loss of bicarbonate
  Ingestion of acids: ammonium chloride, sulfur
  Acid precursors or toxins
    Salicylate
    Ethylene glycol
    Methanol
    Paraldehyde
  Organic acidosis
    Lactic acidosis (D- and L-)
    Ketoacidosis

Table 15.7
Causes of Lactic Acidosis

Tissue hypoxia, e.g., circulatory shock, severe
    hypoxemia, severe heart failure, severe anemia
Acute alcoholism
Drugs and toxins, e.g., phenformin, isoniazid
Diabetes mellitus
Leukemia
Idiopathic
Short bowel syndrome (D-lactic acidosis)

of tissue hypoxia leading to lactic acidosis is circulatory shock, which may be due to sepsis, hypovolemia, or cardiac failure. Generalized convulsion is also a fairly common cause, but the resulting acidosis is transient. Less commonly, tissue hypoxia may result from severe hypoxemia due to respiratory failure, carbon monoxide poisoning, or severe anemia. In type B lactic acidosis, the less common variety, there is no apparent tissue hypoxia, but the possibility of subtle tissue hypoxia must be considered. The causes of type B lactic acidosis include alcoholic intoxication, various drugs (phenformin, isoniazid), leukemia, and diabetes (47, 54). The prognosis of both types of lactic acidosis is dismal.

Ketoacidosis occurs most frequently in diabetes mellitus, but it occasionally occurs in vomiting, binge-drinking chronic alcoholics. When ketoacidosis occurs in the presence of poor mitochondrial oxidation (e.g., ethanol intoxication, septic shock in the diabetic, use of phenformin) the ratio of the reduced form of ketoacid, β-hydroxybutyrate, to the oxidized form, acetoacetate, increases. The usual ratio of β-hydroxybutyrate to acetoacetate in typical diabetic ketoacidosis is about 2.5–3, and the ratio increases to 8 or higher in β-hydroxybutyric acidosis. Since acetoacetate is the only form measured by the nitroprusside reagent (Acetest), the patient with β-hydroxybutyric acidosis may present with a large unexplained anion gap. Lactic acidosis often coexists with β-hydroxybutyric acidosis, because the abnormal redox state of mitochondria leads to increased production of lactic acidosis. Uremic acidosis is most often a result of chronic end-stage renal failure, but in critically ill patients acute renal failure is a common cause. Lactic acidosis also commonly coexists in this setting.

MANAGEMENT

Restoration of normal blood pH and bicarbonate concentration is the ultimate aim of therapy for metabolic acidosis. Rapid restoration of normal pH is usually unnecessary and may be undesirable for several reasons. When the pH is increased acutely, there may be insufficient time for restoration of a normal concentration of the red blood cell 2,3-DPG (37). In addition, a sudden increase in extracellular pH may cause a paradoxical CSF acidosis (51). Rapid restoration of a normal serum bicarbonate level in metabolic acidosis would be undesirable, because persistent hyperventilation produces a very high blood pH, simulating respiratory alkalosis (50).

The initial aim in the treatment of severe metabolic acidosis should be to increase the blood pH to a level at which adverse cardiovascular effects of severe acidemia can be avoided. Although the risk of acidosis varies with the agent and the cardiovascular status of patients, it is considered prudent, at least in older subjects, to keep blood pH above 7.1–7.2. The blood pH may be increased by the administration of alkali or by allowing alkali to be produced endogenously by metabolism of retained organic anions (OA^-):

$$OA^- + H_2CO_3 \longrightarrow OAH + HCO_3^-$$
$$\downarrow$$
$$CO_2 + H_2O$$

Successful treatment of the cause of organic acidosis increases the serum bicarbonate concentration by the latter mechanisms. When ketoacidosis is treated with insulin and fluid, the outcome is usually predictable: a substantial increase in the plasma bicarbonate concentration with a concomitant increase in arterial pH. Exogenous alkali is rarely necessary in ketoacidosis.

In contrast to the favorable outcome in ketoacidosis, response to treatment in lactic acidosis is usually poor. In lactic acidosis induced by hypoxia (type A), the prognosis depends on the cause of tissue hypoxia. In most cases of circulatory shock, the prognosis is extremely poor, but with seizure-induced lactic acidosis, recovery is usually complete within hours after the control of the seizure (45). Improvement in the microcirculation with the infusion of sodium nitroprusside may be effective in a patient with idiopathic lactic acidosis (75).

Rapid recovery is the rule with alcohol-induced lactic acidosis, but the prognosis of other type B lactic acidosis is usually bad. Treatment for type B lactic acidosis has consisted of the administration of alkali in the hope of spontaneous recovery, but administration of bicarbonate tends to be self-defeating because it may also lead to increased production of lactic acid (20).

Discouraged by the poor results of bicarbonate therapy and offering theoretical arguments against alkali therapy as discussed above, some authors have recommended against the use of bicarbonate in the treatment of all types of lactic acidosis (70). In contrast, others feel that the judicious use of bicarbonate is still beneficial to patients with severe metablic acidosis (39). Dichloroacetate, an experimental drug, offers some hope in the treatment of type B lactic acidosis (55, 71). Its main action is stimulation by pyruvate dehydrogenase, the enzyme responsible for conversion of pyruvate to acetyl CoA. Increased conversion of pyruvate to acetyl CoA results in a decrease in pyruvate concentration, which in turn increases utilization of lactate as well as alanine. Despite the theoretical prediction that lactic acidosis due to hypoxia should respond only to the supply of sufficient oxygen, dichloroacetate also causes a striking increase in serum bicarbonate concentration in patients with type A lactic acidosis. A major drawback of the drug appears to be the frequent occurrence of CNS side effects when it is used chronically (72).

D-Lactic acidosis is a disorder that occurs in patients with the short bowel syndrome. The acidosis is caused by production of D- and L-lactic acids by the colonic bacteria; L-lactic acid that is absorbed is rapidly metabolized and there is no accumulation, but D-lactate accumulates in the body fluids. Accumulation of D-lactate has been attributed to its slow metabolism, but a recent study showed that the rate of D-lactate metabolism in humans is quite fast, suggesting that there may be an additional defect in the mechanism of D-lactate in those who develop D-lactate acidosis (44). A neurological syndrome characterized by mental confusion, disorientation, and staggering gait commonly accompanies the disease. Treatment consists of sterilization of the gut with an antibiotic (42).

The response to the administration of alkali depends on the type of metabolic acidosis. In nonorganic acidosis, the alkali requirement can be estimated with reasonable accuracy. In organic acidosis, in contrast, the alkali requirement is usually much more than predicted in lactic acidosis, whereas it is much less than predicted in ketoacidosis. In lactic acidosis, almost continuous administration of bicarbonate may be needed to maintain serum bicarbonate at a reasonable level, whereas in ketoacidosis administration of insulin and fluid usually suffices.

There are three types of alkali that can be used for the treatment of metabolic acidosis: bicarbonate, salts of organic acids, and tromethamine (THAM). Organic salts used as a bicarbonate substitute include lactate, acetate, and citrate. Each milliequivalent of the organic salts produces 1 mEq of bicarbonate. Thus, the milliequivalent doses of organic salts are the same as those of bicarbonate. However, because they require metabolism, an increase in bicarbonate concentration is delayed. Furthermore, when metabolism is impaired (e.g., in lactic acidosis) administration of an organic salt may have no effect on the serum bicarbonate concentration. The amount and speed of administration of bicarbonate and organic salts vary widely depending on the severity of acidosis. Shohl's solution (citric acid and sodium citrate) contains 1 mEq of alkali (as citrate) per milliliter and is tkaen orally.

In contrast to the delayed and sometimes uncertain responses to organic salts, THAM increases serum bicarbonate concentration promptly and predictably in the following reaction:

$$\text{THAM} + H_2CO_3 \longrightarrow \text{THAM-H}^+ + HCO_3^-$$
$$\downarrow$$
$$CO_2 + H_2O$$

Because formation of bicarbonate by THAM occurs at the expense of carbonic acid, rapid infusion of THAM results in a marked reduction in PCO_2, and therefore it should be given slowly, not exceeding the rate of 2 mmol/minute.

For a given quantity of bicarbonate administration, the rise in serum bicarbonate is less in severe than in mild metabolic acidosis (i.e., the apparent volume of distribution of bicarbonate is greater in severe than in mild metabolic acidosis). However, the absolute increase in pH for a given dose of bicarbonate administered is greater in more severe metabolic acidosis than in mild acidosis, because the proportionate increase in serum bicarbonate is greater with severe acidosis. In practice, however, there is no need to estimate the bicarbonate requirements to achieve a certain specific level. Since pH is determined by the ratio of bicarbonate/PCO_2 and a change in ventilation and PCO_2 following acute increase in serum bicarbonate cannot be accurately predicted, it is difficult to predict what the pH will be, even if the increase in bicarbonate concentration were accurately predicted. The best approach is to administer two to three ampules of sodium bicarbonate (44.5 or 50 mEq/ampule) by direct intravenous bolus injection, and then repeat the blood-gas measurement 20–30 minutes after bicarbonate injection to determine the need for further bicarbonate administration.

For treatment of chronic acidosis, citrate is more palatable than bicarbonate and citrate is available as Shohl's solution. For treatment of uremic acidosis, sodium acetate is the most commonly used alkali in hemodialysis fluids, and sodium lactate in peritoneal dialysis fluids. Administration of THAM probably has no advantage in treatment of metabolic acidosis in most situations (7), but would be more advantageous than bicarbonate in treating metabolic acidosis complicated by respiratory acidosis. THAM is available as a 0.3 M solution, and the rate of infusion of THAM should not exceed 30 ml/minute.

METABOLIC ALKALOSIS

Metabolic alkalosis is defined as an increase in extracellular pH caused by an increase in the serum bicarbonate concentration. Normally, the kidney's ability to excrete the excess bicarbonate when the serum bicarbonate is high is so great that it is virtually impossible to maintain metabolic alkalosis by a mechanism that simply causes increased generation of bicarbonate; another mechanism must coexist that prevents the rapid renal loss of bicarbonate. Hence, there are always two abnormalities for sustained metabolic alkalosis: an abnormality that increases the extracellular bicarbonate concentration and an abnormality that causes increased renal bicarbonate threshold.

Mechanisms for Increase in Serum Bicarbonate

There are several mechanisms for increasing the extracellular bicarbonate concentration. These include: loss of HCl (from the stomach or, rarely, in the stool), administration of bicarbonate or bicarbonate precursors, metabolism of bicarbonate precursors, shift of $H+$ into the cell, contraction of extracellular volume by loss of sodium chloride and water, and increased renal excretion of acid (Table 15.8).

Table 15.8
Mechanisms and Causes of Increasing Extracellular Bicarbonate Concentration

Loss of HCl from the stomach, e.g., gastric suction, vomiting

Administration of bicarbonate or bicarbonate precursors, e.g., sodium lactate, sodium acetate, sodium citrate

Shift of H^+ into the cell, e.g., K^+ depletion

Rapid contraction of extracellular volume by loop diuretics

Increased renal excretion of acid, e.g., diuretic therapy, hypermineralocorticoid state, potassium depletion, high PCO_2, secondary hypoparathyroidism

Of these, the two most frequent causes of metabolic alkalosis are increased renal generation of bicarbonate and loss of HCl from the stomach.

Gastric suction is a particularly frequent cause of metabolic alkalosis in critically ill patients, because acid secretion is often markedly stimulated in these patients owing to the stress of severe illness. Considerable loss of acid may still occur in these patients even when gastric acid secretion is inhibited by cimetidine or ranitidine. Diuretic therapy with complicating hypokalemia is also a common cause of metabolic alkalosis in critically ill patients. Sometimes, metabolic alkalosis is a complication of the treatment of metabolic acidosis; administration of bicarbonate to a patient with lactic acidosis increases the production of lactic acid, which is retained as lactate following titration by bicarbonate. The subsequent metabolism of the lactate can lead to a rapid increase in the serum bicarbonate concentration.

Mechanisms for Maintaining High Serum Bicarbonate

Since the kidney is the organ responsible for excreting the excess bicarbonate when the concentration is abnormally high (77), renal failure would be the most effective mechanism for maintaining excess bicarbonate. However, in mild to moderate renal failure, the ability to excrete bicarbonate is still well preserved (30). Other mechanisms of maintaining a high serum bicarbonate concentrate include contraction of EAV, potassium deficiency, high PCO_2, and secondary hypoparathyroidism. Chloride deficiency is usually listed among the causes of increased renal bicarbonate threshold, but chloride deficiency without reduced

Table 15.9
Mechanisms and Causes of Maintaining High Serum Bicarbonate Concentration

Reduced effective arterial volume, e.g., diuretic therapy, vomiting, heart failure and other edema forming states
Potassium deficiency
Chloride deficiency accompanied by low effective arterial volume, e.g., vomiting
High PCO_2
Secondary hypoparathyroidism, e.g., milk-alkali syndrome, certain malignancy-induced hypercalcemia
Severe renal failure

EAV does not increase the bicarbonate threshold (Table 15.9). For example, in severe hyponatremia due to SIADH, total-body chloride content might be reduced, but renal bicarbonate threshold is not increased because EAV is not reduced.

The commonest causes of increased renal bicarbonate threshold encountered clinically are low EAV and potassium deficiency. These two and severe renal failure are probably the mechanisms responsible for maintenance of over 95% of cases of metabolic alkalosis. In most patients who develop metabolic alkalosis due to gastric suction or vomiting, the high renal bicarbonate threshold is caused by low EAV and hypokalemia. Thus if the renal threshold of bicarbonate is maintained normal by prevention of volume depletion and potassium depletion, large losses of gastric fluid will not lead to metabolic alkalosis.

Management

Since the increased renal bicarbonate threshold in metabolic alkalosis is most often caused by reduced EAV and hypokalemia, correction of these abnormalities leads to rapid restoration of bicarbonate concentration in most patients. Correction of low EAV is accomplished by administration of normal saline or half-normal saline. Sometimes discontinuation of an offending agent (e.g., a diuretic) and restoration of normal salt intake is sufficient. If volume depletion is to be avoided, chloride must be given to replace the excreted bicarbonate; it can be given as either sodium chloride or potassium chloride. In certain clinical situations such as edema-forming states, treatment of reduced EAV with salt solution may not be feasible. A logical and effective choice in such situations is acetazolamide (Diamox),

a carbonic anhydrase inhibitor, which will treat metabolic alkalosis as well as edema. Diamox can be given either intravenously or orally. The starting dose is 250 or 500 mg and can be repeated at 6–hour intervals until a desired serum bicarbonate concentration is achieved. Acetazolamide administration usually reduces the renal bicarbonate threshold to a subnormal level, but when it is administered to patients with severe volume depletion, it may not be able to reduce bicarbonate threshold to even a normal level.

Correction of metabolic alkalosis by renal excretion of bicarbonate requires adequate renal function. In renal failure, metabolic alkalosis can be treated by administration of dilute HCl or acidifying salts or by dialysis; the latter has an advantage in that it treats uremia as well as alkalosis. HCl can be administered in 0.1 or 0.05 N solution into a central vein (78). Acidifying salts include ammonium chloride, arginine chloride, and lysine chloride. Metabolism of these salts results in release of HCl, which then titrates bicarbonate. The amount of acidifying salts to be administered depends on the severity of metabolic acidosis. When they are given by intravenous infusion, the optimal rate is about 1 mEq/minute. If continuous acid loss from the stomach is the cause of metabolic alkalosis, an inhibitor of acid secretion such as cimetidine or ranitidine may be useful. Considerable acid secretion, however, may still occur in some patients even with the maximal dose of these drugs.

References

1. Adrogue HJ, Wilson H, Boyd AE, et al: Plasma acid-base patterns in diabetic ketoacidosis. *N Engl J Med* 307:1603, 1982.
2. Arieff AL: Hyponatremia, convulsions, respiratory arrest, and permanent brain damage after elective surgery in healthy women. *N Engl J Med* 314:1529, 1986.
3. Adlinger KA, Samaan NA: Hypokalemia with hypercalcemia. Prevalence and significance in treatment. *Ann Intern Med* 87:571, 1977.
4. Bartter FC, Schwartz WB: The syndrome of inappropriate secretion of antidiuretic hormone. *Am J Med* 42:651, 1967.
5. Beck LH: Hypouricemia in the syndrome of inappropriate secretion of antidiuretic hormone. *N Engl J Med* 301:528, 1979.
6. Bismuth C, Gaultier M, Conso F, et al: Hyperkalemia in acute digitalis poisoning: prognostic significance and therapeutic implications. *Clin Toxicol* 6:153, 1973.
7. Bleich HL, Schwartz WB: Tris buffer (THAM). An appraisal of its physiological effects and clinical usefulness. *N Engl J Med* 274:782, 1966.
8. Bode HH, Harley BM, Crawford JD: Restoration of normal drinking behavior by chlorpropamide in patients

with hypodipsia and diabetes insipidus. *Am J Med* 51:304, 1971.

9. Bronson WR: Pseudohyperkalemia due to release of potassium from white blood cells during clotting. *N Engl J Med* 274:369, 1966.

10. Brown JJ, Chin RR, David DL, et al: Falsely high serum potassium levels in patients with hyperaldosteronism. *Br Med J* 2:18, 1970.

11. Carrilho F, Bosch J, Arroyo V, et al: Renal failure associated with demeclocycline in cirrhosis. *Ann Intern Med* 87:195–197, 1977.

12. Carroll HJ, Oh MS: Electrolyte physiology and body composition in *Water, Electrolyte and Acid-Base Metabolism.* Philadelphia, JB Lippincott, 1978, p 1.

13. Carroll HJ, Tice DA: The effects of epsilon aminocaproic acid upon potassium metabolism in the dog. *Metabolism* 15:499, 1966.

14. Cooperman LH: Succinylcholine-induced hyperkalemia in neuromuscular disease. *JAMA* 213:1867, 1970.

15. Cowell DC, McGrady PM: Direct-measurement ion-selective electrodes. Analytical error in hyponatremia. *Clin Chem* 31:2009, 1985.

16. Decaux, Genette F, Mockel J: Hypouremia in the syndrome of inappropriate secretion of antidiuretic hormone. *Ann Intern Med* 93:716, 1980.

17. DeFronzo RA, Goldberg M, Agus ZS: Normal diluting capacity in hyponatremic patients. *Ann Intern Med* 84:538, 1976.

18. Forrest JN, Cohen AD, Torretti J, et al: On the mechanism of lithium-induced diabetes insipidus in man and rat. *J Clin Invest* 53:1115–1123, 1974.

19. Forrest JN, Cox M, Hong C, et al: Superiority of demeclocycline over lithium in the treatment of chronic syndrome of inappropriate secretion of antidiuretic hormone. *N Engl J Med* 298:173–177, 1978.

20. Fraley DS, Adler S, Bruns FJ, et al: Stimulation of lactate production by administration of bicarbonate in a patient with a solid neoplasma and lactic acidosis. *N Engl J Med* 303:1100–1102, 1980.

21. Francisco LL, Sawin LL, DiBona GF: Mechanism of negative potassium balance in the magnesium deficient rat *Proc Soc Exp Biol Med* 168:382, 1981.

22. Frick PG, Schmid JR, Kistler HJ, et al: Hyponatremia associated with hyperproteinemia in multiple myeloma. *Helv Med Acta* 33:317–329, 1967.

23. Furhman SA, Eckfeldt JH: Hyponatremia and ion-selective electrodes. *Ann Intern Med* 102:872, 1985.

24. Graettinge JS, Muenster JJ, Checchia CS, et al: A correlation of clinical and hemodynamic studies in patients with hypothyroidism. *J Clin Invest* 37:502, 1958.

25. Granerus AK, Jagenburg R, Svanborg A: Kaliuretic effect of L-dopa treatment in Parkinsonian patients. *Acta Med Scand* 201-291-297, 1977.

26. Hartman RC, Auditore JC, Jackson DP: Studies in thrombocytosis. I. hyperkalemia due to release of potassium from platelets during coagulation. *J Clin Invest* 37:699, 1958.

27. Hantman D, Rossier B, Zohlman R, et al: Rapid correction of hyponatremia in the syndrome of inappropriate secretion of antidiuretic hormone. *Ann Intern Med* 78:870, 1973.

28. Hertz P, Richardson JA: Arginine-induced hyperkalemia in renal failure patients. *Arch Intern Med* 130:778, 1972.

29. Hoffbrand BI, Steward JD: Carbenecillin and hypokalemia. *Br Med J* 4:746, 1970.

30. Husted FC, Nolph KD, Maher JF: NaHCO$_3$ and NaCl tolerance in chronic renal failure. *J Clin Invest* 56:414, 1975.

31. Gennari FJ: Current concepts: Uses and limitations. *N Engl J Med* 310:102, 1984.

32. Kestens PJ, et al: The effect of insulin on the uptake of potassium and phosphate by the isolated perfused canine liver. *Metabolism* 12:941, 1963.

33. Ladenson JK, Apple FS, Koch DD: Misleading hyponatremia due to hyperlipemia: A method-dependent error. *Ann Intern Med* 95:707, 1981.

34. Linas SL, Berl T, Robertson GL, et al: Role of vasopressin in the impaired water excretion of glucocorticoid deficiency. *Kidney Int* 18:58–67, 1980.

35. Mattar JA, et al: Cardiac arrest in the critically ill. Hyperosmolar states following cardiac arrest. *Am J Med* 56:162, 1974.

36. Mir MA, Brabin B, Tinag OT, et al: Hypokalemia in acute myeloid leukemia. *Ann Intern Med* 82:54–57, 1972.

37. Mitchell JH, Sildenthal K, Johnson RL: The effects of acid-base disturbances on cardiovascular and pulmonary function. *Kidney Int* 1:375, 1972.

38. Moses AM, Howanitz J, vanGemert M, et al: Clofibrate-induced antidiuresis. *J Clin Invest* 52:535, 1973.

39. Narins RG, Cohen JJ: Bicarbonate therapy for organic acidosis: the case for its continued use. *Ann Intern Med* 106:615, 1987.

40. Norenberg MD, Leslie KO, Robertson AS: Association between rise in serum sodium and central pontine myelinolysis. *Ann Neurol* 11:128, 1982.

41. Oh MS: Selective hypoaldosteronism. *Resident Staff Physician* 28:46S–62S, 1982.

42. Oh MS, Phelps K, Traube M, et al: D-Lactic acidosis in a man with the short bowel syndrome. *N Engl J Med* 301:249, 1979.

43. Oh MS, Uribarri J, Barrido D, et al: Central pontine myelinolysis following isotonic saline infusion: is 0.5 NS better than NS in treating hypotonic dehydration? *Kidney Int* 31:212, 1987.

44. Oh MS, Uribarri J, Alveranga D, et al: Metabolic utilization and renal handling of D-lactate in man. *Metabolism* 34:621, 1985.

45. Orlinger CE, Estace JC, Wunsch CD, et al: Natural history of lactic acidosis after grand mal seizures. *N Engl J Med* 297:796–799, 1977.

46. Olster JR, Perez GO, Vaamonde CA: Relationship between blood pH and phosphorus during acute metabolic alkalosis. *Am J Physiol* 235:F345–F351, 1978.

47. Park R, Arieff AL: lactic acidosis. *Adv Intern Med* 25:33, 1980.

48. Phelps KR, Lieberman RL, Oh MS, et al: The syndrome of hyporeninemic hypoaldosteronism. *Metabolism* 29:186, 1980.

49. Phelps KR, Oh MS, Carroll HJ: Heparin-induced hyperkalemia: report of a case. *Nephron* 25:254–258, 1980.

50. Pierce NF, et al: The ventilatory response to acute base deficit in humans. Time course during development and correction of metabolic alkalosis. *Ann Intern Med* 172:633, 1970.

51. Posner JB, Plum E: Spinal fluid and pH and neurological symptoms in acidosis. *N Engl J Med* 277:605, 1967.

52. Rado JP: Combination of carbamezepine and chloropropamide in the treatment of "hyporesponder" pituitary diabetes insipidus. *J Clin Endo Metab* 38:1, 1974.

53. Raskind M, Burns RF: Water metabolism in psychiatric disorders. *Semin Nephrol* 4:316, 1984.

54. Relman AS: lactic acidosis. In Brenner BM, Stein JH: *Contemporary Issues in Nephrology. Acid-Base and Potassium Homeostasis.* New York, Churchill Livingstone, 1978, vol 2, p 65.

55. Relman ASD: Lactic acidosis and a possible new treatment. *N Engl J Med* 298:564–565, 1978.

56. Robinson AG: DSDAVP in the treatment of central diabetes insipidus. *N Engl J Med* 294–507, 1976.

57. Roza O, Berman LB: The pathophysiology of barium: hypokalemic and cardiovascular effects. *J Pharmacol Exp Ther* 177:433–439, 1971.

58. Santensanio F, et al: Evidence for a role of endogenous insulin and glucagon in the regulation of potassium homeostasis. *J Lab Clin Med* 81:809, 1973.

59. Schambelan M, Sebastian A, Rector FC Jr: Mineralocorticoid-resistant renal hyperkalemia without salt wast-

ing (type II pseudohypoaldosteronism): role of increased renal chloride reabsorption. *Kidney Int* 19:716, 1981.

60. Schrier RW: Treatment of hyponatremia: Editorial. *N Engl J Med* 312:1121, 1985.

61. Schrier RW, Lehman D, Zacherle B, et al: Effect of furosemide on free water excretion in edematous patients with hyponatremia. *Kidney Int* 3:30, 1973.

62. Scribner BH, Burnell JM: Interpretation of serum potassium concentration. *Metabolism* 5:468, 1956.

63. Sebastian A, McSherry E, Morris RC: Renal potassium wasting in renal tubulatr acidosis (RTA). Its occurrence in types I and II RTA despite sustained correction of systemic acidosis. *J Clin Invest* 50:667, 1971.

64. Sebastian A, McSherry Z, Morris RC: Metabolic acidosis with special reference to the renal acidosis. In Brenner BM, Rector FC: *The Kidney*. Philadelphia, WB Saunders, 1976, p 615.

65. Singer I, Rotenberg D, Puschett JB: Lithium-induced nephrogenic diabetes insipidus. *J Clin Invest* 51:1081, 1972.

66. Singer I, Rotenberg D: Demeclocyline-induced nephrogenic diabetes insipidus. In vivo and in vitro studies. *Ann Intern Med* 79:679, 1973.

67. Skowsky WR, Kikuchi TA: The role of vasopresin in the impaired water excretion of myxedema. *Am J Med* 64:613, 1978.

68. Spencer PW, Voyce MA: Familial hypomagnesemia and hypokalemia. *Acta Paediatr Scand* 65:505, 1976.

69. Sperlakis N, Schneider MF, Harris EJ: Decreased K^+ conductance produced by Ba^{++} in frog sartorius fibers. *J Gen Physiol* 50:1565–1583, 1967.

70. Stacpoole PW: The lactic acidosis: the case against bicarbonate therapy (editorial). *Ann Intern Med* 105:276, 1986.

71. Stacpoole PW, Moore GW, Korhauser DM: Metabolic effects of dichloroacetate in patients with diabetes mellitus and hyperlipoproteinemia. *N Engl J Med* 298:526–530, 1978.

72. Stacpoole PW, Harman EM, Curry SH, et al: Treatment of lactic acidosis with dichloroacetate. *N Engl J Med* 309:390, 1983.

73. Sterns RH, Riggs JE, Schochet SS, Jr: Osmotic demyelinating syndrome following correction of hyponatremia. *N Engl J Med* 314:1535, 1986.

74. Szatalowicz VL, Arnold PE, Chaimovitz L, et al: Radioimmunoassay of plasma arginine vasopressin in hyponatremic patients with congestive heart failure. *N Engl J Med* 305:203, 1981.

75. Taradash MR, Jacobson LB: Vasiodilatory therapy of idiopathic lactic acidosis. *N Engl J Med* 293:468, 1975.

76. Uribarri J, Oh MS, Carroll HJ: Salt-losing nephritis. *Am J Nephrol* 3:193, 1983.

77. Van Goidsenhoven GMT, et al: The effect of prolonged administration of large doses of sodium bicarbonate in man. *Clin Sci* 13:383, 1954.

78. Wilson RF, Gibson D, Percivel AK: Severe alkalosis in critically ill surgical patients. *Arch Surg* 105:197, 1972.

16

Parenteral Nutrition

Laurence H. Ross, M.D.
John P. Grant, M.D.

The healthy adult is in a state of nitrogen equilibrium where daily dietary nitrogen intake equals nitrogen loss. When dietary intake is limited or interrupted, the human adapts by reducing physical activity and lowering core body temperature with a reduction in metabolic rate. The term "basal metabolic rate" (BMR) describes the minimal energy expenditure of a trained subject at rest after an overnight fast. In chronic uncomplicated starvation, the body reduces energy expenditure by up to 5–10% below the BMR. If starvation is complicated by stress or sepsis, however, energy expenditure markedly increases and may approach 200% BMR. When dietary intake does not meet an individual's energy requirement, the human resorts to catabolism of body mass to generate energy. Proteins are broken down for gluconeogenesis and lipids are mobilized for lipid oxidation. This catabolic state is not without serious consequences and cannot be sustained indefinitely. The fat mass is relatively expendable. However, there are no known protein reserves in the body; each protein molecule serves some biological function. During acute and chronic starvation, protein is derived from all parts of the body with preservation only perhaps of the brain. Seven-day fasting in rats produces a 30% body weight loss with 30–40% decrease in liver, kidney, lung, gastrointestinal tract, and heart masses with similar losses of organ protein content (2, 79). Similar data are reported in humans (101). Associated with the loss of organ mass and protein content is an impairment of organ function (47). In particular, skeletal muscle function is decreased as starvation progresses as demonstrated by the Minnesota Experiment in 1944 (89). More acute starvation in hospitalized patients also decreases muscle function independent of measured muscle mass (113a). Respiratory muscle function is also impaired in chronic malnutrition as measured by pulmonary function tests (90). Acute starvation decreases maximal inspiratory vacuum and maximal expiratory pressures in hospitalized patients (129). Doekel et al. (33) demonstrated that a short period of semistarvation in normal volunteers impaired the ventilatory response to hypoxia. Likewise Weissman et al. demonstrated loss of chemoreceptor sensitivity to hypercarbic gas mixtures following short periods of protein-free diets in normal volunteers (203). Catabolism of the gastrointestinal tract leads to loss of villous height and absorptive surface with depletion of brush border enzymes and malabsorption (118). Loss of normal gastric acid secretion is associated with bacterial overgrowth of the upper gastrointestinal tract contributing to diarrhea (45). Delayed gastric emptying with small bowel hypermotility also occurs. Hepatic function is markedly impaired with undernutrition both with respect to the microsomal enzyme system as well as the protein synthetic pathways (98, 163). On the other hand, some enzyme systems, including the gluconeogenic series, increase in activity with progressive starvation. Changes in renal function during starvation include loss of concentrating ability with progressive diuresis in the face of dehydration and impaired ability to excrete titrable acid leading to metabolic acidosis (99, 100). In children, impaired clearance of aminoglycosides may occur due to altered glomerular and tubular function with severe protein depletion (16). Cardiac reserves and function are depressed (1, 68). Immune system function becomes impaired as starvation progresses, causing loss of chemotactic and phagocytic activity of the lymphocyte, anergy to common skin test antigens, and impairment of the humoral response (10, 175).

Because of these alterations in organ function, as well as other complex interactions, undernourished patients have an increased incidence of morbidity and mortality. Prognostic relationships exist between morbidity and mortality and serum albumin and transferrin concentrations, delayed-type hypersensitivity skin test reactions, percent weight loss from usual weight, and various combinations of these parameters (27, 62a, 104a, 131, 156a, 159). Surveys of infectious complications in patients undergoing clean surgical procedures demonstrate malnutrition (defined as weight loss and a low serum albumin concentration) to be as important a factor as old age, obesity, diabetes, and infections in other parts of the body (22, 27). It therefore behooves the physician in the critical care unit to consider the patient's nutritional status in the initial patient evaluation. The need for immediate and intensive nutritional support must be considered whenever a patient's nutritional status is threatened by disease or when significant preillness malnutrition is present. Whenever possible the enteral route should be utilized to reduce costs and risks. If the enteral route cannot or should not be utilized for nutritional support, there should be no hesitancy in providing intravenous nutrition. At no time should nutritional support be withheld until some parameter indicates the presence of malnutrition. Instead, emphasis should be placed on prophylactic nutritional support to avoid the occurrence of malnutrition and its complications. As a rule, patients admitted to critical care units for evaluation and treatment should be receiving adequate nutritional support within the first 36 hours of admission.

ENDOCRINE RESPONSE TO STRESS

The endocrine response to stress is a complex feedback system that is intimately related to the metabolic response to stress. In this section only a brief discussion of the endocrine response is presented, and for simplification a division is made between the hormones of catabolism, anabolism, and fluid-electrolyte balance.

Catabolic Hormones

GLUCOCORTICOIDS

Immediately after injury there is a rapid increase in cortisol secretion lasting for 24–48 hours (39). However, even with minor injuries, up to two to five times normal excretion of urinary hydroxycorticoids is found for 7–10 days (77, 124, 125). With severe or prolonged stress, elevations of urinary hydroxycorticoids are detected for weeks to months and may be associated with hypertrophy of the adrenal cortex. Cortisol acts in concert with the catecholamines to stimulate lipolysis (109), to inhibit protein synthesis, to facilitate amino acid mobilization from muscle (21), to induce the enzymes of gluconeogenesis (170, 204), to enhance secretion of glucagon while inhibiting insulin secretion (117, 151), and to stimulate conversion of lactic acid to glycogen (137).

CATECHOLAMINES

Epinephrine and norepinephrine are secreted within seconds of injury (22). Although their biologic half-lives are short, their continued secretion for several days and, in severe stress, several weeks, results in a prolonged metabolic effect (52, 123). Epinephrine induces the enzymes of hepatic glycogenolysis and gluconeogenesis, stimulates glucagon secretion, inhibits insulin secretion, stimulates lipolysis, enhances amino acid release from skeletal muscle, and inhibits the uptake of glucose by peripheral tissues (93, 154). In addition, epinephrine leads to the secretion of pituitary ACTH, which stimulates glucocorticoid secretion (39).

GLUCAGON

Glucagon is a potent catabolic hormone secreted by the pancreatic cells in response to trauma, and is in part mediated by cortisol and catecholamine secretion. It acts predominately on the hepatocyte to prevent hypoglycemia by stimulating gluconeogenesis and glycogenolysis. In the periphery it may enhance lipolysis and proteolysis (192).

Anabolic Hormones

INSULIN

Insulin is a potent anabolic hormone secreted by pancreatic β cells. It plays a central role in the regulation of glucose metabolism by inhibiting gluconeogenesis and glycogenolysis in the hepatic cells through the stimulation of glucokinase and UDPG-glycosyl transferase, and the inhibition of pyruvate carboxylase and phosphorylase. Insulin also promotes glucose and potassium uptake by peripheral tissues, inhibits lipolysis, and favors protein synthesis (125). The stress reaction (largely catecholamine mediated) leads to a marked depression in insulin production and secretion that results in a disproportionately and persistently low serum insulin level (121, 154). With the increase in serum glucagon, the molar insulin:glucagon ratio is depressed resulting in an increase in gluconeogenesis and glycogenolysis.

GROWTH HORMONE

Stress is a strong stimulant of growth hormone secretion (208). Growth hormone stimulates nitrogen, phosphorus and potassium retention, fatty acid oxidation, and ketogenesis. It also inhibits insulin action and promotes amino acid uptake with protein synthesis (108).

ANDROGENS

Testosterone, in addition to its other roles, is a potent anabolic hormone. It stimulates protein synthesis and decreases amino acid catabolism. Retention of nitrogen, potassium, phosphorus, and calcium are manifestations of its anabolic effect. Stress and catecholamines suppress testosterone production (125).

Fluid and Electrolyte Hormones

ANTIDIURETIC HORMONE

Antidiuretic hormone (ADH) is a powerful hormone responsible for maintaining a proper solute/solvent ratio in the serum. Hypovolemia and hypertonicity during stress are strong stimulants for ADH release from the posterior pituitary gland (125). Its primary site of action is the kidney where it promotes water reabsorption.

ALDOSTERONE

Aldosterone hormone promotes reabsorption of sodium bicarbonate while increasing potassium and hydrogen losses. Aldosterone secretion in stress is augmented by catecholamines and hyponatremia. In addition, isotonic hypovolemia, by increasing renin production, leads to angiotensin release that in turn stimulates aldosterone secretion (180). The endocrine response to stress can be graphically displayed as in Figure 16.1.

METABOLIC RESPONSE TO STRESS

The metabolic response to stress and injury as first described by Cuthbertson (29) in the

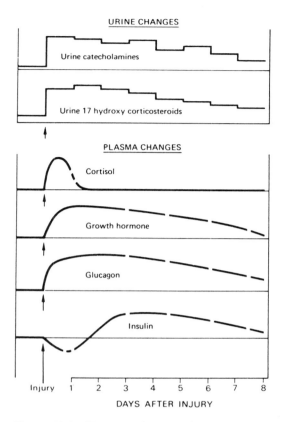

Figure 16.1. Hormone changes after injury. (Reprinted with permission. From Fleck A: Metabolic response to injury. Ledingham IM, Mackay G: *Jamieson and Kay's Textbook of Surgical Physiology.* New York, Churchill Livingstone, 1978, pp 45.)

1930s can be divided into several phases that do not have sharp demarcations but rather gradual transitions.

The acute phase begins immediately following injury and lasts for 12–36 hours. It is characterized by a rapid secretion of the stress hormones (catecholamines, glucocorticoids, glucagon, growth hormones, etc.), marked fluid shifts, acid-base imbalances, and a decrease in energy expenditure, oxygen consumption, and core temperature (94). Therapeutic priorities are to provide hemostasis, cardiovascular stability, and electrolyte balance. If the injury is severe there is an accompanying metabolic acidosis from anaerobic carbohydrate metabolism, development of oxygen deficit, a rise in the acute phase proteins, hyperglycemia due to insulin resistance, and an elevation in serum free fatty acids (39). Vigorous nutritional support during this initial phase in not indicated due to other priorities.

After the first 12–36 hours, the acutely stressed patient enters the catabolic phase when aggressive nutritional support is needed. During this phase there is an increase in urea production and urinary urea nitrogen excretion due to protein catabolism. Uncomplicated starvation does not increase urinary urea nitrogen excretion, instead it is associated with normal or decreased excretion (5–7 g/day) (126). With stress, however, the urinary urea nitrogen excretion may increase to 7–40 g/day depending upon the degree of stress (20 g nitrogen/day = 175 g protein/day = 0.5 kg lean tissue/day) (127). Other potential sources of nitrogen loss during stress include blood, transudates, exudates, and wound drainage. Protein catabolism supplies the carbon skeletons for gluconeogenesis not obtainable from fat oxidation and also provides substrates acutely needed for the synthesis of blood, structural proteins, and enzymes. Prior to the development of intravenous feeding, it was felt that net nitrogen loss was mandatory and irreversible during this phase (29). However, the advent of nonvolitional tube feeding and total parenteral nutrition (TPN) has shown that although the catabolic response cannot be suppressed, the negative nitrogen balance and subsequent body wasting can be reduced and at times overcome by infusion of specially formulated intravenous solutions (19b, 88a, 116a, 165).

The catabolic phase is associated with marked increases in daily caloric expenditure and nitrogen excretion. The two tend to parallel each other with increasing degrees of stress except in severe stress, where the caloric expenditure increases more than nitrogen excretion (111). An equation for estimation of BMR in healthy individuals was first developed by Harris and Benedict in 1919 (62). This equation is still valid but must be adjusted by a factor of approximately 10% to obtain the clinically more useful value of resting metabolic expenditure (RME). In stress the energy expenditure is markedly increased above the predicted RME (Fig. 16.2). After extensive metabolic studies, Long et al. (111) modified the original Harris-Benedict equation to better estimate daily caloric expenditure by adding a stress and activity factor (Table 16.1).

In times of stress, when an individual is usually unable or unwilling to eat, the body adapts by converting from exogenous to endogenous sources of carbohydrate, fat, and protein. Carbohydrates are stored mainly as glycogen (500 g) (126). Mobilization by glycogenolysis can provide only about 1700 kcal, which is exhausted after 8 hours. Certain organs require glucose as their caloric source early in starvation (CNS, heart, renal medulla, leukocytes, fibroblasts). To provide glucose, the body converts protein into glucose in the liver and kidney by gluconeogenesis. The conversion of body protein is an inefficient and

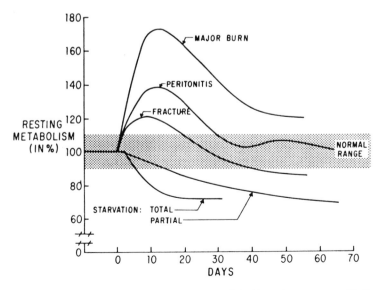

Figure 16.2. Changes in resting metabolic expenditure (RME) in six patient groups with time. (Reprinted with permission. From Long CL et al.: Metabolic response to illness and injury: estimation of energy and protein needs from indirect calorimetry and nitrogen balance. *J Paren Enter Nutr* 3:452–456, 1979.)

Table 16.1
Calculation of Actual Energy Expenditure (AEE)[a]

AEE (men)	= (66.47 + 13.75W + 5.011 − 6.76A) × (activity factor) × (injury factor)
AEE (women)	= (6.55.10 + 9.56W + 4.8511 − 4.68A) × (activity factor) × (injury factor)
Where AEE	= actual energy expenditure, W = weight in kg, 11 = height in cm, A = age in years

Activity factor	Use	Injury factor	Use
Confined to bed	1.2	Minor operation	1.20
Out of bed	1.3	Skeletal trauma	1.35
		Major sepsis	1.60
		Severe thermal burn	2.10

[a] Modified from Long CL *et al.* Metabolic response to injury and illness: estimation of energy and protein needs from indirect calorimetry and nitrogen balance. *J Paren Enter Nutr* 3:452–456, 1979.

expensive process as it yields few calories (20 kcal gained for each gram of nitrogen excreted = 6.25 g of protein = 30 g of wet muscle tissue) (126). Other tissues can use fatty acids for energy, which are a rich and expendible source. Up to 300–500 g/day of fat may be oxidized, providing 2700–4500 kcal/day (126). Even by providing large amounts of exogenous glucose through TPN, the stressed body prefers to convert excess glucose to glycogen while the endogenous fat stores continue to be oxidized (6). In the unstressed depleted patient, however, extra glucose is converted into fat, and fat oxidation is suppressed. When excess glucose is given to the hypermetabolic, stressed patient, gluconeogenesis is not suppressed and protein catabolism continues (112).

The electrolyte and acid-base derangements that occur during the catabolic phase are largely due to losses from, or shifts between, compartments and reflect cellular destruction, proteolysis, and the body's effort to maintain an effective circulating blood volume. In the urine, excretion of potassium, phosphorus, sulfate, magnesium, creatinine, creatine, and uric acid are elevated (128). Bicarbonate and sodium are retained by the kidney through the effect of aldosterone, which results in kaluresis, acidic urine, and mild metabolic alkalosis that can be aggravated by blood transfusions (citrate metabolized to bicarbonate) and nasogastric suction (hydrogen ion loss).

If the clinical course progresses without complications, the catabolic phase gradually gives way to an anabolic phase (126). There is a decrease in urinary nitrogen excretion that reflects a decrease in protein catabolism, a diuresis of salt and water, a normalization of serum potassium and sodium, and a change in the endocrine pattern from the stress hormones (catecholamine, glucocorticoids, and glucagon) to the growth hormones (insulin, androgens, and growth hormone). The state of convalescence may continue for weeks to months depending on the body protein and fat lost during catabolism. During recovery, essential amino acids, total protein, and caloric requirements are greater than normal, but less than during the stressed period, and appropriate adjustments must be made. Nutritional support is very important during this period, but since the patient is no longer critically ill, an oral diet is usually resumed and intensive intravenous or enteral nutritional support is usually not necessary.

SUBSTRATE REQUIREMENTS FOR NUTRITIONAL SUPPORT

Fluid Requirements

Fluid requirements for patients on total nutritional support are somewhat greater than for patients on 5% dextrose solutions. The standard formulas used to calculate fluid requirements based either on body weight or body surface area assume a catabolic state with release of 300–500 ml of water a day from oxidation of fat and release of intracellular water. When a patient is converted to an anabolic state with nutritional support, the released intracellular water is no longer available and indeed, in the anabolic state, new cells are being formed and requirements for new intracellular water can be marked. The standard formulas therefore underestimate fluid requirements by 500–800 ml/day. To assure adequate fluid supplementation, one must give consideration to basic fluid requirements, requirements of an anabolic state, the replacement of measured losses, and replacement of estimated insensible and third-space fluid losses. Insensible fluid loss estimates must be increased by 360 ml/°C/day in febrile patients. fluid administration must also be appropriately adjusted in patients with congestive heart failure, renal failure, pulmonary edema, and those receiving humidified air.

Caloric Requirements

An interaction exists between calorie and nitrogen substrates (133, 206). If one increases caloric support to a patient, less nitrogen is required to achieve nitrogen balance. On the other hand, if one increases nitrogen intake, fewer calories are required to achieve nitrogen balance. The optimal ratio of calories-to-nitrogen in the patient requiring intensive care remains to be determined. Usually an estimate of optimal nitrogen supplementation is made and then caloric supplementation is given to assure nitrogen balance. This often results in a calorie-to-nitrogen ratio between 100:1 and 200:1. The caloric source is typically 25–50% glucose providing 0.86–1.72 kcal/ml. Other sugars have been utilized with no improvement in clinical effect.

Recent studies utilizing insulin and glucose clamp techniques show reduced glucose utilization in stressed patients (6.23±.87 mg/kg/minute) compared with normals (9.46±.79 mg/kg/minute) (11). Furthermore, increases in glucose infusions above 5.0 mg/kg/minute fail to improve protein synthesis and are not associated with increased glucose oxidation (16a).

With limitation on glucose utilization during stress, attention has been given to the use of alternate fuels during stress including lipid, branched chain amino acids, and ketone bodies. In mild stress, clearance of lipids from the blood is increased (56b). One cannot assume, however, that uptake and clearance documents utilization. Goodenough et al. (44a) found only about 8% of infused lipids to be immediately oxidized, with the remainder stored as neutral fats for later use. In addition, Long et al. (113) found less nitrogen-sparing effect with substitution of carbohydrate in a stressed animal model. With severe stress, Lindholm and Rossner (110a) found significant impairment of lipid clearance, especially when multiple organ failure was present.

Difficulty with lipid utilization during stress may in part be related to its dependence on carnitine for transport into the mitochondria for β oxidation. Carnitine deficiency, although rare, has been reported in patients with renal failure, liver disease, cardiac or skeletal muscle disease, patients with stress, and in clinical settings of inadequate intake of carnitine or its precursors (13a, 184a). A new lipid emulsion, the so-called structured lipid emulsion, which is composed of both long-chain fatty acids and medium-chain fatty acids, has been found by Maiz et al. to be more effective in sparing nitrogen in the stressed animal model (116a). The product they used contained 60% medium-chain fatty acids. These fatty acids can be readily metabolized even in the absence of carnitine and may be of great use in the future as commercial products become available.

Some early investigations with ketone bodies have also been promising. These intermediates of fat metabolism enter the energy cycle more easily than either long-chain fatty acids or medium-chain fatty acids. Sherwin et al. (176a) have demonstrated reasonable tolerance of a conjugated solution in monkeys and some nitrogen-sparing capabilities, however the product is far from being clinically useful.

Another alternate fuel that has attracted much interest recently is branched-cain amino acids. These three amino acids are unique in that they appear to be the preferred fuel of skeletal muscle during stress and are not metabolized by the liver. Infusions of branched chain amino acid–enriched solutions to patients in varying degrees of stress suggest their greatest benefit to be in selected patients with marked stress mainly early during the first week or so (11a, 19b, 88a, 133a). These products are currently available both for enteral and parenteral infusion.

A final alternate fuel of perhaps great importance is the amino acid glutamine. This amino acid is the preferred fuel of the gastrointestinal tract, especially during stress. Currently available amino acid solutions for intravenous use do not contain glutamine, and concern has been raised that the lack of this fuel may result in wasting of the gastrointestinal tract with breakdown of the mucosal barrier and increase risks of sepsis and multiple organ failure. Grant and Snyder (48a) have recently shown preservation of the rat intestine when 1 or 2% glutamine is added to intravenous nutrition solutions compared with wasting when it was not.

Current practice is to attempt to provide stressed patients with their estimated, or preferably measured, caloric needs. Caloric needs can be estimated from the Harris-Benedict equation as in Table 16.1 (95, 111, 207). Roughly, mild stress is associated with a 35–37 kcal/kg/day caloric requirement, moderate stress with 37/42 kcal/kg/day, and severe stress with 42–50 kcal/kg/day. Activity such as vigorous exercise increases requirements by up to 5 kcal/kg/day. Actual measurement of caloric expenditure can be accomplished with one or several metabolic carts available that measure oxygen consumption and carbon dioxide production. An onboard computer calculates energy expenditure, along with several other useful parameters such as respiratory quotient and substrate utilization. Up to 1500–1800 kcal are given daily as carbohydrate with the rest being given as long-chain fatty acids, while one watches carefully to assure lipid clearance from the blood. If the stress is moderate to severe, branched-chain enriched amino acid solutions are used as the protein source. It is hoped that structured lipid emulsions and glutamine supplements will be available soon.

Attempts to improve glucose tolerance with insulin infusion during stress has met with limited success (207). When used, only monocomponent, and preferable recombinant insulin should be given. Although insulin can increase uptake of glucose by peripheral tissues and therefore lower blood glucose concentrations in stress, studies have failed to demonstrate increase in glucose oxidation or nitrogen sparing. Potential adverse effects of insulin must be considered. It has been proposed that increased serum insulin and free fatty acids associated with the neuroendocrine response to stress inhibit and activity or pyruvate dehydroginase, thereby limiting the entry of glucose into the Krebs cycle for oxidative metabolism (194a). The increase in pyruvate favors fat synthesis, which requires energy and produces carbon dioxide. In general, use of insulin beyond 50–75 U/day is not recommended. If intolerance persists, an alternate fuel source should be sought and carbohydrate infusion reduced to 5 mg/kg/day or less.

Nitrogen Requirements

Minimal nitrogen supplementation to maintain nitrogen balance with adequate caloric support is estimated to be between 0.5 and 0.75 g/kg/day. However, to achieve optimal nitrogen utilization and preserve lean body mass, it is recommended that between 1.0 and 1.5 g/kg be administered to the unstressed patient (4). During mild to moderate stress up to 2 g/kg/day should be given, and with severe stress 2.5 g/kg/day may be required. Patients with protein-losing enteropathies or nephropathies, those with exudative wound losses, or those undergoing hemodialysis or peritoneal dialysis may have markedly increased requirements due to excessive loss of nitrogen. In practice, a level of nitrogen supplementation is selected along with adequate caloric support, and if in doubt, patients are then monitored for nitrogen balance by comparing total nitrogen input to total losses. Either caloric or nitrogen support is increased until the appropriate nitrogen balance is achieved (0.0 for maintenance of body cell mass, ±0.04–0.07 g/kg/day for body cell mass repletion). Use of amino acid solutions enriched with branched-chain amino acids may have some advantage in the stressed patient and their use is under investigation (11a, 19b, 88a, 133a).

Electrolyte Requirements

Requirements for electrolytes are markedly different in the anabolic state compared with the catabolic state. In particular, those electrolytes in high concentrations within cells are required to a greater extent during total nutritional support than during administration of 5% dextrose solutions. Therefore, supplementation with adequate potassium, phosphorus and magnesium (the anabolic electrolytes) is critical for safe and effective total nutritional support. Rudman et al. (164) demonstrate that not only must all the electrolytes be given, but they must be given in appropriate amounts to establish optimal nitrogen repletion. Requirements occur in three phases. Phase I is during the first 12–24 hours, when anabolic electrolyte deficits must be replaced. Patients who are severely malnourished often have normal serum concentrations of anabolic electrolytes. The true total body deficiency is not apparent until feeding is initiated. Phase II occurs between 12 and 40 hours and follows conversion to an anabolic state. In this phase, increased anabolic electrolyte requirements are due to formation of new intracellular water and the loss of release due to breakdown of body cell mass. Phase III of anabolic electrolyte requirements occurs when patients become stable after repletion of deficits and establishment of the anabolic state. In this phase, anabolic electrolyte shifts are uncommon and requirements are fairly constant. The requirements for other electrolytes, including sodium, chloride, and calcium are not changed from routine 5% dextrose solutions as these are predominantly extracellular ions.

Vitamin Requirement

Requirements for vitamins during intravenous feeding in patients requiring intensive support are not adequately determined. The American Medical Association (AMA) has established guidelines for infusion of vitamins to nonstressed patients receiving intravenous support (Table 16.2) (132). Both B-complex and fat-soluble vitamin deficiencies occur during both short-term and extended periods of nutritional support and must be considered.

Mineral Requirements

The need to provide calcium, phosphorus, and magnesium during total nutritional support is well recognized. Phosphorus is an important component in normal immune function as well as oxygen transport. Routine supplementation with 20 mM phosphorus per 1000 kcal should be modified based on serum concentrations. Deficiency of magnesium is associated with a syndrome similar to hypocalcemia with tetany and muscle fasiculations as well as altered mental status. Routine supplementation ranges between 0.3 and 0.45 mEq/kg/day. Adequate calcium supplementation ranges between 0.2 and 0.3 mEq/kg/day.

Trace Element Requirements

There is controversy over requirements for various trace elements during TPN. Recent AMA guidelines suggest administration of zinc, copper, manganese, and chromium to the unstressed patient (Table 16.3) but offer no advice as to requirements of the critical care patient (55). Deficiency syndromes are identified in patients receiving TPN for zinc, chromium, copper, manganese, selenium, iron and iodine. Preparation and stability of these elements in the TPN solution presents a major challenge to the pharmaceutical industry. However, single components as well as combination solutions are now available. Interactions between various trace elements are well known. Further discussion of calcium, phosphorus, magnesium, and zinc requirements and toxicity as well as deficiency syndromes is included later in this chapter.

Other Additives

Many other additives are often included in the intravenous nutritional solution including 1000 or more units of heparin per liter, up to 25 g of albumin per liter, hydrochloric acid, cimetidine, and even occasionally antibiotics and steroids. As can be appreciated from the above discussion, intravenous nutritional solutions can be extremely complex. The chance of precipitate formation or adverse interactions is good and expertise in formulation and meticulous monitoring is critical for safe and effective nutritional support.

VASCULAR ACCESS, SOLUTION PREPARATION, AND ADMINISTRATION

Solutions formulated to provide calorie, nitrogen, electrolyte, trace element, and vitamin requirements by necessity are quite hypertonic, a quality that prohibits their administration through peripheral veins. Central access via the superior vena cava or inferior vena cava is therefore necessary for total nutritional support. In clinical practice, catheters are typically placed percutaneously into the superior vena cava by either the infraclavicular or supraclavicular approach to the subclavian vein, or, less commonly, via the external or internal jugular veins. Occasionally, when there is no access in the neck or shoulder due to skin lesions or draining infections, catheters are placed in an antecubital vein and advanced into the superior vena cava. If the superior vena cava is not available due to thrombosis, access can be achieved through a small anterior thoracotomy with placement of tubes directly into the right atrium through the right atrial appendage. In addition, catheters have been placed through the femoral system and they are advanced well into the inferior vena cava, although this carries the risk of venous thrombosis. More recently long-term access catheters have been utilized for nutritional support. These catheters are made of silastic and are anchored to the subcutaneous tissues by a Dacron cuff. They are placed percutaneously in the operating room via the subclavian vein or through a small cutdown over the internal or external jugular vein, advanced into the right atrium, and then tunneled subcutaneously to exit on the anterior chest wall. The long subcutaneous tract appears to reduce infectious complications. Newer catheters now

Table 16.2
Recommended Daily Allowances of Vitamins[a]

Method	Fat-Soluble Vitamins				Water-Soluble Vitamins							
	A (IU)	D (IU)	E (IU)	K (mg)	B$_1$ (mg)	B$_2$ (mg)	B$_3$ (mg)	B$_5$ (mg)	B$_6$ (mg)	B$_9$ (mg)	B$_{12}$ (mg)	C (mg)
Oral												
FAO/WHO	2500	100			0.9[b]/1.2	1.3/1.8		14.5/19.8		200	2.0	30
NRC	5000	400	12/15		1.2/1.5	1.4/1.8	5–10	14/20	2.0	400	3.0	45
Normal serum concentration per 100 ml	90–233	112–168	0.5–1.2		0.001–0.006		0.015–0.04	0.3–0.6	0.003–0.008	0.4–2.0	0.02–0.09	0.4–1.0
Intravenous	3300	200	10.0		3.0	3.6	15.0	40.0	4.0	400.0	5.0	100.0

[a]Modified from Grant JP: *Handbook of Total Parenteral Nutrition.* Philadelphia, WB Saunders, 1980, p 172.
[b]Top figure is daily allowance for females; bottom figure is for males.

Table 16.3
Trace Elements

Element	Excretion	RDA[a]	Body Stores	Measured Level
Iron	0.1 mg urine 0.3–0.5 mg feces ± sweat/skin Total = 0.5–1.0 mg/day	16–18 mg/day p.o. 0.5–1.0 mg/day i.v.	3–5 g (50% Hgb, 35% bone marrow, 15% tissues and enzymes)	Serum: 45–160 µg/dl
Zinc	0.3–0.7 mg/d urine (8 mg/day stress) 17.1 mg/kg stool or ileostomy 12.2 mg/kg UGI drainage	10–15 mg p.o. 2.5–4.0 mg i.v.	1–2.3 g	Plasma: 80 µg/dl Hair: 103 PPM
Copper	25 ± 13 µg/kg/day via vile	30 µg/kg/day p.o. 20 µg/kg/day i.v.	75–150 mg (brain, liver, heart, spleen, kidney, blood)	Serum: 75–150 µg/dl
Manganese	Mainly via bile and pancreatic juice	0.7–22 mg/day p.o. 2–10 µg/kg/day i.v.	12–20 mg (brain, kidney, pancreas, liver, bone)	Serum: 0.8 µg/dl
Selenium	?	? 120 µg/day i.v.		Serum: 2–22 µg/dl
Iodine		1 µg/kg/day		Plasma: 3.6–6.0 µg/dl
Chromium	7–10 µg/d urine	70–80 µg/day p.o. 0.14–0.2 µg/kg/day i.v.	6 mg (skin, muscle, fat, testes, bone, liver, spleen)	Serum: 0.3–0.72 µg/dl
Molybdenum	?	2.0 µg/kg/day p.o.	?	?

[a]RDA, recommended daily allowance.

have double or triple lumens, allowing general access while one lumen is reserved for nutritional support. On rare occasions a port of the Swan Ganz catheter or the central port of a dual lumen percutaneous subclavian vein dialysis catheter can be employed for feeding, but because of infectious complications these methods should be avoided unless absolutely necessary. Care of central venous catheters must be meticulous to avoid infectious complications. With appropriate care, catheter related infections should be less than 1%. Complications of catheter insertion can be significant but are generally preventable with proper knowledge of anatomy and care during insertion.

Solutions Used for Intravenous Support

Multiple protein sources are now available for intravenous infusion. Initially these sources were casein or fibrin hydrolysates. More recently, crystalline amino acid solutions have replaced the hydrolysate solutions and are available as 3.5–10% solutions. Protein and electrolyte content of these solutions vary widely, and each solution should be carefully evaluated prior to mixing a patient's formula. Although various solutions have slightly different amino acid compositions, there are no apparent clinical differences between products. Specialized amino acid solutions for renal failure and liver failure are available and branched-chain amino acid enriched solutions are available for use in critically ill patients.

Carbohydrate is provided as a 10% to 70% solution and is mixed in various ratios with the protein solutions. Patients with volume intolerance may have special formulas mixed with 70% dextrose and 10% amino acids to reduce free water.

Since 1973 fat emulsions have been available for intravenous use. They are particularly useful in meeting essential fatty acid requirements of patients during long-term intravenous nutrition and are useful as a caloric source as well, especially during acute stress and sepsis. Fat emulsions are available in 10% and 20% concentrations.

Multiple additives are available in combination or singly so that all electrolytes, trace elements, and minerals can be added with little danger of contamination and pyrogenicity. Solutions of multivitamins that contain both fat-soluble and water-soluble vitamins are also available. Vitamin K must be given orally or by intramuscular injection.

These solutions must be mixed in a specific order to avoid complexing and precipitation. Exposure to light may result in vitamin and amino acid deterioration. Interactions between vitamin C and heparin and the various trace elements, although rarely clinically important, are theoretically possible.

Writing Orders for Parenteral Nutrition

Patients requiring TPN should begin on approximately 2000 ml a day of a 25% dextrose solution with approximately 4% amino acids. This will provide approximately 500 g of carbohydrate, which is generally well tolerated during initiation of intravenous support, and 80 g of protein. In patients with volume restrictions, either the solutions should be concentrated, or the starting volume of the standard solution should be reduced. If glucose intolerance on 5% dextrose solutions or diabetes is present, insulin should be added to the initial order. If the blood glucose concentration is above 150 mg/dl, 10 U of insulin should be added per 250 g of carbohydrate. If the blood glucose concentration is greater than 200 mg/dl, 20–25 units of insulin should be added and if greater than 250 mg/dl, 30–50 units insulin per 250 g carbohydrate are called for. If after the first 24 hours, the patient is stable on the 2-liter infusion, the infusion rate should be advanced to the required caloric support, increasing by 1000 kcal/day. If glucose intolerance is observed even with the addition of insulin, lipid calories should be substituted for carbohydrate. When the feeding solution is discontinued, the amount infused should be reduced by 1000 kcal/day until the patient is receiving 2000 kcal in 24 hours. At this point the solution is converted overnight to 5% dextrose and then discontinued the following morning. Whenever the solution must be suddenly interrupted, it is recommended that a 5% dextrose solution with appropriate electrolytes be substituted via a peripheral vein to run at the same rate as the previous intravenous nutrition solution. At no time is 10% dextrose necessary. When converting to 5% dextrose by a peripheral vein, one must be careful be taken to assure adequate insulin coverage in those patients who are glucose intolerant.

Patient Monitoring

Patients in the critical care unit should have serum electrolytes, urea nitrogen, and glucose concentrations evaluated daily until stability is achieved. Serum calcium, phosphorus and magnesium concentrations should be initially monitored every other day and the prothrombin time and white blood count two to three times a week. After stability has been reached, electrolytes and minerals should be monitored twice a week for the next week and then, depending on the degree of stability, reduced to once a week. Patients are observed carefully for evidence of sepsis, which may be heralded by glucose intolerance 12–24 hours before obvious clinical sepsis. In addition, body weight is monitored carefully to avoid fluid overload with the expectation of no more than 0.5-kg weight gain per day in malnourished patients receiving intensive support. Finally, careful observation of the access catheter with routine dressing changes is necessary to avoid septic complications.

Other Techniques of Administration

New innovations in nutritional support are being evaluated in the critical care setting. The first of these is cyclic intravenous feeding, whereby for 12–16 hours a day patients receive intensive nutritional support and during the remaining 8–12 hours a day they are either on protein solutions alone or converted to a heparin lock (50, 116). Whether cyclic feeding is more advantageous from a metabolic viewpoint remains to be determined. Another method to consider in the critical care unit is modular feeding in which some nutrition substrates are given enterally and the rest are given parenterally through intravenous catheters. An example might be the administration of amino acids and fats through a peripheral vein with glucose via an enteric feeding tube. This is especially useful when the gastrointestinal tract is only partially usable and one wishes to avoid the risks of central venous cannulation.

CATHETER-RELATED COMPLICATIONS OF TPN

Subclavian catheter insertion has the potential for numerous complications and should be performed or directly supervised only by experienced physicians. Full knowledge of the subclavian vein anatomy and attention to minute details minimizes the occurrence of pneumothorax, arterial puncture, hemomediastinum, hemothorax, hydrothorax and hydromediastinum, and virtually eliminates brachial plexus injury, thoracic duct injury, air embolism, and catheter emboli. In large-series catheter insertion complications occur between 1% and 5% of the time, with 1% or less being major complications (13, 17, 30, 166).

The majority of pneumothoraces are small and nonprogressive and usually resolve over several days without treatment. However, some are large and progressive, requiring chest tube placement. If after tube placement an air leak persists for several days, it may be necessary to remove the catheter as it may be passing through lung and pleura which would cause a bronchopleural fistula. A pneumothorax is an especially serious problem in the patient receiving mechanical ventilation. The positive pressure ventilation can delay closure of a small leak, and if the pneumothorax is not recognized, the patient can develop a tension pneumothorax.

Arterial puncture is a risk associated with most approaches to the great veins. Usually puncture of an artery does not pose a serious problem if the needle is carefully removed as normal muscular contraction of the artery prevents significant leakage of blood. If the direction of the needle is altered during insertion or withdrawal, however, the artery and/or vein may be lacerated resulting in development of hemothorax or hemomediastinum with possible cardiac tamponade requiring emergent surgical decompression.

Air embolism is a completely avoidable and potentially lethal complication (24). Aspiration of air may occur during insertion of the catheter (84), during changing of the intravenous tubing (49), upon accidental separation of the intravenous tubing (142), or through the subcutaneous tract, which may fail to close after removal of the catheter (145). Treatment consists of placing the patient in a head-down, left lateral decubitus position (141). Needle aspiration of the right ventricle and even emergency thoracotomy may be necessary to remove the air in the pulmonary outflow tract (178).

Catheter shearing and embolization may occur if the catheter is unwisely manipulated in and out through a metal insertion needle. If the catheter is severed, it may embolize to the subclavian or inominant vein, right atrium, right ventricle, or pulmonary artery. In any case, it should be removed promptly by vascular radiology or by surgery to avoid thrombus formation, infection, cardiac arrhythmias, and possible perforation of the vessels or heart. Use of a smaller needle and guidewire in the Seldinger technique greatly reduces all of the above risks.

With the development of newer and more pliable catheter materials great vein perforation, leading to hemothorax and hemomediastinum or the perforation of the right atrium, is very infrequent.

Another difficulty related to placement of the TPN catheter is improper catheter tip location. The catheter should be a few centimeters superior to the right atrium in the superior vena cava. Improper location can lead to thrombophlebitis, atrial or ventricular perforation, and cardiac arrhythmias. Subclavian vein phlebitis and thrombosis can result in edema of the arm, face, and neck and can be a cryptic source of infection or pulmonary emboli (17, 46). Treatment consists of removal of the catheter, blood and catheter cultures, and initiation of intravenous heparin therapy. If infection is present, vigorous antibiotic therapy is warranted.

Sepsis is a serious complication of TPN. Patients who require TPN are already at high risk due to malnutrition, broad-spectrum antimicrobial therapy, use of corticosteroids, and concominant infection in the lungs, urine, and wounds. Most septic problems related to TPN can be eliminated by scrupulous attention to aseptic catheter placement, solution preparation, and administration (55, 166, 167). Primary catheter sepsis is defined as a septic episode in which no other source is found and the septic episode resolves upon catheter removal with culture-positive identification of the same microorganism on the catheter or in blood drawn through the catheter as is present in the peripheral blood (46). Management of patients who become febrile while receiving TPN begins with a detailed investigation for a possible etiology of the fever. An effort should be made to preserve the central catheter. If the etiology of the fever is still elusive, and there is a fever of .38.5°C often with shaking chills every 4–8 hours, leukocytosis with increased polymorphonucleocytes, and glucose intolerance, the catheter should be removed and blood, catheter tip, and feeding solution cultures obtained. If the clinical condition is not urgent and the diagnosis of catheter-related sepsis is not obvious, cultures can be obtained through the catheter and the administration of the TPN solution can be continued until the culture results are available (115). If the patient's fever is greater than 38.5°C with shaking chills while the medical staff is waiting for the culture results, peripheral infusion of 5% dextrose should be initiated and the central catheter removed and cultured.

METABAOLIC COMPLICATIONS OF TPN

Hyperglycemia

The normal adult in good health is able to metabolize 400–500 g carbohydrate/day and, if increased gradually over several days, upward to 1500 g/day. Attention must be paid to patients with stress, extremes of age, malnutrition, diabetes, and sepsis. Often these patients need nutrition the most, but are the least tolerant to glucose loading, often developing severe hyperglycemia and glucosuria. If 2 g glucose/100 ml urine is permitted to continue, a vigorous osmotic diuresis will ensue, leading to a syndrome of hyperglycemic, hyperosmolar, nonketotic acidosis with an associated mortality approaching 40–50% (32). Optimal therapy is obviously prevention, but survival is improved by early intervention, with rapid fluid replacement with 0.5 N saline (½ NS) + 20 mEq KCl at 250 ml/hour. Insulin should be added to the intravenous solution at 15–20 units/hour while carefully monitoring blood glucose and potassium concentrations. Correction of the acidosis with sodium bicarbonate should be gradual. The goal is to achieve a slow return to normal serum glucose therapy permitting equilibration between the blood and the cerebral spinal fluid, preventing cerebral edema.

Normal serum glucose concentrations during TPN should be less than 200 mg/dl with no more than 2+ or 1% glucosuria. Values greater than 200 mg/dl should be treated. Normal insulin supplementation was discussed earlier but if a patient is glucose tolerant and suddenly develops glucose intolerance, the following should be evaluated as a potential source of hyperglycemia and/or glucosuria:

1. MEDICATION CHANGE. Many medications interfere with the urinary sugar determination by standard Clinitest or Tes-Tape techniques (Table 16.4). There are some medications that effect glucose metabolism directly

Table 16.4
Drug Interference with Urine Glucose Determinations[a]

Drug	Effect on Copper Reduction (Clinitest)	Effect on Glucose Oxidase (Tes-Tape)	Dealing with Potential Interferences

Cephalosporins
  Keflin
  Keflex
  Kefzol, Ancef
  Kafocin
  Loridine
	False positive (black-brown color)	No effect	Use glucose oxidase test

Vitamin C (in large doses)	False positive	False negative	Also may monitor blood glucose[a]
Aspirin and other salicylates (in very large doses)	False positive	False negative	Also may monitor blood glucose[a]
Aldomet (methyldopa) (in very large doses)	False positive	No effect	Use glucose oxidase test
Benemid (probenecid)	False positive	No effect	Use glucose oxidase test
Achromycin (tetracycline, injection only)	False positive	False negative	Also may monitor blood glucose[a]
Pyridium (phenazopyridine)	No effect	False positive and false negative	Use copper reduction method
Chloromycetin (chloramphenicol)	False positive (potentially)	No effect	If in doubt, use glucose oxidase test
Levodopa (in large doses)	False positive	False negative	Also may monitor blood glucose[a]

[a] Note: Potential interferences with glucose oxidase tests (Tes-Tape) can be eliminated by careful testing. While interfering substances will prevent color development in the part of the paper actually dipped into the urine sample, they will not prevent accurate development in a band across the very highest portion of the wetted tape. A true-negative test occurs when the band remains the same color as the rest of the tape, and a true-positive test occurs when the band changes to one of the colors shown on the color chart. (Reprinted with permission. From Grant JP: *Handbook of Total Parenteral Nutrition.* Philadelphia, WB Saunders, 1980.)

(corticosteroids, certain diuretics, phenytoin, and phenothiazines).

2. ERROR IN RATE OF FLUID ADMINISTRATION. A sudden increase in the infusion rate commonly leads to glucose intolerance.

3. IMPENDING SEPSIS. Glucosuria, hyperglycemia, and hyperkalemia may occur up to 12 hours before a temperature elevation or any other sign of sepsis.

4. INSULIN NEEDS. A change in insulin requirements with persistently elevated serum glucose may indicate the formation of antibodies to insulin or resistance of peripheral tissues to the effects of insulin possibly due to chromium deficiency (82). Some patients who tolerate low doses of glucose will, as doses are increased, exhibit evidence of a diabetic state and require insulin during TPN.

Hypoglycemia

Administration of a hypertonic dextrose solution to a nondiabetic patient is associated with a rapid rise in serum insulin, which reaches a steady state four to six times greater than basal within 6 hours (168). As the infusion continues, serum glucose and insulin concentrations gradually decrease. With interruption of the carbohydrate infusion, serum insulin falls to basal levels within 60 minutes and blood glucose decreases to below previous basal levels, but seldom to less than 60 mg/dl. In spite of a rapid decline in serum insulin, reactive hypoglycemia is occasionally observed with abrupt discontinuance of TPN (35). It may occur if the infusion is interrupted for as little as 15–30 minutes. Therefore, in patients receiving greater than 2000 kcal/day of TPN, the solution should be tapered by 1000 kcal/day to 2000 kcal, then changed to 5% dextrose at 100–125 ml/hour for 12–24 hours, at which time the catheter can safely be removed. If abrupt cessation of TPN is necessary,

a peripheral infusion of 5% dextrose with appropriate electrolytes at the same rate as the TPN should be given for 12–24 hours.

Anabolic Electrolytes

POTASSIUM

Potassium is the most abundant intracellular cation. Ninety-eight percent of the total body potassium is within the intracellular fluid pool with an average intracellular concentration of 150 mEq/liter. Intravascular potassium is a mere 2% of total body potassium, 3.5–5.0 mEq/liter. Serum concentrations are, therefore, a poor indicator of total body potassium. The kidneys are the major route of potassium excretion, eliminating approximately 100 mEq/day in the normal healthy person. In certain situations, the kidneys can preserve potassium, but not as efficiently as it can preserve sodium. Potassium is essential to the function and operation of the cell, to the maintenance of the resting potential of the cell membrane by maintaining an extracellular/intracellular gradient, to various enzyme systems, to carbohydrate metabolism, and to protein metabolism (7, 23, 41).

Hypokalemia (Table 16.5) reflects a decrease in extracellular potassium, and is usually the result of insufficient administration or gastrointestinal or urinary losses. The lost potassium should be replaced with either the chloride, acetate, or phosphate salts at 10 mEq/hour to a maximum of 40 mEq/hour.

Hyperkalemia is usually the result of excessive exogenous administration or decreased urinary output. On rare occasions hyperkalemia is factitious, resulting from red cell lysis or forearm acidosis caused by improper blood-drawing techniques. Hyperkalemia is especially prominent in renal failure when the glomerular filtration rate is below 5 ml/min, but may also result from transfusion of aged blood, Addison's disease, tissue trauma, or

Table 16.5
Clinical Symptoms of Potassium Alterations

System	Hyperkalemia	Hypokalemia
Neuromuscular	Diarrhea, weakness, intestinal colic	Paralytic ileus, muscular weakness, possible paralysis
Cardiac	Ventricular arrhythmias, ECG changes: peaked T waves, prolonged PR interval, possible cardiac arrest	Atrial and ventricular premature contractions, myocardial fibrosis, ECG changes: flat T waves, U waves
Metabolic		Abnormal carbohydrate metabolism, negative nitrogen balance

potassium-sparing diuretics (triamterene or spironolactone). Treatment should be rapid and aggressive as hyperkalemia can lead to cardiac arrest. Specific treatment consists of glucose and insulin administration to increase intracellular transport of potassium; correction of metabolic acidosis with sodium bicarbonate transporting potassium, intracellularly; kaluretic diuretics; ion exchange resins; dialysis; and intravenous calcium which lowers the threshold away from the resting potential of the cell membrane (42).

PHOSPHORUS

The phosphate ion is an integral modulator of human metabolism. It participates in energy transfer through high energy phosphates (ATP), oxygen transport and release, leukocyte phagocytosis and microbial resistance (26, 61). Approximately 80% of the adult body's phosphorus is located in bones and teeth, while 9% is within skeletal muscle. Serum phosphorus is a small fraction of total body phosphorus (2.5–4.3 mg/100 ml) and is normally inversely related to serum calcium. Serum phosphate concentrations are regulated by the kidneys and excretion is directly related to phosphate ingestion, as well as serum parathormone level.

Hypophosphatemia may result from insufficient administration in the TPN fluid, alkalosis due to increased phosphorylation of carbohydrate (respiratory greater than metabolic), Gram-negative bacteremia, salicylate intoxication, impaired absorption (phosphate binding antacids—Mg^{2+}, A^{2+}), increased renal clearance (hyperparathyroidism, vitamin D deficiency, Fanconi syndrome, hypomagnesemia, hypokalemia), metabolic acidosis, and alcoholism. Phosphate deficiency may develop within the first 24 hours of TPN if inadequate or no supplemental phosphate is given (179, 190). Glucose administration stimulates insulin secretion, which facilitates transport of glucose and phosphate into the liver and skeletal muscle thus acutely lowering blood concentrations. In addition phosphorus is taken up rapidly in skeletal muscle upon initiation of nutritional support following starvation leading to hypophosphatemia. Renal losses and amino acid binding of phosphate are minimal.

Clinical symptoms of phosphate depletion usually appear when the inorganic phosphate concentration is less than 1.0 mg/100 ml. Symptoms and signs include weakness of the muscles of extremities, neck, mastication, and respiration. There may be paresthesias, absent deep tendon reflexes, anisocoria, hyperventilation, mental obtundity, and an abnormal EMG (179, 190). Bone pain may mimic ankylosing spondylitis. There is a depletion of ATP that conformationally affects RBC membranes leading to rigid spherocytes. Also seen are abnormal red blood cell and platelet survival times, shift of the oxyhemoglobin curve to the left, and impaired white blood cell chemotaxis and phagocytosis (80, 190).

Phosphate replacement can be accomplished by adding sodium or potassium phosphate to the TPN solution in excess of maintenance until normal serum inorganic phosphate concentrations are re-established. To avoid a rapid decrease in calcium and associated tetany, phosphate supplements should be accompanied with 0.2–0.3 mEq/liter calcium infusion.

Hyperphosphatemia is usually the result of renal failure. In this setting a large portion of the phosphate becomes nonultrafilterable and forms colloidal complexes with calcium. This usually occurs when the glomerular filtration rate is 20–25 ml/minute. These complexes may be responsible for the development of metastatic calcifications in soft tissues and organs. Other etiologies of hyperphosphatemia include neoplastic diseases treated with cytotoxic agents, oral phosphate, and phosphate-containing enemas. Hyperphosphatemia may lead to hypocalcemia with possible tetany. Effective treatment consists of the administration of phosphate binding antacids (aluminum hydroxide), which decreases the gastrointestinal absorption of phosphate.

MAGNESIUM

Magnesium is the second most abundant intracellular cation, exceeded only by potassium. The average adult body contains about 330 mEq magnesium per kilogram, of which 60% is bound to the bony skeleton. Most of the remaining magnesium is concentrated in the body cells, particularly the liver, muscle, and heart. Only about 1% of the body's magnesium is in serum (1.4–2.2 mEq/liter). In magnesium deprivation, the kidney can reduce losses to less than 1 mEq/day.

Magnesium has vital metabolic functions important in the activation of many metabolic enzyme systems (especially the ATPases) (197). Many cellular energy processes are catalyzed by magnesium (196). Magnesium is essential in protein synthesis as well as synthesis of nucleic acids (15). Magnesium is of special importance to the normal function of nervous tissue, skeletal muscle, and the heart (174).

Hypomagnesemia may be the result of inadequate intake, impaired absorption, or excessive losses. Inadequate intake can result from prolonged administration of magnesium-free TPN solutions or severe starvation. Magnesium depletion may be associated with various malabsorption syndromes, extensive small bowel resections, intestinal or biliary tract fistulas, prolonged vomiting or nasogastric suction, chronic alcoholism, pancreatitis, parathyroid disease, and diabetes, especially if large insulin doses are required. Renal losses of magnesium may be secondary to diuretic abuse with mercurials, ammonium chloride, and thiazides; the diuretic phase of acute renal failure; or various intrinsic renal diseases such as glomerulonephritis, pyelonephritis, and nephrosclerosis (3). Clinical manifestations are usually present when the serum concentration is less than 1.0 mEq/liter. Many signs and symptoms resemble hypocalcemia and differentiation is essential as tetany from hypocalcemia is only temporarily corrected by magnesium administration and vice versa. Most clinical signs of hypomagnesemia are related to increased neuromuscular irritability such as confusion, hyperactive deep tendon reflexes, convulsions, tetany, positive Chvostek's sign, tremor, clonus, nystagmus, muscle fasiculation, paresthesias, and weakness (177). Magnesium deficiency also affects the cardiovascular system as evidenced by depression of ST segments and inverted T waves in precordial leads and tachycardia. Finally, magnesium deficiency can result in severe potassium wasting in the urine. Treatment is by administration of up to 40 mEq of magnesium sulfate per day, the rate of administration depending on the clinical situation.

Hypermagnesemia is rare during TPN except in patients with renal failure, diabetic acidosis, aldosterone deficiency, hyperparathyroidism, and those who use magnesium-containing laxatives and enemas excessively (3, 46). The clinical spectrum of hypermagnesemia usually involves impairment of neuromuscular transmission as reflected by hypotension, nausea, vomiting, lethargy, drowsiness, hyporeflexia, weakness, respiratory depression, coma, and cardiac arrest. ECG changes reveal QT prolongations, a prolonged PR interval, and various degrees of atrioventricular block. Intravenous calcium can temporarily reverse the depressant effects of excess magnesium. Cardiac and pulmonary support may be necessary, but the best therapy is prevention. Dialysis can be used to lower the serum magnesium concentration.

TRACE ELEMENT DEFICIENCY

Trace element metabolism during nutritional support is a new and largely unexplored area. The term "trace element" refers to those elements present in such small quantities that their precise concentrations can not be measured accurately using conventional equipment. Usually the elements are present in concentrations less than 100 μg/g (122). With the development of TPN and the refinement of highly purified constituents, various deficiency syndromes have been recognized (54). Trace element deficiencies develop during TPN for several reasons: There may be reduced intake, increased utilization, decreased plasma binding of the elements secondary to either a decrease in synthesis or an increase in loss of the plasma binding proteins, or there may be increased excretion of the trace elements through primary or secondary routes of elimination. Iron, zinc, copper, manganese, selinium, iodine, chromium, cobalt, and molybdenum are essential to human nutrition. Fluorine, vanadium, nickel, silicon, and tin are felt to be only possibly important during TPN. Administration of these elements must be individualized because toxic concentrations and manifestations have yet to be recognized. In patients with renal and hepatic dysfunction, appropriate adjustments in dosage must be made. Table 16.3 details the route of excretion, recommended daily supplementation, body stores, and measured levels of the nine essential trace elements (53). Often clinical symptoms may take months to become evident because of large body stores of the trace elements.

IRON

Iron is necessary for the production of hemoglobin and myoglobin as well as for the functioning of some essential metabolic enzymes (148). Deficiency is demonstrated by a hypochromic, microcytic anemia, low serum iron, and high total iron binding capacity. Its deficiency leads to increased susceptibility to helminth infections, depression of cellular immunity, and a decrease in bactericidal activity of leukocytes (20, 85, 201). To calculate replacement of a preexisting iron deficiency the following formula is useful:

Iron (mg) needed $= 0.3$ (wt in lb)
$$\times \frac{100\text{-Hgb} \times 100}{14.8}$$

ZINC

Zinc was first shown to be essential in 1934 (188). It is required for both RNA and DNA synthesis, as well as for the proper functioning of a number of zinc-dependent metabolic enzymes including aldolases, dehydrogenases, peptidases, and thymidine kinases (119). Much of our knowledge of zinc comes from the various manifestations of zinc deficiency such as growth retardation (57), impaired wound healing (153), alopecia (87, 88), depressed cellular immunity (150), acrodermatitis enteropathica-like skin lesions (58), anorexia with impairment of taste and smell, hypogonadism, diarrhea, and glucose intolerance (155). Patients prone to zinc deficiency include those on long-term corticosteroid therapy, those with bilateral adrenalectomies, major surgical, traumatized, and septic patients, and those with malabsorption syndromes, fistulous disease, and low dietary intake (40, 66, 198). Zinc toxicity results in fever, nausea, vomiting, and diarrhea.

COPPER

Copper deficiency in adults during TPN typically presents as a hematological abnormality usually consisting of anemia, leukopenia, and neutropenia (195). The precise mechanism for these changes is unclear, but it is known that in copper deficiency iron stores are not effectively utilized for heme formation. Zidar et al. (209) show an inappropriately low level of erythropoietin for the degree of anemia and demonstrate ineffective granulopoesis. In children, copper deficiency may lead to osteoporosis by an unknown mechanism (65). In addition, copper is important in the electron transport system (110), connective tissue integrity, and wound healing (92). Acute copper toxicity follows ingestion of greater than 15 mg of elemental copper and is associated with nausea, vomiting, intestinal cramps, diarrhea, intravascular hemolysis, and renal impairment.

MANGANESE

Manganese participates in the activation of many enzyme systems (136), such as chondroitin sulfate synthesis (105) and protein synthesis via stimulation of RNA, and DNA polymerase activity. Doisy et al. report a case of manganese deficiency manifested by weight loss, dermatitis, slow growth, change in hair color, alteration of protein synthesis, and hypocholesterolemia (34). Manganese is also possibly involved in glucose utilization. Toxicity of manganese is rare but it may damage the extrapyirmidal system causing symptoms resembling Parkinson's disease.

SELENIUM

In experimental animals, selenium deficiency can cause liver necrosis, pancreatic atrophy, and a form of muscular dystrophy (171). In the human, several case reports have been published describing severe muscle pain, thigh tenderness and cardiomyopthy (15a, 39a, 156a, 193, 198a). Most importantly, selenium is involved as a catalyst for the important enzyme glutathione peroxidase (183). This enzyme protects against oxidative stress and cellular damage by peroxides. Selenium can function as an antioxidant and probably important in drug metabolizing systems.

IODINE

Much has been written about iodine and its deficiency syndrome of thyroid goiter. Iodine is an integral part of the thyroid hormones thyroxine and triiodothyronine, and therefore is important in the regulation of body metabolism.

CHROMIUM

Chromium has only recently been recognized as an important element in carbohydrate metabolism through its close association with the glucose tolerance factor (GTF). Chromium through GTF, appears to exert its effect peripherally by potentiating the effect of insulin upon muscle and fat calls. Jeejeebhoy et al. (82) describe a case of chromium deficiency in a patient receiving home TPN for 3 years. Symptoms included weight loss, hyperglycemia, abnormal glucose tolerance, and a diabetic-like peripheral neuropathy.

COBALT

The only human requirement for cobalt is the amount necessary for the structure of vitamin B_{12}. Humans are unable to incorporate cobalt into the corrinoid ring of this vitamin, therefore the cobalt is absorbed in total with vitamin B_{12}. Deficiency of B_{12} is described later.

MOLYBDENUM

This metal is essential in xanthine oxidase (160). There are no documented deficiency syndromes in humans.

FLUROINE

Fluorine may play an important role in fertility, growth, and maintenance of a normal hematocrit (191). It also benefits maintenance of teeth and the skeleton.

NICKEL

In animals, deficiency has led to impairment of reproduction, hair loss, and hepatocyte dysfunction (134). There has been no documented deficiency in humans.

SILICON

Silicon appears to be involved in bone calcification, structure of cartilage matrix, and possibly mucopolysaccharide metabolism (19). No human deficiency syndrome is known.

VANADIUM

In animals, deficiency of this element reduces body growth, increases packed red blood cell values, increases plasma triglycerides, impairs reproduction, and impairs bony development (172). No human deficiency is documented.

TIN

Tin may contribute to the tertiary structure of proteins. No deficiency syndrome is documented.

VITAMIN DEFICIENCIES

Vitamins are essential components in the metabolism of carbohydrates, protein, and fat. It is only over the past 40–50 years that the symptoms of various vitamin deficiencies have been well delineated. Recommended daily allowances (Table 16.2) for each vitamin are established by the World Health Organization (146) and others (31, 132). Unfortunately, these values are based on oral not intravenous intake and changes in requirements with disease and injury are unknown. When work was first started in vitamin research it was convenient to divide them into two groups: fat-soluble and water-soluble.

Fat-Soluble Vitamins (A, D, E, K)

VITAMIN A

The activity of vitamin A is measured in international units (IU) where 1 IU is equal to 0.3 μg of crystalline vitamin A alcohol or 0.6 μg of β-carotene. The decreased biological activity of carotene is due to the less efficient absorption from the intestine and to a low efficiency in converting carotene to vitamin A (147). In the normal healthy person stores of vitamin A (600,000 IU) can support the body for 3 months to a year. However, infection, hypothermia and other stresses rapidly decrease the supply of vitamin A. Serum vitamin A levels are not a good reflection of total body stores (161). The functions of vitamin A include contributions to vision, growth, and reproduction. Deficiencies usually arise because of interference with absorption or storage, inadequate dietary intake, interference with conversion from carotene to vitamin A, and rapid loss of vitamin A from the body (161). Deficiencies of vitamin A are associated with nyetalopia, xerophthalmia, phyrnoderma, decreased resistance to infection, retardation of growth, depressed production of corticosteroids, and mild leukopenia with a decrease in polymorphonuclear leukocytes and an increase in juvenile forms. Prevention of vitamin A deficiency is possible by maintenance therapy. The recommended oral intake of vitamin A is 2500–5000 IU/day. Suggestions for intravenous infusion of vitamin A are slightly higher, 2500–8000 IU/day, due to binding to glass and plastic (132).

VITAMIN D

The activity of vitamin D is also measured in international units, where 1 mg vitamin D equals 40,000 IU. Vitamin D stores are maintained normally by both dietary intake and conversion of vitamin D from the action of ultraviolet light on the skin. It is transported to the liver, where it is hydroxylated to 25-$(OH)D_3$ and then converted by the renal mitochondria to the highly active form $1,25\text{-}(OH)_2D_3$. In this form vitamin D regulates calcium and phosphorus homeostasis in conjunction with parathormone and thyrocalcitonin (139). Vitamin D increases the absorption of calcium and phosphate from the intestine and also regulates the rate of reabsorption of phosphates by the renal tubules. Deficiency of vitamin D leads to osteomalacia (rickets), decreased serum calcium and phosphorus, and elevated alkaline phosphatase levels. Tetany due to hypocalcemia may occur. Proposed maintenance therapy for vitamin D is 100–400 IU/day orally or 200–420 IU/day (132).

VITAMIN K

Vitamin K is synthesized by gut flora or acquired from food. Absorption requires the presence of bile salts and pancreatic juices (51). Vitamin K plays an essential role in synthesis of clotting factors (II, VII, IX, X) (184). Deficiency of vitamin K leads to a prolongation of the prothrombin time. There is no recommended daily intake, but 0.7–2.0 mg/day is suggested. While on TPN, Jeejeebhoy et al. (83) suggest 5 mg/week administered intramuscularly.

VITAMIN E

There is much speculation about the function of vitamin E in human nutrition. It may serve primarily as an antioxidant, thereby inhibiting the oxidation of unsaturated free fatty acids (173, 185). Deficiency states of vitamin E are well described and include anemia secondary to hemolysis (74), excessive creatinuria (135), deposition of a ceroid material in smooth muscle, lesions in skeletal muscles similar to muscular dystrophy (8), and increased platelet aggregation (102). The recommended daily oral allowance for vitamin E is 12–15 IU. Suggested intravenous support ranges from 2.1 to 60 IU/day. In our experience, 25–50 IU are needed during TPN. The requirements for vitamin E are increased by the presence of polyunsaturated fatty acids in the diet. Therefore, additional vitamin E should be given when fat is administered during TPN (162).

Water-Soluble Vitamins

The clinical syndromes of water-soluble vitamin deficiencies are often similar and therefore therapy is usually directed towards multiple replacement. The tissue stores of water soluable vitamins are small and deficiencies develop early with dietary restriction. Patients receiving TPN must be supplemented early with these vitamins. Excess water soluable vitamins are excreted in the urine, therefore toxic manifestations are rare.

THIAMINE-VITAMIN B_1

Thiamine functions as a coenzyme for the enzyme transketolase which is important in the phosphogluconate pathway. Thiamine is also believed to be a structural component of nervous system membranes (78). Nutritional deficiencies are common owing to its limited distribution in foods. Mild deficiency leads to peripheral neuropathy characterized by paresthesias, hyperesthesia, anesthesia, and weakness. Muscles become tender with atrophy and there may be foot and wrist drop. With more severe deficiency cardiomegaly may develop especially right sided, along with tachycardia, palpitations, dependent edema, and arterial-venous shunting (138).

Acute pernicious beriberi may occur if a patient becomes thiamine deficient during TPN and is associated with mortality rates up to 50%. High output cardiac failure may be severe. Prolonged thiamine deficiency can lead to Wernicke's encephalopathy (12).

Early recognition and adequate replacement of thiamine deficiency brings rapid recovery. Maintenance requirements for thiamine vary with caloric intake. Recommended doses are approximately 0.5 mg of thiamine/1000 kcal taken orally (169) or 3–21 mg/day during TPN, although intravenous requirements are still unknown.

RIBOFLAVIN-VITAMIN B_2

Riboflavin is a constituent of two coenzymes, riboflavin-5'-phosphate and flavin adenine dinucleotide. These coenzymes are important components of several oxidative enzyme systems involved in electron transport.

There are essentially no stores of riboflavin and deficiency symptoms develop rapidly with dietary restriction (187). Symptoms include inflammation of lips, fissures at the corners of the mouth, scaliness, greasiness, seborrheic dermatitis about nose and scrotum, and vascularization of the cornea. Riboflavin requirements are 1.3–1.7 mg/day orally or 3.6–7.5 mg/day intravenously (132).

PANTOTHENIC ACID-VITAMIN B$_3$

The only functional form of panthothenic acid is coenzyme A which takes part in all acylation reactions. There is no documented deficiency syndrome of pantothenic acid. There is no specified daily allowance, but recommended oral intake is 5–10 mg/day while the suggested intravenous dose is 10–29 mg/day (132).

NIACIN-VITAMIN B$_5$

Niacin plays an important role in body metabolism in the form of coenzymes NAD and NADP. These coenzymes participate in the intracellular respiratory mechanism of all cells by assisting in the stepwise transfer of hydrogen from glycolysis to the flavin mononucleotide. The reduced forms of the coenzymes also participate in many biosynthetic pathways such as fatty acid synthesis.

Clinical symptoms of niacin deficiency include weakness, lassitude, anorexia, dermatitis, inflammation of the mouth, and pellagra. Effective prevention of niacin deficiency is accomplished by providing 14.5–19.8 mg niacin/day orally or 40–140 mg/day intravenously (132).

PYRIDOXINE-VITAMIN B$_6$

Pyridoxine functions as a coenzyme for transaminases, decarboxylases, for the two enzyme systems involved in the metabolism of sulfur-containing amino acids, and phosphorylase. Pyridoxine also functions as a cofactor for hydroxylases, synthetases, and many other enzymes. Deficiency of vitamin B$_6$ is well described. Personality changes, irritability, depression, filiform hypertrophy of the lingual papilla, and stomatitis characterize the deficiency syndrome. There is also a strong tendency to develop genitourinary infections (200). Prolonged vitamin B$_6$ deficiency leads to sideroblastic anemia (202). Vitamin B$_6$ deficiency is accentuated by certain antagonists such as isoniazid, pencillamine, and cycloserine (91). The recommended oral intake pyridoxine is 2.0 mg/day for adult men and 1.5 mg/day for adult women. Intravenous doses of 4.0–6.3 mg are suggested (132).

BIOTIN-VITAMIN B$_7$

Biotin can be synthesized by the intestinal flora, therefore deficiency syndromes are rare (140). The main metabolic activity of biotin is in carboxylation reactions. Deficiencies of biotin lead to a fine-scale desquamation of skin. Adult requirements for biotin are not determined.

FOLIC ACID-VITAMIN B$_9$

Because serum folate concentrations are normally 5–16 ng/ml and body folate stores range from 5–10 mg, serum measurements do not accurately reflect tissue stores. Folate participates in the uptake and transfer of 1-carbon fragments. It is involved in a multitude of metabolic processes such as purine synthesis, pyrimidine nucleotide biosynthesis, and various 3-carbon amino acid conversions. Stores of folate can usually last 3–6 months upon complete dietary restriction (67), but in stressed patients, depletion may be more rapid (37). Deficiencies also result from inadequate absorption secondary to a host of diseases or competing drugs (199); deficiency of vitamin B$_{12}$, which participates in removal of a methyl group to form the active tetrahydrofolic acid; and because of increased requirements associated with pregnancy, malignancy, sepsis, and anemias.

Symptoms include megaloblastic anemia and possibly diarrhea. Recommended daily intake for folate is 200–400 μg/day orally and 0.4–1.0 mg/day intravenously (132).

CYANOCOBALAMIN-VITAMIN B$_{12}$

Vitamin B$_{12}$ absorption is extremely dependent upon two mechanisms: gastric acid and intestinal enzyme separation from food and the gastric intrinsic factor. The normal stores of vitamin B$_{12}$ are 1–10 mg with liver containing 50–90% of total (157). The normal serum concentration is 200–900 g/ml.

Vitamin B$_{12}$ has many metabolic functions, but primarily it acts as a transmethylating agent thereby functioning in biosynthesis of thiamine, methionine, and possibly choline. By an unknown mechanism, vitamin B$_{12}$ assists in movement of folate into cells. It is also involved in seven to eight enzyme reactions and therefore is important in normal fat, carbohydrate, and protein metabolism.

A deficiency of vitamin B$_{12}$ during short-term dietary restriction is rare because of large stores as well as an efficient enterohepatic circulation. When it does occur, it takes 3–6 years to become evident. Deficiencies are characterized by a megaloblastic anemia (pernicious anemia) (25), glossitis, impairment of myelinization of peripheral nerves, and platelet aggregation defects resulting in a prolonged bleeding time (107). Neurological symptoms develop insideously with peripheral paresthesias, decreased vibratory sense, ataxia, central scotomata, confusion, and possibly psychosis.

The recommended daily maintenance for vitamin B_{12} is 2–3 μg/day orally and 5–15 μg/day intravenously. Deficiency symptoms can usually be treated with a single injection of 100–1000 μg of vitamin B_{12} (132). (*Note:* Begin with no more than 100μg as larger doses may cause severe hypokalemia.)

ASCORBIC ACID-VITAMIN C

Vitamin C is active in forming collagen, transporting mitochondrial electrons, metabolizing tyrosine, converting folate to tetrahydrofolic acid, and metabolizing cholesterol. It prevents and cures scurvy, which is characterized by anemia, joint pain, mucous membrane hemorrhages, weakness, and emaciation. Less severe deficiency impairs wound healing, diminishes host immunity, and decreases tyrosine metabolism (46).

No specific daily requirements are known, but 30–45 mg/day orally is recommended while suggested intravenous supplementation is 100–500 mg/day (132). Body stores of vitamin C are minimal, and coupled with increased urinary losses with stress, a deficiency may develop rapidly during TPN if inadequate supplements are given (70). Vitamin C administration interferes with the anticoagulant effects of heparin; 2 mg ascorbic acid neutralizes 1 U of heparin (143).

OTHER COMPLICATIONS OF TPN

Elevated Liver Function Test

Many investigators note a high percentage of patients receiving parenteral nutrition develop elevations of serum bilirubin and hepatic enzymes (SGOT, SGPT, alkaline phosphatase, LDH) (44, 48, 50, 75, 114, 144, 205). Liver biopsies obtained at these times reveal periportal fatty changes with little evidence of inflammation or other abnormalities (75). There is much speculation as to the etiology of these liver changes, but attempted correlation with various parameters has been unsuccessful (48, 64, 149, 152, 176, 189). Changes are seen with equal frequency when casein or protein hydrolysates or crystalline amino acids are used

as protein sources. The liver enzyme elevations also do not correlate with the initiation of feeding preoperatively versus postoperatively, with the mean serum glucose level, or with the amount of exogenous insulin administered.

It has been proposed that early changes are secondary to toxic conversion products of the amino acid tryptophan in the presence of sodium bisulfite (48). Sheldon et al. (176) found evidence of progressive intrahepatic cholestases, bile duct proliferation, and bile plugs associated with serum hepatic enzyme changes, and felt that this was due to an imbalance in the caloric:nitrogen ratio. Langer et al. (103) theorized that the changes were secondary to lack of essential fatty acids, whereas others have reported these changes while patients received intravenous fat. Kaminski et al. (86) postulated that fatty infiltration was associated with a decreased ability to transport lipid away from the liver due to a deficiency of lipotropic factors and Hall et al. (56a) documented abnormalities in fat synthesis, fat oxidation, fat uptake, and fat mobilization by the liver. Others feel that changes are secondary to protein allergies (64, 149, 189). The precise etiology of these changes remains to be determined. Most investigators feel it is due to glucose overloading (50, 114, 162a).

Elevation of Blood Urea Nitrogen (BUN)

Almost all patients receiving parenteral nutrition demonstrate some elevations of BUN regardless of renal function. The elevation rarely exceeds normal limits in patients with normal renal function; if it does it usually plateaus at less than 80 mg/dl. Some of the elevation can be attributed to dehydration. However, in patients with compromised renal function (creatine clearance < 20 ml/minute) the BUN may progressively increase, thereby limiting the amount of nitrogen that can be infused. In patients with a creatinine clearance > 20 ml/minute, usually 9 g or more of nitrogen per day will be well tolerated. In more severe renal failure, special formulas may be required to reduce nitrogen support to 6–9 g or less per day (1a, 46).

Essential Fatty Acid Deficiency

There are three polyunsaturated fatty acids that cannot be synthesized by humans (linoleic, arachidonic, and linolenic); however, only linoleic acid is essential in the adult diet. Arachidonic acid can be synthesized when linoleic acid is present. The precise role and need for linolenic acid in the adult is undetermined. The average daily intake of fat in the human diet is approximately 100–180 g, approximately 12–125 g of which are essential fatty acids (EFA). The RDA for EFA is not established, but suggested intravenous supplementation ranges from 1% to 4% of the total caloric intake or 25–100 mg/kg/day of linoleic acid (18, 59, 72, 186).

EFA play a primary role in the structure and maintenance of cell membranes, prostaglandin synthesis, and various transport mechanisms (106). EFA deficiency leads to a decrease in the efficiency of calorie utilization, and possibly the dissociation of oxidative phosphorylation and the impairment of production of high-energy phosphate bonds. The clinical symptoms of EFA deficiency include diarrhea, dryness of skin, hair loss, impaired wound healing, and brittle and osteoporotic bones (18, 59, 72). Biochemical changes include decreased cholesterol levels thrombocytopenia, increased platelet aggregation, increased capillary permeability, anemia, increased RBC fragility, elevations of serum hepatic enzymes, and fatty infiltration of the liver (181, 186).

EFA deficiency can be documented by an elevated serum 5,8,11-eicosatrienoic: arachiodonic acid ratio that is normally less than 0.4 (72, 73). All symptoms can be reversed with the administration of linoleic acid. If the oral route is available, oils high in linoleic acid such as corn oil or safflower oil may be administered (5 ml twice or three times a day). Other available routes include topical administration of corn oil or safflower oil (15 ml three times a day) (156), or intravenous administration of 25–100 mg/kg/day of linoleic acid as a 10% or 20% fat emulsion (60). Biochemical signs of EFA deficiency may develop early over the first few days of fat-free TPN, whereas clinical symptoms may require several weeks to become obvious, in any case, fat administration should be started early in the course of TPN therapy.

Hypoalbuminemia

Albumin is a major synthetic product of the liver, and averages about 130–200 mg/kg/day, but may be as high as 860 mg/kg/day during maximum synthesis. Depressed serum albumin concentrations may result from decreased synthesis, increased degradation, or altered fluid status.

Depressed synthesis is associated with many conditions including malnutrition, cancer, acute stress, cirrhosis, hypothyroidism, and exposure to hepatic toxins. The main clinical condition associated with increased degradation is catabolism (36). Because of the redistribution of extravascular albumin into the plasma pool, serum concentrations of albumin decrease slowly and do not always reflect the total body pool. When the serum albumin concentration is 2.5 mg/100 ml, the total exchangeable albumin pool may be less than one-half its normal level.

Hypoalbuminemia has been associated with impairment of soft and bony tissue healing (43), decreased immune defense (104), depressed gastrointestinal motility (120), and impaired intestinal absorption of water and electrolytes (130). A major function of albumin is regulating the distribution of body water through its osmotic properties (76). We therefore try to reestablish normal total body albumin content rapidly in catabolic patients by adding up to 25 g albumin/liter TPN. The approximate amount of total body albumin deficit can be determined by the formula: grams albumin deficit $= (4.0 - Alb)BW(kg)$. When albumin is given alone without adequate nutritional support, it is used as a calorie substrate but when given with adequate caloric support, its half-life approaches normal. In patients who have acute respiratory distress or possible damage to pulmonary capillary integrity, it may be wise not to administer albumin because it may leak into the perivascular pulmonary tissues (71). Use personal judgement in deciding whether to administer albumin during TPN.

Acid-Base Derangements

Acid-base balance is an extremely complex system involving multiple feedback mechanisms. An in-depth discussion is beyond the scope of this section.

Parenteral nutrition has the potential for either causing or magnifying acid-base disturbances. Most enzymatic and metabolic processes in the human are pH sensitive and the body strives to preserve acid-base homeostasis. Therefore frequent monitoring of the serum pH is made in critically ill patients receiving parenteral nutrition.

Metabolic acidosis can usually be attributed to either abnormal production of acid or to excessive loss of base. Diseases or processes leading to excess production of acid include diabetes mellitus, hyperthryoidism, high fat diets, hepatitis, anesthesia, sepsis, low cardiac output syndromes leading to lactic acidosis, and many others. Disease states which may lead to excess loss of bicarbonate include diarrhea, pancreatic, biliary, or small intestinal drainage, renal insufficiency and the administration of acidifying salts.

There are, however, two other potential causes which should be considered in patients receiving TPN:

1. Synthetic L-amino acids contain one-third to one-fifth the titratable acidity of the older protein hydrolysates, but they too can induce metabolic acidosis due to an increased amount of cationic amino acids compared to anionic amino acids (63).
2. Metabolic acidosis may result from excessive chloride administration (56, 158). An increased quantity of chloride ions are filtered at the renal glomerulus, thereby providing more chloride to be reabosrbed in the distal renal tubules with sodium. This increased sodium chloride reabsorption inversely effects hydrogen ion secretion into the tubules leading to a hyperchloremic metabolic acidosis.

Metabolic alkalosis may result from gastric suctioning, vomiting, diarrhea, diuretic intake, excessive administration of potassium-free solution, excessive ingestion of antacids, and hyperadrenocorticism. However, during parenteral nutrition, special attention should be paid to patients on prolonged nasogastric suctioning. In addition to the loss of hydrogen ions, the loss of chloride ions leads to less chloride filtration by the renal glomerulus and therefore greater amounts of H^+ ion secreted in the distal tubule in exchange for sodium.

Prevention of acid-base disturbances is the best treatment. To avoid difficulties of excess chloride infusion, the Na:Cl ratio is adjusted to 1:1 and additional anions are given as acetate, lactate, or phosphate. Nasogastric losses are replaced carefully with appropriate electrolyte solutions. If acid losses are extreme, it may be necessary to administer an H_2 blocker or even to infuse dilute hydrochloric acid intravenously. Hydrochloric acid up to 0.2 N is compatible with crystalline amino acid solutions or standard dextrose solutions and can be administered via central venous line. It is suggested that trace elements, vitamin, and other low-priority additives be removed when hydrochloric acid is added to prevent untoward reactions.

Lethargy

Patients will occasionally become weak, tired, lethargic, and even semicomatose upon initiation of TPN. The cause of this lethargy is unknown. One suggestion is that the change from starvation to full nutritional support may result in metabolic or hormonal changes that lead to sedation (108). An increase in serum tryptophan enhances its passage into the brain, which leads to serotonin production and lethargy. There is no specific therapy and symptoms usually diminish after 6–10 days. Exercise may be safely encouraged.

Alopecia

Excessive or complete loss of hair is common during TPN but is usually not due to the nutrition solution. The most common cause is an interruption of the normal hair cycle in response to a stressful event (trauma, sepsis, malnutrition). Hair undergoes three phases of growth. The anagen phase is the period of intense mitotic activity, formation of the hair root, and growth of the hair shaft. The catagen phase is a short period of transition when the hair follicle stops growing and regresses to a state similar to the embryologic follicle germ. The final resting stage, the telogen phase, is when the keratinized hair shaft and hair bulb are lying within the resting follicle. At some point the follicles are reactivated and the old hair is shed. Normally, 85% of hairs in the scalp are in the anagen phase while 15% are in the telogen phase. With stress, many hair follicles simultaneously enter the telogen phase (97). Shortly thereafter, the hair is shed and the follicles start over in the anagen phase. Hair loss is therefore a common but temporary event. Other causes of hair loss include severe protein depletion and zinc deficiency.

NUTRITIONAL SUPPORT IN SPECIAL CLINICAL SETTINGS

Renal Failure

Renal failure is a frequent complication in the critically ill patient. Metabolic requirements of these patients are no different than requirements of patients without renal failure (182). Any initial attempt to reduce metabolic support to avoid volume or protein tolerance is avoided. Rather, effective hemodialysis or peritoneal dialysis is established early to permit aggressive TPN. If dialysis is established, no reduction need be made in the routine supply of nutrients as dialysis will clear any excesses or waste by-products. Indeed, it must be recognized that there is a loss of nitrogen during dialysis that requires replacement. Hemodialysis results in loss of up to 9 g amino acids and 3–4 g peptides over 4 hours while in peritoneal dialysis up to 15 g of amino acids and 40 g of protein may be lost. Only in cases in which dialysis is contraindicated or not available should consideration be given to modification of nutritional support reducing both volume and protein content. In this setting, if intravenous protein support is reduced below 30–40 g a day (the minimum protein support providing adequate essential amino acids in currently available solutions) administration of essential amino acids as supplements or essential amino acids alone should be considered. Renal failure solutions containing only essential amino acids are commercially available. They are packaged in 200- to 250-ml volume and provide approximately 6 g of protein as essential amino acids plus histadine. These are mixed with 500 ml of 70% dextrose to provide calories. One or two bottles are administered daily until renal function recovers adequately or dialysis becomes available, permitting administration of more balanced solutions. The routine supplementation of vitamins, essential fatty acids, trace elements, and minerals must be emphasized during the feeding program whether specialized renal failure formulas or standard products are used. Morbidity and mortality of renal failure is in part due to the subsequent metabolic alteration and nutritional depletion that results when nutritional support is inadequate. Aggressive nutritional support coupled with adequate dialysis offers significantly improved care for these high-risk patients.

Hepatic Failure

Providing adequate nutritional support to patients with hepatic failure poses a major metabolic problem. These patients often manifest protein intolerance, which is characterized by increased serum ammonia concentra-

tions and hepatic encephalopathy. Studies by Fischer et al. (38) suggest the onset of hepatic encephalopathy may be due to abnormal amino acid profiles due to the altered hepatic function. In particular, straight-chain and aromatic amino acids are increased in the blood and brain, whereas branched-chain amino acids are decreased. The resulting abnormal ratio between aromatic and branched-chain amino acids contributes to altered amino acid transport through the blood-brain barrier and an abnormal neurotransmitter profile (81). Experimentation in the animal as well as clinical trials in humans have demonstrated that products containing high concentrations of branched-chain amino acids and low concentrations of aromatic amino acids improve or prevent hepatic encephalopathy while permitting aggressive protein supplementation of up to 100–150 g per day (73a). Coupled with adequate caloric, vitamin, electrolyte, mineral, and trace element supplementation, anabolism can often be achieved even in the patient with significant hepatic failure. Recent studies, however, have not confirmed the earlier findings (19a, 122a, 197a). Current recommendations are to provide routine protein loading until or unless encephalopathy is present at which time use of branched-chain enriched products may be useful.

Respiratory Failure

Respiratory failure due to malnutrition is manifested in two ways. The first and most common is a decrease in respiratory skeletal and diaphragmatic muscle function with a subsequent decrease in ventilatory effort. In these cases, nutritional support must be aggressive and complete in hopes of regenerating skeletal and diaphragmatic muscle mass. Excessive carbohydrate administration in patients with respiratory failure leads to increased carbon dioxide production and perhaps respirator dependency (5). In these situations it is perhaps best to continue the administration of a nutrient solution until muscle mass is regenerated, and then either interrupt the feeding solution or convert to a more balanced carbohydrate-fat caloric substrate in order to reduce carbon dioxide production, allowing for ventilation weaning.

The second form of respiratory failure results from loss of chemoreceptor sensitivity as outlined earlier. Receptors sensitive to hypoxic states are impaired by combined protein-caloric depletion, whereas chemoreceptors sensitive to hypercarbia are impaired mainly by protein depletion. Sensitivity of both receptors is rapidly restored with nutritional support.

Frequently, critically ill patients also have chronic obstructive pulmonary disease. In selected cases, these patients can be weaned from respirators and gradually advanced to a significantly improved quality of life with instigation of aggressive intravenous nutritional support coupled with an active physical therapy program (73a).

Cardiac Failure

Cardiac dysfunction in the malnourished, critically ill patient can occur by two mechanisms (69). In the first, patients have intrinsic cardiac disease such as valvular or coronary artery disease, which leads to progressive cardiac failure and subsequent decreased nutritional intake and cardiac cachexia. Attempts at nutritional rehabilitation without correction of the intrinsic cardiac disease, and sometimes even after correction of their cardiac disease, can be catastrophic. The additional burden on the myocardium of regenerated body cell mass can lead to irreversible cardiac failure. Maintenance of body cell mass should be the priority rather than restoration of normal body cell mass. Only as myocardial function improves should one attempt to increase body mass.

Other patients present with malnutrition as a primary diagnosis with subsequent nutritional injury to the myocardium and cardiac failure. They demonstrate the same picture of cardiac cachexia but require nutritional support as specific therapy. Nutritional support is begun slowly and advanced gradually, allowing time for recovery of myocardial function. Patients should be observed carefully for tachycardia and congestion as they are quite prone to develop congestive heart failure. An exercise program is important during nutritional rehabilitation.

Cancer

The value of nutritional support of patients with malignant processes remains controversial (14). Although it does not improve survival, there is evidence of improved tolerance and response to therapy and improved quality of life. Cancer patients often demonstrate a marked increase in metabolic rate and altered metabolic pathways probably because of an effect of the cancer on the host. Failure to meet the increased metabolic demands results in rapid development of cachexia. Hospitalized patients who undergo intensive chemotherapy, radiotherapy, or surgical therapy should be nutritionally supported during their therapy to afford the best change of response. On the other hand, patients who have no further effective therapeutic intervention available and who are terminally ill should not have intravenous nutritional support initiated.

Burns

Data are now available supporting the use of intensive nutritional support in patients with extensive body burns (28). The increase in metabolic rate is well documented and complications resulting from rapid nutritional decay are extensively reported. Often nutritional support is administered solely via the gastrointestinal tract, but at times supplementation via the intravenous route is also required. As with volume supplementation in burn patients, formulas have been developed to calculate nitrogen and caloric requirements based on the degree and percent of body burn.

Spinal Cord Injury

Little is known of the metabolic requirements of the patient with spinal cord injury. Psychological stress is felt to increase basal metabolic rate, whereas neurological injury eliminates much muscular activity. Denervation of skeletal muscles results in mandatory wasting of skeletal muscle mass, rendering nitrogen balance studies of little value. Of some value is actual measurement of oxygen consumption and carbon dioxide production to determine the RME.

References

1. Abel RM, Fischer JE, Buckley ML, et al: Malnutrition in cardiac surgical patients. *Arch Surg* 111:45–50, 1976.
1a. Abel RM, Shik VE, Abbott WM, et al: Amino acid metabolism in acute renal failure: Influence of intravenous essential L-amino acid hyperalimentation therapy. *Ann Surg* 180:350–355, 1974.
2. Addis P, Poo LJ, Lew W: The quantities of proteins lost by the various organs and tissues of the body during a fast. *J Biol Chem* 115:111–116, 1936.
3. Alfrey AC: Disorders of magnesium metabolism. In Shrier RW: *Renal and Electrolyte Disorders* Boston, Little, Brown, 1976, pp 223–242.

4. Anderson GH, Patel DG, Jeejeebhoy KN: Design and evaluation by nitrogen balance and blood aminograms of an amino acid mixture for total parenteral nutrition of adults with gastrointestinal disease. *J Clin Invest* 53:904–912, 1974.

5. Askanazi J, Weissman C, Rosenbaum SH, et al: Nutrition and the respiratory system. *Crit Care Med* 10:163–172, 1982.

6. Askanazi J, Carpentier YA, Elwyn DH, et al: Influence of total parenteral nutrition on fuel utilization in injury and sepsis. *Ann Surg* 191:40–46, 1980.

7. Beal JM, Frost PM, Smith JL: The influence of caloric and potassium intake on nitrogen retention in man. *Ann Surg* 138:842–845, 1953.

8. Binder HJ, Hertin DC, Hurst V, et al: Tocopherol deficiency in man. *N Engl J Med* 273:1287–1297, 1965.

9. Bingham JG, Krischer JP, Shuster JJ et al: Effects of nutrition on length of stay and survival for burned patients. *Burns* 7:252–257, 1981.

10. Bistrian BR, Sherman M, Blackburn GL, et al: Cellular immunity in adult marasmus. *Arch Intern Med* 137:408–412, 1977.

11. Black PR, Brooks DC, Bessey PQ, et al: Mechanisms of insulin resistance following injury. *Ann Surg* 196:420–435, 1982.

11a. Blackburn GL, Moldawer LL, Usui S, et al: Branched chain amino acid administration and metabolism during starvation, injury and infection. *Surgery* 86:307–315, 1979.

12. Blennow G: Wernicke's encephalopathy following prolonged artificial nutrition. *Am J Dis Child* 129:1456, 1975.

13. Borja AR: Current status of infraclavicular subclavian vein catheterization. *Ann Thorac Surg* 13:615–624, 1972.

13a. Borum PR (ed): Role of carnitine supplementation in clinical nutrition. In *Clinical Aspects of Human Carnitine Deficiency.* Pergamon Press, NY, 1986.

14. Brennan MF: Total parenteral nutrition in the cancer patient. *N Engl J Med* 305:375–382, 1981.

15. Brenner S, Jacob F, Meselson M: An unstable intermediate carrying information from genes to ribosomes for protein synthesis. *Nature (Lond)* 190:576–581, 1961.

15a. Brown MR, Cohen HJ, Lyons JM, et al: Proximal muscle weakness and selenium deficiency associated with long term parenteral nutrition. *Am J Clin Nutr* 43:549–554, 1986.

16. Buchanan N, Davis MD, Eyberg C: Gentamycin pharmacokinetics in kwashiorkor. *Br J Clin Pharmacol* 8:451–453, 1979.

16a. Burke JF, Wolfe RR, Mullany CJ, et al: Glucose requirements following burn injury. *Ann Surg* 190:274–285, 1979.

17. Burni C, Krischak G: Techniques and complications of administration of total parenteral nutrition. In Manni C, Magalini SI, Scrascia E: *Total Parenteral Nutrition.* New York, American Elsevier, 1976, pp 306–315.

18. Caldwell MD, Jonsson HT, Othersen HB Jr: Essential fatty acid deficiency in an infant receiving prolonged parenteral alimentation. *J Pediatr* 81:894–898, 1972.

19. Carlisle EM: Silicon: an essential element for the chick. *Science* 178:619–521, 1972.

19a. Cerra FB: A multi-center trial of branched chain enriched amino acid infusion (FO80) in hepatic encephalopathy. *Hepatology* 2:699, 1982.

19b. Cerra FB, Mazuski JE, Chute E, et al: Branched chain metabolic support. A prospective, randomized, double-blind trial in surgical stress. *Ann Surg* 199:286–291, 1984.

20. Chandra RK: Reduced bactericidal capacity of polymorphs in iron deficiency. *Arch Dis Child* 48:864–866, 1973.

21. Clark I: Effect of cortisone upon protein synthesis. *J Biol Chem* 200:69–76, 1953.

22. Committee on Trauma, National Academy of Sciences-National Research Council: Postoperative wound, infections: the influence of ultraviolet irradiation of the operating room and of various other factors. *Ann Surg (Suppl)* 16:1–192, 1964.

23. Conn J: Hypertension, the potassium ion and impaired carbohydrate tolerance. *N Engl J Med* 273:1135–1142, 1965.

24. Coppa GF, Gouge TH, Hofstetter SR: Air embolism: a lethal but preventable complication of subclavian vein catheterization. *J Parent Enter Nutr* 5:116–168, 1981.

25. Cooper BA, Lowenstein L: Relative folate deficiency of erythrocytes in pernicious anemia and its correction with cyanocobalamin. *Blood* 24:502–521, 1964.

26. Craddock PR, Yawata Y, Van Santen L, et al: Acquired phagocyte dysfunction. A complication of the hypophosphatemia of parenteral hyperalimentation. *N Engl J Med* 290:1403–1407, 1974.

27. Cruse PJE, Foord R: A five-year prospective study of 23,649 surgical wounds. *Arch Surg* 107:206–210, 1973.

28. Curreri PW: Nutritional support of burn patients. *World J Surg* 2:215–221, 1978.

29. Cuthbertson DP: The disturbances of metabolism produced by bony and non-bony injury, with notes on certain abnormal conditions of bone. *Biochem J* 24:1224–1263, 1930.

30. Daly JM, Lawson M, Speir A: Intravenous access in chemotherapy patients. *Int Adv Surg Oncol* 4:59–82, 1981.

31. Dietary Allowances Committee and Food and Nutrition Board: *Recommended Dietary Allowances,* ed 8. Washington, DC, National Academy of Sciences, 1974.

32. Docomal M, Cantos JW: Hyperosmolar nonketotic coma complicating intravenous hyperalimentation. *Surg Gynecol Obstet* 136:729–732, 1973.

33. Doekel RC, Zwillich CW, Scoggin CH, et al: Clinical semi-starvation: depression of the hypoxic ventilatory response. *N Engl J Med* 295:358–361, 1976.

34. Doisy EA Jr: Micronutrient control on biosynthesis of clotting proteins and cholesterol. In Hemphill DD: *Proceedings of the University of Missouri's 6th Annual Conference on Trace Substances in Environmental Health.* Columbia, MO, University of Missouri Press, 1973, p 193.

35. Dudrick SJ, MacFaydyen BV Jr, Van Buren CT, et al: Parenteral hyperalimentation. Metabolic problems and solutions. *Ann Surg* 176:259–264, 1972.

36. Eckart J, Tempel G, Schreiber V, et al: The turnover of I-125-labeled serum albumin after surgery and injury. In Wilkinson AW: *Parenteral Nutrition.* Edinburgh, Churchill Livingstone, 1972, pp 288–298.

37. Eichner ER, Pierce HI, Hillman RS: Folate balance in dietary-induced megaloblastic anemia. *N Engl J Med* 284:933–938, 1971.

38. Fischer JE, Rosen HM, Ebeid AM, et al: The effect of normalization of plasma amino acids on hepatic encephalopathy in man. *Surgery* 80:77–91, 1976.

39. Fleck A: Metabolic response to injury. In Ledingham IM, Mackay G: *Jamieson and Kay's Textbook of Surgical Physiology.* New York, Churchill Livingstone, 1978.

39a. Fleming CR, Lie JT, McCall JT, et al: Selenium deficiency and fatal cardiomyopathy in a patient on home parenteral nutrition. *Gastroenterology* 83:689–693, 1982.

40. Flynn A, Strain WH, Pories WJ, et al: Zinc deficiency with altered adrenocortical function and its relation to delayed healing. *Lancet* 1:789–791, 1973.

41. Fourman PS: Experimental observations of the tetany of potassium deficiency. *Lancet* 2:575, 1954.

42. Gabow P: Disorders of potassium metabolism. In Schrier RW: *Renal and Electrolyte Disorders.* Boston, Little, Brown, 1976, pp 143–165.

43. Garrow JS: Protein nutrition and wound healing. *Proc Nutr Soc* 28:242–248, 1969.

44. Ghadimi H, Abaci F, Kumar S, et al: Biochemical aspects of intravenous alimentation. *Pediatrics* 48:955–965, 1971.

44a. Goodenough RD, Wolfe RR: Effect of total parenteral nutrition on free fatty acid metabolism in burned patients. *J Parent Enter Nutri* 8:357–360, 1984.

45. Gracey M, Suharjono S, Stone DE: Microbial contamination of the gut: another feature of malnutrition. *Am J Clin Nutr* 26:1170–1174, 1973.

46. Grant JP: *Handbook of Total Parenteral Nutrition.* Philadelphia, WB Saunders, 1980.

47. Grant JP: Clinical impact of protein malnutrition on organ mass and function. In Blackburn GL, Grant JP, Young VR: *Amino Acids Metabolism and Medical Applications.* Boston, John Wright PSG Inc., 1983, pp 347–358.

48. Grant JP, Cox CE, Kleinman LM: Serum hepatic enzyme and bilirubin elevations during parenteral nutrition. *Surg Gynecol Obstet* 145:573–580, 1977.

48a. Grant J, Snyder P: Use of L-glutamine in TPN. *J Surg Res* (in press).

49. Green HL, Nemir P Jr: Air embolism as a complication during parenteral alimentation. *Am J Surg* 121:614–616, 1971.

50. Greenlaw C: Liver enzyme elevations associated with total parenteral nutrition. *Drug Intell Clin Pharm* 14:702–709, 1980.

51. Gross L, Brotman M: Hypoprothrombinemia and hemorrhage associated with cholestyramine therapy. *Ann Intern Med* 72:95–96, 1970.

52. Groves AC, Griffiths J, Leung F, et al: Plasma catecholamines in patients with serious postoperative infection. *Ann Surg* 178:102–107, 1973.

53. Guidelines for Essential Trace Element Preparations for Parenteral Use: A statement by the Nutrition Advisory Group *J Paren Enter Nutr* 3:263–267, 1979.

54. Guidelines for Essential Trace Element Preparations for Parenteral use. AMA Department of Foods and Nutrition. *JAMA* 241:2051–2054, 1979.

55. Guidelines for Infectious Control in Hyperalimentation Therapy: National Nosocomial Infection Study Quarterly Report, May, 1972, p 22.

56. Guyton AC: *Textbook of Medical Physiology*, ed 4. Philadelphia, WB Saunders, 1971, p 437.

56a. Hall RI, Grant JP, Ross HL, et al: Pathogenesis of hepatic steatosis in the parenterally fed rat. *J Clin Invest* 74:1658–1668, 1984.

56b. Hallberg D: Studies on the elimination of exogenous lipids from the bloodstream. The effect of fasting and surgical trauma in man on the elimination rate of a fat emulsion injected intravenously. *Acta Physiol Scand* 65:151–163, 1965.

57. Hambidge RM, Hambidge C, Jacobs M, et al: Low levels of zinc in hair, anorexia, poor growth, and hypogeusia in children. *Pediatr Res* 6:868–874, 1972.

58. Hambidge KM, Neldnes KH, Walravens PA: Zinc and acrodermatitis, enteropathica. In Hambidge KM, Nichols BL (eds): *Zinc and Copper in Clinical Medicine.* New York, Spectrum Publications, 1978, pp 81–98.

59. Hansen AE, Haggard ME, Boeloche AN, et al: Essential fatty acids in infant nutrition. III. Clinical manifestations of linoleic acid deficiency. *J Nutr* 66:565–576, 1958.

60. Hansen LM, Hardie WR, Hidalgo J: Fat emulsion for intravenous administration: clinical experience with intralipid 10%. *Ann Surg* 184:80–88, 1976.

61. Harken AH, Woods M: The influence of oxyhemoglobin affinity on tissue oxygen consumption. *Ann Surg* 183:130–135, 1976.

62. Harris JA, Benedict FG: Biometric studies of basal metabolism in man. Carnegie Institution of Washington, Publication No. 279, 1919.

62a. Harvey KB, Moldawer LL, Bistrian BR, et al: Biological measures for the formation of a hospital prognostic index. *Am J Clin Nutr* 34:2013–2022, 1981.

63. Heird WC, Dell RB, Driscoll JM Jr, et al: Metabolic acidosis resulting from intravenous alimentation mixtures containing synthetic amino acids. *N Engl J Med* 287:943–948, 1972.

64. Heird WC, Driscoll JM, Schullinger JN, et al: Intravenous alimentation in pediatric patients. *J Pediatr* 80:351–372, 1972.

65. Heller RM, Kirchner SG, O'Neill JA Jr, et al: Skeletal changes of copper deficiency in infants receiving prolonged total parenteral nutrition. *J Pediatr* 92:947–948, 1978.

66. Henzel JH, DeWeese MS, Pories WJ: Significance of magnesium and zinc metabolism in the surgical patient. *Arch Surg* 95:991–999, 1967.

67. Herbert V: Experimental nutritional folate deficiency in men. *Trans Assoc Am Physicians* 75:307–320, 1962.

68. Heymsfield SB, Bethel RA, Ansley JD, et al: Cardiac abnormalities in cachectic patients before and during nutritional repletion. *Am Heart J* 95:584–594, 1978.

69. Heymsfield SB, Smith J, Redd S, et al: Nutritional support in cardiac failure. *Surg Clin North Am* 61:635–652, 1981.

70. Hodges RE, Hood J, Canham JE, et al: Clinical manifestations of ascorbic acid deficiency in man. *Am J Clin Nutr* 24:432–443, 1971.

71. Holcroft JW, Trunkey DD: Pulmonary extravasation of albumin during and after hemorrhagic shock in baboons. *J Surg Res* 18:91–97, 1975.

72. Holman RT: The ratio of trienoic-tetraenoic acids in tissue lipids as a measure of essential fatty acid requirement. *J Nutr* 70:405–410, 1960.

73. Holman RT: Essential fatty acid deficiency. *Prog Chem Fats Other Lipids* 9:329–331, 1971.

73a. Horst D, Graze N, Conn HO: A double-blind randomized comparison of dietary protein and an oral branched chain amino acid (BCAA) solution in cirrhotic patients with chronic portal-systemic encephalopathy. *Hepatology* 2:184, 1982.

74. Horwitt MK, Harvey CC, Duncan GD, et al: Symposium on the role of some of the newer vitamins in human metabolism and nutrition; effects of limited tocopherol intake in man with relationships to erythrocyte hemolysis and lipid oxidations. *Am J Clin Nutr* 4:408–419, 1956.

75. Host WR, Serlin O, Rush BF Jr: Hyperalimentation in cirrhotic patients. *Am J Surg* 123:57–62, 1971.

76. Howland WS, Schweizer O, Ragasa J, et al: Colloid oncotic pressure and levels of albumin and total protein during major surgical procedures. *Surg Gynecol Obstet* 143:592–596, 1976.

77. Hume DM: The neuro-endocrine response to injury: present status of the problem. *Ann Surg* 138:548–557, 1953.

78. Itokawa Y, Schultz RA, Cooper JR: Thiamine in nerve membranes. *Biochim Biophys Acta* 266:293–299, 1972.

79. Jackson CM: Effect of acute and chronic inanition upon the relative weights of the various organs and systems of adult albino rats. *Am J Anat* 18:75–116, 1915.

80. Jacob HS, Amsden T: Acute hemolytic anemia with rigid red cells in hypophosphatemia. *N Engl J Med* 285:1446–1450, 1971.

81. James JH, Jeppsson B, Ziparo V, et al: Hyperammonaemia, plasma amino acid imbalance, and blood-brain amino acid transport: A unified theory of portal-systemic encephalopathy. *Lancet* 2:772–775, 1979.

82. Jeejeebhoy KN, Chu RC, Marliss EB, et al: Chromium deficiency, glucose intolerance, and neuropathy reversed by chromium supplementation in a patient receiving long-term total parenteral nutrition. *Am J Clin Nutr* 30:531–538, 1977.

83. Jeejeebhoy KN, Langer B, Tsallas G, et al: Total parenteral nutrition at home: studies in patients surviving 4 months to 5 years. *Gastroenterology* 71:943–953, 1976.

84. Johnson CL, Lazarchick J, Lynn HI: Subclavian venipuncture: preventable complications; report of two cases. *Mayo Clin Proc* 45:712–719, 1970.

85. Joynson DHM, Walker DM, Jacobs A, et al: Defect of cell-mediataed immunity in patients with iron-deficiency anaemia. *Lancet* 2:1058–1059, 1972.

86. Kaminski DL, Adams A, Jellinek M: The effect of hyperalimentation on hepatic lipid content and lipogenic enzyme activity in rats and man. *Surgery* 88:93–100, 1980.

87. Kay RG, Tasman-Jones C, Pybus J, et al: A syndrome of acute zinc deficiency during total parenteral alimentation in man. *Ann Surg* 183:331–340, 1976.

88. Kay RG, Tasman-Jones C: Acute zinc deficiency in man during intravenous alimentation. *Aust NZ J Surg* 45:325–330, 1975.

88a. Kern KA, Bower RJ, Atamian S, et al: The effect of a new branched chain-enriched amino acid solution on postoperative catabolism. *Surgery* 92:780–785, 1982.

89. Keys A, Brozek J, Henschel A, et al: *The Biology of Human Starvation*. Minneapolis, University of Minnesota Press, 1950, pp 714–748.

90. Keys A, Brozek J, Henschel A, et al: *The Biology of Human Starvation*. Minneapolis, University of Minnesota Press, 1950, pp 601–606.

91. Kilsell ME: Vitamin B_6 in metabolism of the nervous system. *Ann NY Acad Sci* 166:1–364, 1969.

92. Kim CS, Hill CH: The interrelationship of dietary copper and amine oxidase in the formation of elastin. *Biochem Biophys Res Commun* 24:395–400, 1966.

93. Kinney JM, Long CL, Duke JH: Carbohydrate and nitrogen metabolism after injury. In Porter R, Knight J: *Injury Metabolism in Trauma*. London, J & A Churchill, 1970, p 103.

94. Kinney JM: The metabolic response to injury. In Richards JR, Kinney JM: *Nutritional Aspects of Care in the Critically Ill*. New York, Churchill Livingstone, 1977.

95. Kinney JM: *Energy requirements of the surgical patient*. In American College of Surgeons, Committee on Pre- and Postoperative Care: *Manual of Surgical Nutrition*. Philadelphia, WB Saunders, 1975, pp. 233–234.

96. Klein PD, Johnson RM: Phosphorus metabolism in unsaturated fatty acid deficient rats. *J Biol Chem* 211:103–110, 1954.

97. Klingman AM: Pathologic dynamics of human hair loss. *Arch Dermatol* 83:175–198, 1961.

98. Krishnaswamy K, Naidu AN: Microsomal enzymes in malnutrition as determined by plasma half life of antipyrine. *Br Med J* 1:538–540, 1977.

99. Klahr S, Tipathy K, Garcia FT, et al: On the nature of the renal concentrating defect in malnutrition. *Am J Med* 43:84–95, 1967.

100. Klahr S, Tipathy K, Lotero H: Renal regulation of acid-base in malnourished man. *Am J Med* 48:325–331, 1970.

101. Krieger M: Ueber die Atrophie der menschlichen Organe bei Inanition. *Z Angew Anat Konstitutional* 7:87–134, 1921.

102. Lake AM, Stuart MJ, Oski FA: Vitamin E deficiency and enhanced platelet function. Reversal following E supplementation. *J Pediatr* 90:722–725, 1977.

103. Langer B, McHattie JD, Zohrab WJ, et al: Prolonged survival after complete bowel resection using intravenous alimentation at home. *J Surg Res* 15:226–233, 1973.

104. Law DK, Dudrick SJ, Abdou HI: Immunocompetence of patients with protein-calorie malnutrition: the side effects of nutritional repletion. *Ann Intern Med* 79:545–550, 1973.

104a. Lawson LJ: Parenteral nutrition in surgery. *Br J Surg* 52:795–800, 1965.

105. Leach RM Jr, Muenstes AM, Wien EM: Studies on the role of manganese in bone formation. II. Effect upon chondroitin sulfate syntheses in chick epiphyseal cartilage. *Arch Biochem Biophys* 133:22–28, 1969.

106. Lehninger AL: The enzymatic and morphologic organization of the mitochondria. *Pediatrics* 26:466–475, 1960.

107. Levin PH: A qualitative platelet defect in severe vitamin B_{12} deficiency. Response, hyperresponse, and thrombosis after vitamin B_{12} therapy. *Ann Intern Med* 78:533–539, 1973.

108. Levine R: Analysis of the actions of the hormonal antagonists of insulin. *Diabetes* 13:362–365, 1964.

109. Levine R, Haft DE: Carbohydrate homeostasis. *N Engl J Med* 283:175–183, 1970.

110. Linder MC, Munro HN: Iron and copper metabolism during development. *Enzyme* 15:111–138, 1973.

110a. Lindholm M, Rossner S: Rate of elimination of the Intralipid fat emulsion from the circulation in ICU patients. *Crit Care Med* 10:740–746, 1982.

111. Long CL, Schaffel N, Geiger JW, et al: Metabolic response to injury and illness: estimation of energy and protein needs from indirect calorimetry and nitrogen balance. *J Paren Enter Nutr* 3:452–456, 1979.

112. Long CL, Kinney JM, Gerger JW: Nonsuppressability of gluconeogenesis by glucose in septic patients. *Metabolism* 25:193–201, 1976.

113. Long JM III, Wilmore DW, Mason AD Jr, et al: Effect of carbohydrate and fat intake on nitrogen excretion during total parenteral feeding. *Ann Surg* 185:417–422, 1977.

113a. Lopes J, Russell D, Whitwell J, et al: Skeletal muscle function in malnutrition. *Am J Clin Nutr* 36:602–610, 1982.

114. Lowry SF, Brennan MF: Abnormal liver function during parenteral nutrition: relation to infusion excess. *J Surg Res* 26:300–307, 1979.

115. Macht SD: A technique for evaluating sepsis in TPN patients. *J Paren Enter Nutr* 1:92–99, 1977.

116. Maini B, Blackburn GL, Bistrian BR: Cyclic hyperalimentation: an optimal technique for preservation of visceral protein. *J Surg Res* 20:515–525, 1976.

116a. Maiz A, Yamazaki K, Sobrado J, et al: Protein metabolism during total parenteral nutrition in injured rats using medium-chain triglycerides. *Metabolism* 33:901–909, 1984.

117. Marco J, Calle C, Roman D, et al: Hyperglucagonism induced by glucocorticoid treatment in man. *N Engl J Med* 288:128–131, 1973.

118. Mayoral LG, Tripathy K, Bolanos O, et al: Intestinal, functional, and morphologic abnormalities in severely protein-malnourished adults. *Am J Clin Nutr* 25:1084–1091, 1972.

119. McClain CJ: Trace metal abnormalities in adults during hyperalimentation. *J Paren Enter Nutr* 5:424–429, 1981.

120. Mecray PM Jr, Barden RP, Ravdin IS: Nutritional edema: its effect on gastric emptying time before and after gastric operations. *Surgery* 1:53–64, 1927.

121. Meguid M, Brennan MF, Aoki TT, et al: Hormone-substrate interrelationships following trauma. *Arch Surg* 109:776–783, 1974.

122. Meurling S, Plantin LO: The concentrations of trace elements in blood from healthy newborn infants. *Acta Chir Scand* 147:481–485, 1981.

122a. Millikan WJ, Henderson JM, Warren WD, et al: Total parenteral nutrition with FO80 in cirrhotics with subclinical encephalopathy. *Ann Surg* 52:294–304, 1983.

123. Moore FD: *Metabolic Care of the Surgical Patient*. Philadelphia, WB Saunders, 1959, p 460.

124. Moore FD, Steenburg RW, Ball MR, et al: Studies in surgical endocrinology. I. The urinary excretion of 17-hydroxycorticoids, and associated metabolic changes in cases of soft tissue trauma of varying severity and in bone trauma. *Ann Surg* 141:145–174, 1955.

125. Moore FD, Megurd MM: Homeostasis and nutrition in the surgical patient: The metabolic and endocrine re-

sponse to injury. In Byrne JJ, Goldsmith HS: *General Surgery I.* Philadelphia, Harper & Row, 1982.

126. Moore FD: *Metabolic Care of the Surgical Patient.* Philadelphia, WB Saunders, 1959.

127. Moore FD, Ball MR: *The Metabolic Response to Surgery.* Springfield, IL, Charles C Thomas, 1952.

128. Moore FD: Homeostasis: bodily changes in trauma and surgery. In Sabiston DC: *Davis-Christopher Textbook of Surgery,* ed 11. Philadelphia, WB Saunders, 1977, pp 27–64.

129. Moran LR, Thurlow J, Custer P, et al: Nutritional assessment as a predictor of physical performance (abstr). *J Paren Enter Nutr* 3:514, 1980.

130. Moss G: Postoperative metabolism. The role of plasma albumin in the absorption of water and electrolytes. *Pacific Med Surg* 75:355–358, 1967.

131. Mullen JL: Consequences of malnutrition in the surgical patient. *Surg Clin North Am* 61:465–487, 1981.

132. Multivitamin Preparations for Parenteral Use: A statement by the Nutrition Advisory Group. *J Paren Enter Nutr* 3:258–262, 1979.

133. Munro HN: General aspects of the regulation of protein metabolism by diet and hormones. In Munro HN, Allison JB: *Mammalian Protein Metabolism.* New York, Academic Press, 1964, vol 1, pp 381–481.

133a. Nachbauer CA, James JH, Edwards LL, et al: Infusion of branched chain-enriched amino acid solutions in sepsis. *Am J Surg* 147:743–752, 1984.

134. Nielsen FH, Ollerich DA: Nickel: a new essential trace element. *Fed Proc* 33:1767–1772, 1974.

135. Nitowsky HM, Tildon JT, Levin S, et al: Studies of tocopherol deficiency in infants and children. VII. The effect of tocopherol on urinary, plasma, and muscle creatine. *Am J Clin Nutr* 10:368–378, 1962.

136. O'Dell BL, Campbell BJ: Trace elements: metabolism and metabolic function. In Florkin M, Stotz E: *Comprehensive Biochemistry.* New York, Elsevier North-Holland, 1971, p 223.

137. Oji N, Shreeve WW: Gluconeogenesis from 14-C and 3-H-labeled substrates in normal and cortisone-treated rats. *Endocrinology* 78:765–772, 1966.

138. Olson RE: Proceeding of a conference on beriberi. *Fed Proc* 17 (Suppl 2):24–27, 1958.

139. Omdahl JL, Deluca HF: Vitamin D. In Goodheart RS, Shils ME: *Modern Nutrition in Health and Disease,* ed 5. Philadelphia, Lea & Febiger, 1973, pp 158–165.

140. Oppel TW: Studies of biotin metabolism in man; excretion of biotin in human urine, relationship between biotin content of diet and its output in urine and feces; excretion of 2 biotin-like substances in urine. *Am J Med Sci* 204:856–875, 1942.

141. Oppenheimer MJ, Durant TM, Lynch P: Body position in relation to venous air embolism and the associated cardiovascular respiratory changes. *Am J Med Sci* 225:362–373, 1953.

142. Ordway CB: Air embolus via CVP catheter without positive pressure: presentation of case and review. *Ann Surg* 179:479–481, 1974.

143. Owen CA Jr, Tyce GM, Glock EV, et al: Heparin-ascorbic acid antagonism. *Mayo Clin Proc* 45:140–145, 1970.

144. Parsa MH, Habif DV, Ferrer JM, et al: Intravenous hyperalimentation: Indications, technique and complications. *Bull NY Acad Med* 48:920–942, 1972.

145. Paskin DL, Hoffman WS, Tuddenham WJ: A new complication of subclavian vein catheterization. *Ann Surg* 179:266–268, 1974.

146. Passmore R, Nicol BM, Rao MN, et al: Handbook of human nutritional requirements. *WHO Monogr Ser* 0(61):1–66, 1974.

147. Patel SM, Mehl JW, Denel HJ Jr: Studies on carotenoid metabolism; site of conversion of cryptoxanthen to vitamin A in the rat. *Arch Biochem Biophys* 30:103–109, 1951.

148. Peden JC: Present knowledge of iron and copper. *Nutr Rev* 25:321–324, 1967.

149. Peden VH, Witzelben CL, Skelton MA: Total parenteral nutrition. *J Pediatr* 78:180, 1971.

150. Pekarek RS, Sandstead HH, Jacob RA, et al: Abnormal cellular responses during acquired zinc deficiency. *Ann J Clin Nutr* 32:1466–1471, 1979.

151. Perley M, Kipnis DM: Effects of glucocorticoids on plasma insulin. *N Engl J Med* 274:1237–1241, 1966.

152. Popper H: Cholestasis. *Am Rev Med* 19:39–56, 1968.

153. Pories WJ, Strain WH: Zinc and wound healing. In Prasad AS: *Zinc Metabolism.* Springfield, IL, Charles C Thomas, 1966, p 378.

154. Porte D, Robertson RP: Control of insulin secretion by catecholamine, stress, and the sympathetic nervous system. *Fed Proc* 32:1792–1796, 1973.

155. Prasad AS, Miale A Jr, Farid Z, et al: Zinc metabolism in patients with the syndrome of iron deficiency anemia, hepatosplenomegaly, dwarfism, and hypogonadism. *J Lab Clin Med* 61:537–549, 1963.

156. Press M, Hartop PJ, Prottey C: Correction of essential fatty acid deficiency in man by the cutaneous application of sunflower seed oil. *Lancet* 1:597–599, 1974.

156a. Quercia RA, Korn S, O'Neill D, et al: Selenium deficiency and fatal cardiomyopathy in a patient receiving long-term home parenteral nutrition. *Clin Pharmacol* 3:531–535, 1984.

157. Rappazzo ME, Salmi HA, Hall CA: The content of vitamin B_{12} in adult and foetal tissue: a comparative study. *Br J Haematol* 18:425–433, 1970.

158. Rector FC JR: Acidification of the urine. In Orloff J, Berline RW, Geiger SR: *Handbook of Physiology.* Washington, DC, American Physiological Society, 1973, p 447.

159. Reinhardt GF, Myscofski JW, Wilkens DB, et al: Incidence and mortality of hypoalbuminemic patients in hospitalized veterans. *J Paren Enter Nutr* 4:357–359, 1980.

160. Richert DA, Westerfeld WW: Isolation and identification of the xanthene oxidase factor as molybdenum. *J Biol Chem* 203:915–923, 1953.

161. Roels OA, Lui NST: The vitamins. Vitamin A and carotene. In Goodheart RS, Shils ME: *Modern Nutrition in Health and Disease,* ed 5. Philadelphia, Lea & Febiger, 1973, pp 142–157.

162. Roels OA: Present knowledge of vitamin E. In *Present Knowledge in Nutrition,* ed 3. New York, Nutrition Foundation, 1967, pp 86–88.

162a. Ross LH, Griffeth L, Hall RI, et al: Elimination of hepatotoxicity of total parenteral nutrition using fat-carbohydrate mixture. *Surg Forum* 35:97–99, 1984.

163. Rothschild MA, Oratz M, Schreiber SS: Albumin synthesis. *N Engl J Med* 286:748–757, 816–821, 1972.

164. Rudman D, Millikan WJ, Richardson TJ, et al: Elemental balances during intravenous hyperalimentation of underweight adult subjects. *J Clin Invest* 55:94–104, 1975.

165. Rush BF Jr, Richardson JD, Griffen WO: Positive nitrogen balance immediately after abdominal operations. *Am J Surg* 119:70–76, 1970.

166. Ryan JA, Abel RM, Abbott WM, et al: Catheter complications in total parenteral nutrition. *N Engl J Med* 290:757–761, 1974.

167. Sanderson I, Deitel M: Intravenous hyperalimentation without sepsis. *Surg Gynecol Obstet* 136:572–585, 1973.

168. Sanderson I, Deitel M: Insulin response in patients receiving concentrated infusions of glucose and casein hydrolysate for complete parenteral nutrition. *Ann Surg* 179:387–394, 1974.

169. Sauberlich HE, Herman YF, Stevens CO: Thiamine requirements of the adult human. *Am J Clin Nutr* 23:671–672, 1970.

170. Schumner W: The metabolic effects of trauma. *Contemp Surg* 1:39–45, 1972.

171. Schwartz K: Essentiality and metabolic functions of selenium. In Burch RE, Sullivan JF: *The Medical Clinics of North America Symposium on Trace Metals.* Philadelphia, WB Saunders, 1976, pp 745–758.

172. Schwarz K, Milne DB: Growth effect of vanadium in the rat. *Science* 174:426–428, 1971.

173. Schwarz K: Role of vitamin E, selenium, and related factors in experimental nutritional liver diseases. *Fed Proc* 20:58–67, 1965.

174. Seelig MS, Heggtveit HA: Magnesium interrelationships in ischemic heart disease: a review. *Am J Clin Nutr* 27:59–79, 1974.

175. Selvaraj RJ, Bhat KS: Phagocytosis and leukocyte enzymes in protein-calorie malnutrition. *Biochem J* 127:255–259, 1972.

176. Sheldon GF, Peterson SR, Sanders R: Hepatic dysfunction during hyperalimentations. *Arch Surg* 113:504–508, 1978.

176a. Sherwin RS, Hendler RG, Felig P: Effect of ketone infusions on amino acid and nitrogen metabolism. *J Clin Invest* 55:1382–1390, 1975.

177. Shils ME: Experimental human magnesium depletion. *Medicine* 48:61–81, 1969.

178. Shires T, O'Banion J: Successful treatment of massive air embolism producing cardiac arrest. *JAMA* 167:1483–1484, 1958.

179. Silvis SE, Paragas PD Jr: Paresthesias, weakness, seizures, and hypophosphatemia in patients receiving hyperalimentation. *Gastroenterology* 62:513–520, 1972.

180. Skillman JJ, Lauler DP, Hickler RB, et al: Hemorrhage in normal man: effect on renin, cortisol, aldosterone, and urine composition. *Ann Surg* 166:865–885, 1967.

181. Soderhjelm L, Wiese HF, Holman RT: The role of polyunsaturated acids in human nutrition and metabolism. *Prog Chem Fats Other Lipids* 9:555–585, 1970.

182. Steffee WP: Nutritional support in renal failure. *Surg Clin North Am* 61:661–670, 1981.

183. Sunde RA, Hoekstra WG: Structure, synthesis and function of glutathione peroxidase. *Nutr Rev* 38:265–273, 1980.

184. Suttie JW: Mechanism of action of vitamin K: demonstration of a liver precursor of prothrombin. *Science* 179:192–194, 1973.

184a. Tao RC, Yoshimura NN: Carnitine metabolism and its application in parenteral nutrition. *J Parent Enter Nutr* 4:469–486, 1980.

185. Tappel AL: Free-radical lipid peroxidation damage and its inhibition by vitamin E and selenium. *Fed Proc* 20:58–67, 1965.

186. Tashiro T, Ogata H, Yokoyama H, et al: The effects of fat emulsion on essential fatty acid deficiency during intravenous hyperalimentation in pediatric patients. *J Pediatr Surg* 10:203–213, 1975.

187. Tillotson JA, Baker EM: An enzymatic measurement of the riboflavin status in man. *Am J Clin Nutr* 25:425–431, 1972.

188. Todd WR, Elvehjem CA, Hart EB: Zinc in the nutrition of the rat. *Am J Physiol* 107:146–156, 1934.

189. Touloukian RJ, Downing SE: Cholestasis associated with long term parenteral hyperalimentation. *Arch Surg* 106:56–62, 1973.

190. Travis SF, Sugerman JH, Ruberg RL, et al: Alterations of red cell glycolytic intermediates and oxygen transport as a consequence of hypophosphatemia in patients receiving intravenous hyperalimentation. *N Engl J Med* 285:763–768, 1971.

191. Underwood EJ: *Trace Elements in Human and Animal Nutrition,* ed 3. New York, Academic Press, 1971, p 369.

192. Unger RH, Orci L: Physiology and pathophysiology of glucagon. *Physiol Rev* 56:778–826, 1976.

193. Van Rij AM, McKenzie JM, Thomson CD, et al: Selenium supplementation in total parenteral nutrition. *J Paren Enter Nutr* 5:120–124, 1981.

194. Van Rij AM, Thomson CD, McKenzie JM, et al: Selenium deficiency in total parenteral nutrition. *Am J Clin Nutr* 32:2076–2085, 1979.

194a. Vary TC, Siegel JH, Nakatani T, et al: Regulation of glucose metabolism by altered pyruvate dehydrogenase activity. I. Potential site of insulin resistance in sepsis. *JPEN* 10:351–355, 1986.

195. Vilter RW, Bozian RC, Hess EV, et al: Manifestations of copper deficiency in a patient with systemic sclerosis on intravenous hyperalimentation. *N Engl J Med* 291:188–191, 1974.

196. Vitale JJ, Nakamura M, Hegsted DM: The effect of magnesium deficiency on oxidative phosphorylation. *J Biol Chem* 228:573–576, 1957.

197. Wacker WEC, Parisi AF: Magnesium metabolism. *N Engl J Med* 278:658–662, 712–717, 772–776, 1968.

197a. Wahren J, Jacques D, Desurmont P, et al: Is intravenous administration of branched chain amino acids effective in the treatment of hepatic encephalopathy? *Hepatology* 3:475–480, 1983.

198. Walker BE, Dawson JB, Kelleher J, et al: Plasma and urinary zinc in patients with malabsorption syndromes or hepatic cirrhosis. *Gut* 14:943–948, 1973.

198a. Watson RD, Cannon RA, Kurland GS, et al: Selenium responsive myositis during prolonged home total parenteral nutrition in cystic fibrosis. *J Paren Enter Nutr* 9:58–60, 1985.

199. Waxman S, Corcino JJ, Herbert V: Drugs, toxins, and dietary amino acids affecting vitamin B_{12} or folic acid absorption or utilization. *Am J Med* 48:599–608, 1970.

200. Wayne L, Well JJ, Friedman BI, et al: Vitamin B_6 in internal medicine. *Arch Intern Med* 101:143–155, 1958.

201. Weinberg ED: Iron and susceptibility to infectious disease. *Science* 184:952–956, 1974.

202. Weintraub LR, Conrad ME, Crosby WH: Iron-loading anemia. Treatment with repeated phlebotomies and pyridoxine. *N Engl J Med* 275:169–176, 1966.

203. Weissman C, Askanazi J, Rosenbaum SH: Amino acids and respiration (in press).

204. Welt IO, Stetten D Jr: Effect of cortisone upon rates of glucose production and oxidation in the rat. *J Biol Chem* 197:57–66, 1952.

205. Wigger JH: Hepatic changes in premature infants receiving intravenous alimentation (abstr). Toronto, Pediatric Pathology Club, 1971.

206. Wilmore DW: *The Metabolic Management of the Critically Ill.* New York, Plenum Press, 1977, p 197.

207. Wilmore DW, Moylan JA, Bristow BF, et al: Anabolic effects of human growth hormone and high caloric feedings following thermal injury. *Surg Gynecol Obstet* 138:875–884, 1974.

208. Wright PD, Johnson IDA: The effect of surgical operation on growth hormone levels in a plasma. *Surgery* 77:479–486, 1975.

209. Zidar BL, Shaddus RK, Zeigler Z, et al: Observations on the anemia and neutropenia of human copper deficiency. *Am J Hematol* 3:177–185, 1977.

17

Divalent Ions: Calcium, Magnesium, and Phosphorus

Gary P. Zaloga, M.D., F.A.C.P., F.A.C.N.
Bart Chernow, M.D., F.A.C.P., F.C.C.P.

Calcium (Ca^{2+}), magnesium (Mg^{2+}), and phosphorus (PO_4) are divalent ions that are essential for normal body function. Disorders involving these ions are common in critically ill patients due to their underlying illnesses and the effects of administered drugs. This chapter discusses the pharmacology, homeostasis, causes, clinical features, and treatment of disorders involving these ions. The emphasis is placed upon those disorders most commonly seen in the critical care setting.

CALCIUM

Ca^{2+} is important in humans for both structural and biochemical integrity. The normal adult body contains approximately 1000–1400 g of Ca^{2+} of which 99% is in the skeleton and 1% is in the soft tissues and extracellular spaces. Ca^{2+} is the most abundant electrolyte in the human body. Skeletal Ca^{2+} supports and protects body tissues and serves as a storehouse, providing Ca^{2+} for physiologic requirements when dietary Ca^{2+} is unavailable. Loss of skeletal Ca^{2+} with aging (e.g., osteoporosis) is responsible for loss of height and fractures.

Ca^{2+} movement into the cell and release from intracellular sites is vital for the coupling of receptor-stimulated cell surface events to cellular responses (i.e., stimulus-response coupling). Ca^{2+} is required for muscle contraction (e.g., excitation-contraction coupling), hormonal and neurotransmitter secretion (i.e., stimulus-secretion coupling), cell division, cell motility, axonal flow, enzyme activity, cell membrane structure, and blood coagulation. It also plays a vital role in the cardiac action potential and is essential for cardiac pacemaker automaticity.

Measurement of Blood Calcium

Ca^{2+} circulates in the blood in three forms: an ionized fraction (50%), a protein bound (mostly to albumin) fraction (40%), and a diffusible but nonionized fraction in chelates with other circulating ions (10%). It is the ionized fraction that is thought to be physiologically active and homeostatically regulated. A determination of the total serum calcium concentration is the measurement that is performed in most hospital laboratories. However, alterations in the amount of protein present, the percentage of Ca^{2+} bound to protein, and the amount of Ca^{2+} bound in chelates may affect the total Ca^{2+} value independent of the ionized Ca^{2+} concentration (94, 109, 132, 133, 135).

A variety of factors can alter the serum total and ionized Ca^{2+} levels (15, 133). Protein bound Ca^{2+} (primarily albumin) represents a large proportion (40%) of the total serum Ca^{2+} concentration. Thus, alterations in a patient's serum albumin concentration can change that person's total serum Ca^{2+} measurement. Critically ill patients with low serum albumin levels characteristically have a low total serum Ca^{2+} value, while serum ionized Ca^{2+} measurements may be normal (135). On the other hand, a normal total serum Ca^{2+} level in the face of hypoalbuminemia may indicate ionized hypercalcemia. Elevations in serum protein levels (e.g., from albumin infusions, venostasis as a consequence of prolonged tourniquet use during phlebotomy, and rarely, myeloma) may also raise the total serum Ca^{2+} value and mask hypocalcemia.

Blood pH alters Ca^{2+} binding to serum proteins: acute acidosis decreases protein binding (increases the serum ionized Ca^{2+} concentration) while alkalosis increases protein binding (decreases ionized Ca^{2+}). Measurement of the total serum Ca^{2+} concentration in critically ill patients with acid-base changes may therefore give deceiving results. For example, a patient being therapeutically hyperventilated (e.g., in an attempt to reduce cerebral blood flow following head injury) may develop ionized hypocalcemia, without abnormalities in the total serum Ca^{2+} concentration, due to an alkalosis-induced increase in Ca^{2+} binding to proteins. Patients given bicarbonate for control of metabolic acidosis can also develop acute ionized hypocalcemia. Shifts in ionized Ca^{2+} induced by changes in arterial pH are usually small; however, occasionally, they may be associated with clinically important hypocalcemia. Patients most susceptible to hypocalcemia are those with an underlying abnormality in parathyroid hormone (PTH) and vitamin D metabolism.

Free fatty acids (FFA) constitute a major metabolic fuel for the body and are carried in the circulation bound to the albumin molecule. We (143) and others (3) have found that FFAs increase Ca^{2+} binding to albumin. Serum FFA levels increase during critical illness due to illness-induced elevations in plasma concentrations of epinephrine, glucagon, growth hormone, and corticotropin, as well as decreases in serum insulin concentrations. Elevations in FFA levels, sufficient to alter calcium binding, may also occur after the administration of heparin sodium, intravenous lipids, epinephrine, norepinephrine, isoproterenol, or with alcohol ingestion. These pharmacologic agents are commonly used in critically ill patients. Normal individuals have serum FFA concentrations of approximately 250 μmol/liter. Values of FFAs increase to 400–600 μmol/liter after an overnight fast and may rise to 1000 μmol/liter after prolonged fasting (72 hours). Severely stressed patients (e.g., those with acute pancreatitis, diabetic ketoacidosis, sepsis, or acute myocardial infarction) may have serum levels of 3000 μmol/liter. Increases in serum FFA levels in acutely ill and stressed patients may alter the distribution of Ca^{2+} between bound and unbound states. Alterations in Ca^{2+} binding occur in patients with acute pancreatitis, after heparin administration and after intravenous lipid administration (132, 143). FFAs may act as modulators of free Ca^{2+} levels in various pathologic states.

The timing and technique of venipuncture are important in the interpretation of serum Ca^{2+} values. Postprandial increases in serum Ca^{2+} levels of 1–2 mg/dl may occur. Postprandial increases in serum Ca^{2+} are higher and more prolonged in hyperabsorptive states such as hyperparathyroidism, vitamin D excess, and hypothyroidism. To avoid these changes, one should measure serum Ca^{2+} in the fasting state.

Changes in the concentration of chelating ions (e.g., phosphate, bicarbonate, albumin, and citrate) may also lower the circulating ionized Ca^{2+} level. Citrate is used as a blood preservative and anticoagulant. Citrate-induced decreases in ionized Ca^{2+} are usually transient, and without hemodynamic effect in most blood transfusion situations. Howland et al. (61) studied 100 patients who received blood during a variety of surgical procedures. Mean ionized Ca^{2+} levels decreased from 4.06 to 3.22 mg/dl (1.01 to 0.80 mmol/liter) while patients were receiving an average of 18.6 ml of blood per minute. Twenty of the 100 (20%) patients who received blood at this rate had ionized Ca^{2+} levels that fell below 2.5 mg/dl (0.62 mmol/liter) and 10 of the 100 patients (10%) had levels below 2 mg/dl (0.50 mmol/liter). Only one patient (1%) developed hypocalcemia-induced cardiovascular problems (e.g. hypotension). Kahn et al. (68) studied 53 patients undergoing a variety of surgical procedures. Serum-ionized Ca^{2+} levels decreased from a mean of 4.14 to 3.04 mg/dl (1.03 to 0.76 mmol/liter) during transfusion of blood at an average rate of 0.5 ml/kg/minute. However, hemodynamic variables remained stable throughout the period of observation, and ionized Ca^{2+} values returned to normal after discontinuation of the transfusion.

Decreases in ionized Ca^{2+} values during blood transfusion correlate with elevations in circulating citrate levels and speed of transfusion. Denlinger et al. (39) administered citrated blood to anaesthetized patients at rates of 50, 100, and 150 ml/70 kg/minute and found decreases in serum-ionized Ca^{2+} levels of 14%, 31%, and 41%, respectively. After a 5-minute blood transfusion period, ionized Ca^{2+} values returned to normal within 15 minutes, and this normalization correlated with metabolism of the citrate.

The metabolism of citrate is affected by tissue perfusion, acid-base status, and the activity of the rate limiting enzyme, aconitase, which is present in muscle, kidney, and liver. When transfusion rate exceeds citrate metabolism, citrate levels rise and ionized Ca^{2+} levels fall. Citrate may also chelate Mg^{2+}, causing hypomagnesemia, which in turn may accentuate hypocalcemia. Thus, when citrate clearance is impaired (e.g., in hypothermia or with renal or hepatic disease) or blood transfusion is rapid, plasma citrate levels may rise and cause clinically important hypocalcemia and cardiovascular insufficiency. The effect of citrate and other chelators on Ca^{2+} is accentuated in patients with underlying defects of the parathyroid–vitamin D axis. Similar decreases in ionized Ca^{2+} levels may occur after volume resuscitation with albumin, after intravenous injection of radiocontrast media, and after the intravenous administration of phosphates (132).

Heparin is capable of chelating with Ca^{2+}; however, heparin dosages capable of causing Ca^{2+} chelation are not obtained in vivo. However, adding heparin to syringes used to collect blood samples for measurement of ionized Ca^{2+} can significantly lower the ionized Ca^{2+} concentration. Thus, samples used for measurement of plasma or blood Ca^{2+} should use the smallest amount of heparin that will adequately anticoagulate blood. The amount of heparin added should be standardized and each laboratory performing ionized Ca^{2+} measurements should use their own normal values.

The serum-ionized Ca^{2+} value may be altered during hemodialysis, depending on the calcium concentration of the dialysate (58, 90, 132). Patients with renal failure are vulnerable to the hypocalcemic effects of dialysis because they have an impaired ability to hydroxylate vitamin D within the kidney and mobilize calcium. Maynard et al. (90) showed that the drop in blood pressure induced by hemodialysis was reduced when a high Ca^{2+} dialysate was used. Henrich et al. (58) demonstrated that ionized Ca^{2+} values during dialysis were key factors affecting left ventricular contractility, an increase in ionized Ca^{2+} being associated with improved contractility. These studies indicate that the Ca^{2+} composition of the dialysate baths can affect hemodynamics during dialysis. In fact, we have seen hypotensive episodes when critically ill patients were dialyzed against low Ca^{2+} baths. Currently, we recommend use of a high Ca^{2+} bath (7.5 mg/dl) in critically ill patients, unless the patient is hypercalcemic.

Many attempts have been made to mathematically correct the total serum Ca^{2+} concentration for alterations in circulating albumin levels and pH. Despite these attempts, total serum Ca^{2+} and calculated ionized Ca^{2+} levels have been poor predictors of the physiologically active ionized Ca^{2+} fraction (78, 135).

We have found abnormally low total and calculated ionized Ca^{2+} values in 50–60% of critically ill patients (135). However, when ionized Ca^{2+} levels were directly measured, only about 10% of critically ill patients have hypocalcemia. Despite high sensitivity, total serum and calculated ionized Ca^{2+} values lack specificity in predicting ionized hypocalcemia. On the other hand, an elevated total serum Ca^{2+} level in a critically ill patient is usually indicative of ionized hypercalcemia, whereas a normal total serum Ca^{2+} measurement is strong evidence against ionized hypocalcemia (135). We have found that the amount of Ca^{2+} bound to albumin varies widely between patients (e.g., 40–60%) and that alterations in binding that result from blood pH and FFA changes are significantly different between normal and sick patients (implying differences in the physicochemical properties of their binding proteins) (135, 143). At present, we believe that the serum-ionized Ca^{2+} level remains the best measure of Ca^{2+} delivery in critically ill patients, and we recommend that all centers caring for critically ill patients measure ionized Ca^{2+} concentrations. When ionized Ca measurements are not available, an ultrafilterable Ca^{2+} level may be substituted (142). Ultrafilterable Ca^{2+} levels can be easily measured by passing a plasma or serum sample through a small filter, which prevents the passage of protein through it. The Ca^{2+} in the ultrafiltrate can be measured in the hospital laboratory.

Different laboratories have different ways of measuring serum-ionized Ca^{2+} levels. Many laboratories correct the serum pH to 7.4 to correct for losses in carbon dioxide that may have occurred between the time of blood drawing and Ca^{2+} measurement. Since many critically ill patients have alterations in serum pH, we do not correct the pH to 7.4. In addition, we have found that present methods for correcting the pH to 7.4 work poorly in critically ill patients. We are extremely careful to collect our blood samples anaerobically and measure the ionized Ca^{2+} level immediately after drawing.

Calcium Homeostasis

The daily recommended oral dietary intake of Ca^{2+} is 1000–1500 mg. Thirty to 35% of this intake is absorbed primarily in the small intestine by both active (vitamin D–dependent) and passive (concentration–dependent) absorption. Loss of Ca^{2+} via the gastrointes-

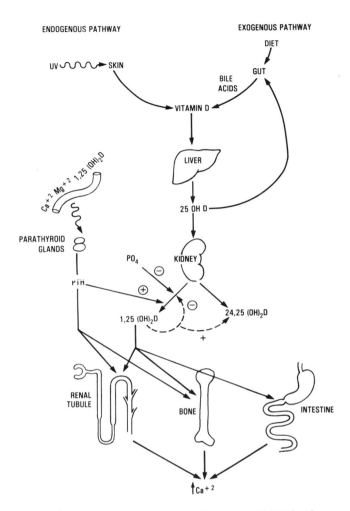

Figure 17.1 Regulation of the serum calcium level.

tinal tract (150–200 mg/day) and urine (150 mg/day) is balanced by gastrointestinal absorption.

The serum Ca^{2+} concentration is maintained within normal limits by the combined effects of PTH and vitamin D (Fig. 17.1). Dietary Ca^{2+} is usually not required, since these hormones can maintain a normal serum Ca^{2+} level via their skeletal effects. However, with chronic Ca^{2+} deficiency the skeletal Ca^{2+} mobilizing response to PTH or 1,25-dihydroxyvitamin D is diminished and predisposes the patient to hypocalcemia. This decrease in PTH and vitamin D responsiveness results from receptor desensitization due to high levels of the hormones and depletion of the mobilizable pool of Ca^{2+} in bone (85). A deficiency in either

hormone, however, may lead to hypocalcemia. Deficiency in PTH may result from parathyroid gland damage (as may occur after neck surgery) or from parathyroid gland suppression. The parathyroid glands may be suppressed by hypercalcemia, hypomagnesemia, hypermagnesemia, or 1,25-dihydroxyvitamin D. PTH increases bone resorption and renal tubular Ca^{2+} reabsorption, and promotes intestinal Ca^{2+} absorption by stimulating the renal conversion of 25-hydroxyvitamin D to 1,25-dihydroxyvitamin D (85). The action of PTH on bone osteoclasts may be mediated through an intermediary monocyte rather than by direct action (85).

Vitamin D can enter the body through the gastrointestinal tract (dietary vitamin D) or can be synthesized in the skin under the influence of ultraviolet light. Either source is sufficient to maintain normal vitamin D levels. However, when sunlight exposure is minimal and dietary intake is poor, vitamin D deficiency may develop. These circumstances are commonly found in elderly, debilitated, and chronically ill patients. Many of these patients are admitted to intensive care units and under the increased metabolic demands of severe illness may be unable to maintain normal serum Ca^{2+} levels. Vitamin D is a fat soluble vitamin, and its absorption is dependent on intact lipolytic activity, biliary secretion, and functional intestinal mucosa. Thus, diseases of the pancreas, liver, biliary system, or intestine may cause vitamin D malabsorption and deficiency (137).

Vitamin D is 25-hydroxylated in the liver and then 1-hydroxylated in the kidneys to 1,25-dihydroxyvitamin D, the active form of the vitamin. Vitamin D's renal hydroxylation is stimulated by both PTH and hypophosphatemia and is suppressed by hyperphosphatemia, acidosis, and 1,25-dihydroxyvitamin D (negative feedback). Synthesis of 25-hydroxyvitamin D within the liver is poorly regulated, and its measurement serves as a good indicator of dietary/skin vitamin D supply. Disease of the kidneys or liver can disrupt Ca^{2+} homeostasis by impairing vitamin D activation. Intestinal and renal tubular Ca^{2+} absorption and bone resorption is stimulated by 1,25-dihydroxyvitamin D. The osteoclast action of 1,25-dihydroxyvitamin D may result from the recruitment and differentiation of precursor cells (85) rather than by action on mature cells.

Thyroid hormone also has effects on the skeleton that affect Ca^{2+} homeostasis. Hyperthyroidism increases bone resorption and may cause hypercalcemia. Hypothyroidism causes a decrease in bone resorption and may cause hypocalcemia.

Hypocalcemia

CAUSES

Hypocalcemia develops when Ca^{2+} leaves the vascular space or is chelated faster than it can be replaced. A frequent underlying problem in critically ill patients who become hypocalcemic is their impaired ability to mobilize skeletal Ca^{2+} because of PTH or vitamin D deficiency. Table 17.1 lists various causes of hypocalcemia.

Table 17.1
Causes of Hypocalcemia

Hypoparathyroidism
  Primary
  Secondary
    After neck surgery
    Radioiodine
    Metastasis
    Hemochromatosis
  Neonatal
Hypomagnesemia or Hypermagnesemia
Hyperphosphatemia
  Iatrogenic
  Tumor lysis
  Rhabdomyolysis
Chelators
  Citrate (e.g., blood)
  Albumin
  Radiocontrast dye
Vitamin D deficiency
  Dietary
  Malabsorption
  Renal insufficiency
  Pseudohypoparathyroidism
Pancreatitis
Sepsis
Hungry bone syndrome
Fat embolism syndrome
Toxic shock syndrome
Burns
Hypothyroidism
Drugs
  Albumin
  Aminoglycosides
  Calcitonin
  Cis-platinum
  Citrate
  Diphosphonates
  EDTA
  Estrogens
  Ethylene glycol
  Gallium nitrate
  Heparin
  Loop diuretics
  Magnesium
  Mithramycin
  Phenobarbital
  Phenytoin
  Phosphates
  Protamine
  Radiocontrast dye
  Sodium fluoride
  Sodium sulfate
  WR-2721

Hypoparathyroidism

Primary (usually autoimmune) hypoparathyroidism is rarely seen, whereas secondary hypoparathyroidism after neck surgery is a common cause of hypocalcemia (98). Hypocalcemia is usually seen when surgery involves removal of a parathyroid adenoma, total or near-total thyroidectomy, or bilateral neck surgery for cancer. Hypocalcemia may occur immediately or 1–2 days after surgery and is transient (lasting less than 5 days) unless permanent parathyroid damage has occurred. Parathyroid insufficiency may result from gland suppression after removal of an adenoma, interference with parathyroid blood supply, or intraoperative release of calcitonin (11). Watson et al. (125) found a close correlation between decrements in serum Ca^{2+} and increases in calcitonin after thyroidectomy; however, no significant changes in PTH levels were observed, which suggests that calcitonin release accounted for the fall in serum Ca^{2+}. Serum Ca^{2+} returned to normal as calcitonin levels fell. With convalescence, there is resolution of edema or revascularization, which results in the reestablishment of parathyroid gland integrity.

Most patients who develop hypocalcemia after neck surgery remain asymptomatic; however, occasionally patients may develop paresthesias, laryngeal spasm, or tetany. We recommend that the serum-ionized Ca^{2+} level be monitored every 12 hours in patients after neck surgery—more frequently if hypocalcemic symptoms develop—until the serum-ionized Ca^{2+} level begins to rise (indicating recovery of the parathyroid glands). Symptomatic or severely hypocalcemic (ionized $Ca^{2+} < 3$ mg/dl) patients should receive supplemental Ca^{2+}. When Ca^{2+} is replaced in these patients, it is important that the Ca^{2+} level be maintained in the low normal ranges so as not to suppress the recovering parathyroid glands. Postoperative hypoparathyroidism may manifest itself late after neck surgery (months to years), and patients at risk should have their serum-ionized Ca^{2+} levels serially monitored. Other patients may have latent hypoparathyroidism after neck surgery, which manifests itself only with stress. Thus, critically ill patients with a previous history of neck surgery should have a serum Ca^{2+} determination performed.

Overt hypoparathyroidism rarely occurs after radioiodine treatment for thyroid disease (98); however, a significant number of these patients may have latent hypoparathyroidism, as measured by a diminished PTH response to ethylene diaminetetraacetic acid (EDTA)-induced hypocalcemia. The serum Ca^{2+} should be monitored in these patients during stress in order to avoid hypocalcemia. Infrequent causes of hypoparathyroidism are metastasis to the parathyroid glands and iron deposition due to hemochromatosis.

Two types of hypocalcemia have been described in newborn infants. The first occurs early after birth (1–3 days) and is called "early neonatal hypocalcemia". It is attributed to parathyroid immaturity and/or physiologic maternal hyperparathyroidism (causing neonatal parathyroid gland suppression) and usually resolves within the first week of life. Neonates have lower serum Ca^{2+} concentrations compared with older infants; the limits for pathologic hypocalcemia have been set at 8 mg/dl in full-term infants and 7 mg/dl in premature infants (98). Predisposing factors for neonatal hypocalcemia include prematurity, maternal diabetes mellitus, perinatal complications, and birth asphyxia. Late-onset neonatal hypocalcemia occurs 6–8 days after birth and is associated with hyperphosphatemia and hypomagnesemia. These infants frequently present with metabolic convulsions and the hypocalcemia likely results from high PO_4 intake (due to milk). High-serum PO_4 levels decrease the serum Ca^{2+} concentration by increasing Ca^{2+} deposition in bone. Hypomagnesemia results from decreased intestinal Mg^{2+} absorption. The hypomagnesemia augments the hypocalcemia via inhibition of PTH secretion and skeletal resistance. Other causes of hypoparathyroidism in infants include maternal hyperparathyroidism and excessive Ca^{2+} or vitamin D intake in the mother (both agents cross the placenta).

Postoperative hypocalcemia may also occur in patients after parathyroid or thyroid surgery, unrelated to hypoparathyroidism. After removal of the stimulus for elevated bone turnover (such as PTH or thyroid hormone) high rates of bone formation may develop and result in a lowering of the serum Ca^{2+} concentration ("recalcification hypocalcemia" or "tetany"). The incidence and severity of symptoms depends on the degree of postoperative bone involvement. These patients also frequently develop hypomagnesemia and hypophosphatemia.

Magnesium

Mg^{2+} abnormalities are common in critically ill patients and may cause hypocalcemia (7, 26, 30, 79, 110, 138, 142). The serum Mg^{2+} level influences both PTH secretion and action. Mild hypomagnesemia stimulates PTH secretion, whereas severe hypomagnesemia

($Mg^{2+} < 1.0$ mg/dl) and hypermagnesemia inhibit PTH secretion. Hypomagnesemia also impairs PTH action at its receptor (i.e., skeletal resistance) and causes vitamin D resistance (11, 92, 93, 110). Since Mg^{2+} is an important cofactor for the activation of adenylate cyclase, it is possible that severe Mg^{2+} deficiency leads to an impairment of the adenylate cyclase receptor resulting in deranged PTH release and skeletal resistance. A variety of diseases and medications can cause hypomagnesemia and hypermagnesemia (see "Magnesium"). Hypomagnesemic hypocalcemia responds poorly to calcium therapy alone but does respond to Mg^{2+} repletion.

Phosphate

Hyperphosphatemia (see "Phosphorus") may cause hypocalcemia as a result of calcium precipitation, inhibition of bone resorption, and suppression of renal 1-hydroxylation of vitamin D (25, 29). The most common causes of this syndrome in the ICU include PO_4 administration (e.g. during the treatment of diabetic ketoacidosis), tumor lysis syndromes following chemotherapy, renal failure, and rhabdomyolysis. Hypocalcemia during rhabdomyolysis is complex and appears to result from a combination of factors which include tissue Ca^{2+} deposition, hyperphosphatemia, impaired 1,25-dihydroxyvitamin D synthesis, and skeletal resistance to PTH (131). The serum PO_4 level should be measured in all hypocalcemic patients, since administration of Ca^{2+} to these patients may increase Ca precipitation and cause further harm. The hypocalcemia in hyperphosphatemic patients is treated by lowering the serum PO_4 level.

Chelators

Chelators are anions that are capable of forming complexes with Ca^{2+}. The most common chelators causing hypocalcemia in critically ill patients are citrated blood, albumin, and radiocontrast dyes.

Vitamin D Deficiency

Vitamin D deficiency is being increasingly recognized as an important cause of hypocalcemia in patients in the ICU. Approximately 20% of the hypocalcemic patients that we see in the ICU have a defect in the vitamin D axis. Many of these patients are chronically ill, malnourished, and have minimal sunlight exposure. They have low-serum 25-hydroxyvitamin D levels, suggestive of dietary vitamin D deficiency. Vitamin D deficiency may also occur in patients with a normal dietary intake as a result of gut malabsorption, defects in fat digestion, impaired biliary secretion or disrupted intestinal integrity (e.g. gastrectomy, gastrojejunostomy, celiac disease, Crohn's disease, intestinal bypass surgery, pancreatic insufficiency, hepatobiliary disease) (137). Excessive amounts of vitamin D bound to its transport protein may be lost in the urine of patients with the nephrotic syndrome.

Acquired defects in the hepatic 25-hydroxylase enzyme have not been shown to cause pathologic vitamin D deficiency (e.g., hypocalcemia). Although hypocalcemia is found in patients with advanced liver disease, the primary cause for low vitamin D levels appears to be malabsorption (failure of biliary secretion) rather than failure of hydroxylation.

Other patients have renal insufficiency with deficiency of the renal 1-hydroxylase system, which is responsible for the production of 1,25-dihydroxyvitamin D. These vitamin D–deficient patients frequently have normal serum Ca^{2+} levels as outpatients; however, they are unable to mobilize sufficient Ca^{2+} to maintain normal circulating levels during critical illness. Pseudohypoparathyroidism (11) is a rare disorder that results from resistance to PTH. Resultant suppression of the 1-hydroxylase system leads to deficiency of 1,25-dihydroxyvitamin D and hypocalcemia.

Pancreatitis

Hypocalcemia is commonly seen in patients with acute pancreatitis and is associated with a poor prognosis (64, 133). The exact etiology of the hypocalcemia in pancreatitis is uncertain. Saponification of Ca^{2+} is inadequate to explain the degree and length of hypocalcemia. PTH has been reported to be elevated (55), normal (53, 108), or decreased (33, 53). Bone and kidney can respond to exogenous PTH when it is given to patients with pancreatitis (108). Although this observation rules out complete end-organ resistance to PTH, it does not rule out partial PTH resistance. Analysis of the data on hypocalcemia in pancreatitis suggests that there are at least two groups of patients who develop hypocalcemia in this disorder. The majority have relative hypoparathyroidism (11) with normal or low PTH during hypocalcemia, whereas the remainder have appropriately increased levels of PTH. The group with elevated PTH levels may suffer from a defect in the vitamin D axis or from tissue resistance to PTH or vitamin D. In one study (55), serum 1,25-dihydroxyvitamin D levels were measured in six pancreatitis patients with hypocalcemia. In these patients serum vitamin D levels were low when the patients were admitted (during hypocalcemia) but increased in parallel with increases in PTH during recovery. Pancreatitis-associated hypomagnesemia and renal failure may also contribute to hypocalcemia.

Sepsis

The hypocalcemia occurring in patients with sepsis appears to have multiple causes (134). Some patients have dietary vitamin D deficiency, while others have acquired parathyroid gland insufficiency, renal 1-hydroxylase insufficiency, or peripheral resistance to 1,25-dihydroxyvitamin D (134). Renal 1-hydroxylase deficiency usually occurs when renal insufficiency accompanies sepsis.

Hungry Bone Syndromes

Hypocalcemia may occur after parathyroidectomy or thyroidectomy in patients with "overactive glands". These patients have accelerated bone resorption and formation. When the stimulus for resorption is removed at surgery, bone formation may exceed mineral supply and hypocalcemia results. The hypocalcemia is usually accompanied by hypophosphatemia and hypomagnesemia. Increased bone formation and hypocalcemia may also occur during osteoblastic metastasis from prostate, breast, and lung malignancies (11).

Fat Embolism Syndrome

Hypocalcemia is occasionally seen in trauma patients with fat embolism. The hypocalcemia probably results from a combination of Ca^{2+} chelation and increases in protein binding of Ca^{2+} induced by release of fatty acids. Transient episodes of ionized hypocalcemia associated with respiratory distress, in a patient after trauma, suggests the presence of this syndrome.

Miscellaneous

Hypocalcemia is associated with the toxic shock syndrome. Although circulating calcitonin levels are elevated in this syndrome, the exact pathogenesis of the hypocalcemia remains undefined (132). Ionized hypocalcemia occurs in patients with burns; however, the etiology remains to be defined. Hypothyroidism affects Ca^{2+} homeostasis by decreasing bone turnover and may also cause hypocalcemia. Hypothyroid patients usually have elevated levels of PTH and 1,25-dihydroxyvitamin D (133). A large number of drugs have been reported to cause hypocalcemia although clear documentation of ionized hypocalcemia is lacking with many. Listed in Table 32.1 are those drugs in which a clear association with hypocalcemia has been documented. Phosphates, citrate, magnesium, radiocontrast dye, albumin and heparin have already been discussed. Aminoglycosides, cis-platinum, and loop diuretics may cause hypocalcemia by producing hypomagnesemia. Cis-platinum also can inhibit bone resorption (24, 76, 77). EDTA and sodium sulfate (57) are potent Ca^{2+} chelators and have been used clinically to treat hypercalcemia. Mithramycin (117), calcitonin (116), estrogens, protamine (103), gallium nitrate (124), and diphosphonates (65, 66, 113) decrease bone resorption and are also used to treat hypercalcemia. WR-2721 is a radioprotective agent that inhibits PTH secretion (49, 50). Anticonvulsants such as phenytoin and phenobarbital have been associated with hypocalcemia and reduced bone mass. Although they increase the hepatic metabolism of vitamin D, this effect does not appear to be adequate to explain the hypocalcemia. These anticonvulsant drugs may also decrease intestinal Ca^{2+} absorption and reduce PTH-induced bone resorption (11). Ethylene glycol intoxication causes hypocalcemia, presumably by oxalate (a metabolic product of ethylene glycol metabolism) complexing with Ca^{2+} (120). Sodium fluoride forms an insoluble salt with Ca^{2+} (54) and may induce hypocalcemia when taken in large doses (as may be used in the treatment of osteoporosis).

CLINICAL MANIFESTATIONS

Hypocalcemia may present with a variety of clinical signs and symptoms (Table 17.2) that relate to increased neuronal irritability (133). Cardiovascular manifestations are the most commonly encountered features of hypocalcemia seen in critically ill patients. Patients may develop hypotension, cardiac insufficiency, bradycardia, arrhythmias (e.g. ventricular fibrillation), and failure to respond to drugs that act through calcium-related mechanisms

Table 17.2
Clinical Manifestations of Hypocalcemia

Cardiovascular
  Hypotension
  Cardiac insufficiency
  Bradycardia
  Arrhythmias
  Insensitivity to catecholamines and digitalis
ECG
      QT and ST interval prolongation
      T wave inversion
Respiratory
  Laryngeal spasm
  Apnea
  Bronchospasm
Neuromuscular
  Tetany
  Chvostek's and Trousseau's signs
  Muscle spasm
  Paresthesias
  Seizures
  Weakness
  Extrapyramidal manifestations
Psychiatric
  Anxiety
  Dementia
  Depression
  Irritability
  Psychosis
  Confusion
Miscellaneous
  Coarse, dry, scaly skin
  Brittle nails
  Thin brittle hair
  Cataracts

(e.g. digoxin, catecholamines, glucagon) (23, 28, 31, 34, 40, 48). Hypocalcemia should always be considered in patients with hypotension that responds poorly to fluids and/or to pressor agents. Restoration of a normal circulating Ca^{2+} level may restore vascular tone and improve cardiac contractility. Ca^{2+} may also be an effective inotropic agent in patients with advanced cardiac disease (18, 48) who have β-adrenergic receptor down-regulation as a result of chronic sympathetic stimulation. In some patients, digitalis may be ineffective, at normal levels, in controlling supraventricular arrhythmias (31) and catecholamines and glucagon (28) may be ineffective in raising blood pressure or heart rate due to hypocalcemia. Agents that decrease cellular Ca^{2+} availability (e.g. β-adrenergic blockers and slow calcium channel antagonists) may exacerbate hypocalcemia-induced cardiac insufficiency. Hypocalcemia may inconsistently cause Q-T and S-T interval prolongation; however, these ECG changes can not be relied upon to exclude a diagnosis of hypocalcemia.

Hypocalcemia may also present as laryngo-spasm or bronchospasm in critically ill patients. We have treated patients who were doing well and were extubated after surgery who required reintubation as a result of hypocalcemia-induced laryngospasm. The laryngospasm resolved with Ca^{2+} repletion.

Tetany and muscle spasms are the classical sign of hypocalcemia, but these signs may be absent in hypocalcemic ICU patients. Chvostek's and Trousseau's signs are nonspecific indicators of hypocalcemia. Chvostek's sign is present in 25% of normal adults while Trousseau's sign is present in 4% of the normal population (11). In addition, Trousseau's sign may be negative in 30% of subjects with hypocalcemia. Anticonvulsant drugs, sedation, and paralyzation may eliminate signs of neuronal irritability. The intubated, sedated or paralyzed patient may be unable to express symptoms such as anxiety and paresthesias. Psychiatric manifestations of hypocalcemia (Table 17.2) are nonspecific and are frequently seen in critically ill patients as a result of their illness.

We routinely monitor serum-ionized Ca^{2+} levels in all critically ill patients and treat all patients with hypocalcemic symptoms or severe hypocalcemia. Life-threatening arrhythmias develop when the ionized Ca^{2+} level approaches 2.0–2.5 mg/dl, and thus we recommend that all patients with an ionized Ca^{2+} concentration below 3.0 mg/dl should receive treatment (Zaloga GP, Flemming S; unpublished data).

TREATMENT

Patients with suspected hypocalcemia should have an ionized Ca^{2+} measured to confirm the diagnosis (Fig. 32.2). Once confirmed these patients should have a blood sample sent for measurement of serum magnesium and phosphorus levels. Blood samples should be saved for plasma PTH and vitamin D levels, should these tests later become necessary (Fig. 17.2).

Acute symptomatic hypocalcemia is a medical emergency that necessitates intravenous Ca^{2+} therapy (Table 17.3). Initial therapy in adults consists of the administration of a Ca^{2+} bolus (100–200 mg of elemental Ca^{2+} over 10 minutes) followed by a maintenance infusion of 1 to 2 mg/kg/hour of elemental Ca^{2+}. A 100–200 mg bolus of elemental Ca^{2+} will usually raise the serum total Ca^{2+} by 1 mg/dl, with levels returning to baseline by 30 minutes after injection. To maintain levels above baseline a continuous infusion or intermittent boluses of

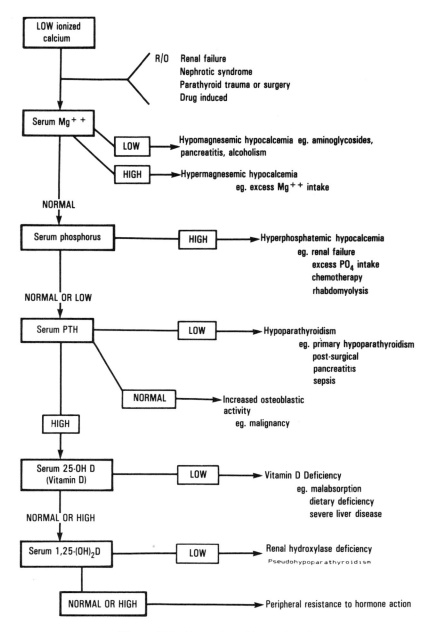

Figure 17.2   Evaluation of hypocalcemia.

Ca^{2+} are necessary. The serum Ca^{2+} usually normalizes in 6–12 hours with this regimen, and the maintenance rate may need to be decreased to 0.3–0.5 mg/kg/hour. Serum Mg^{2+} and PO_4 levels should be measured and restored to normal values. Administration of Ca^{2+} to hyperphosphatemic patients may cause Ca^{2+} precipitation. Hypomagnesemic and hypermagnesemic hypocalcemia responds poorly to

Ca^{2+} therapy, but does respond to normalization of the serum Mg^{2+} level. Potassium deficiency protects the patient from hypocalcemic tetany and arrhythmias, and correction of the hypokalemia without correction of the hypocalcemia may provoke these disorders (54). Administration of drugs that may be aggravating hypocalcemia (e.g., furosemide) should be discontinued or another drug substituted if

Table 17.3
Calcium Preparations

	Size	Contents[a]
Parenteral		
Ca^{2+} Gluconate (10%)	10 ml	93 mg Ca^{2+} (4.6 mEq)
Ca^{2+} Gluceptate	5 ml	90 mg Ca^{2+} (4.5 mEq)
Ca^{2+} Chloride (10%)	10 ml	272 mg Ca^{2+} (13.6 mEq)
Oral		
Ca^{2+} Carbonate, e.g., Os-cal 500	tablets	500 mg Ca^{2+}
Ca^{2+} Gluconate	tablets	500 mg Ca^{2+}
Ca^{2+} Lactate	tablets	650 mg Ca^{2+}
Ca^{2+} Glubionate e.g., Neo-calglucon	syrup	115 mg Ca^{2+}/5 ml

[a] Elemental Ca^{2+}

possible. Intravenous Ca^{2+} preparations are irritating to veins and Ca^{2+} should be diluted in 50–100 ml of 5% dextrose in water. Ca^{2+} chloride should never be injected into tissues; however, Ca^{2+} gluceptate may be given intramuscularly when intravenous access is not possible (54). Ca^{2+} salts should not be administered with bicarbonate, since the two precipitate. Ca^{2+} must be administered cautiously to patients receiving digitalis, since hypercalcemia predisposes to digitalis toxicity. Adequacy of treatment can be monitored at the bedside by following Chvostek's and Trousseau's signs, the ECG, and hemodynamic parameters. Optimal therapy requires frequent monitoring of the serum Ca^{2+}, Mg^{2+}, PO_4, potassium, and creatinine levels. Once serum Ca^{2+} is stable in the low normal range the patient may be started on enteral Ca^{2+} (Table 32.3). Most patients require 2–4 g of calcium per day in divided doses. Ca^{2+} carbonate is converted in the stomach to a soluble calcium salt by hydrochloric acid. It is ineffective in patients with achlorhydria (11).

Table 17.4
Vitamin D Preparations

	Ergocalciferol (Vit D2)	Calcifediol (250HD)	Dihydrotachysterol (1-OHD)	Calcitriol (1,25(OH)2D)
Concentration in serum	10 ng/ml	30 ng/ml		0.03 ng/ml
Physiological dose (μg/day)	10	5	20	0.5
Pharmacological dose (μg/day)	1200	50	200–800	0.25–1
Onset of maximal effect (days)	30	15	15	3
Dosage forms	Tablets 625 μg 1250 μg Solution 8000 U/ml Oil for inject 500,000 U/ml	Capsules 20 μg 50 μg	Tablets 125 μg 200 μg 400 μg Solution 200 μg/ml	Capsules 0.25 μg 0.50 μg
Commercial products	Calciferol	Calderol	Hytakerol	Rocaltrol
Serum half-life (days)	30	15		0.2
Time for reversal of effect (days)	17–60	7–30	3–14	2–10
Advantages	Low cost, prolonged action, parent compound	Liver disease	Renal disease, hypoparathyroidism	Renal disease, liver disease, hypoparathyroidism, rapid onset, rapid offset
Disadvantages	Instability, long toxicity	Expense	Expense	Expense

When Ca^{2+} alone is insufficient in normalizing the serum Ca^{2+} concentration, vitamin D metabolites (Table 17.4) may be added (54). Vitamin D is rarely required during the period of critical illness while the patient is in the ICU. It is usually reserved for chronic treatment of hypocalcemia. The principal effect of vitamin D is to increase gut Ca^{2+} absorption, although it also has effects on bone resorption. The earliest calciferol metabolite that is deficient should be administered first. This approach allows the body to regulate activation of the vitamin and replenishes other vitamin D metabolites, which may have some, as yet unknown, physiologic function. When the 1-hydroxylase enzyme is deficient (as in renal failure) or when patients are resistant to ergocalciferol, they may respond to 1,25-dihydroxyvitamin D. This analogue is more potent than other vitamin D metabolites (Table 17.4), has a quicker onset of action, and a greater tendency to induce hypercalcemia and hypercalciuria, but a shorter duration of toxicity. Vitamin D requirements vary and must be adjusted based on disease activity, interacting drugs, and dietary Ca^{2+} intake. Hypercalciuria with its attendant problems (e.g., nephrocalcinosis and renal stones) may occur before eucalcemia is reached. In these situations, a thiazide diuretic can be helpful in reducing Ca^{2+} excretion. Serum Ca^{2+} and PO_4 levels and urinary Ca^{2+} excretion should be measured at regular intervals. The therapeutic goal is to restore the serum Ca^{2+} to near normal levels (which alleviate symptoms) and avoid complications (e.g., hypercalcemia and hypercalciuria).

Definitive treatment of hypocalcemia involves recognition and correction of the underlying disorder. Frequently, however, acute measures are required to stabilize the serum Ca^{2+} level in safe ranges before addressing the primary problem.

Hypercalcemia

CAUSES

Hypercalcemia occurs when Ca^{2+} enters the vascular space faster than it can be excreted or sequestered. The most common causes (Table 32.5) of hypercalcemia seen in the critical care setting are malignancy, hyperparathyroidism, immobilization, iatrogenic Ca^{2+} administration, hypercalcemia of renal failure, and posthypocalcemic hypercalcemia.

Table 17.5
Causes of Hypercalcemia

Malignancy
Hyperparathyroidism
Immobilization
Iatrogenic calcium administration
Renal causes
   Chronic renal failure
   Recovery from acute renal failure
   After renal transplantation
Posthypocalcemic hypercalcemia
Hypocalciuric hypercalcemia
   Familial
   Hypothyroidism
   Lithium
   Thiazides
   Adrenal insufficiency
   Bartter's syndrome
Granulomatous disease
   Sarcoidosis
   Histoplasmosis
   Coccidiomycosis
   Tuberculosis
Hyperthyroidism
Acquired immune deficiency syndrome (AIDS)
Phosphorus depletion syndrome
Multiple endocrine neoplasia syndromes
Pheochromocytoma
Acromegaly
Drug Induced
   Calcium
   Estrogens or progestins for malignancy
   Lithium
   Milk-alkali syndrome
   Theophylline
   Thiazides
   Vitamin D or A

Malignancy

Hypercalcemia occurs in approximately 10–20% of patients with malignancy because of direct tumor osteolysis of bone and from the secretion of humoral substances that stimulate bone resorption (11). Humoral bone resorbing substances include PTH-like substances (12, 20, 118), 1,25-dihydroxyvitamin D (17, 139), osteoclast activating factor (97), and prostaglandins (115). PTH-like substances cross react in the radioimmunoassay for PTH but are not identical to PTH. They are presently thought to be responsible for most instances of humoral hypercalcemia of malignancy and most likely represent a heterogenous group of molecules. These molecules stimulate bone resorption, and frequently are capable of stimulating the renal adenylate cyclase system and inhibiting phosphate resorption, similar to PTH. They have little activity on the renal 1-hydroxylase enzyme that is responsible for the renal synthesis of 1,25-dihydroxyvitamin D. Tumor synthesis of 1,25-dihydroxyvitamin D is a less common cause of hypercalcemia but has been described in patients with lymphoma (17) and Hodgkin's disease (139). Osteoclast activating factor, a lymphokine released by stimulated peripheral blood leukocytes, may be released into the circulation in neoplasia of lymphoid origin (e.g., multiple myeloma, lymphoma, and leukemia) and, like 1,25-dihydroxyvitamin D, is antagonized by glucocorticoids. Hypercalcemia due to prostaglandins are a rare cause of hypercalcemia, usually occur with solid tumors, and may respond to cyclooxygenase inhibitors. Tumor-related hypercalcemia occurs most commonly with breast, lung, kidney, prostate, and hematologic malignancies. Primary hyperparathyroidism also occurs with a higher frequency in hypercalcemic patients with malignancy (11).

Hyperparathyroidism

Primary hyperparathyroidism is found in the general population with a prevalence that ranges from 0.03% to 0.1% (52, 133). The most common causes of primary hyperparathyroidism are single adenomas (75–87%), hyperplasia of multiple glands (12–22%), and carcinoma of the parathyroid glands (3%). Hypercalcemia in hyperparathyroidism results from the combined effects of both increased PTH and 1,25-dihydroxyvitamin D on the bone, intestine, and kidneys. Many hyperparathyroid patients are asymptomatic and the hypercalcemia is noted only when a serum Ca^{2+} level is measured for other reasons. Most of these patients do not require emergency treatment for their hypercalcemia, but some type of treatment is frequently required to prevent accelerated bone loss. Surgery remains the only definitive treatment for patients with hyperparathyroidism, although some patients may have slight decreases in plasma Ca^{2+} and decreased bone turnover with estrogen or progestogen therapy (47, 60). Estrogens and progestins appear to work by antagonizing PTH action upon the skeleton. When one encounters a patient with hyperparathyroidism due to glandular hyperplasia, a search for other endocrine tumors should be sought as part of the multiple endocrine neoplasia syndromes (e.g. tumors of the pituitary, pancreas, adrenal, and thyroid).

Immobilization

Immobilization hypercalcemia occurs following immobilization in patients with rapid bone turnover. The patients most at risk are children, adolescents, postfracture patients, patients with Paget's disease of bone, and patients with underlying malignancy or hyperparathyroidism. Patients with renal failure are also at risk due to their inability to excrete an increased Ca^{2+} load. Most immobilized patients have increased urinary Ca^{2+} and PO_4 levels but only a few develop hypercalcemia (133). Serum PTH and 1,25-dihydroxyvitamin D levels are usually suppressed and hypercalcemia probably results from a relative increase in osteoclastic activity. Symptoms relate to the degree of hypercalciuria and hypercalcemia. The primary therapeutic modality in these patients is mobilization. Quiet standing for a few hours a day is superior to supine bed exercise. Serum Ca^{2+} levels may also be reduced by saline diuresis, calcitonin, oral phosphates, and diphosphonates. Dietary Ca^{2+} restriction has little effect since most circulating Ca^{2+} is derived from bone.

Renal-Related Causes

Hypercalcemia is occasionally seen in patients with uremia and may be iatrogenic, resulting from excess Ca^{2+} or vitamin D supplementation, from the use of high Ca^{2+} dialysate, or from immobilization. These patients are prone to hypercalcemia because they lack the ability to excrete Ca^{2+} through the kidneys and many have a defect in bone mineralization. Patients with secondary hyperparathyroidism may become hypercalcemic after the institution of dialysis. Dialysis may render the bone more responsive to PTH or may lead to hypercalcemia by lowering PO_4 levels. Other causes of hypercalcemia in these patients include the use of Ca^{2+}-containing cation exchange resins, PO_4 depletion with aluminum hydroxide compounds, or the use of thiazide diuretics. Hypercalcemia may also occur during the recovery phase of acute renal failure or following renal transplantation (11). The cause of hypercalcemia in these patients relates to the presence of secondary hyperparathyroidism, reduction in circulating PO_4 concentrations, tapering of steroids, and perhaps increased sensitivity of bone to PTH during resolution of uremia (11). Hyperplastic parathyroid glands usually involute within 6 months of renal transplantation. At times hyperplastic glands may persist and parathyroidectomy may be necessary to avoid renal graft dysfunction (11).

Posthypocalcemic Hypercalcemia

Transient hypercalcemia is not uncommonly seen in patients after a period of hypocalcemia (45). The hypercalcemia most likely results from increased PTH and 1,25-dihydroxyvitamin D levels that were stimulated by the hypocalcemia. Hypocalcemia resolves faster than the Ca^{2+} mobilizing hormones can readjust, resulting in a transient period of rebound hypercalcemia. A review of six cases of transient hypercalcemia of unknown etiology in our ICU revealed a period of hypocalcemia preceding the hypercalcemia in each case. The hypercalcemia resolved without treatment in all cases.

Hypocalciuric Hypercalcemia

Hypercalcemia may occur in patients associated with decreased urinary Ca^{2+} excretion. The hypercalcemia appears to result from the combination of altered parathyroid gland function and altered ion transport in the kidneys. Marx and associates (84) described the inherited syndrome of familial hypocalciuric hypercalcemia (FHH). This disease rarely causes symptoms and is usually discovered when a serum Ca^{2+} level is obtained for other reasons. Serum Ca^{2+}, PTH, 1,25-dihydroxyvitamin D, and urinary cyclic adenosine monophosphate levels (an index of PTH activity) overlap with normal and hyperparathyroid patients; however, urinary Ca^{2+} excretion is less than 150 mg/day and the Ca^{2+}/creatinine ratio is less than 0.01. These patients generally do well without treatment and do not develop bone disease. Hypocalciuric hypercalcemia may also occur in patients with hypothyroidism (140), with lithium therapy, after thiazide administration, with adrenal insufficiency, and with Bartter's syndrome.

Granulomatous Disease

Hypercalcemia (10–20%) and hypercalciuria (30–50%) are commonly seen in patients with sarcoidosis (11, 52). Most hypercalcemic sarcoid patients have an abnormal chest radiograph, abnormal pulmonary function tests, increased bone turnover, and increased gut absorption of Ca^{2+}. Parathyroid function is suppressed; however, these patients produce excess amounts of 1,25-dihydroxyvitamin D within their granuloma (9, 36, 89). Lymphocytes in granulomata associated with histo-plasmosis, coccidiomycosis, tuberculosis (1), silicone injections, and berylliosis are also capable of producing excessive amounts of active vitamin D metabolites and hypercalcemia. The hypercalcemia in these patients improves with glucocorticoids.

Miscellaneous

Thyroid hormone has direct effects on the skeleton, increasing bone turnover and Ca^{2+} release. Although severe hypercalcemia is rare in patients with hyperthyroidism, mild asymptomatic hypercalcemia is frequently encountered (11). PTH and 1,25-dihydroxyvitamin D levels are suppressed in these patients. Hypercalcemia in patients with hyperthyroidism may respond to calcitonin, glucocorticoids, propranolol, and lowering of thyroid hormone levels. Hypercalcemia associated with suppressed PTH and 1,25-dihydroxyvitamin D levels also may occur in patients with the acquired immune deficiency syndrome (AIDS) and probably results from increased bone turnover (136). Phosphorus depletion may occur in patients given phosphate-binding antacids. Stimulation of 1,25-dihydroxyvitamin D synthesis may lead to increased gut Ca^{2+} absorption and bone resorption and thereby cause hypercalcemia. Catecholamines may increase PTH secretion and stimulate bone turnover. In fact, hypercalcemia is occasionally seen in patients with pheochromocytoma (11). These patients may respond to therapy with β-adrenergic blockers. Growth hormone can enhance the formation of 1,25-dihydroxyvitamin D and hypercalcemia has been reported in patients with acromegaly (11). Patients with breast cancer may rarely develop progressive hypercalcemia after receiving treatment with estrogens or progestins, as a result of tumor necrosis with release of bone-resorbing substances. A variety of drugs may cause hypercalcemia (Table 17.5). Vitamin D or A administration increases bone turnover and causes hypercalcemia. Vitamin D also increases intestinal Ca^{2+} absorption. Hypervitaminosis D- or A-induced hypercalcemia responds to glucocorticoid administration. The milk-alkali syndrome (102, 120) consists of hypercalcemia, alkalosis, and renal impairment and is seen in patients who ingest excessive amounts of Ca^{2+} and alkali (e.g. Ca^{2+} carbonate or milk plus sodium bicarbonate for treatment of peptic ulcers). The alkali lowers the urine solubility for Ca^{2+}, decreases Ca^{2+} excretion, and may cause progressive hypercalcemia and renal insufficiency. Ca^{2+} depresses PTH secretion and increases renal bicarbonate reabsorption, further worsening alkalosis. Thiazides and lithium enhance renal Ca^{2+} resorption and decrease renal Ca^{2+} excretion (11). Lithium may also stimulate parathyroid gland activity. Theophylline causes an elevation of the serum Ca^{2+} level that is mediated through adrenergic mechanisms and is compatible with enhancement of PTH action (91). Serum Ca^{2+} levels fall after the administration of beta-adrenergic blockers.

CLINICAL MANIFESTATIONS

Hypercalcemia causes a variety of effects on multiple organ systems (Table 17.6). Ca^{2+} may form stones within the kidneys or disrupt tubular or glomerular function. Reduction in glomerular filtration results from volume depletion and a reduction in the ultrafiltration coefficient (11). Impairment of sodium reabsorption results from inhibition of sodium-potassium ATPase in the ascending limb of Henle and distal tubules. Ca^{2+} antagonism of antidiuretic hormone activity within the kidney can lead to a state of nephrogenic diabetes insipidus (impaired renal concentration), progressive dehydration, and further hypercalcemia. Neuromyopathic manifestations are common and may contribute to the failure to wean a hypercalcemic patient from the ventilator. Neuropsychiatric changes are frequent but are not specific for hypercalcemia.

The cardiovascular effects of hypercalcemia include hypertension and arrhythmias. These may respond to Ca^{2+} channel antagonists (141). Electrocardiographic changes are not reliable indicators of the degree of hypercalcemia and QT shortening is seen in only a minority of cases (43). Hypercalcemia increases cardiac sensitivity to digitalis and may lead to digitalis-related toxicity. Ca^{2+} administration in rats decreases cardiovascular responses to epinephrine (Zaloga GP, Willey SC, Malcolm D, Chernow B, Holaday J; unpublished data). Ca^{2+} may work in this situation by inhibiting adenyl cyclase activity. The clinical implications of this work await further studies in humans.

Anorexia is common in hypercalcemic patients. These patients are also prone to the development of pancreatitis and peptic ulcer disease. Skeletal disease may occur secondary to direct tumor invasion or secretion of bone-resorbing substances. Hypomagnesemia may result from Ca^{2+}-induced inhibition of Mg^{2+}

Table 17.6
Clinical Features of Hypercalcemia

Cardiovascular
  Hypertension
  Arrhythmias
  Digitalis sensitivity
  Catecholamine resistance
  QT shortening
Urinary system
  Nephrocalcinosis
  Nephrolithiasis
  Tubular dysfunction
    Renal tubular acidosis
    Impaired Na reabsorption
    Free water loss
  Glomerular disorders
  Interstitial nephritis
Gastrointestinal
  Peptic ulcers
  Pancreatitis
  Constipation
  Anorexia
  Nausea/vomiting
Neuromuscular
  Weakness, atrophy
  Hyporeflexia
Neuropsychiatric
  Depression
  Personality change
  Psychomotor retardation
  Memory impairment
  Psychosis
  Disorientation
  Obtundation
  Coma
  Seizures
  EEG abnormalities
Skeletal
  Osteopenia
  Osteitis fibrosa cystica
Miscellaneous
  Skin necrosis
  Corneal calcification
  Conjunctivitis
  Pruritis
  Decreased bronchial clearance of secretions
  Hypomagnesemia

reabsorption in the renal tubules (11). The threshold for the development of hypercalcemic symptoms varies; however, most asymptomatic patients have a total serum Ca^{2+} level below 12 mg/dl (with a normal albumin concentration). Factors such as the rapidity with which the serum Ca^{2+} rises, accompanying renal failure, electrolyte disturbances, cardiovascular status, and the general state of debilitation of the patient can alter the threshold for symptoms. The most common causes of death as a result of hypercalcemia relate to renal failure, arrhythmias, and central nervous system impairment.

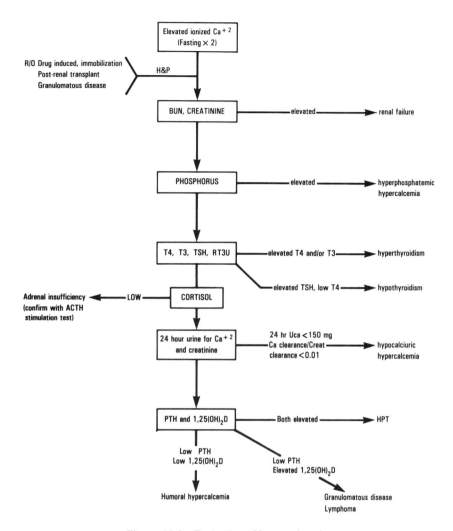

Figure 32.3 Evaluation of hypercalcemia.

EVALUATION

Hypercalcemia should be documented by measuring a fasting serum calcium level (Fig. 17.3) to exclude exogenous causes of hypercalcemia (e.g., orally or intravenously administered Ca^{2+}). Once established, a careful history, physical examination, and review of the patient's chart, including drugs, may uncover the cause of the hypercalcemia in most cases. Renal function and phosphate levels should be measured to rule out renal causes. Measurement of thyroid hormone and TSH concentrations can detect hypothyroidism or hyperthyroidism. A 24-hour urine collection for Ca^{2+} and creatinine determinations helps to separate hypocalciuric from hypercalciuric

syndromes. Frequently, one must differentiate between primary hyperparathyroidism and malignancy (Table 17.7). The best tests that distinguish between these two entities are PTH and 1,25-dihydroxyvitamin D measurements. PTH is elevated in primary hyperparathyroidism and normal or low in patients with hypercalcemia of malignancy. The 1-hydroxylase enzyme is stimulated by PTH and 1,25-dihydroxyvitamin D levels are usually high in patients with hyperparathyroidism. On the other hand, 1,25-dihydroxyvitamin D values are low in malignancy unless due to rare tumors that contain a 1-hydroxylase enzyme. PTH and factors released from certain tumors are both capable of raising nephrogenous cAMP levels (85). An elevated nephrogenous cAMP level

Table 17.7
Primary Hyperparathyroidism Versus
Hypercalcemia of Malignancy

	Hyper-parathyroidism	Malignancy
Clinical course	Chronic	Acute
Serum Ca^{2+}	<12.5 mg/dl	>12.5 mg/dl
Serum Cl	>102 mEq/liter	<102 mEq/liter
Serum PO_4	Normal or low	Normal or high
Cl/PO_4	>33	<33
Acid-base	Hyperchloremic acidosis	Metabolic alkalosis
Renal calculi	Frequent	Rare
Osteitis fibrosa	Present	Absent
Urinary Ca^{2+}	High	Very high
PTH	Elevated	Low or normal
1,25(OH)2D	High	Low
TmP/GFR	Low	Variable
Nephrogenous cAMP	High	Variable

cannot distinguish between hypercalcemia due to hyperparathyroidism or malignancy; however, low levels can help to exclude hyperparathyroidism. A careful search for malignancy using chest roentgenograms, bone and liver scans, and computed tomography scanning may also help to establish a definitive diagnosis. If no malignancy can be found after a careful search and laboratory data are compatible with primary hyperparathyroidism, then neck exploration should be performed. In high-risk patients, selective venous catheterization with analysis of serum for PTH or nuclear medicine scanning may help to localize the site of overactive parathyroid tissue.

TREATMENT

Definitive treatment of hypercalcemia lies in the correction of the cause (e.g., surgery for hyperparathyroidism or chemotherapy, surgery or radiotherapy for malignancy); however, while evaluation is taking place it may be necessary to treat the patient to avoid complications and symptoms of hypercalcemia. Ca^{2+} enters and exits the circulation from the gastrointestinal, skeletal or renal routes. The goal of therapy is to minimize Ca^{2+} entry and maximize Ca^{2+} exit. General measures of treatment (Table 17.8) include hydration, correction of electrolyte abnormalities, removal of offending drugs, dietary Ca^{2+} restriction, and mobilization of the patient. Concomitant electrolyte disturbances (e.g. potassium, Mg^{2+}, PO_4) are common in patients with hypercalcemia. Aldinger and Samaan (5) found a 16.9% incidence of hypokalemia in patients with primary

hyperparathyroidism and a 52.3% incidence in patients with hypercalcemia of malignancy. Serum potassium levels were lowest in patients with the highest serum Ca^{2+} concentrations. Hypokalemia or hypomagnesemia increase the arrhythmogenic potential of hypercalcemia. Diuresis may further lower the serum Mg^{2+} and potassium concentrations.

Renal Ca^{2+} excretion can be enhanced with the use of saline (inhibits proximal tubule reabsorption) and furosemide (inhibits distal Ca^{2+} reabsorption) (Table 17.8). Sodium competes with Ca^{2+} in the kidney and inhibits its reabsorption. In addition, expansion of intravascular volume dilutes the Ca^{2+} concentration in the blood and promotes renal flow. Furosemide and saline are adjusted to main-

Table 17.8
Treatments of Hypercalcemia: Alternatives

General Measures
  Hydration
  Remove offending drugs
  Dietary Ca^{2+} restriction
  Treat underlying disorder
  Mobilization
Increase Renal Ca^{2+} Excretion
  Saline: 2–3 liters over 3–6 hr, maintain urine output >200–300 ml/hr
  Furosemide: 10–40 mg i.v. every 2–4 hr
  Dialysis
Decrease Bone Resorption
  Calcitonin: 1–2 MRC U/kg i.v. or i.m. every 6 hours
  Mithramycin: 25 μg/kg i.v. over 4 hours every 2–7 days
  Glucocorticoids: Hydrocortisone 3 mg/kg/day in divided doses every 6 hours or prednisone 40–60 mg/day
  Indomethacin: 25 mg p.o. every 6 hours
  Etidronate disodium: 7.5 mg/kg/day i.v. in 250-ml saline over 2 hours for 1–4 days or 5–10 mg/kg/day p.o.
  Cis-platinum: 100 mg/m² over 24 hours
  Gallium nitrate: 200 mg/m²/day by continuous infusion for 5–7 days
Ca^{2+} Chelators
  Phosphates
    p.o.: 500–1000 mg every 6 hours
    i.v.: 50 mM PO_4 over 8–12 hours
    Rectal: Phosphosoda 5 ml every 6 hours; Fleets enema 100 ml twice daily
  EDTA: 10–50 mg/kg over 4 hours
  Sodium citrate
  Sodium sulfate
Ca^{2+} Antagonists
  Verapamil 5–10 mg i.v.
  Nifedipine 10–20 mg sublingually
PTH Antagonists
  WR-2721 430–910 mg/m² over 20–60 minutes

tain a urine output of 200–300 ml/hour. Sodium, Mg^{2+}, PO_4, and potassium should be monitored and replaced as necessary. Central hemodynamic monitoring may be necessary in patients with heart or renal disease. Ca^{2+} may also be removed from the plasma with dialysis (22) in patients with oliguric renal disease. Hemodialysis can clear up to 682 mg of Ca^{2+} per hour as compared with 124 mg/hour for peritoneal dialysis and 82 mg/hour for forced diuresis (22).

Ca^{2+} may be lowered by agents which decrease bone resorption (Table 17.8). These agents work best in patients with hyperresorptive diseases such as hyperparathyroidism, Paget's disease, and malignancy. Calcitonin (116) inhibits osteoclastic bone resorption and can be given to patients with hyperphosphatemia and before hydration is complete. It is particularly useful in treating patients with congestive heart failure or renal failure in whom large quantities of saline or PO_4 cannot be used. A hypocalcemic effect (average decrease of 2–3 mg/dl) may be seen in 6–10 hours. Calcitonin has low toxicity but occasionally may cause nausea, vomiting, abdominal cramps, skin rash, flushing, and diarrhea. The major disadvantages of calcitonin are its unpredictability (25% do not respond) and drug resistance. Calcitonin resistance frequently develops in patients after 48–72 hours of use as a result of receptor down-regulation and uncoupling of adenyl cyclase (11); resistance may be delayed by the coadministration of glucocorticoids (20–40 mg prednisone every 6 hours) or oral phosphates. Discontinuation of the drug for 24–48 hours can also restore effect.

Osteoclastic bone resorption may be decreased by mithramycin (117) Table 17.8. This drug is almost always effective but takes 12–24 hours to produce a hypocalcemic effect, and its maximal hypocalcemic effect occurs at 5–7 days. If a response is not seen within 24–48 hours the dose may be repeated until a response is seen. Hypocalcemia may be seen following its use and it has renal, hepatic, and hematologic toxicities (especially thrombocytopenia).

Cisplatinum is able to lower serum Ca^{2+} levels in cancer-associated hypercalcemia in animals (76) and humans (77). Lad et al. (77) treated 13 patients with severe cancer-induced hypercalcemia refractory to rehydration with a 24-hour infusion of cisplatinum (100 mg/m² of body surface area). Nine patients achieved normocalcemia. The maximal lowering oc-

curred 10 days after treatment and persisted for a mean duration of 38 days. Cisplatinum inhibits PTH and tumor extract-induced osteolysis in vitro in the mouse calvarium bone resorption assay (24), suggesting that it controls hypercalcemia by inhibiting bone resorption. Gallium nitrate (124) is an antitumor compound that decreases Ca^{2+} resorption from bone and causes hypocalcemia. Warrell et al. (124) treated 10 patients with cancer-related hypercalcemia with gallium nitrate (200 mg/m²/day by continuous infusion for 5–7 days). Total serum Ca^{2+} concentrations decreased from 13.8 mg/dl to 8.0 mg/dl. Gallium nitrate produced few side effects although nephrotoxicity has been reported. Nausea and myelosuppression do not occur.

Glucocorticoids decrease osteoclastic bone resorption, inhibit osteoclast activating factor, block prostaglandin synthesis, and antagonize vitamin D action. They are the agents of choice in vitamin D excess states and in treating hypercalcemia due to granulomatous disease (e.g., sarcoidosis). Glucocorticoids are also effective in control of hypercalcemia in patients with multiple myeloma and lymphoid malignancies. They are ineffective in patients with hyperparathyroidism.

Indomethacin has been used to treat hypercalcemia in patients with some tumors that produce prostaglandins (e.g. hypernephroma and lung cancer). Propranolol has been used to treat hypercalcemia in patients with pheochromocytoma. Hypercalcemia in patients with hyperthyroidism responds to treatment of the thyroid disease. Diphosphonates decrease bone resorption by binding to hydroxyapatite and by inhibiting osteoclast function (65, 66, 113). Etidronate disodium (113), 7.5 mg/kg/day administered intravenously reduced Ca^{2+} to normal in 3 days in 19 of 26 patients with hypercalcemia of malignancy (mean decrease in Ca^{2+} of 2.2 mg/dl). It is the only diphosphonate approved for clinical use in the United States. We have also used this agent orally with some success. Side effects may occasionally occur and include nausea, vomiting, diarrhea, hyperphosphatemia, renal dysfunction, and defective bone mineralization. Oral and intravenous dichloromethylene diphosphonate is also effective in lowering serum Ca^{2+} levels in patients with malignancy and hyperparathyroidism (11, 65, 66). However, this drug is not approved for use in the United States. Large doses of protamine cause acute hypocalcemia in animals by blocking efflux of Ca^{2+} from bone (100). Further studies are needed to examine its potential clinical utility in control of hypercalcemia due to diseases associated with increased bone turnover.

Chelators (e.g., phosphates and EDTA) are indicated for the management of life-threatening hypercalcemic emergencies when an immediate lowering of the ionized Ca^{2+} level is required (Table 17.8). Phosphates (oral, rectal, or intravenous) are extremely effective agents for lowering circulating Ca^{2+}. They work by binding and precipitating Ca^{2+}, inhibiting bone resorption, and decreasing renal activation of vitamin D. Their major disadvantage is the potential for extraskeletal calcification in vital structures (e.g., heart, retina, and kidney). Orally and rectally administered phosphates are safer than intravenously administered phosphates but require several days for maximal effect. Intravenous phosphates work rapidly (maximal effect 6–24 hours) but should not be given in doses exceeding 50 mM over 6–8 hours. Serum Ca^{2+} may fall from 1 to 6 mg/dl depending upon the dose of PO_4 administered. Patients should be well hydrated and blood pressure and electrolytes should be monitored closely. Phosphates are contraindicated in the hyperphosphatemic hypercalcemic patient and should be withheld if the total serum $Ca^{2+} \times PO_4$ product exceeds 60–70. EDTA (ethylenediamine tetraacetic acid) forms complexes with Ca^{2+} as well as Mg^{2+} and is excreted in the urine. It is very effective in lowering circulating Ca^{2+} levels. Hydration is important so as to minimize renal toxicity. It is best given centrally and should be diluted in saline. A dose of EDTA of 50 mg/kg usually lowers the serum Ca^{2+} concentration by 2–3 mg/dl. Infusion of albumin, sodium citrate (19), or sodium sulfate (57) can also be used to acutely lower the ionized Ca^{2+} level. However, these agents have not been tested in clinical trials for the treatment of hypercalcemia and should not be used as primary therapy.

The chemoprotective and radioprotective agent, WR-2721, lowers serum Ca^{2+} when administered to patients with malignancy (49, 50). Reduction of PTH secretion plays a role in the hypocalcemic action of WR-2721, and this agent has been used to treat refractory hypercalcemia in a patient with parathyroid cancer (50). Further studies are needed before widespread use of this agent is recommended. Conjugated estrogens (1.25 mg daily) and norethindrone (5 mg daily) may lower serum Ca^{2+} and inhibit bone resorption by antagonizing PTH in patients with mild hyperparathyroidism (60, 83).

Ca^{2+} may have toxic life-threatening effects upon the cardiovascular system (e.g., arrhythmias, heart block, and cardiac arrest). These effects may be antagonized by calcium channel blockers such as verapamil (141) while awaiting definitive therapy.

Saline, furosemide, phosphates, EDTA, sodium citrate, sodium sulfate, and dialysis have a rapid hypocalcemic effect (within hours) and should be used for life-threatening hypercalcemic emergencies. WR-2721 and protamine are experimental agents that also work within hours of administration. Calcitonin and mithramycin work within 1–3 days of administration while glucocorticoids, prostaglandin inhibitors, gallium nitrate, diphosphonates, and cis-platinum take 4–7 days to elicit a hypocalcemic effect.

MAGNESIUM

Magnesium is the second most common intracellular cation, next to potassium. It is essential for the activity of many metabolic pathways and is vital to a number of enzyme systems. It is required for the activity of phosphatases, which are essential for splitting high-energy ATP bonds and providing energy for the sodium-potassium ATPase pump, proton pump, calcium ATPase pump, neurochemical transmission, muscle contraction, glucose-fat-protein metabolism, oxidative phosphorylation, and DNA synthesis (104). Mg^{2+} is also required for the activity of adenylate cyclase.

The total body content of Mg^{2+} in the average adult is 2000 mEq, about 50–60% of which is in the skeleton and 20% in muscle (104). Less than 1% of total body Mg^{2+} is found in the serum, and thus, serum levels may not accurately reflect intracellular stores (79). The total serum Mg^{2+} concentration ranges from 1.7 to 2.4 mg/dl (1.4–2.0 mEq/liter) in normal adults and is composed of three fractions: a protein-bound fraction (30%), a chelated fraction (15%), and an ionized fraction (55%). It is the ionized fraction that is physiologically active and homeostatically regulated. Although no reliable method is clinically available for the measurement of ionized Mg^{2+} concentrations, a simple filter method is available for measuring ultrafilterable (ionized plus chelated) levels (142). Ultrafilterable levels adjust the Mg^{2+} concentration for variations in serum protein levels.

The normal dietary intake of Mg^{2+} is approximately 25–30 mEq/day (0.3–0.4 mEq/kg/day), which is close to the amount required to maintain Mg^{2+} balance (16). Mg^{2+} is ubiquitous in foods, and dietary Mg^{2+} deficiency is rare unless food intake is severely limited. Mg^{2+} is absorbed in the small intestine and excreted in the urine and stool (104). Normally 30–40% of dietary Mg^{2+} is absorbed; however, this amount may increase during deficiency states. Gut Mg^{2+} absorption occurs by both a vitamin D dependent and independent mechanism. Mg^{2+} homeostasis is primarily regulated in the kidney by tubular reabsorption (35, 88, 104, 111, 123). The kidneys possess a remarkable ability to conserve Mg^{2+} and can decrease excreted Mg^{2+} to less than 1–2 mEq/day in deficiency states. Failure of the kidneys to conserve Mg^{2+} during hypomagnesemia suggests that the cause is renal Mg^{2+} wasting. Mg^{2+} reabsorption in the renal tubule is enhanced by PTH, vitamin D, extracellular fluid depletion, Mg^{2+} depletion, hypothyroidism, and hypocalcemia (104). Renal Mg^{2+} excretion is increased by extracellular fluid expansion, hypermagnesemia, hypercalcemia, loop and osmotic diuretics, PO_4 depletion, metabolic acidosis, and protein and alcohol intake (104). However, the majority of reabsorption is independent of hormonal influences. Urinary Mg^{2+} reabsorption is linked to reabsorption of Ca^{2+} and sodium and renal loss of either of these electrolytes causes Mg^{2+} loss. A tubular maximum (Tm) for Mg^{2+} reabsorption occurs at serum concentrations of 1.5–2.0 mg/dl. This Tm is close to the normal serum Mg^{2+} concentration and small changes in the serum level rapidly alter renal Mg^{2+} excretion. Thus, in Mg^{2+} overload, the kidneys can rapidly excrete excess Mg^{2+}. During correction of Mg^{2+} deficiency, despite cellular Mg^{2+} depletion, much of the administered Mg^{2+} is lost in the urine and repletion usually takes 5–7 days (e.g., to replete intracellular stores). With a normal functioning kidney, obligate loses of Mg^{2+} in stool, sweat, urine, and secretions amount to about 0.3 mEq/kg/day.

Although PTH and vitamin D can increase renal and gastrointestinal absorption of Mg^{2+}, this ion also has potent effects upon the parathyroid glands (7, 26, 30, 79, 110, 138). Hypermagnesemia and severe hypomagnesemia decrease PTH secretion, whereas mild hypomagnesemia stimulates secretion. Hypomag-

nesemia may also impair end-organ response to PTH (79, 110).

Hypomagnesemia

CAUSES

Hypomagnesemia usually occurs when Mg^{2+} losses exceed dietary intake and usually results from a defect in renal Mg^{2+} conservation or excessive stool losses (Table 17.9). Since there is an obligate daily Mg^{2+} loss, severe malnutrition or inadequate supplementation in parenteral nutrition or intravenously administered fluids may also cause hypomagnesemia. Hypomagnesemia may also develop when Mg^{2+} requirements are increased but intake remains constant (e.g., in pregnancy). Decreased gut absorption of Mg^{2+} and/or excessive stool losses may occur in a variety of diseases (e.g., inflammatory bowel disease, gastroenteritis, pancreatic insufficiency, fistulas, short bowel syndromes, ileal bypass, intestinal resection, and cholestatic liver disease). Hypomagnesemia results from a combination of reduced mucosal surface area, increased intestinal secretion, and formation of insoluble Mg^{2+} soaps in the stool due to complexing with unabsorbed fat. Secretions from the lower gastrointestinal tract are richer in Mg^{2+} (10–14 mEq/liter) than secretions from the upper tract (1–2 mEq/liter).

Acute hypomagnesemia can result from internal redistribution of Mg^{2+}. Mg^{2+} shifts into cells following the administration of glucose or amino acids (13, 16). This shift is more pronounced when intracellular Mg^{2+} depletion is coupled to an anabolic state, as may occur with refeeding after starvation or protein-calorie malnutrition, with administration of parenteral nutrition to depleted patients, and with insulin treatment of hyperglycemic disorders. Increased catecholamines from endogenous or exogenous sources, correction of acidosis, and hungry bone syndromes may also lower the serum Mg^{2+} levels by shifting Mg^{2+} into cells.

A large number of diseases may disrupt renal conservation of Mg^{2+} and result in hypomagnesemia. However, when advanced renal disease develops, hypermagnesemia usually occurs. Medications that alter renal Mg^{2+} conservation (Table 17.9) include the diuretics, aminoglycoside antibiotics, amphotericin B, cisplatinum, cardiac glycosides, calcium,

Table 17.9
Causes of Hypomagnesemia

Gastrointestinal Losses
   Reduced absorption
     Malabsorption
     Laxative abuse
     Fistulas
     Prolonged NG suction
   Reduced Intake
     Malnutrition
     Hyperalimentation
     Prolonged i.v. therapy
Drug-Induced Losses
   Diuretics
     Furosemide
     Thiazides
     Mannitol
     Glucose
     Urea
   Aminoglycosides
   Amphotericin B
   Cis-platinum
   Carbenicillin
   Thyroid hormone
   Digoxin
   Calcium
   Ethanol
   Insulin[a]
   Saline
   Citrate (blood)
   Catecholamines[a]
Renal Losses
   Renal disease
     Glomerulonephritis
     Tubular disorders
     Interstitial nephritis
     Diuretic phase of ATN
   Hypercalcemia
   Hyperaldosteronism
   Hyperthyroidism
   PO_4 deficiency
   Diabetic ketoacidosis
   SIADH
Miscellaneous Losses
   Lactation
   Pregnancy
   Severe sweating
   Hungry bone syndrome[a]
   Burns
   Sepsis
   Hypothermia
   Cardiopulmonary bypass
   Administration of glucose, amino acids, and insulin[a]
   Mg^{2+} free dialysis
   Refeeding after starvation[a]

[a] Redistribution of Mg^{2+}.

and saline (79). Aminoglycosides cause hypomagnesemia in 38% of patients receiving a standard intravenous course (138). Cardiac glycosides may cause hypomagnesemia by blocking the action of the sodium-potassium

ATPase pump in the renal tubule. This effect is important in view of the fact that hypomagnesemia may also potentiate digitalis toxicity. Thyroid hormone excess causes loss of Mg^{2+} in the urine because of increases in glomerular filtration and may also shift Mg^{2+} intracellularly. Citrate (found in blood products) can lower the serum ionized Mg^{2+} concentration by chelation.

Hypomagnesemia is frequently encountered in patients admitted to the hospital for ethanol withdrawal. Although acute ethanol intake results in increased renal Mg^{2+} excretion, chronic ethanol exposure has no lasting effect. Hypomagnesemia in alcoholic patients results primarily from poor dietary intake, ketosis, emesis, diarrhea, and hyperaldosteronism. Many alcoholic patients have a normal serum Mg^{2+} level on admission, which decreases during hospitalization because of metabolic changes induced during hospitalization (e.g., insulin secretion induced by dextrose infusion and anabolism). These patients may benefit from careful monitoring of the serum Mg^{2+} concentration. Despite the occurrence of hypomagnesemia in many patients with delirium tremens, there are no convincing data to suggest a cause-and-effect relationship. Mg^{2+} supplementation has not been shown to prevent delirium tremens.

CLINICAL MANIFESTATIONS

Signs and symptoms of Mg^{2+} deficiency (Table 17.10), like hypocalcemia, relate to increased neuronal irritability and tetany. Symptoms are rare when the total serum Mg^{2+} concentration is above 1.5 mg/dl and most symptomatic patients have levels below 1.0 mg/dl. Most symptomatic patients with hypomagnesemia have concomitant hypocalcemia or hypokalemia, and it is unclear whether hypomagnesemia alone causes symptoms (70). Hypomagnesemic patients may complain of muscle spasms, paresthesias, and weakness. Correction of hypomagnesemia can improve respiratory muscle strength (94). Central nervous system effects range from coma, disorientation, apathy, and depression to irritability and seizures.

Cardiovascular consequences of Mg^{2+} depletion may include heart failure, coronary artery spasm, arrhythmias, and hypotension (13, 21, 63). Hypomagnesemia increases cardiac sensitivity to the effects of digitalis and pressor agents (16) and can lead to toxicity at

Table 17.10
Clinical Manifestations of Hypomagnesemia

Cardiovascular
  Heart failure
  Arrhythmias
  Coronary artery spasm
  Vasospasm
  Hypertension
  Digitalis sensitivity
  Decreased pressor response
  ECG: Prolonged PR and QT interval, ST
    depression, Tall peaked T-waves (early),
    Broadening and decreased amplitude of T
    waves (late), wide QRS (late)
Gastrointestinal
  Dysphagia
  Anorexia
  Nausea
  Abdominal cramps
Neuromuscular
  Tetany
  Muscle spasm, tremor
  Seizures
  Confusion, disorientation
  Obtundation, coma
  Ataxia, nystagmus
  Apathy
  Depression
  Paresthesias
  Irritability
  Weakness
  Psychosis
Miscellaneous
  Hypokalemia
  Hypocalcemia
  Hypophosphatemia

lower serum digitalis levels (10). This effect may result from the synergistic effects of magnesium and digitalis on the cardiac sodium-potassium pump. Mg^{2+} deficiency is thought to lead to increased vascular tone and reactivity by modulating uptake, content, and distribution of Ca^{2+} in the smooth muscle cell (13). Hypomagnesemia may contribute to vasospasm and hypertension. Standard antiarrhythmic therapy and defibrillation may be ineffective in controlling ventricular arrhythmias associated with Mg^{2+} deficiency (63).

Hypomagnesemia may cause hypokalemia and intracellular potassium depletion. Repletion of intracellular and extracellular potassium may be impaired unless concurrent Mg^{2+} deficits are simultaneously treated (13, 16, 127, 128). Hypomagnesemic hypokalemia results from impaired renal potassium conservation due to diminished activation of the sodium-potassium adenosine triphosphatase pump and altered cell membrane permeability to potassium (126, 138). Hypomagnesemia-induced hypocalcemia results from impaired PTH se-

cretion, end-organ resistance to PTH, and vitamin D resistance (7, 92, 93, 110). Impaired Mg^{2+} dependent adenyl cyclase generation of cyclic AMP may be responsible for some of these effects (13). These patients present with clinical features of hypocalcemia (Table 17.2). Hypocalcemia may be difficult to correct until Mg^{2+} is replaced.

EVALUATION

Hypomagnesemia is usually diagnosed when the serum Mg^{2+} level is below normal limits. However, since Mg^{2+} is 30% protein bound, low total serum levels may occur in patients with hypoalbuminemia despite the occurrence of normal ionized concentrations (142). There is an easy method for normalizing serum Mg^{2+} for alterations in serum protein values through the use of protein retaining filters (142). Mg^{2+} is primarily an intracellular ion, and circulating levels may not always reflect the status of the intracellular environment. However, most patients with chronic hypomagnesemia have Mg^{2+} depletion (16). At present, we remain dependent upon the serum level, until new methods become available for assessing intracellular Mg^{2+} activity.

Measurement of urine Mg^{2+} excretion (24-hour urine measurement) is helpful in separating renal from nonrenal causes of hypomagnesemia. Normal kidneys are capable of decreasing Mg^{2+} excretion to 1–2 mEq/day in deficiency states. High urinary Mg^{2+} excretion (>3 mEq/day) in the presence of a low-serum Mg^{2+} level suggests increased renal loss of Mg^{2+} as the mechanism for Mg^{2+} depletion. Low urinary Mg^{2+} excretion ($<1–2$ mEq/day) in the presence of hypomagnesemia suggests renal conservation of Mg^{2+} and a Mg^{2+} deficient state because of decreased intake, redistribution, or nonrenal losses. If Mg^{2+} depletion is suspected in patients with a normal serum Mg^{2+} concentration and low Mg^{2+} excretion (e.g., intact renal Mg^{2+} conservation), a Mg^{2+} load test can be helpful. After a baseline 24-hour urine collection, 30 mmol of Mg^{2+} sulfate is administered in 500 ml of 5% dextrose in water over 12 hours; urine is collected for 24 hours from the beginning of the infusion. Individuals with normal Mg^{2+} stores excrete more than 60–80% of the administered load within 24 hours, whereas Mg^{2+} deficient patients excrete less than 50% (13, 14, 16). Decreased fractional Mg^{2+} excretion occurs in Mg^{2+} deficiency as a result of enhanced reabsorption of Mg^{2+} in the renal tubules because of resetting of Mg^{2+} transport (104). This test should be used with caution in patients with renal insufficiency, disturbances in cardiac conduction, or advanced respiratory insufficiency. Careful review of the clinical situation and medications usually reveals the cause.

TREATMENT

Mg^{2+} deficiency is treated by the administration of Mg^{2+} supplements (Table 17.11). Mild deficiency may be treated with diet alone. Mg^{2+} requirements range from 0.3 to 0.4 mEq/kg/day orally or 12–30 mEq/day during parenteral nutrition. These requirements assume no unusual losses and must be augmented accordingly. For maintenance intravenous therapy or parenteral nutrition, we give the sulfate salt so as to provide needed sulfate ions as well (27). Overt or severe hypomagnesemia ($Mg^{2+} < 1$ mg/dl) should be treated with intravenous Mg^{2+} (35, 44, 56, 79, 111). We recommend giving an initial dose of 600 mg of elemental Mg^{2+} over 3 hours followed by a maintenance dose of 600–900 mg of elemental Mg^{2+} per 24 hours. In emergency situations the loading dose of Mg^{2+} should not exceed 15 mg/minute, and the patient should receive continuous ECG monitoring to avoid cardiac toxicity (see "Hypermagnesemia"). Replacement therapy should be carried out over 5–7 days to allow time for intracellular stores to be replenished. Mg^{2+} sulfate may be given intramuscularly, however, it is painful. During therapy, patients require monitoring of the serum Mg^{2+} level, neurologic status, respiratory status, renal function, ECG, and blood pressure. Patellar reflexes should be monitored at the bedside during Mg^{2+} repletion, and therapy stopped if the reflexes become suppressed. If the patient is hypocalcemic, we prefer to use the chloride salt, since the sulfate salt can chelate with Ca^{2+} and further lower its level. If the patient has renal insufficiency, replacement should be closely guided by the serum Mg^{2+} level so as to avoid toxicity. Hypocalcemia may occur during therapy if the patient develops hypermagnesemia.

Once the patient is stable, Mg^{2+} can be replaced by the oral route (Table 17.11). Mg^{2+} oxide is the preferred Mg^{2+} preparation. Mg^{2+}-containing antacids are poorly absorbed and should not be used to replace Mg^{2+} unless other preparations are not available.

Magnesium and the Heart

Intractable ventricular arrhythmias associated with hypomagnesemia may respond to Mg^{2+} therapy (16, 42, 63, 82). Mg^{2+} therapy has also been useful in suppressing ventricular tachycardia and fibrillation in patients with ischemic heart disease who have normal serum Mg^{2+} levels (2, 62). Abraham et al. (2) treated a group of patients with acute myocardial infarction with Mg^{2+} sulfate (2.4 g administered intravenously over 20 minutes daily for 3 days). Potentially lethal arrhythmias were reduced from 34.8% to 14.6%, when compared with placebo. We have used Mg^{2+} sulfate (1 g administered intravenously over 20 minutes every 6 hours) effectively in the ICU to treat refractory ventricular tachycardias and ventricular fibrillation. Mg^{2+} depletion interferes with the sodium-potassium ATPase and causes ionic imbalance and electrical instability. Mg^{2+} administration prolongs the effective refractory period, depresses conduction, increases the membrane potential (makes it more negative), and can control ventricular tachyarrhythmias. Thus, when ventricular fibrillation or malignant ventricular arrhythmias cannot be controlled with conventional antiarrhythmic drugs,

Table 17.11
Magnesium Supplements[a]

Parenteral	
Mg^{2+} Chloride	Loading: 600 mg elemental Mg^{2+} in D5W over 3 hours
1 g = 118 mg Mg^{2+} = 9 mEq	Maintenance: 600–900 mg Mg^{2+} per day
Mg^{2+} Sulfate	Same as for Mg^{2+} Chloride
1 g = 98 mg Mg^{2+} = 8 mEq	(intramuscularly: 200 mg every 4 hours for 24 hours then 100 mg every 4 hours)
Enteral	
Mg^{2+} Oxide tablets	20–80 mEq/day in divided doses
tablet = 111 mg Mg^{2+} = 9 mEq	
Mg^{2+} Gluconate tablets	20–80 mEq/day in divided doses
500 mg tablet = 32 mg Mg^{2+} = 2.4 mEq	

[a] 1 mEq = 0.5 mmol = 12.3 mg Mg^{2+}

we recommend infusing Mg^{2+}. Iseri et al. (62) give 16 mEq slowly over 1 minute followed by 80 mEq over the next 5 hours. Potassium chloride at 10 mEq/hour is also infused since there is evidence that Mg^{2+} and potassium depletion frequently occur together. It may be necessary to continue a maintenance infusion of Mg^{2+} to prevent recurrence of arrhythmias. We usually aim for a serum Mg^{2+} concentration of 3–4 mg/dl.

Intravenous administration of Mg^{2+} (50 mmol $MgCl_2$ in 1000 ml isotonic dextrose at 100 ml/hour for 6 hours followed by 22 ml/hour for 18 hours) has been reported to reduce both mortality and arrhythmias (106) when given to patients with acute myocardial infarction. Placebo (n = 74) and Mg^{2+} treated (n = 56) patients had similar admission serum Mg^{2+} levels. However, 4 weeks after myocardial infarction the patients given Mg^{2+} had a lower mortality (7% versus 19%). The proportion of patients requiring treatment for arrhythmias was also lower (21% versus 47%). In another study, Rasmussen et al. (105) found that patients with acute myocardial infarctions dropped their serum Mg^{2+} concentrations over the first 32 hours after infarction. The drop appeared to result from an extracellular to intracellular shift in Mg^{2+}. Kafka et al. (67) noted a 6% incidence of hypomagnesemia in patients with acute myocardial infarction, whereas Dyckner (41) reported a 46% incidence. Hypomagnesemia was associated with a higher frequency of major ventricular arrhythmias. Kafka et al. (67) also found a 17% incidence of hypokalemia in their patients with myocardial infarction. Ventricular arrhythmias occurred in all patients with both hypokalemia and hypomagnesemia.

Whang and colleagues (129) found a 19% incidence of hypomagnesemia and 9% incidence of hypokalemia in patients receiving digitalis. Hypomagnesemia and hypokalemia are important since both predispose to digitalis toxicity (13, 63, 114). Mg^{2+} deficiency may also enhance digoxin uptake by myocardial cells (51). Iseri et al. (63) reported the efficacy of intravenously administered Mg^{2+} in treating hypomagnesemic patients with toxic reactions to digitalis and recurrent ventricular tachycardia. Mg^{2+} responsive ventricular arrhythmias may also occur in normomagnesemic patients receiving digitalis (32, 62). A decrease in serum Mg^{2+} after cardiopulmonary bypass surgery has been reported (21). Suppression of cardiac arrhythmias after heart surgery may be assisted by Mg^{2+} therapy.

Magnesium and Bronchospasm

Relief of dyspnea and stridor after Mg^{2+} infusion has been observed on occasion. The Mg^{2+} ion has an inhibitory action on smooth muscle contraction, histamine release from mast cells, and on acetylcholine release from cholinergic nerve terminals (6, 101). Okayama et al. (101) studied the bronchodilating effect of Mg^{2+} sulfate infusion (0.5 mmol/minute for 20 minutes) in 10 patients with mild asthma. Serum Mg^{2+} concentration rose from 2.1 mg/dl (0.86 mmol/l) to 5.1 mg/dl (2.08 mmol/l) with this dose. Mg^{2+} infusion decreased respiratory resistance by 30%, improved forced vital capacity by 17%, and improved forced expiratory volume at 1 second by 18%. There were no adverse effects on blood pressure or heart rate. The magnitude of these effects were similar to those found with albuterol inhalation. These authors also administered Mg^{2+} to three patients with severe asthma who were treated with dexamethasone, aminophylline, and inhaled albuterol. They noted an improvement in wheezing, dyspnea, and sputum expectoration. More studies (prospective, blinded, and randomized) are needed before this therapy can be recommended, but Mg^{2+} infusion may provide yet another new drug for the treatment of reactive airway disease. Extreme caution must be used since hypermagnesemia can depress neuromuscular and cardiovascular function.

Hypermagnesemia

Spontaneous hypermagnesemia is rare in clinical practice and most cases result from iatrogenic causes (27, 30, 79, 96, 111). The most common etiology of hypermagnesemia is the administration of Mg^{2+} containing antacids, enemas, or parenteral nutrition to patients with renal insufficiency. Other causes of hypermagnesemia include hypothyroidism, Addison's disease, lithium intoxication, familial hypocalciuric hypercalcemia, and the administration of Mg^{2+} to patients with premature labor or preeclampsia/eclampsia. Hypermagnesemia may also occur in infants born to mothers who received Mg^{2+} for these problems.

Hypermagnesemia diminishes neuromuscular transmission and can depress skeletal muscle function and cause neuromuscular blockade (Table 17.12). Mg^{2+} excess inhibits prejunctional release of acetylcholine and de-

Table 17.12
Clinical Manifestations of Hypermagnesemia

	Serum Mg^{2+} Level (mg/dl)
Normal level	1.7–2.4
Decrease in DTR	4–5
ECG Changes	
e.g., prolonged PR, QRS, ST	4–6
Bradycardia	4–7
Hypotension	5–7
Somnolence	6–8
Respiratory insufficiency	10–12
Heart block	15
Respiratory paralysis	18
Cardiac arrest	15–24

creases motor end plate sensitivity to acetylcholine (104). Excess Mg^{2+} may also cause vasodilation and hypotension. Hypermagnesemia increases neuromuscular sensitivity to the effects of skeletal muscle relaxants and can result in more prolonged and potent effects of these drugs. Hypocalcemia may result from hypermagnesemia-induced parathyroid gland suppression (30).

The neuromuscular and cardiac toxicity of hypermagnesemia can be transiently antagonized by the administration of intravenous Ca^{2+} (5–10 mEq). Definitive therapy to lower the serum Mg^{2+} level consists of stopping all drugs and supplements containing Mg^{2+} and administering saline and furosemide to enhance renal excretion. In patients with renal failure, Mg^{2+} may be removed by dialysis.

PHOSPHORUS

The adult body contains about 700–800 g of PO_4. PO_4 is the major intracellular anion and is essential for a large variety of biochemical processes. It is required in protein, fat, and carbohydrate metabolism and is the source of high-energy bonds in adenosine triphosphate and phosphocreatine. PO_4 high energy bonds provide the energy for maintenance of cellular integrity, muscle contraction, neurologic function, hormonal secretion, and cell division. PO_4 is also a component of 2,3-diphosphoglycerate, which functions as a regulator of oxygen release from hemoglobin. PO_4 is a component of cyclic nucleotides, nicotinamide diphosphate, phospholipids, nucleic acids, and participates in the urinary buffering of acids.

The normal serum PO_4 level is 4.0–7.1 mg/dl in children and 2.7–4.5 mg/dl in adults (29). The average dietary intake of PO_4 ranges from 800–1200 mg/day, with most being absorbed in the small intestine by both passive (50%) and active (vitamin D dependent) transport. Thus, even in vitamin D deficient states the gut is able to absorb enough PO_4 to maintain normal serum levels. PO_4 is excreted in the urine and stool. PO_4 is primarily regulated by the kidneys, with most PO_4 reabsorption occurring in the proximal tubules. Tubular reabsorption increases to a maximum (TmP), with further increases in PO_4 being excreted in the urine. This system is analogous to that which is seen with glucose. The set point for the TmP determines one's fasting serum PO_4 level and is affected by a large number of drugs. It is reduced by aminohippurate sodium, amino acids, dextrose, acetoacetate, sodium bicarbonate, saline, acute hypercapnia, thyroid hormone, estrogen, digoxin, long-term corticosteroids, and renal vasodilation (29, 87). Infusion of dextrose in amounts sufficient to cause glycosuria decrease tubular reabsorption of PO_4 by 20% and both may share a common reabsorptive pathway (87). Extracellular volume expansion is associated with decreases in the proximal tubular reabsorption of both PO_4 and sodium (87), resulting in phosphaturia. Growth hormone increases the TmP and thus decreases the amount of PO_4 excreted in the urine. Higher growth hormone levels in children may explain their higher serum PO_4 concentrations.

The amount of PO_4 in excreted urine also depends upon PTH and its effects upon tubular PO_4 reabsorption. PTH produces phosphaturia by decreasing TmP via the adenyl cyclase system. This phosphaturic effect is important in Ca^{2+} homeostasis. PTH increases bone resorption and releases Ca^{2+} and PO_4. Hyperphosphatemia is avoided by the renal action of PTH. Acute hypercalcemia and hypermagnesemia decrease the renal excretion of PO_4 by inhibiting PTH secretion, whereas hypocalcemia and hypomagnesemia do the reverse. PO_4 has no direct effect upon the parathyoid glands, but rather affects PTH secretion through its affects upon the ionized Ca^{2+} level.

PO_4 affects the 1-hydroxylation of 25-hydroxyvitamin D within the kidney and this effect is independent of PTH. Hypophosphatemia stimulates the 1-hydroxylase, whereas hyperphosphatemia inhibits it. 1,25-Dihydroxyvitamin D can stimulate PO_4 mobilization from bone and enhance absorption from the intestine. It plays a minor role in regulating renal PO_4 reabsorption.

Insulin causes glucose and PO_4 to move into

cells and is responsible for hypophosphatemia seen during insulin administration or high carbohydrate feedings. PO_4 is trapped in the cell when glucose is converted to glucose-6-phosphate.

Hypophosphatemia

CAUSES

Hypophosphatemia results from three primary mechanisms (Table 17.13): intracellular shift of PO_4, increased loss of PO_4 through the kidneys, and decreased gastrointestinal absorption of PO_4.

Carbohydrate loading (e.g., intravenous dextrose solutions and pareneteral nutrition) causes hypophosphatemia by shifting PO_4 into the cell and accounts for about half of the cases of hypophosphatemia seen in hospitalized patients. PO_4 is trapped in the cell when glucose is converted to glucose-6-phosphate (29, 72). Inadequate PO_4 in parenteral nutrition or rapid refeeding of severely starved patients elicits a similar response. Acute respiratory and metabolic alkalosis stimulates intracellular glycolysis, consuming PO_4 in the process (15). Sepsis, central nervous system disorders, and salicylate poisoning cause hyperventilation and respiratory alkalosis. Salicylate poisoning may also stimulate glycolysis directly. Treatment of hypothermia causes a shift of PO_4 into the cell and may also cause hypophosphatemia (81). Hypophosphatemia is common after severe burns and results from a combination of increased metabolism, respiratory alkalosis, sepsis, inappropriate phosphaturia, excess catecholamine and cortisol secretion, and hyperalimentation.

Epinephrine and glucagon, like insulin, can also cause a reduction in the circulating PO_4 level, presumably by stimulating the cellular utilization of glucose and accelerating the formation of intracellular PO_4 esters. The intravenous infusion of epinephrine at a rate of 10 μg/min for 10 minutes, results in a 25% fall in the serum PO_4 concentration (86).

Hypomagnesemia augments renal PO_4 excretion; however, hypomagnesemia alone rarely causes hypophosphatemia since it also suppresses parathyroid hormone secretion, causing hypocalcemia and a reduction in PO_4 excretion. The two effects balance out. However, hypophosphatemia may occur in these patients when magnesium is replaced without PO_4, resulting in a surge in parathyroid hormone release and augmented phosphaturia.

Table 17.13
Causes of Hypophosphatemia

Transcellular Shift
  Recovery from malnutrition[a]
  Carbohydrate loading[a]
  Recovery from hypothermia[a]
  Recovery from burns[a]
  Acute alkalosis[a]
  Alcoholism[a]
  Diabetic ketoacidosis[a]
  Sepsis
  Salicylate poisoning
  Hungry bone syndrome
  Anabolic steroids
Gastrointestinal Losses
  Malabsorption
  Emesis
  Diarrhea
  Prolonged NG suction
  PO_4 binding resins
  Vitamin D deficiency
Drug-Induced
  Anabolic steroids
  Antacids[a]
  Calcitonin
  Corticosteroids
  Diuretics
  Epinephrine
  Glucagon
  Insulin[a]
  Sodium bicarbonate
  Saline diuresis
  Salicylates
Renal Losses
  Renal tubular defects e.g., myeloma, heavy metals, RTA, Fanconi syndrome
  Hyperparathyroidism
  Hypomagnesemia
  Hypokalemia
  Acidosis
  Pregnancy
  Vitamin D deficiency or resistance
  Reye's syndrome
  Recovery from ATN
  After renal transplant
  Diuresis
  Oncogenic hypophosphatemia
Miscellaneous
  Hemodialysis
  Inadequate PO_4 in i.v. fluids

[a]Most common causes of severe hypophosphatemia (PO_4 <1 mg/dl).

Diuretic therapy, renal tubular defects (e.g., from myeloma or heavy metals), primary and secondary hyperparathyroidism, vitamin D deficiency, and acidemia are other causes of renal PO_4 wasting and hypophosphatemia. Vitamin D deficiency causes hypophosphatemia via its effects on increasing PTH secretion (induced by hypocalcemia) and reduced intestinal PO_4 absorption. Posttransplantation hypophosphatemia develops in over 50% of patients with a transplanted kidney and results from a combination of renal phosphaturia, persistent hyperparathyroidism, glucocorticoid therapy, 1,25-dihydroxyvitamin D deficiency, and use of antacids (15). Hypophosphatemia has also been associated with a variety of tumors (15). These tumors appear to elaborate substances that interfere with renal PO_4 reabsorption, bone mineralization, and renal 1,25-dihydroxyvitamin D synthesis.

Inadequate PO_4 intake alone rarely causes hypophosphatemia. However, hypophosphatemia may occur in patients on a marginally adequate PO_4 intake when another cause for hypophosphatemia occurs (Table 17.13). A frequently seen clinical situation is that of a chronically ill patient admitted to the hospital and placed on intravenous dextrose solutions (containing little PO_4) or given nonabsorbable PO_4 binding antacids. PO_4 binding antacids, such as aluminum or magnesium hydroxide, are common causes of hypophosphatemia. These antacids bind PO_4 that is found in enteral nutrition as well as PO_4 that is secreted into the gut. Thus, they produce hypophosphatemia even in patients who are not fed enterally. Malabsorption states, such as is seen with pancreatic disease or diarrhea, may also cause hypophosphatemia by impairing PO_4 absorption and increasing gut losses.

Hypophosphatemia is commonly seen during the treatment of diabetic ketoacidosis and hyperglycemic hyperosmolar nonketotic syndromes. Serum PO_4 levels are usually normal at the time the patient is admitted, despite total body depletion of PO_4 (73, 74). After the initiation of insulin therapy, PO_4 shifts into the cells along with glucose and potassium. Plasma levels may decrease to less than 1 mg/dl within 24 hours of initiation of therapy (73, 107). PO_4 deficiency is associated with insulin resistance, decreased levels of 2,3-DPG, and decreased intracellular ATP. Low 2,3-DPG shifts the hemoglobin dissociation curve to the left, decreasing oxygen off-loading to the tissues. This alteration in the oxyhemoglobin dissociation curve may be important clinically in some patients, since elevated levels of glycosylated hemoglobin (found in diabetics) also impairs oxygen off-loading. As acidosis is corrected during the treatment of ketoacidosis, the ability of hemoglobin to release oxygen is even further decreased. PO_4 supplementation can more quickly restore 2,3-DPG levels and intracellular ATP concentrations to normal. Although deleterious effects of hypophosphatemia on the clinical course of diabetic ketoacidosis have not been conclusively shown (69, 130), we have seen a number of patients develop complications believed to be secondary to hypophosphatemia (e.g., seizures and respiratory failure). In addition, if one looks

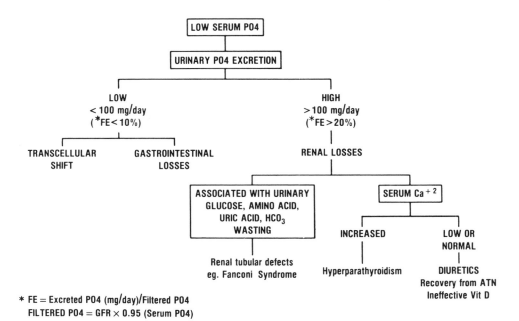

Figure 17.4. Evaluation of hypophosphatemia.

at all patients with hypophosphatemia, diabetic ketoacidosis is a common cause. For the above reasons, we recommend administering PO_4 for the treatment of hyperglycemic states, provided that hyperphosphatemia can be avoided.

Hypophosphatemia is common in alcoholics admitted to the hospital (15, 112). These patients are frequently malnourished and suffer from malabsorption processes. When admitted to the hospital, they are given intravenous or oral carbohydrate loads that shift PO_4 into the cells. Respiratory alkolosis may develop, especially during withdrawal, and further exacerbate hypophosphatemia. Hypomagnesemia, hypokalemia, alcohol, and acidosis may lead to impaired renal conservation of PO_4.

Hypophosphatemia (PO_4 <2.4 mg/dl) occurs in approximately 29% of surgical patients (119). Hypophosphatemia develops 24 hours after surgery and results from glucose infusions, increased tissue metabolism, increased catecholamine secretion, and renal PO_4 losses (15, 59, 119). It is not known whether routine PO_4 supplementation in these patients would improve outcome.

The cause of hypophosphatemia can usually be determined from the medical history and clinical setting. When in doubt, measurement of urinary PO_4 excretion may be helpful (Fig. 17.4). Transcelluar shifts of PO_4 and gastrointestinal loss of PO_4 evoke avid renal PO_4 reabsorption, decreasing the fractional excretion of PO_4 in the urine to less than 10%. Renal causes of hypophosphatemia result in PO_4 wasting in the urine and a fractional excretion of PO_4 greater than 20%.

Table 17.14
Clinical Features of Hypophosphatemia

General
  Weakness
  Malaise
Myocardial Insufficiency
Impaired Pressor Responses
Respiratory Insufficiency
Rhabdomyolysis
Hepatocellular Damage
Hematologic
  Hemolysis
  Platelet dysfunction
  Leukocyte dysfunction
Skeletal
  Osteomalacia
  Fractures
  Increased bone resorption
Metabolic
  Impaired glucose tolerance
  Impaired gluconeogenesis
  Impaired phospholipid synthesis
  Hypercalciuria
  Hypermagnesemia
Neurological
  Ataxia
  Confusion
  Obtundation
  Coma
  Delirium
  Dysarthria
  Encephalopathy
  Muscle weakness
  Irritability
  Myopathy
  Paresthesias
  Seizures
  Tremor
Gastrointestinal
  Anorexia
  Nausea
  Vomiting

CLINICAL MANIFESTATIONS

Severe hypophosphatemia is associated with decreased levels of PO_4 containing metabolites (e.g., ATP, 2,3DPG) and membrane phospholipids and may cause a variety of clinical problems (Table 32.14). Patients may develop cardiac insufficiency (15, 37, 46, 100). The cause for cardiac insufficiency is uncertain but may relate to depleted intracellular PO_4 stores (e.g., ATP, creatine phosphate), impaired action of the sodium potassium ATPase pump, decreased calcium flux, or impaired catecholamine action (15, 75).

Patients with serum PO_4 levels of less than 2 mg/dl may complain of muscle weakness, anorexia, or tremor. As PO_4 levels approach 1 mg/dl, respiratory weakness or insufficiency may occur (8, 99, 122). Respiratory failure is more likely to occur in patients with underlying lung disease. In addition, hypophosphatemia may decrease muscle strength and impair weaning from ventilators. PO_4 supplementation in these patients may improve muscle strength (8, 122). We have treated a few patients with advanced pulmonary disease whom we could not wean off the ventilator because of respiratory muscle fatigue. After PO_4 supplementation, these patients were weaned from the ventilator. Hypophosphatemia has been reported to produce a large number of neurologic symptoms that include ataxia, tremor, paresthesias, myopathy, seizures, coma, and death.

Muscle cell integrity depends upon PO_4 and severe hypophosphatemia (< 1 mg/dl) may injure the cell and cause rhabdomyolysis. Severe hypophosphatemia may also affect blood cells and cause hemolysis, platelet dysfunction, and leukocyte dysfunction. Hemolytic anemia is rarely seen unless the plasma PO_4 falls below 0.5 mg/dl. Depressed erythrocyte levels of 2,3DPG shift the oxyhemoglobin dissociation curve to the left (reduces P_{50}), decreasing oxygen delivery to the tissues. Depressed leukocyte chemotaxis, phagocytosis, and bactericidal activity may impair recovery from infection. Metabolic consequences of hypophosphatemia include insulin resistance (38), impaired gluconeogenesis, impaired bone mineralization, and liver dysfunction. Hypercalciuria results from release of Ca^{2+} from bone in an attempt to maintain normal serum PO_4 concentrations (15) and decreased renal absorption of Ca^{2+}. Hypermagnesemia also results from increased mobilization of Mg^{2+} from bone and reduced Mg^{2+} reabsorption in the kidney (15).

PO_4 depletion is associated with three major alterations in renal acid-base regulation: proximal tubular bicarbonate wasting, impaired distal acidification, and decreased buffer excretion (diminished renal ammoniagenesis and hypophosphaturia) (15). Acid-base stability is usually well preserved because of the balance of acidifying and alkalinizing forces (e.g., alkali released from bone). However, prolonged and severe PO_4 depletion may exhaust bone stores of alkali and result in a metabolic acidosis.

THERAPY

The potential consequences of severe hypophosphatemia necessitate prompt recognition and treatment so as to avoid potentially devastating consequences. Serious life-threatening consequences usually do not occur until the serum PO_4 concentration falls below 1 mg/dl. Primary therapy should be oriented towards preventing hypophosphatemia. Serum PO_4 levels, like other primarily intracellular ions, may not adequately reflect body stores. Thus, initial therapy is usually empiric and one must monitor the serum level to avoid hyperphosphatemia.

Initially, one should stop all drugs (if possible) that are contributing to hypophosphatemia. The list of drugs must include PO_4-binding antacids, intravenous glucose, and diuretics.

For immediate correction of profound hypophosphatemia (< 1 mg/dl) or symptomatic hypophosphatemia, intravenous therapy (71, 80, 121) is necessary (Table 32.15), since oral PO_4 preparations when given in large amounts usually cause diarrhea. The rate of administration of PO_4 varies in the literature from 0.3 mg/kg/hour to 4 mg/kg/hour (71, 80, 121).

Based upon our experience we recommend the following: If depletion is recent and uncomplicated give 0.6 mg (0.02 mmol)/kg/hour; if prolonged and multifactorial give 0.9 mg (0.03 mmol)/kg/hour. Check the serum PO_4 level every 6–12 hours until the level has stabilized,

Table 17.15
Phosphate Preparations

Preparation	PO_4 Content[a]	Daily Dose
Enteral		
Whole milk	1 mg/ml	1200 ml
Skim milk	0.9 mg/ml	1330 ml
Neutro-Phos[b]	250 mg/capsule	1–2 t.i.d.
Potassium-PO_4 (K-Phos)	125 mg tablet	3–4 t.i.d.
	250 mg tablet	1–2 t.i.d.
Parenteral		
Potassium-PO_4	93 mg/ml	1000 mg/day
	(4 mEq/ml K^+)	
Sodium-PO_4	93 mg/ml	1000 mg/day
	(4 mEq/ml Na^+)	
Neutral Sodium-PO_4	2.8 mg/ml	1000 mg/day
	(0.16 mEq/ml Na^+)	
Neutral Sodium		
Potassium-PO_4	3.1 mg/ml	1000 mg/day
	(0.16 mEq/ml Na^+;	
	0.02 mEq/ml K^+)	

[a]31 mg PO_4 = 1 mmol PO_4
[b]Also available as a solution.

so as to avoid hyperphosphatemia. Hyperkalemia may result from excessive administration of potassium phosphate, especially in patients with impaired renal function. If the patient is also hypocalcemic or hypercalcemic, PO_4 should be administered at a slower rate and both PO_4 and Ca^{2+} monitored. Risks of treatment include hyperphosphatemia, hypocalcemia, hypotension, hyperkalemia (with potassium PO_4), hypomagnesemia, hyperosmolality, metastatic calcification, and renal failure. Extreme caution must be used when administering PO_4 to patients with renal insufficiency or failure, since these patients have a diminished ability to excrete PO_4. Parenteral solutions of PO_4 are hypertonic and should be diluted before use or given by central line. The addition of calcium to PO_4-containing solutions or administration through the same intravenous line may cause precipitation. Parenteral PO_4 may be discontinued and enteral therapy (Table 17.15) started when the serum PO_4 level exceeds 2 mg/dl. Repletion should be carried out over 5–7 days to replace intracellular stores and then the patient placed on a maintenance dose (e.g., 1200 mg/day orally or 1000 mg/day intravenously in the adult). Additional PO_4 may be required if excess losses are present. Hypomagnesemia is common in patients with PO_4 deficiency and should always be measured and replaced as needed (121).

Hyperphosphatemia

CAUSES

Hyperphosphatemia results from three basic mechanisms (Table 17.16): reduced renal excretion, increased entrance of PO_4 into the extracellular space from the intracellular space, and increased PO_4 or vitamin D intake.

Levels of PO_4 remain within normal ranges until the glomerular filtration rate falls below 20–25 ml/minute. Hyperphosphatemia, as well as renal failure, impair the renal conversion of 25-hydroxyvitamin D to 1,25-dihydroxyvitamin D. Impaired synthesis of 1,25-dihydroxyvitamin D contributes to hypocalcemia and secondary hyperparathyroidism. PO_4 rises in patients with acute renal failure and frequently occurs before the rise in blood urea nitrogen or creatinine. Elevated PO_4 levels are also seen in patients with hypoparathyroidism due to the loss of the phosphaturic action of parathyroid hormone. Hyperphosphatemia and

Table 17.16
Causes of Hyperphosphatemia

Reduced Renal Excretion
  Renal insufficiency
  Hypoparathyroidism
  PTH resistance
  Hyperthyroidism
  Acromegaly
  Diphosphonates
  Tumoral calcinosis
Increased PO_4 or Vitamin D Intake
  Ingestion of PO_4 (e.g., laxatives)
  Intravenous PO_4
  PO_4 enemas
  Vitamin D
Increased PO_4 Entrance into Extracellular Fluid
  Acidosis
  Chemotherapy
  Rhabdomyolysis
  Sepsis
  Malignant hyperpyrexia
  Fulminant hepatitis
  Severe hypothermia
  Hemolysis

hypercalcemia occur in hyperthyroidism as a result of increased bone resorption, parathyroid gland suppression, and increased tubular reabsorption of PO_4. Diphosphonates are used to treat patients with Paget's disease of bone and hypercalcemia. These agents cause hyperphosphatemia by reducing PO_4 excretion and altering its distribution between cellular compartments.

Hyperphosphatemia may occur when PO_4 enters the extracellular space after cellular damage induced by chemotherapy (tumor lysis syndrome), rhabdomyolysis, malignant hyperthermia, hypothermia, sepsis, or hepatic necrosis. The hyperphosphatemia is exaggerated when there is concomitant renal insufficiency. Hyperphosphatemia may also occur from overzealous administration of PO_4-containing compounds (25) or from laxative abuse. PO_4 deficiency is common in patients with diabetic ketoacidosis. However, since potassium deficits are usually twice that of PO_4 deficits, potassium should be replaced with a combination of KCl and K_2PO_4 so that hyperphosphatemia is avoided. Serum PO_4 levels may be artificially increased as a result of hemolysis during blood drawing.

Measurement of glomerular filtration and urinary PO_4 excretion are helpful in evaluating the etiology of hyperphosphatemia (Fig. 17.5). A glomerular filtration rate less than 20–25 ml/minute suggests renal failure as the cause. Relatively normal glomerular filtration with a PO_4 excretion greater than 1500 mg/day sug-

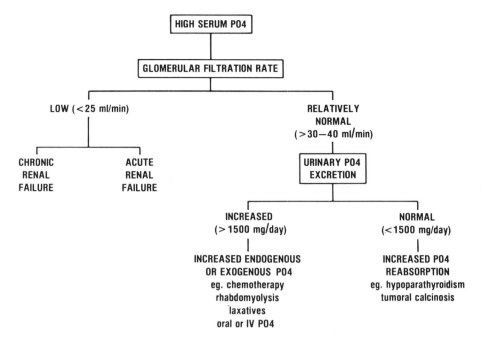

Figure 17.5 Evaluation of hyperphosphatemia.

gests increased PO4 loading from either endogenous or exogenous sources. Normal renal filtration with a PO4 excretion less than 1500 mg/day indicates increased PO4 reabsorption as the cause.

Symptoms of hyperphosphatemia relate primarily to the hypocalcemia that it induces and ectopic calcification. Soft tissue calcification usually occurs when the calcium-phosphate product exceeds 75. In addition, alkalosis favors calcification.

THERAPY

The therapy of hyperphosphatemia is aimed at eliminating the PO4 source, removing PO4 from the circulation, and at correcting any associated hypocalcemia. Dietary PO4 intake should be restricted. PO4 excretion in the urine can be increased by saline (250–500 ml/hour) and acetazolamide (500 mg every 6 hours) (4). Intestinal PO4 absorption can be minimized and PO4 can be removed from the body via the gastrointestinal tract with oral PO4 binders (e.g., aluminum hydroxide), which are of benefit even if no oral PO4 is given. If renal insufficiency is not a problem, alternating aluminum hydroxide with magnesium salts can decrease aluminum-induced constipation. If symptomatic hypocalcemia is present the patient

should be given calcium. Hemodialysis or peritoneal dialysis are effective in removing PO4 in renal failure.

References

1. Abbasi AA, Chemplavil JK, Farah S, et al: Hypercalcemia in active pulmonary tuberculosis. *Ann Intern Med* 90:324–328, 1979.
2. Abraham AS, Rosenmann D, Kramer M, et al: Magnesium in the prevention of lethal arrhythmias in acute myocardial infarction. *Arch Intern Med* 147:753–755, 1987.
3. Aguanno JJ, Ladenson JH: Influence of fatty acids on the binding of calcium to albumin. *J Biol Chem* 257:8745–8748, 1982.
4. Agus ZS, Goldfarb S, Wasserstein A: Disorders of calcium and phosphate balance. In Brenner BM, Rector FC (eds): *The Kidney*, 2nd ed. Philadelphia, WB Saunders 1981, pp 940–1022.
5. Aldinger KA, Samaan NA: Hypokalemia with hypercalcemia. *Ann Intern Med* 85:571–573, 1977.
6. Altura BM, Altura BT, Carella A: Magnesium deficiency induced spasms of umbilical vessels: Relation to preeclampsia, hypertension, growth retardation. *Science* 221:376–378, 1983.
7. Anast CS, Winnacker JL, Forte LR, et al: Impaired release of parathyroid hormone in magnesium deficiency. *J Clin Endocrinol Metal* 42:707–717, 1976.
8. Aubier M, Murciano D, Lecocguic Y, et al: Effect of hypophosphatemia on diaphragmatic contractility in patients with acute respiratory failure. *N Engl J Med* 313:420–424, 1985.
9. Bell NH, Stern PH, Pantzer E, et al: Evidence that increased circulatory 1α, 25-dihydroxyvitamin D is the

probable cause for abnormal calcium metabolism in sarcoidosis. *J Clin Invest* 64:218–225, 1979.

10. Beller GA, Hood WB, Smith TW, Abelmann WH, Wacker WEC: Correlation of serum magnesium levels and digitalis intoxication. *Am J Cardiol* 33:225–229, 1974.

11. Benabe JE, Martinez-Maldonado: Disorders of calcium metabolism. In Maxwell MH, Kleeman CR, Narins RG: *Clinical Disorders of Fluid and Electrolyte Metabolism*, 4th ed. New York, McGraw Hill, 1987, pp 759–788.

12. Benson RC, Riggs BL, Pickard BM, Arnaud DC: Radioimmunoassay of parathyroid hormone in hypercalcemic disease. *Am J Med* 56:821–826, 1974.

13. Berkelhammer C, Bear RA: A clinical approach to common electrolyte problems: hypomagnesemia. *Can Med Assoc J* 132:360–368, 1985.

14. Bohmer T, Mathiesen B: Magnesium deficiency in chronic alcoholic patients uncovered by an intravenous load test. *Scand J Clin Lab Invest* 42:633–636, 1982.

15. Brauthbar N, Kleeman CR: Hypophosphatemia and hyperphosphatemia: clinical and pathophysiologic aspects. In Maxwell MH, Kleeman CR, Narins RG: *Clinical Disorders of Fluid and Electrolyte Metabolism*, 4th ed. New York, McGraw Hill, 1987, pp 789–830.

16. Brautbar N, Massry SG: Hypomagnesemia and hypermagnesemia. In Maxwell MH, Kleeman CR, Narins RG: *Clinical Disorders of Fluid and Electrolyte Metabolism*, 4th ed. New York, McGraw Hill, 1987, pp 831–849.

17. Breslau NA, McGuire JL, Zerwekh JE, et al: Hypercalcemia associated with increased serum calcitriol levels in three patients with lymphoma. *Ann Intern Med* 100:1–7, 1984.

18. Bristow MR, Ginsburg R, Minobe W, et al: Decreased catecholamine sensitivity and beta-adrenergic receptor density in failing human hearts. *N Engl J Med* 307:205–211, 1982.

19. Bristow MR, Schwartz D, Binetti G, Harrison DC, Daniels JR: Ionized calcium and the heart. *Circ Res* 41:565–574, 1977.

20. Buckle R: Ectopic PTH syndrome, pseudohyperparathyroidism, hypercalcemia of malignancy. *J Clin Endocrinol Metab* 3:237–251, 1974.

21. Burch GE, Giles TD: The importance of magnesium deficiency in cardiovascular disease. *Am Heart J* 94:649–657, 1977.

22. Cardella CJ, Birkin BL, Roscoe M, Rapoport A: Role of dialysis in the treatment of severe hypercalcemia: report of two cases successfully treated with hemodialysis and review of the literature. *Clin Nephrol* 12:285–290, 1979.

23. Chaimovitz C, Abinader E, Benderly A, et al: Hypocalcemic hypotension. *J Am Med Assoc* 222:86–87, 1972.

24. Chang J, Abramson EC, Mayer M, et al: The effects of cisplatin on parathyroid hormone and tumor-induced bone resorption. *Clin Res* 33:888A, 1985.

25. Chernow B, Rainey TG, Georges LP, et al: Iatrogenic hyperphosphatemia: a metabolic consideration in critical care medicine. *Crit Care Med* 9:772–774, 1981.

26. Chernow B, Smith J, Rainey TG, et al: Hypomagnesemia: implications for the critical care specialist. *Crit Care Med* 10:193–196, 1982.

27. Chernow B, Zaloga GP: SCCM - ions for society members (sulfate, chloride calcium, magnesium). In *Critical Care - State of the Art*. Fullerton, CA, Society of Critical Care Medicine, 1984, vol 4, pp K1–43.

28. Chernow B, Zaloga GP, Malcolm D, Clapper M, Holaday JW: Glucagon's chronotropic action is calcium dependent. *J Pharmacol Exp Ther* (in press)

29. Chester WL, Zaloga GP, Chernow B: Phosphate metabolism in the critically ill patient. In Geelhoed G, Chernow B (eds): *Endocrine Aspects of Acute Illness: Clinics in Critical Care Medicine*. New York, Churchill Livingstone, 1985, vol 5, pp 205–216.

30. Cholst IN, Steinberg SF, Tropper PJ, et al: The influence of hypermagnesemia on serum calcium and parathyroid hormone levels in human subjects. *N Engl J Med* 310:1221–1225, 1984.

31. Chopra D, Janson P, Sawin CT: Insensitivity to digoxin associated with hypocalcemia. *N Engl J Med* 296:917–918, 1977.

32. Cohen L, Kitzes R: Magnesium sulfate and digitalis-toxic arrhythmias. *JAMA* 249:2808–2810, 1983.

33. Condon JR, Ives D, Knight MJ, Day J: The aetiology of hypocalcemia in acute pancreatitis. *Br J Surg* 62:115–118, 1975.

34. Connor TB, Rosen BL, Bleaustein MP et al: Hypocalcemia precipitating congestive heart failure. *N Engl J Med* 307:869–872, 1982.

35. Cronin RE, Knochel JP: Magnesium deficiency. *Adv Intern Med* 28:509–533, 1983.

36. Cushard WG, Simon AB, Canterbury JM, et al: Parathyroid function in sarcoidosis. *N Engl J Med* 286:395–398, 1972.

37. Darsee JD, Nutter DO: Reversible severe congestive cardiomyopathy in three cases of hypophosphatemia. *Ann Intern Med* 89:867–870, 1978.

38. DeFronzo RA, Lang R: Hypophosphatemia and glucose intolerance. Evidence for tissue insensitivity to insulin. *N Engl J Med* 303:1259, 1980.

39. Denlinger JK, Nahrwold ML, Gibbs PS, et al: Hypocalcemia during rapid blood transfusion in anaesthetized man. *Br J Anaesth* 48:995–999, 1976.

40. Drop LJ: Ionized calcium, the heart and hemodynamic function. *Anesth Analg* 64:432–451, 1985.

41. Dyckner T: Serum magnesium in acute myocardial infarction. Relation to arrhythmias. *Acta Med Scand* 207:59–66, 1980.

42. Dycker T, Weater PO: Relation between potassium, magnesium and cardiac arrhythmias. *Acta Med Scand* (Suppl) 647:163–169, 1981.

43. Ellman H, Dembin H, Seriff N: The rarity of shortening of the QT interval in patients with hypercalcemia. *Crit Care Med* 10:320–322, 1982.

44. Flink EB: Therapy of magnesium deficiancy. *Ann NY Acad Sci* 162:901–905, 1969.

45. Forster J, Querusio L, Burchard KW, Gann DS: Hypercalcemia in critically ill surgical Patients. *Ann Surg* 202:512–517, 1985.

46. Fuller TJ, Nichols WW, Brenner BJ, et al: Reversible depression in myocardial performance in dogs with experimental phosphorus deficiency. *J Clin Invest* 62:1194, 1978.

47. Gallagher JC, Wilkinson R: The effect of ethinyloestradiol on calcium and phosphorus metabolism of postmenopausal women with primary hyperparathyroidism. *Clin Sci* 45:785–802, 1973.

48. Ginsburg R, Esserman LJ, Bristow MR: Myocardial performance and extracellular ionized calcium in a severely failing heart. *Ann Intern Med* 98:603–606, 1983.

49. Glover D, Riley L, Carmichael K, et al: Hypocalcemia and inhibition of parathyroid hormone secretion after administration of WR-2721 (a radioprotective and chemoprotective agent). *N Engl J Med* 309:1137–1141, 1983.

50. Glover DJ, Shaw L, Glick JH, et al: Treatment of hypercalcemia in parathyroid cancer with WR-2721, S-2-(3-aminopropylamino) ethyl-Phosphorothioic Acid. *Ann Intern Med* 103:55–57, 1985.

51. Goldman RH, Klelger RE, Schweizer E, et al: The effect on myocardial ^{3}H-digoxin in magnesium deficiency. *Proc Soc Exp Biol Med* 136:747–749, 1971.

52. Habener JF, Potts JT: Parathyroid physiology and primary hyperparathyroidism. In Avioli LV, Krane M (eds): *Metabolic Bone Disease*, vol 2. New York, Academic Press, 1978, pp 1–147.

53. Haldimann B, Goldstein DA, Akmal M, Massry SG: Renal function and blood levels of divalent ions in acute pancreatitis. *Mineral Electrolyte Metab* 3:190–199, 1980.

54. Haynes RC, Murad F: Agents affecting calcification: calcium, parathyroid hormone, calcitonin, vitamin D, and other compounds. In Gilman AG, Goodman LS, Rall TW, Murad F (eds): *The Pharmacological Basis of Therapeutics*, New York, Macmillan, 1985, pp 1517–1543.

55. Hauser CJ, Kamrath RO, Sparks J, Shoemaker WC: Calcium homeostasis in patients with acute pancreatitis. *Surgery* 94:830–835, 1983.

56. Heath DA: The emergency management of disorders of calcium and magnesium. *Clin Endocrinol Metab* 9:487–502, 1980.

57. Heckman BA, Walsh JH: Hypernatremia complicating sodium sulfate therapy for hypercalcemic crisis. *N Engl J Med* 276:1082–1083, 1967.

58. Henrich WL, Hunt JM, Nixon JV: Increased ionized calcium and left ventricular contractility during hemodialysis. *N Engl J Med* 310:19–23, 1984.

59. Hessov I, et al: Prevention of hypophosphatemia during post-operative routine glucose administration. *Acta Clin Scand* 146:109, 1980.

60. Horowitz M, Wishart J, Need A, Morris H, Philcox J, Nordin C: Treatment of postmenopausal hyperparathyroidism with norethindrone. *Arch Intern Med* 147:681–685, 1987.

61. Howland WS, Schweizer O, Jascott D, et al: Factors influencing the ionization of calcium during major surgical procedures. *Surg Gynecol Obstet* 143:895–900, 1976.

62. Iseri LT, Chung P, Tobis J: Magnesium therapy for intractable ventricular tachyarrhythmias in normomagnesemic patients. *Western J Med* 138:823–828, 1983.

63. Iseri LT, Freid J, Barnes AR: Magnesium deficiency and cardiac disorders. *Am J Med* 58:837–846, 1975.

64. Jacobs ML, Daggett WM, Civetta JM, et al: Acute pancreatitis: analysis of factors influencing survival. *Ann Surg* 185:43–51, 1977.

65. Jacobs TP, Siris ES, Bilezikian JP, Baquiran DC, Shane E, Canfield RE: Hypercalcemia of malignancy: treatment with intravenous dichloromethylene diphosphonate. *Ann Intern Med* 94:312–316, 1981.

66. Jung A: Comparison of two parenteral diphosphonates in hypercalcemia of malignancy. *Am J Med* 72:221–226, 1982.

67. Kafka H, Langevin L, Armstrong PW: Serum magnesium and potassium in acute myocardial infarction. *Arch Intern Med* 147:465–469, 1987.

68. Kahn RC, Jascott D, Carlon GC, et al: Massive blood replacement: correlation of ionized calcium, citrate, and hydrogen ion concentration. *Anesth Analg* 58:274–278, 1979.

69. Keller V, Berger W: Prevention of hypophosphatemia by phosphate infusion and during treatment of diabetic ketoacidosis and hyperosmolar coma. *Diabetes* 29:87, 1980.

70. Kingston ME, Al-Siba'i MB, Skooge WC: Clinical manifestations of hypomagnesemia. *Crit Care Med* 14:950–954, 1986.

71. Kingston M, Al-Siba'i MB: Treatment of severe hypophosphatemia. *Crit Care Med* 13:16–18, 1985.

72. Fitzgerald FT: Hypophosphatemia. *Adv Internal Med* 23:137, 1978.

73. Knochel JP: The pathophysiology and clinical characteristics of severe hypophosphatemia. *Arch Intern Med* 137:203–220, 1977.

74. Kreisberg RA: Diabetic ketoacidosis. New concepts and trends in pathogenesis and treatment. *Ann Intern Med* 88:681, 1978.

75. Kreusser W, Vetter HO, Mittmann U, Horl WH, Ritz E: Haemodynamics and myocardial metabolism of phosphorus depleted dogs: effect of catecholamines and angiotensin II. *Eur J Clin Invest* 12:219, 1982.

76. Kukla LJ, Abramson EC, McGuire WP, et al: Cis-platinum treatment for malignancy-associated humoral hypercalcemia in an athymic mouse model. *Calcif Tissue Int* 36:559–562, 1984.

77. Lad TE, Mishoulam HM, Shevrin DH, Kukla LJ, Abramson EC, Kukreja SC: Treatment of cancer-associated hypercalcemia with cisplatin. *Arch Intern Med* 147:329–332, 1987.

78. Ladenson JH, Lewis JW, Boyd JC: Failure of total serum calcium corrected for protein, albumin, and pH to correctly assess free calcium status. *J Clin Endocrinol Metab* 46:986–993, 1978.

79. Lee C, Zaloga GP: Magnesium metabolism. *Semin Resp Med* 7:75–80, 1985.

80. Lentz RD, Brown DM, Kjellstrand CM: Treatment of severe hypophosphatemia. *Ann Intern Med* 89:941, 1978.

81. Levy LA: Severe hypophosphatemia as a complication of the treatment of hypothermia. *Arch Intern Med* 140:128, 1980.

82. Loeb HS, Petras RM, Gunrar RM, et al: Paroxysmal ventricular fibrillation in two patients with hypomagnesemia. *Circulation* 37:210–215, 1967.

83. Marcus R, Madvig P, Crim M, et al: Conjugated estrogens in the treatment of postmenopausal women with hyperparathyroidism. *Ann Intern Med* 100:633–640, 1984.

84. Marx SJ, Attie MJ, Levine MA, et al: The hypocalciuric or benign variant of familial hypercalcemia: clinical and biochemical features in fifteen kindreds. *Medicine* 60:397–412, 1981.

85. Marx SJ, Bourdeau JE: Calcium metabolism. In Maxwell MH, Kleeman CR, Narins RG: *Clinical Disorders of Fluid and Electrolyte Metabolism*, 4th ed. New York, McGraw Hill, 207–244, 1987.

86. Massara F, Camanni F: Propranolol block of adrenaline-induced hypophosphatemia in man. *Clin Sci Mol Med* 38:245, 1970.

87. Massry SG, Friedler RM, Coburn JW: Excretion of phosphate and calcium. *Arch Intern Med* 131:828, 1973.

88. Massry SG, Silby MS: Hypomagnesemia and hypermagnesemia. *Clin Nephrol* 7:147–153, 1977.

89. Mason RS, Frankel T, Chan YL, et al: Vitamin D conversion by sarcoid lymph node homogenate. *Ann Intern Med* 100:59–61, 1984.

90. Maynard JC, Cruz C, Kleerekoper M, et al: Blood pressure response to changes in serum ionized calcium during hemodialysis. *Ann Intern Med* 104:358–361, 1986.

91. McPherson ML, Prince SR, Atamer ER, Maxwell DB, Ross-Clunis H, Estep HL: Theophylline-induced hypercalcemia. *Ann Intern Med* 105:52–54, 1986.

92. Medalle R, Waterhouse C, Hahn TJ: Vitamin D resistance in magnesium deficiency. *Am J Clin Nutrition* 29:854–858, 1976.

93. Miravet L, Ayigbede O, Carre M, Rayssiguier Y, Larvor P: Lack of vitamin D action on serum calcium in magnesium deficient rats. In Catin M, Seelig MS (eds): *Magnesium in Health and Disease*. New York, SP Medical and Scientific Books, 1980, pp 281–289.

94. Molloy DW, Dhingra S, Solven F, Wilson A, McCarthy DS: Hypomagnesemia and respiratory muscle power. *Am Rev Respir Dis* 129:497–498, 1984.

95. Moore EW. Ionized calcium in normal serum, ultrafiltrates and whole blood determined by ion exchange electrodes. *J Clin Invest* 49:318–334, 1970.

96. Mordes JP, Wacker WE: Excess magnesium. *Pharmacol Rev* 29:273–300, 1978.

97. Mundy GR, Raisz LG, Cooper RH, et al: Evidence for the secretion of an osteoclast stimulating factor in myeloma. *N Engl J Med* 291:1041–1046, 1974.

98. Nagant De Deuxchaisnes C, Krane SM: Hypoparathy-

roidism. In Avioli LV, Krane SM (eds): *Metabolic Bone Disease.* Orlando, FL, Academic Press, 1978, vol 2, pp 217–445.

99. Newman JH, Neff TA, Ziporin P: Acute respiratory failure associated with hypophosphatemia. *N Engl J Med* 296:1101, 1977.

100. O'Connor LR, Wheeler WS, Bethune JR: Effect of hypophosphatemia on myocardial performance in man. *N Engl J Med* 297:901, 1977.

101. Okayama H, Aikawa T, Okayama M, Sasaki H, Mue S, Takishima T: Bronchodilating effect of intravenous magnesium sulfate in bronchial asthma. *J Am Med Assoc* 257:1076–1078, 1987.

102. Orwoll ES: The milk-alkali syndrome: current concepts. *Ann Intern Med* 97:242–248, 1982.

103. Potts M, Doppelt S, Taylor S, Folkman J, Neer R, Potts JT: Protamine: A powerful in-vivo inhibitor of bone resorption. *Calcif Tissue Int* 36:189–193, 1984.

104. Quamme GA, Dirks KJ: Magnesium metabolism. In Maxwell MH, Kleeman CR, Narins RG: *Clinical Disorders of Fluid and Electrolyte Metabolism,* 4th ed. McGraw Hill, New York, 1987, pp 297–316.

105. Rasmussen HS, Aurup P, Hojberg S, Jensen EK, McNair P: Magnesium and acute myocardial infarction. *Arch Intern Med* 146:872–874, 1986.

106. Rasmussen HS, Norregard P, Lindeneg O, et al: Intravenous magnesium in acute myocardial infarction. *Lancet* 1:234–235, 1986.

107. Riley MS, Schade DS, Eaton RP: Effects of insulin infusion on plasma phosphate in diabetic patients. *Metabolism* 28:191, 1979.

108. Robertson GM, Moore EW, Switz DM, Sizemore GW, Estep HL: Inadequate parathyroid response to acute pancreatitis. *N Engl J Med* 294:512–516, 1976.

109. Robertson WG: Measurement of ionized calcium in body fluids - a review. *Ann Clin Biochem* 13:540–548, 1976.

110. Rude RK, Oldham SB, Singer FR: Functional hypoparathyroidism and parathyroid hormone end-organ resistance in human magnesium deficiency. *Clin Endocrinol* 5:209–224, 1976.

111. Rude RK, Singer FR: Magnesium deficiency and excess. *Annu Rev Med* 32:245–259, 1981.

112. Ryback R, Eckardt MJ, Paulter MA: Clinical relationship between serum phosphorus and other blood chemistry values in alcoholics. *Arch Intern Med* 140:673, 1980.

113. Ryzen E, Martodam RR, Troxell M, Benson A, Paterson A, Shepard K, Hicks R: Intravenous etidronate in the management of malignant hypercalcemia. *Arch Intern Med* 145:449–452, 1985.

114. Seller RH, Cangiano J, Kim KE, et al: Digitalis toxicity and hypomagnesemia. *Am Heart J* 79:57–68, 1970.

115. Seyberth HW, Segre GV, Morgan JL, et al: Prostaglandins as mediators of hypercalcemia associated with certain types of cancer. *N Engl J Med* 293:1278–1283, 1975.

116. Silva OL, Becker KL: Calcitonin in the treatment of hypercalcemia. *Arch Intern Med* 132:337–339, 1973.

117. Singer FR, Neer RM, Murray TM, et al: Mithramycin treatment of intractable hypercalcemia due to parathyroid carcinoma. *N Engl J Med* 283:634–636, 1970.

118. Stewart AF, Horst R, Deftos LJ, Cadman EC, Lang R, Broadus PE: Biochemical evaluation of patients with cancer-associated hypercalcemia. *N Engl J Med* 303:1377–1383, 1980.

119. Swaminathan R, et al: Hypophosphatemia in surgical patients. *Surg Gynecol Obstet* 148:448, 1979.

120. Turk J, Morrell L, Avioli L: Ethylene glycol intoxication. *Arch Intern Med* 146:1601–1603, 1986.

121. Vannatta JB, Whang R, Papper S: Efficacy of intrave- nous phosphorus therapy in the severely hypophos- phatemic patient. *Arch Intern Med* 141:885, 1981.

122. Varsano S, Shapiro M, Taragan R, Bruderman I: Hypophosphatemia as a reversible cause of refractory ventilatory failure. *Crit Care Med* 11:908–909, 1983.

123. Wacker WEC, Parisi AF: Magnesium metabolism. *N Engl J Med* 278:658–663, 712–717, 772–776, 1968.

124. Warrell RP, Bockman RS, Coonley CJ, Isaacs M, Staszewski H: Gallium nitrate inhibits calcium resorption from bone and is effective treatment for cancer-related hypercalcemia. *J Clin Invest* 73:1487–1490, 1984.

125. Watson CG, Steed DL, Robinson AG, Deftos LJ: The role of calcitonin and parathyroid hormone in the pathogenesis of post-thyroidectomy hypocalcemia. *Metabolism* 30:588–589, 1981.

126. Webb S, Schade DS: Hypomagnesemia as a cause of persistent hypokalemia. *J Am Med Assoc* 233:23–24, 1975.

127. Whang R, Flink EB, Dyckner T, Wester PO, Aikawa JK, Ryan MP: Magnesium depletion as a cause of refractory potassium repletion. *Arch Intern Med* 145:1686–1689, 1985.

128. Whang R, Morosi HJ, Rodgers D, et al: The influence of continuing magnesium deficiency on muscle K repletion. *J Lab Clin Med* 70:895–902, 1967.

129. Whang R, Oei TO, Watanabe A: Frequency of hypomagnesemia in hospitalized patients receiving digitalis. *Arch Intern Med* 145:655–656, 1985.

130. Wilson R, Kever SP, Lee AS, et al: Phosphate therapy in DKA. *Arch Intern Med* 142:517, 1982.

131. Zaloga GP, Chernow B: Hypocalcemia and rhabdomyolysis. *J Am Med Assoc* 257:626, 1987.

132. Zaloga GP, Chernow B: Hypocalcemia in critical illness. *J Am Med Assoc* 256:1924–1929, 1986.

133. Zaloga GP, Chernow B: Stress-induced changes in calcium metabolism. *Sem Respir Med* 7:52–68, 1985.

134. Zaloga GP, Chernow B: The multifactorial basis for hypocalcemia during sepsis: studies of the PTH-vitamin D axis. *Ann Intern Med* 107:36–41, 1987.

135. Zaloga GP, Chernow B, Cook D, et al: Assessment of calcium homeostasis in the critically ill patient. The diagnostic pitfalls of the McLean Hastings Nomogram. *Ann Surg* 202:587–594, 1985.

136. Zaloga GP, Chernow B, Eil C: Hypercalcemia and disseminated cytomegalovirus infection in the acquired immune deficiency syndrome. *Ann Intern Med* 102:331–333, 1985.

137. Zaloga GP, Chernow B, Hodge J, Eil C: Hypocalcemia and altered vitamin D metabolism in patients with small intestinal disease. *Military Med* 153:34–37, 1988.

138. Zaloga GP, Chernow B, Pock A, et al: Hypomagnesemia is a common complication of aminoglycoside therapy. *Surg Gynecol Obstet* 158:561–565, 1984.

139. Zaloga GP, Eil C, Medberry CA: Humoral hypercalcemia in Hodgkin's disease associated with elevated 1,25(OH)$_2$D levels and subperiosteal bone resorption. *Arch Intern Med* 145:155–157, 1985.

140. Zaloga GP, Eil C, O'Brian JT: Reversible hypocalciuric hypercalcemia associated with hypothyroidism. *Am J Med* 77:1101–1104, 1984.

141. Zaloga GP, Malcolm DS, Holaday J, Chernow B: Verapamil reverses calcium cardiotoxicity. *Ann Emerg Med* 16:637–639, 1987.

142. Zaloga GP, Wilkens R, Tourville J, Wood D, Klymer DM: A simple method for determining physiologically active calcium and magnesium concentrations in critically ill patients. *Crit Care Med* 15:813–816, 1987.

143. Zaloga GP, Willey SC, Chernow B: Free fatty acids alter calcium binding. A cause for misinterpretation of serum calcium values and hypocalcemia in critical illness. *J Clin Endocrinol Metab* 64:1010–1014, 1987.

18

Pharmacologic Approach to Gastrointestinal Disease in Critical Illness

David A. Johnson, M.D., F.A.C.P., F.A.C.G.
Edward L. Cattau, Jr., M.D., F.A.C.P., F.A.C.G.

A broad spectrum of gastrointestinal diseases may be manifested in an intensive care unit (ICU). A bleeding peptic or variceal lesion may be the primary reason for a patient's admission to the ICU, or a secondary complication, for example hepatic insufficiency, stress ulceration, or bowel ischemia, may develop during the course of an ICU stay. A working knowledge of the pharmacokinetic properties of drugs used to treat such conditions, as well as the indications and complications implicit with their use, is paramount in maximizing the care afforded to these patients during an ICU stay. The goal of this chapter is to discuss the gastrointestinal medications that may be used by the intensive care physician and to focus on special considerations that may be of importance in select patients.

ANTACIDS

The numerous antacids available differ in chemical composition, neutralizing capacity (39, 52), cost effectiveness (39, 52), potential side effects (171), and palatability. The major mechanisms of action of these agents, how-

Table 18.1
Neutralizing Capacity, Sodium Content, and Cost Effectiveness of Liquid Antacids

Antacid	Acid Neutralizing Capacity (mEq/ml)	Volume Containing 140 mEq (ml)[a]	Sodium Content (mg/5 ml)	Comparative Monthly Cost of Therapy ($)	Composition
Maalox TC	4.2	33	1.2	44	Aluminum hydroxide, magnesium hydroxide
Titralac	4.2	33	11.0	35	Calcium carbonate, glycine
Delcid	4.1	34	1.5	57	Aluminum hydroxide, magnesium hydroxide
Mylanta-II	3.6	39	1.1	63	Aluminum hydroxide, magnesium hydroxide, simethicone
Camalox	3.2	44	2.5	55	Aluminum hydroxide, magnesium hydroxide, calcium carbonate
Gelusil-II	3.0	47	1.3	74	Aluminum hydroxide, magnesium hydroxide, simethicone
Basaljel ES	2.9	48	23.0	101	Aluminum carbonate
ALternaGEL	2.5	56	2.0	71	Aluminum hydroxide
Digel	2.5	56	8.5	51	Aluminum hydroxide, magnesium hydroxide
Mylanta	2.4	58	0.7	67	Aluminum hydroxide, magnesium hydroxide, simethicone
Maalox Plus	2.3	61	2.5	68	Aluminum hydroxide, magnesium hydroxide, simethicone
Gelusil	2.2	64	0.7	80	Aluminum hydroxide, magnesium hydroxide, simethicone
Riopan Plus	1.8	78	0.3	78	Magaldrate, simethicone
Amphojel	1.4	100	7.0	114	Aluminum hydroxide

[a] 140 mEq, seven times per day.

ever, are similar, with the reduction of hydrogen ion concentration by neutralization and reduction of pepsin activity. Antacids range in the strength of acid neutralization (Table 18.1) from the oxyaluminum compounds, which raise the gastric pH to 3–4, to magnesium hydroxide, which can raise the pH to 9.

Antacids suppress pepsin activity when given in sufficient quantity to elevate the pH of gastric contents above 2.3, and irreversibly inactivate the enzyme at a pH above 6.9 (144). Antacids, however, do not appear to have direct antipepsin activity (92, 125).

The most commonly used antacids include calcium carbonate, aluminum hydroxide, and magnesium hydroxide, either alone or in combination. Each compound has some unique physical and chemical properties. A common feature of antacids is that they all contain sodium, although the content varies (Table 18.1). Antacids also cause alkalinization of the urine, which can alter renal excretion of several drugs. The tubular reabsorption of drugs that are weak bases such as quinidine, procainamide, or ephedrine may be increased, resulting in higher serum levels. In contrast, the reabsorption of drugs that are weak acids such as salicylates, phenobarbitone, and sulfonamides may be less, increasing their urinary excretion and lowering serum levels (171). Antacids also have a potential for influencing the gut absorption of various drugs (Table 18.2).

Calcium-Containing Antacids

Calcium carbonate has a relatively rapid onset and prolonged duration of action. The amount of calcium absorbed is dependent on the amount of gastric acid. After a single 2-g dose, 0–2% is absorbed in achlorhydric patients, 9–16% in normal subjects, and 11–34% in patients with peptic ulcers (74). Moreover, the fraction of calcium absorbed is the same during chronic therapy with daily doses of 20 g. A dose-absorption curve is not available; however, the amount absorbed probably reaches a plateau at a single dose of 40–50 g (63). Although there is a transient rise in serum calcium after a single oral 4-g dose of calcium carbonate, chronic hypercalcemia does not develop with daily doses as high as 20 g in patients with normal renal function. In patients with azotemia, hypercalcemia can develop with doses as low as 3.4 g/day. Calcium excretion varies directly with the creatinine clearance, and less than 1–9% of the amount absorbed is excreted in normal subjects, even after weeks of therapy (28).

Aluminum-Containing Antacids

Commercial preparations of aluminum hydroxide have varying low efficacy, partly because of nonreactive bulk (H_2O and fixed CO_2),

Table 18.2
Effect of Antacids on Drug Absorption and Excretion

Drugs *not affected* by concomitant antacid administration:	Drugs with *decreased absorption* during antacid administration:	Drugs with *increased absorption* during antacid administration:
Carbenoxolone[a]	Ampicillin	Aspirin[b]
Cimetidine	Carbenoxolone[a]	Bishydroxycoumarin
Chlordiazepoxide	Chlorpromazine	Levodopa
Ethionamide	Digitoxin	Nalidixic acid
Fenoprofen	Digoxin	Naproxen[a]
Glucocorticoids[a]	Glucocorticoids[a]	Pseudoephedrine hydroxide
Naproxen[a]	Iron	Sulfadiazine acid[a]
Theophylline	Isoniazid	
Quinidine sulfate	Naproxen[a]	
Warfarin sodium	Oral contraceptives	
	Pentobarbital	
	Phenytoin	
	Quinine sulfate	
	Sulfadiazine sodium[a]	
	Tetracyclines	
	Tolbutamide	
	Vitamin A	

[a] Presence in more than one group indicates conflicting data.
[b] Simultaneous alterations that may result in decreased serum levels.

but also because of the formation of polymers that dissolve very slowly. Moreover, proteins, peptides, amino acids, and certain dietary organic acids impair the neutralizing capacity of this antacid (58). A study of the ingestion of four aluminum-containing compounds (aluminum hydroxide, carbonate, aminoacetate, and phosphate) by normal volunteers revealed a significant increase in urinary aluminum levels with three of the four compounds (no rise with aluminum phosphate) (81). In renal failure, administration of aluminum hydroxide can elevate serum aluminum to potentially dangerous levels (8). Excessive aluminum intake in patients with renal failure may contribute to the development of dialysis encephalopathy (2), myopathy, and an osteomalacia provoked by undetected hypophosphatemia and compensating skeletal demineralization (4). High doses of aluminum hydroxide, even without renal failure, can lead to a phosphorus depletion syndrome (98), particularly if low phosphate intake or malabsorption is present. Aluminum hydroxide may also produce constipation and fecal impaction, especially in elderly patients (68).

Magnesium-Containing Antacids

Although magnesium hydroxide is classified as a nonabsorbed antacid, 5–33% of magnesium is absorbed (39, 101) and can lead to hypermagnesemia and death in patients with renal insufficiency (63). Supersaturation of the urine with magnesium may predispose patients to nephrolithiasis. Additionally, siliceous nephrolithiasis may be seen with use of magnesium trisalicylate.

The pathogenesis of the cathartic effect of magnesium may be multifactorial. The primary cause is the formation of magnesium salts, which are delivered as an osmotic load to the bowel and stimulate both secretion and motility (174). Another possible factor is that magnesium is a weak stimulant of gallbladder contraction and pancreatic secretion, although the clinical significance of this stimulation is not defined (102).

HISTAMINE H$_2$-ANTAGONISTS

With the synthesis of Burimamide in 1972, Black and coworkers (9) demonstrated the existence of two classes of histamine receptors: H$_1$ and H$_2$. In contrast to the H$_1$ type, H$_2$-receptors are not antagonized by conventional antihistamines and are involved in the action of histamine on the gastric parietal cell. Metiamide was the first H$_2$-blocker used clinically, but it caused agranulocytosis. Cimetidine was the first H$_2$-blocker to receive widespread use. The subsequent introduction of ranitidine and more recently famotidine has given the clinician several options directed at gastric acid suppression.

Cimetidine has an imidazole ring as does histamine, but has a much less basic and longer side chain. Cimetidine has a cyanoguanidine group whereas metiamide, its forerunner, had a thiourea group. This structural difference may explain why cimetidine has not been associated with the same incidence of severe agranulocytosis seen with metiamide.

The H$_2$-receptors have been identified in many sites including the atrium, stomach, uterus, ileum, mesenteric and cutaneous vascular beds, bronchial musculature, parathyroid cells, adipocytes, and T suppressor cells (55). The clinical importance of H$_2$-receptor blockade in organs other than the stomach is not clearly defined.

Cimetidine

MECHANISM OF ACTION

Cimetidine, acting as a reversible competitive antagonist of the action of histamine on H$_2$-receptors, predictably inhibits histamine-stimulated acid secretion on parietal cells. The mechanism by which cimetidine inhibits the acid secretion promoted by the other two endogenous secretagogues (acetylcholine and gastrin) is less well understood. The previously held view that histamine is the "final common mediator" of acid secretion has largely been replaced with the current concept that the parietal cell has separate receptors for each of the secretagogues. The interaction of histamine with its receptors increases the affinity of the parietal cell for gastrin and acetylcholine and thereby potentiates their effects (156). Since cimetidine and anticholinergics inhibit acid secretion by different mechanisms, their effects are synergistic (46).

Cimetidine is a potent inhibitor of all phases of gastric secretion. Both basal and nocturnal basal acid secretion are reduced 90–95% by a 300-mg dose (6). Pepsin output is reduced by cimetidine in humans, probably as a result of decreased secretion of gastric juice (6). Cimetidine-induced reduction in stimulated (but not basal) intrinsic factor secretion has been demonstrated and is related to decreased gastric volume (6, 149). The effects of H_2-antagonists on gastric mucus secretion in humans is less clear, although it seems unlikely that mucus secretion is mediated by H_2-receptors.

Fasting serum gastrin levels are unaffected by cimetidine; however, postprandial levels are raised because of the reduction in acid feedback and inhibition of gastrin release (97). There have been no reports of a "rebound" increase in peak acid output following therapy. Cimetidine has no apparent action on gastric emptying (97) or bile acid composition or secretion (97, 115).

PHARMACOKINETICS

Cimetidine can be administered orally, intravenously, and intramuscularly. Food delays absorption of the drug, so peak serum levels are lower but the duration of effect is prolonged when given with meals. Parenterally administered cimetidine achieves higher peak drug levels than those obtained by oral administration; however, the clinically effective drug level is maintained for approximately 4 hours, similar to the time achieved with the oral route. Measurement of blood cimetidine levels is not clinically useful (49).

Approximately 15% of cimetidine is metabolized in the liver and most of the drug is excreted unchanged in the urine. Use of cimetidine in patients with liver disease is not contraindicated, but reduced dosages may be necessary with severe liver impairment. In renal failure drug accumulation may occur, and

Table 18.3
Cimetidine Dosage in Patients with Impaired Renal Function

Estimated Creatinine Clearance[a] (ml/min/1.73 m^2)	Appropriate Dosing Regimen
>40 (mild)	300 mg/6 hr
20–40 (moderate)	300 mg/8 hr
0–20 (severe)	300 mg/12 hr

[a]Estimated creatinine clearance is calculated as follows:

Males:

$$Cl_{cr} = \frac{140 - age}{serum\ creatinine} \times \frac{weight\ (kg)}{72}$$

Females:

$$Cl_{cr} = \frac{140 - age}{serum\ creatinine} \times \frac{weight\ (kg)}{72} \times 0.85$$

therefore the lowest frequency of dosing compatible with an adequate patient response should be used (Table 18.3). Hemodialysis lowers the level of circulating drug by at least 50% and the dosage schedule should be adjusted so that the timing of a scheduled dose coincides with the end of hemodialysis (99, 168). A dosage of 400 mg/day on nondialysis days and 800 mg/day on dialysis days has been used effectively in acute duodenal ulceration, with 200 mg/day continued thereafter as maintenance therapy (37). Insufficient amounts of cimetidine are removed during peritoneal dialysis to warrant a postdialysis supplemental dose (71, 169). With advancing age, plasma cimetidine half-life and the volume of distribution tend to increase so that even in the absence of severe renal failure, reducing standard doses of oral cimetidine by one-third to one-half appears justified (139).

Experience with gross overdosage of cimetidine is limited. In the few cases that have been reported in humans, doses up to 10 g have not been associated with any untoward effects (110). The usual measures should be taken to remove unabsorbed material from the gastrointestinal tract, in addition to clinical monitoring and supportive therapy. Studies in animals indicate that toxic doses are associated with respiratory failure and tachycardia, which may be controlled by assisted respiration and administration of a β-blocker (142).

Small amounts of cimetidine are excreted in bile and, with unabsorbed drug, excreted in the feces. The drug crosses the placental barrier, is excreted in milk, and is widely distributed in almost all tissues except the brain (38). The blood-brain barrier may become more permeable to cimetidine, however, in patients with severe medical illnesses, especially uremia (114).

DOSAGE AND INDICATIONS

Cimetidine is approved for use in the short-term treatment of active duodenal or benign gastric ulcer as well as the long-term prevention thereof. Effective oral dosage regimens include 300 mg four times daily, 400 mg twice daily, or 800 mg at bedtime. For use in pathologic hypersecretory conditions, such as Zollinger-Ellison syndrome, dosage and dosing interval may need to be adjusted but should not exceed 2400 mg/day. For parenteral administration, cimetidine may be given as a 300-mg dose every 6–8 hours intramuscularly or intravenously. It may also be delivered by a continuous intravenous infusion starting at 40–50 mg/hr and adjusted to maintain a desired target gastric pH.

SPECIAL CONSIDERATIONS

The effect of H_2-blockers on hepatic function and hepatic drug metabolism needs consideration. Contrary to previous impressions, cimetidine does not cause a fall in hepatic blood flow. Cimetidine does, however, affect type I biotransformation and reduces microsomal mixed function oxidase activity, so there is a potential effect on other drugs that are metabolized by the microsomal cytochrome P-450 enzyme system. For example, it is generally accepted that blood levels of warfarin and theophylline rise when either is given simultaneously with cimetidine. Reduction of the doses of these agents by approximately one-third is advised, along with regular monitoring of serum theophylline concentrations and prothrombin

time. Other drugs that should be reduced when cimetidine is administered, particularly in the elderly, are benzodiazepines such as diazepam and chlordiazepoxide, since cimetidine inhibits the N-demethylation of these drugs. In contrast, lorazepam and oxazepam have limited hepatic biotransformation (glucuronide conjugation) that is not influenced by cimetidine, and doses need not be altered. A complete list of H_2-receptor drug interactions is shown in Table 18.4 (147).

Cimetidine inhibits gastric acid secretion and causes an increase in the pH of the stomach and proximal small bowel. An increased pH could lead to differences in the rate and extent of absorption of drugs that are destroyed at a low pH or require low pH for disintegration or dissolution. The known effects of H_2-antagonists on absorption of several orally administered drugs are shown in Table 18.5.

Cimetidine has decreased effectiveness in

Table 18.4
Drug Interactions with Cimetidine and Ranitidine

Drug	Comments	References
Antiarrhythmics	Inhibition of procainamide and quinidine metabolism have been reported.	62, 157
Anticoagulants (oral)	Cimetidine competitively inhibits metabolism, and a marked increase in prothrombin time has been demonstrated.	118, 148, 153
Anticonvulsants	Increased serum phenytoin and carbamazepine levels have been reported when used with cimetidine.	5, 66, 163, 176
Benzodiazepines	Potentiated sedation by inhibited metabolism of those agents metabolized by glucuronidation. Reduction in dose not required for oxazepam, lorazepam, temazepam.	87, 120, 140
β-Blockers	Clearance of propranolol is reduced by cimetidine by inhibition of drug-metabolizing enzymes and reduced hepatic blood flow.	45, 65
Carmustine (BCNU)	Increased bone marrow toxicity has been reported with concomitant use.	143
Chlormethiazole	Cimetidine alters the disposition of drug and results in increased pharmacologic effect.	150
Lidocaine HCl	Cimetidine increases serum levels by reducing systemic clearance; 50% reduction in maintenance infusion recommended following standard loading dose.	53, 88
Narcotic analgesics	Cimetidine may enhance activity of morphine, meperidine, methadone, and fentanyl citrate.	51, 95
Nifedipine	Both cimetidine and ranitidine increase the hypotensive activity of this drug.	85
Theophylline	Cimetidine inhibits clearance; 50% reduction in dose of theophylline should be considered when given together.	24, 75, 129

Table 18.5
Effects of H$_2$-Antagonists on Absorption of Orally Administered Drugs

	References
Increased absorption	
Aspirin	82
Decreased absorption	
Ketoconazole	167
Insignificant or inconsistent effects on absorption	
Penicillin	44, 136, 146
Furosemide	137
Digoxin	80
Cotrimoxazole	136
Tetracycline	146

Table 18.7
Comparison of Reported Adverse Effects for Cimetidine and Ranitidine

Adverse Effect, by System	Cimetidine	Ranitidine
Central nervous system		
Malaise	+	+
Confusion	+	+
Insomnia	+	+
Agitation	+	+
Hallucinations	+	+
Depression	+	+
Cardiovascular		
Bradycardia	+	
Tachycardia	+	+
Ectopy	+	+
Dermatologic		
Rash	+	+
Alopecia	+	+
Endocrine		
Gynecomastia	+	
Reversible impotence	+	
Prolactin elevation	+	
Chylomicronemia	+	
Gastrointestinal		
Diarrhea	+	+
Constipation	+	+
Hepatitis	+	+
Pancreatitis	+	
General		
Fever	+	+
Hematopoietic		
Leukopenia	+	+
Pancytopenia	+	+
Thrombocytopenia	+	
Musculoskeletal		
Arthralgias	+	+
Myalgias	+	
Renal		
Elevation in creatinine	+	+
Interstitial nephritis	+	

burn patients and possibly other surgical patients (78). Increased clearance of cimetidine has been demonstrated, the total clearance correlating with the size of the burn. Trauma and surgical patients may be pharmacologically different from nonsurgical patients because of inflammation-induced alterations in hemodynamic and organ functions. Increased renal and hepatic blood flow occur as part of the response to tissue trauma and injury (78). Dosage schedules may need to be altered in this patient population to compensate for the enhanced clearance of cimetidine.

Cimetidine is stable in parenteral nutrition fluids. It is effective when administered via continuous intravenous infusion rather than intermittent intravenous injection, and continuous infusion is considerably less expensive overall (35). Incompatibility with certain drugs has been described (Table 18.6), and administration via separate intravenous lines is suggested when cimetidine is to be given simultaneously with these drugs (141, 180).

SIDE EFFECTS

Numerous adverse reactions have been attributed to cimetidine (Table 18.7), which is understandable in view of the attention and scrutiny the drug has received, its widespread use, and its systemic effects. The reported frequency of side effects has differed considera-

Table 18.6
Cimetidine Hydrochloride Incompatibilities

Aerosporin
Aminophylline
Amphotericin B
Barbiturates
Cephalosporins
Garamycin
Fat emulsions

bly but is low in all studies (109, 178). A worldwide reporting system showed the incidence of adverse effects to be as follows: 7.3/100,000 patients treated (1.1/100,000 with mental confusion); gastrointestinal-hepatobiliary system abnormalities, 4.8/100,000; skin and musculoskeletal disturbances, 3.1/100,000; abnormal hematologic findings, 2.3/100,000; and interstitial nephritis, <0.1/100,000 (54).

Symptoms of central nervous system (CNS) toxicity are among the commonest of cimetidine's unwanted effects. Cimetidine crosses the blood-brain barrier, and the CNS symptoms tend to be more frequent in elderly and very young patients, those receiving high dosages, and those with renal or hepatic disease. The effects on the CNS may be due to blockage of the H$_2$-receptors and consequent partial inhibition of the neurotransmitter properties of histamine (181). Cimetidine may also interfere with the function of endogenous enkephalins (22). Physostigmine reverses cimetidine-induced confusion (114), but experience with use of this drug is limited and it is recommended only in the presence of life-threatening CNS toxicity.

Pharmacologic studies in humans show that both the myocardium and peripheral blood vessels possess H_2-receptors (162). Stimulation of cardiac H_2-receptors causes positive chronotropic and inotropic responses. Stimulation of H_2-receptors in peripheral vessels causes vasodilation. The physiologic role of these receptors has not been established. Bolus injection of cimetidine in critically ill patients is associated with a decrease in blood pressure, particularly in patients requiring vasoconstrictor support (84). This hypotension is probably induced by arterial vasodilation. Cardiac dysrhythmias may occur with cimetidine use, although such reactions have not been reported after oral or slow intravenous administration in normal subjects (14, 15).

Cimetidine has a weak antiandrogen effect. Gynecomastia may be caused by blockade of androgen receptors that mediate the normal suppression of breast tissue (160). Serum prolactin levels do not rise after oral administration of cimetidine, but bolus intravenous administration results in dose-dependent prolactin elevations (32). Chylomicronemia has been described with cimetidine use in a patient with hypertriglyceridemia (3). The clinical picture included musculoskeletal pain, abdominal pain, and splenomegaly on two separate occasions during cimetidine administration. This potentially treacherous complication should be considered, therefore, when prescribing cimetidine for patients with known hyperlipidemia.

Mild, self-limited elevations in liver transaminases may occur with cimetidine, and hepatitis of the idiosyncratic or hypersensitivity type has been described. Cholestasis is rare, and hepatotoxicity with cimetidine is uncommon and appears to be reversible (54).

Fever is an infrequent idiosyncratic effect of cimetidine use. The onset of fever varies from 5 to 13 days, persists the entire course of treatment, and is gone within 12–72 hours after stopping the drug (3). Rechallenges lead to new onset of fever within 12–24 hours. The range of temperature reported is 38.5–39.5°C. Associated findings include malaise, night sweats, epigastric pain, and leukopenia.

The hematologic effects of cimetidine have been scrutinized in view of the profound effects of metiamide. Several cases of granulocytopenia, thrombocytopenia, and pancytopenia have been reported, but are rare (56). Bone marrow suppression appears to occur by a dose-dependent idiosyncratic mechanism.

Cimetidine may have immunologic effects by influencing a subclass of human thymic-dependent suppressor T lymphocytes that have H_2-receptors. Histamine stimulates these suppressor cells and may thereby serve a local immunoinhibitory role. Blockage of these receptors conceivably could interfere with this inhibitory function and result in augmented cell-mediated immune responses. Skin reactivity to common antigens improves with cimetidine therapy in patients with chronic mucocutaneous candidiasis and Crohn's disease. Remission of symptoms also occurred in some patients with herpes virus infections. Cimetidine does not, however, appear to influence the function of grafts or increase the number or severity of rejection episodes (79, 138).

Small increases in serum creatinine occur commonly during cimetidine therapy. The values rarely exceed 2 mg/dl, are not associated with changes in blood urea or urinalysis, and return rapidly to baseline values on discontinuance of the drug. These mild elevations in creatinine are not regarded as an adverse reaction and do not require discontinuance of therapy. Acute interstitial nephritis has been described and appears to be an idiosyncratic or hypersensitivity reaction. Clinical features include fever, malaise, mild eosinophilia, and decreased renal function developing after several weeks of cimetidine therapy (108).

Ranitidine

Ranitidine is an H_2-receptor antagonist that was released 6 years after cimetidine was introduced. In contrast to cimetidine, which contains the same imidazole ring found in histamine, ranitidine includes a furan ring, which is not chemically related to histamine and does not occur naturally in the human body. Studies with ranitidine indicate that it is 5–12 times as potent as cimetidine (on a molar basis) in inhibiting stimulated gastric acid secretion in humans (18).

PHARMACOKINETICS

The pharmacokinetic profile of ranitidine is similar to that of cimetidine. Neither product is inherently long-acting and they have similar half-lives of 2.0–3.0 hours. If equipotent doses of cimetidine and ranitidine are administered, the duration of action is essentially the same. The bioavailability of oral ranitidine is about 50%, compared with 70% for cimetidine (182). The bioavailability of ranitidine is influenced by hepatic function. The drug is taken up and metabolized by the liver by "first pass" kinetics. Up to 30% of the drug is metabolized by the liver to nitrogen oxide, sulfuric oxide, and demethyl derivatives, and at least 50% is excreted by the kidney unchanged (18). When given orally, ranitidine is rapidly absorbed from the gastrointestinal tract, and absorption is not influenced by food ingestion.

DOSAGE AND INDICATIONS

Ranitidine has essentially the same indications as cimetidine. Oral dosage schedules for active peptic ulcer disease include 150 mg twice daily or 300 mg at bedtime. Ranitidine is very rapidly absorbed after intramuscular injection, with bioavailability of 90–100% compared with intravenous administration. The dosage for intramuscular or intravenous delivery is 50 mg every 8 hours, and the drug may also be given as a continuous infusion starting at 150 mg/day with dosage adjusted as required to attain the desired target gastric pH. When given as an intravenous bolus, the volume should be injected over a period of not less than 5 minutes.

OVERDOSAGE

There is no experience to date with deliberate overdosage. As with cimetidine, the usual measures to remove unabsorbed material from the gastrointestinal tract should be employed. Studies in dogs receiving ranitidine in excess of 225 mg/kg/day have shown muscular tremors, vomiting, and rapid respiration. Single oral doses of 1000 mg/kg in mice and rats were not lethal; intravenous LD_{50} values were 83 mg/kg and 77 mg/kg, respectively (124).

SPECIAL CONSIDERATIONS

The drug interaction potential for ranitidine was initially thought to be considerably less than for cimetidine, since ranitidine has a lesser effect on cytochrome P-450–mediated drug metabolism. As experience using ranitidine increases, more drug interactions have been defined. There are reports of interactions between ranitidine and warfarin (133), benzodi-

azepine (41), fentanyl (95), metoprolol (159), nifedipine (18), acetaminophen (133), and theophylline (48). Interaction with acetaminophen is particularly significant in view of hepatic dependence on glutathione for detoxification of acetaminophen, and suggests that ranitidine, like other furans, may have finite glutathione requirements for safe elimination and freedom from hepatotoxicity. Some drug interactions may also develop from the ability of ranitidine, like cimetidine, to reduce hepatic blood flow by 20–40%. As with cimetidine, strong antacids may reduce absorption of ranitidine.

In geriatric patients, the half-life of ranitidine is prolonged by about 50%, presumably as a result of a decrease in the glomerular filtration rate (68). The bioavailability of ranitidine in patients with liver disease is increased, and the serum half-life is slightly prolonged because of decreased hepatic metabolism and a slight reduction in glomerular filtration rate (179). It is probably not necessary to change the usual therapeutic dose in patients with mild hepatic disease, although caution should be observed in all patients with hepatic dysfunction. In patients with serious renal disease, therapeutic levels can be obtained with lower doses. The recommended dose in patients with a creatinine clearance below 50 ml/min is 50 mg every 18–24 hours. Should the patient's condition require, the frequency of dosing may be increased with caution. Hemodialysis reduces the level of circulating ranitidine. Ideally, the dosage schedule should be adjusted so that the timing of a scheduled dose coincides with the end of hemodialysis.

SIDE EFFECTS

Initially, ranitidine was thought to have fewer side effects than cimetidine; however, more reports are continually being generated as the experience with ranitidine increases. Unlike cimetidine, ranitidine binds minimally if at all to androgen receptors, the hepatic mixed function oxidase system, and peripheral lymphocytes (182). It once was believed that ranitidine, less lipophilic than cimetidine, would not enter the cerebrospinal fluid or cause the neurologic problems occasionally seen with cimetidine. However, ranitidine does enter the cerebrospinal fluid, and the lesser lipophilicity is offset by greater potency in the CNS. An overview of the side effects for both cimetidine and ranitidine is shown in Table 18.7.

Famotidine

Famotidine, another H_2-receptor antagonist drug, was released for clinical use in late 1986. As a result, the clinical data that come from widespread use are limited. Famotidine is a guanidinathiazole derivative containing neither the imidazole ring of cimetidine nor the furan ring of ranitidine. It acts as a reversible competitive H_2-receptor inhibitor, with an antisecretory potency in animal studies that is 30–100 times greater than that of cimetidine and 6–10 times greater than that of ranitidine (27).

PHARMACOKINETICS

Famotidine is incompletely absorbed, with bioavailability of 40–45% for orally administered dosages. There is a minimal first pass metabolism. Drug elimination is 65–70% renal and 30–35% metabolic (155).

DOSAGE AND INDICATIONS

Famotidine is likely to have the same indications as cimetidine and ranitidine, although at the time of its release, famotidine was indicated only for the short-term treatment of active duodenal ulcers, maintenance therapy for healed duodenal ulcers, and treatment of pathologic hypersecretory conditions, e.g., Zollinger-Ellison syndrome. The adult oral dosage is 40 mg at bedtime or 20 mg twice daily. The starting dose for hypersecretory conditions is 20 mg orally every 6 hours, with doses up to 160 mg every 6 hours having been administered to some patients with severe Zollinger-Ellison syndrome (69, 170).

OVERDOSAGE

There are no reported cases of deliberate overdosage, but the approach to treatment would be similar to that for cimetidine and ranitidine overdose. The oral LD_{50} of famotidine in rats and dogs is 3000 mg/kg and 2000 mg/kg, respectively (40).

SPECIAL CONSIDERATIONS

In patients with severe renal insufficiency (creatinine clearance <10 ml/min), the half-life of famotidine exceeds 20 hours and is approximately 24 hours if the patient is anuric. The dose should be reduced to 20 mg at bedtime or the dosing interval prolonged to 36–48 hours as indicated by the patient's clinical response (27). No drug interactions have yet been defined in controlled studies. Specific clinical interaction studies have shown no interference with compounds metabolized by hepatic microsomal enzyme processes, including diazepam, phenytoin, theophylline, and warfarin (155). In elderly patients, there are no clinically important age-related changes in pharmacokinetics.

SIDE EFFECTS

As was learned with ranitidine, the true incidence of side effects is not known until after several years of widespread clinical use. In the controlled trials to date, the reported side effects of famotidine include headache (4.7%), dizziness (1.3%), constipation (1.2%), and diarrhea (1.7%) (23, 40, 155). Other adverse reactions may be defined as drug exposure increases. Safety studies conducted in healthy volunteers have shown no famotidine-induced actions on the cardiovascular, endocrine, or renal systems (23).

OTHER DRUGS USED IN SUPPRESSION OF GASTRIC ACID SECRETION AND ULCER HEALING

Omeprazole

Omeprazole (5-methoxy-2-[4-methoxy-(3,5-dimethyl-2-pyridinyl)-methyl]-sulfinyl-1h-benzimidazole) is a substituted benzimidazole and a potent inhibitor of gastric acid secretion. This class of drugs is new and currently undergoing phase trials for clinical use in the United States. The agents act by selective noncompetitive inhibition of the hydrogen-potassium ATPase enzyme in the parietal cell. This action interferes with the hydrogen-potassium ATPase proton pump (the final common pathway of gastric acid secretion) and therefore abolishes all responses to all types of stimulation (172).

PHARMACOKINETICS

Omeprazole is a weak base ($pK_a = 4$) that is absorbed from the small bowel at an alkaline pH. In the parietal cell, the drug is trapped in the acid secretory canaliculus. The acid environment allows formation of a sulfoxide metabolite that binds to hydrogen-potassium

ATPase, irreversibly inactivating the enzyme and thereby inhibiting gastric acid secretion. Plasma concentrations of drug do not correlate with gastric acid inhibition because the drug irreversibly inactivates hydrogen-potassium ATPase with single-dose inhibition of secretion for up to 3 days (60 hours after the drug is cleared from the circulation) The bioavailability of oral omeprazole increases with repeated doses because absorption improves as gastric pH increases. After 7 days of treatment with 30 or 60 mg daily, there is almost 100% inhibition of basal and stimulated acid secretion (70).

DOSAGE AND INDICATIONS

Neither dosage nor indications for omeprazole have yet been established in the United States. With oral dosages in the range of 20–40 mg/day, omeprazole does appear to heal ulcers more rapidly than H_2-receptor antagonists. In addition, at 4 weeks following therapy more patients appear to have ulcer healing with omeprazole (94). For gastric ulcers, in limited trials omeprazole appears to be as effective as H_2-receptor blockers (29). Omeprazole is highly effective in treating patients with Zollinger-Ellison syndrome for prolonged periods (105).

SPECIAL CONSIDERATIONS

The dramatic effects of omeprazole in the suppression of gastric acid secretion have caused some concern about its long-term use. Of most concern is the possible relationship between omeprazole-induced achlorhydria, elevated serum gastrin concentrations, and gastric carcinoid tumors in rats (42). In humans, the treatment of duodenal and gastric ulcer patients for several weeks produces modest reversible elevations in serum gastrin concentrations. No changes in the number of gastric endocrine cells have been noted. Serum gastrin concentrations and endocrine cell numbers in the gastric mucosa of Zollinger-Ellison syndrome patients apparently do not change following treatment with omeprazole. Further concern has been raised about the long-term use of omeprazole and the development of bacterial overgrowth. To date, however, there have been no reports of illness related to bacterial overgrowth in patients treated with omeprazole for weeks or years. Omeprazole also inhibits drug metabolism by the hepatic microsomal P-450 monooxygenase system (61). Dosage adjustment of such drugs should be considered if omeprazole is used concomitantly.

Sucralfate

Sucralfate is a nonabsorbable salt of sucrose octasulfate and aluminum hydroxide that is effective in gastroduodenal ulcer healing (128). When the drug reaches the acidic environment (pH <3–4) of the stomach, some aluminum hydroxide dissociates from sucrose octasulfate molecules and the residual compound becomes negatively charged. Polymerization of the sucrose octasulfate molecule occurs and simultaneously, a paste-like substance is formed, which is the active form of sucralfate. This paste-like material binds to necrotic ulcer tissue in both the stomach and duodenum. The mechanism for this attachment is, in part, related to the binding of negatively charged sucralfate molecules to positively charged proteins such as albumin, fibrinogen, damaged mucosal cells, and dead leukocytes in the ulcer base (135).

There are two possible mechanisms to explain sucralfate's effectiveness in promoting ulcer healing. First, the adherent complex that sucralfate forms with protein at the ulcer site acts as an effective barrier against acid, pepsin, and bile (117). Second, since large doses of sucralfate increase prostaglandin release into gastric juice in rats, a cytoprotective effect may be due to prostaglandin release (67). It has also been suggested that the gastric protection afforded by sucralfate is related to a prostaglandin-independent increase in mucus production (151). Sucralfate has minimal acid-neutralizing capability and in vitro studies indicate that it absorbs bile acids (117).

PHARMACOKINETICS

Sucralfate is only minimally absorbed from the gastrointestinal tract. The small amounts of the sulfated disaccharide that are absorbed are excreted primarily in the urine.

DOSAGE AND INDICATIONS

The recommended adult oral dosage of sucralfate, when used for treatment of duodenal ulcer, is 1 g four times a day on an empty stomach. Alternatively, a dose of 2 g twice a day appears to be equally effective in the short-term treatment of duodenal ulcer (17). The tablet may be dissolved in 15–30 ml of water or 5–15 ml of glycerol, although the clinical efficacy of this dosing form has not been well studied. Although currently approved only for use in duodenal ulcer disease, this drug may also be effective in gastric ulcer, esophageal sclerotherapy–induced ulcers, and esophagitis, and for mucosal damage due to nonsteroidal antiinflammatory drugs (20).

SPECIAL CONSIDERATIONS

Although sucralfate appears to be most effective at low pH, prior administration of cimetidine had little effect on binding of sucralfate to ulcer tissue in rats. Despite this finding, if both drugs are to be used concomitantly, we recommend staggering the dosing intervals so that the sucralfate is given 60 minutes before the cimetidine. Animal studies have shown that simultaneous administration of sucralfate with tetracycline, phenytoin, digoxin, or cimetidine results in a statistically significant reduction in the bioavailability of these agents. This reduction may be prevented by separating the administration of these agents and sucralfate by 2 hours. The interaction appears to be nonsystemic and presumably results from sucralfate binding of these agents within the gastrointestinal tract. The clinical importance of these animal studies is unknown at present, but separate administration of sucralfate and these other agents is recommended when alterations in bioavailability are thought to be critical for the concomitantly administered drugs. Although sucralfate is only minimally absorbed from the gastrointestinal tract, it seems prudent to monitor for signs of aluminum toxicity when the drug is to be administered chronically to dialysis patients with end-stage renal disease. Concomitant dosing with antacids may be prescribed as needed for relief of pain, but should not be taken within one-half hour before or after sucralfate since it may impede sucralfate tissue binding.

SIDE EFFECTS

Because of minimal absorption, side effects are rare. Constipation is the most common (2.3%), followed by oral dryness (0.7%) and dizziness (0.4%) (73). There is no experience with overdosage in humans. Animal data with dosings of up to 12 mg/kg have not shown a lethal effect.

Prostaglandins

Prostaglandins (particularly those of the E and I series) exert pronounced effects on various functions of the digestive system. In the stomach, these agents stimulate bicarbonate secretion and also have antisecretory, antiulcer, and cytoprotective effects (90).

Several prostaglandins of the E type are being evaluated for the treatment of gastric and duodenal ulcer and gastroduodenal side effects of nonsteroidal antiinflammatory drugs, and for the management of upper gastrointestinal bleeding (16, 89). The release of these agents in the United States has been prevented because of concern over the uterotonic effects of certain prostaglandins and the possible abortive sequelae in child-bearing females. Diarrhea is another common side effect, but appears to be less if lower doses are used. The role of prostaglandins in the treatment of gastrointestinal disease may be limited in the United States if approval by the Food and Drug Administration is not granted.

PROKINETIC AGENTS

Metoclopramide

Metoclopramide is a methoxychlorinated derivative of procainamide and a dopamine antagonist. This drug has a prokinetic effect, most effective in the upper gastrointestinal tract. It has little, if any, effect on the gallbladder or colon. The esophagogastric effects of this drug include increases in acid clearance, esophageal peristaltic amplitude, lower esophageal sphincter pressure, gastric emptying, and gastric contraction rate and amplitude (1, 145). In the small bowel, metoclopramide induces the equivalent of a migrating motor complex, inasmuch as the increase in gastric motility that it induces extends into the duodenum and small bowel.

PHARMACOKINETICS

Metoclopramide is well absorbed when given orally, with an onset of action of 30–60 minutes and duration of pharmacologic effect of 1–2 hours. The onset of action following an intravenous dose is 1–3 minutes and following an intramuscular dose is 10–15 minutes (145). Approximately 85% of a radioactive dose appears in the urine within 72 hours, with approximately one-half present as free or unconjugated metoclopramide.

DOSAGE AND INDICATIONS

Metoclopramide may be administered in doses of 10–15 mg before meals and at bedtime. If symptoms occur intermittently or at specific times, the use of metoclopramide in doses of 20 mg may be preferred. Caution should be observed in using doses in excess of 40 mg/day, although larger doses have been used by oncologists in treating nausea and vomiting associated with emetogenic cancer chemotherapy.

The gastrointestinal uses of this drug include treatment of gastroesophageal reflux, diabetic gastroparesis, slowed gastric emptying after gastric resection, gastroparesis, and idiopathic gastric stasis (106). In patients with postoperative ileus, metoclopramide improves nausea and vomiting and abdominal pain, and facilitates return of bowel sounds and passage of flatus and stools. As mentioned above, the effects in the colon are less than those in the upper gastrointestinal system, and although metoclopramide may be helpful in some patients with colonic hypomotility, clinical evidence is lacking.

SPECIAL CONSIDERATIONS

The effects of metoclopramide on gastrointestinal motility are antagonized by anticholinergic drugs and narcotic analgesics. Additive sedative effects can occur when given with alcohol, sedatives, hypnotics, narcotics, or tranquilizers. Absorption of certain drugs from the stomach may be diminished (e.g., digoxin) by metoclopramide, whereas absorption of other drugs from the small bowel may be accelerated (e.g., acetaminophen, tetracycline, levodopa, ethanol). Diabetic gastroparesis may be responsible for poor glucose control in some patients, since administered insulin may begin to act before food has left the stomach, leading to hypoglycemia. Adjustment of insulin dosages may be necessary, therefore, if gastric stasis improves with the use of metoclopramide. Dosages in children, elderly patients, and those with renal failure must be carefully monitored. Metoclopramide elevates serum prolactin levels in all patients, some of whom may develop associated breast enlargement, nipple tenderness, galactorrhea, or menstrual irregularity. Metoclopramide is incompatible with the following intravenous admixtures: cephalothin sodium, chloramphenicol sodium, and sodium bicarbonate (123). Contraindications to the use of metoclopramide include use whenever stimulation of gastrointestinal motility might be dangerous, as in the presence of mechanical obstruction or perforation. Metoclopramide is contraindicated in patients with pheochromocytoma because the drug may cause a hypertensive crisis, probably due to release of catecholamines from the tumor. Phentolamine may be used to control such crises if they occur (123). Metoclopramide should also not be used in epileptics or patients receiving other drugs that are likely to cause extrapyramidal reactions, since the frequency and severity of seizures or extrapyramidal reactions may be increased.

SIDE EFFECTS

The incidence of side effects due to metoclopramide is approximately 20% (145). The main problems are drowsiness, restlessness, and anxiety. Dry mouth, depression, lightheadedness, constipation, and diarrhea are less commonly reported. Extrapyramidal reactions such as oculogyric crises, opisthotonos, trismus, and torticollis occur in about 1% of patients. Rarely, dystonic reactions may present as stupor and dyspnea. These effects can be reversed with intramuscular administration of 50 mg of diphenhydramine hydrochloride and discontinuance of the drug.

Domperidone

Domperidone is another prokinetic agent currently in clinical trials in the United States. This drug is a specific dopamine antagonist that stimulates the gastrointestinal tract and has antiemetic properties, but does not cross the blood-brain barrier and rarely causes extrapyramidal side effects (57).

PHARMACOKINETICS

Peak plasma concentrations of domperidone are attained 10–30 minutes after intramuscular and oral administration, and 1–2 hours after rectal administration of suppositories. The bioavailability of intramuscular domperidone is 90%, whereas that of oral domperidone is 13–17% because of "first pass" hepatic and gut wall metabolism. The elimination half-life of domperidone is 7.5 hours in healthy subjects, but can be prolonged up to 20.8 hours in patients with severe hepatic insufficiency.

DOSAGE AND INDICATIONS

Dosage recommendations have not been established pending completion of clinical trials. Daily dosage regimens have ranged from 40 to 120 mg/day in divided doses. The drug has some promise for treatment of gastroesophageal reflux and gastric stasis. High concentrations of the drug are found in the esophagus, stomach, and small intestine. Domperidone probably has minimal effect on colonic motility.

SIDE EFFECTS

Domperidone is well tolerated and seldom causes important side effects. It has a potent effect in stimulating prolactin secretion. Other reported side effects include dry mouth, pruritus, headache, diarrhea, and nervousness. Extrapyramidal and true dystonic reactions are rare, and CNS effects have not been reported.

Cisapride

Cisapride is a new prokinetic agent currently under clinical investigation in both the United States and Europe. This agent is thought to facilitate acetylcholine release at the myenteric plexus without affecting the secretory gland level. In vitro, it stimulates ileal contractility, increases gastric tonic and phasic motility, and furthers antroduodenal coordination. In vivo, it stimulates digestive and interdigestive antroduodenal motility and improves gastric emptying. Animal data support a prokinetic effect on the esophagus, stomach, small bowel, and colon (106) Unlike metoclopramide and domperidone, cisapride has no dopamine antagonist properties.

PHARMACOKINETICS

In humans, the plasma level of cisapride decays triexponentially with a half-life of 19.4 hours after intravenous administration. The bioavailability after oral administration is in the range of 35–40%. Plasma levels after oral administration of a 10-mg tablet peak at 1.5–2.0 hours (106).

DOSAGE AND INDICATIONS

Dosage recommendations are not established pending completion of clinical trials. In humans, cisapride in doses of 2, 4, and 8 mg intravenously and 4, 10, and 16 mg orally increase gastric emptying, antral peristalsis, lower esophageal sphincter pressure, small bowel transit, and colonic transit (106, 107). Preliminary reports suggest that cisapride may be useful in patients with idiopathic gastric stasis, gastroparesis diabeticorum, and intestinal pseudoobstruction (47, 106). This agent appears to have the most pronounced colonic effect of the prokinetic agents studied to date and also holds special promise for use in patients with colonic ileus and idiopathic constipation.

ANTIDIARRHEAL AGENTS

Several agents may be used in the ICU for management of diarrhea. There are no absolute dosage recommendations for any one of these agents and dosages should be titrated to effect in each patient. Bismuth subsalicylate is commonly used as an over-the-counter treatment for diarrhea for adults; 2 tablespoons every ½–1 hours can be given (not to exceed eight doses a day). Signs of salicylism may be noted. Caution is advised when administering to patients taking medication for anticoagulation, diabetes, or gout. Opiates such as codeine (15–60 mg up to every 4 hours) or belladonna tincture (0.3–1.0 ml up to every 8 hours) are frequently used for treatment of diarrhea. The pharmacokinetics of opiates are altered with age, resulting in increased plasma levels in the older patient. Loperamide hydrochloride is a long-acting antidiarrheal agent given as a 4-mg dose initially, followed by a 2-mg dose after each unformed stool, not to exceed a maximum dose of 16 mg/day. It is relatively devoid of central effects and no specific side effects have been reported in the elderly. Diphenoxylate hydrochloride with a small amount of atropine is also commonly used for treatment of diarrhea. It is extensively metabolized before it is excreted, mostly in bile. The drug is chemically similar to meperidine and thus may potentiate the actions of barbiturates, tranquilizers, and alcohol. Respiratory depression can occur when excessive doses are administered, and concomitant administration of monoamine oxidase inhibitors are contraindicated. The adult dosage recommended is 2.5–5.0 mg, three to four times per day.

α-Adrenergic agonists stimulate sodium and chloride absorption in the intestine and the use of such agents may therefore have a potent antidiarrheal effect. Ion transport in the intestine is mediated by an α_2-adrenergic receptor.

Clonidine, a widely prescribed antihypertensive medication, is a specific α_2-adrenergic agonist. Both clonidine and lidamine, a structurally similar analogue, can stimulate water and electrolyte absorption and thereby inhibit diarrhea (104).These medications, however, have prominent cardiovascular and central nervous system effects. At present, they probably should be used to control diarrhea only in patients unresponsive to conventional treatment or unable to use opiate compounds.

Somatostatin is a 14-amino acid peptide found in the D cell, one of the endocrine cells of the gut. It stimulates water and electrolyte absorption in the intestine and inhibits diarrhea in patients with carcinoid tumors and short bowel syndrome. A synthetic analogue has been recently developed for use in controlling diarrhea in patients with carcinoid syndrome (93).

LAXATIVES

Successful management of constipation requires knowledge of normal bowel physiology, conditions with which constipation is associated, and potential complications. Table 18.8 shows some of the agents and conditions with which constipation is associated. Laxatives should be used in critically ill patients only after the differential diagnostic concerns have been fully considered.

Osmotic or Saline Laxatives

Osmotic or saline laxatives contain slowly absorbable or nonabsorbable salts, especially magnesium. These salts are hyperosmotic, drawing water into the lumen of the small intestine and causing a large quantity of fluid to enter the ascending colon producing a fluid overload with loose, easily passed stools. The most widely used saline laxative is magnesium hydroxide (milk of magnesia). Dosages of 1–2 tablespoons/day are usually effective. Magnesium citrate is useful, usually in doses of 5–10 oz/day. Care must be taken when giving magnesium salts to patients with renal insufficiency (hypermagnesemia may result) and when giving sodium salts to those with congestive heart failure.

Lactulose is an especially effective laxative. It is a carbohydrate that is not digested and therefore serves as an osmotic load, stimulating water secretion in the bowel. Lactulose

Table 18.8
Drugs and Abnormalities Associated with Constipation

Drugs
  Aluminum-containing antacids
  Anticholinergics
  Barium sulfate
  Calcium channel blockers (especially verapamil)
  Cholestyramine
  Chronic laxative abuse
  Chronic lead exposure
  Opiates
  Phenothiazines
  Tricyclic antidepressants
  Vincristine
Mechanical obstruction
Metabolic abnormalities
  Diabetes mellitus
  Hypercalcemia
  Hypothyroidism
  Porphyria
Muscular or connective tissue disorders
  Myotonic dystrophy
  Primary muscle abnormalities
  Scleroderma
Neurologic abnormalities
  Autonomic neuropathy
  Multiple sclerosis
  Parkinson's disease
  Spinal cord abnormalities
  Tabes dorsalis
Rectal disorders
  Anal fissures
  Hemorrhoids
  Ulcerative proctitis

syrup can be given in a dosage of 15–30 ml/day as needed, with increasing dosages of up to 60 ml/day.

Other Laxative Agents

Osmotic or stimulant laxatives include cascara sagrada, senna, bisacodyl, phenolphthalein, and castor oil. Suppositories, e.g. glycerol, act directly on the rectal mucosa to stimulate peristalsis. Small-dose (4-oz) phosphate solution enemas may be used, although serum phosphate may rise with repeated usage. Tap water enemas may be used with lukewarm water without soap. The volume should be less than 500 ml (16 oz). Several instances of soapsud-colitis have been reported (86). An electrolyte-polyethylene glycol solution (Colyte; GoLYTELY) used for preparation for colonoscopy or barium enema (43) can be used in constipated patients as long as there is no evidence of obstruction.

Table 18.9
Drugs Used for Pharmacologic Therapy of Portal Hypertension

Vasoconstrictors
Vasopressin
Somatostatin
β-Adrenergic blockers
Nonselective
Selective
Vasodilators
Nitroglycerin
Isosorbide dinitrate
Prazosin
Sodium nitroprusside
Clonidine
Ketanserin
Calcium channel blockers
Miscellaneous
Pentagastrin
Domperidone
Metoclopramide

DRUGS FOR THE TREATMENT OF PORTAL HYPERTENSION

Pharmacologic efforts to treat portal hypertension are directed toward reducing the increased blood flow in the portal collateral system and reducing the increased intrahepatic resistance, thereby reducing variceal pressure (127, 134). Vasoconstrictors reduce splanchnic blood flow and therefore portal flow. Vasodilators dilate the intrahepatic vasculature, reducing vascular resistance to portal blood flow. Additionally, there are other drugs that reduce the blood flow or pressure in the gastroesophageal-variceal system by mechanisms other than active vasoconstriction or vasodilation (Table 18.9).

Vasoconstrictors

VASOPRESSIN

Vasopressin is a peptide produced by the posterior pituitary gland. When infused at pharmacologic doses, it causes splanchnic vasoconstriction with a consequent reduction in portal blood flow and portal pressure. Vasopressin may be given intraarterially as well as by intravenous infusion. Since the intraarterial administration requires special skills and facilities and superimposes complications related to catheterization and the maintenance of catheter position, continuous intravenous infusion is the route of choice with portal hypertensive bleeding.

Vasopressin infusion should be begun at a dose of 0.2–0.4 U/min intravenously. Dosages of up to 1.0 U/min are sometimes necessary to control bleeding, but this dose significantly increases the risk of toxicity. Tapering of the dose before discontinuation appears to be unnecessary because vasopressin does not prevent rebleed from varices.

The list of potential adverse effects of vasopressin is lengthy (127, 134). Vasopressin produces increased gut motility, presumably by stimulation of smooth muscle, with attendant abdominal cramps and occasionally diarrhea. The vasoconstrictive effects may result in bowel ischemia and necrosis. An increase in cardiac afterload, baroreceptor-mediated bradycardia, decreased coronary blood flow, and direct impairment of cardiac contractibility are responsible for the decreased cardiac output and myocardial performance observed with this agent (183). Severe arrhythmias and myocardial infarction may occur with the use of vasopressin in humans; therefore, close supervision and cardiac monitoring are advised during infusion. The drug is contraindicated in patients with known coronary artery disease and should be used cautiously in alcoholics who may have a subclinical cardiomyopathy. Vasopressin has also been associated with respiratory arrest and cerebral hemorrhage. Nonhemodynamic effects of vasopressin include antidiuresis and stimulation of endothelial release of plasminogen activator and factor VIII (25). Administration of vasopressin to nonbleeding patients with cirrhosis is not, however, associated with chemical evidence of fibrinolysis (132).

β-ADRENERGIC BLOCKADE

Propranolol, a universal β-blocker, reduces portal pressure both acutely and chronically when administered to patients with portal hypertension. The mechanism of effect seems to be via a reduction in splanchnic blood flow. This action is the result of both a reduction in cardiac output (β_1-blockade) and splanchnic vasoconstriction, the latter probably due to β_2-blockade with unopposed α-adrenergic–mediated constrictive effects on splanchnic blood flow in humans (e.g., 29% reduction) (130). The principal application of propranolol therapy has been in the prevention of variceal bleeding, although the results of clinical studies are mixed and further controlled studies are required to define the place of propranolol in prevention of variceal bleeding (30).

SOMATOSTATIN

The hormone somatostatin reduces splanchnic blood flow, although the mechanism is unclear. In cirrhotic patients, hepatic blood flow decreases progressively with somatostatin infusion rates of 2.5 and 7.5 μg/min, but there is no further decrease with larger doses. The effect on portal pressure in cirrhotic patients is controversial (158). In contrast to vasopressin, somatostatin has minimal systemic effects at the dose used.

Vasodilators

Nitrates by themselves are mild portal hypotensive agents. Portal blood flow actually rises rather than falls in response to these vasodilators. Portal pressure is presumably reduced because the fall in portal inflow pressure, secondary to systemic vasodilation, is greater than the fall in hepatic vein pressure. Direct dilation of the portal vein is another possible mechanism of action. Oral, transdermal, and intravenous administration of nitrates reduces portal pressure. The primary use of nitrates at present appears to be in conjunction with vasopressin. Nitroglycerin reverses the cardiotoxic effects of vasopressin. It enhances the portal hypotensive effects by reducing the increase in portal venous resistance induced by vasopressin. Hemodynamic studies supported the favorable results observed in clinical trials (60, 166).

The effects of several other vasodilators on portal pressure have been studied. Prazosin, an α-adrenergic blocker, at a dose of 5 mg twice a day produced a sustained decline of 17% in portal pressure without a mean change in arterial pressure or cardiac output (113). Clonidine, a centrally acting α-adrenergic agonist, has been evaluated in one report in which intravenously administered clonidine (2.5 mg/kg) lowered the hepatic venous pressure gradient by 25% (177). Ketanserin, a selective 5-hydroxytryptamine–blocking agent, reduces portal pressure in animals, suggesting a specific role for serotonin in the maintenance of portal hypertension (33). The effects of all of these agents require clinical confirmation, and their use in portal hypertension remains investigational.

Miscellaneous Agents

Several agents selectively increase lower esophageal sphincter pressure and contract the esophageal musculature and decrease blood flow through the esophageal vessels, supposedly by compression of collateral vessels feeding the varices. Agents such as pentagastrin, domperidone, and metoclopramide may have a future role in the medical therapy of portal hypertension (103).

Sclerosant Solutions

Injection sclerotherapy has become a first-line treatment modality for bleeding varices of the esophagus in many patients. A brief review of the pharmacology of the different sclerosing agents is included here. A common denominator among sclerosing agents is their ability to induce an inflammatory reaction within or outside the vascular endothelium, resulting in a fibrotic, varicopenic esophagus. The amount of sclerosant injected into each varix is approximately 1–2 ml with an average total of 15–25 ml used per session. The most commonly used variceal sclerosing agents in the United States are sodium morrhuate and sodium tetradecyl sulfate.

Sodium morrhuate is a mixture of sodium salts of cod liver oil. Preparation may be nonuniform, and allergic reactions ranging from rash to anaphylaxis may be seen. Fever, chest pain, pleural effusion, and deep postsclerosis ulceration are more common than with sodium tetradecyl sulfate. Acute respiratory distress syndrome has been reported in two patients within 24 hours of sclerotherapy with sodium morrhuate (116). A more recent study, however, has shown that only 20% of injected sodium morrhuate reaches the pulmonary circulation and as a result, pulmonary endothelium is exposed to only small amounts of this agent with no change in diffusing capacity (31).

Sodium tetradecyl sulfate is a synthetic anion detergent. The surface activity of the fatty acid anions of the soap is thought to be responsible for the physical properties leading to variceal thrombosis. The effect of long-term esophageal variceal sclerotherapy using this agent have recently been evaluated; no serious long-term or short-term impairment of lung function was noted (91). Sodium tetradecyl sulfate is commercially available in 1% and 3% solutions.

Ethanolamine oleate, although not commercially available in the United States, is a widely used effective sclerosing agent. It is derived from oleic acid and is similar in physical properties to sodium morrhuate—in fact, sodium oleate is one of the chief constituents of the fatty acids in sodium morrhuate. Ethanolamine produces rare allergic reactions and has resulted in one such death. Data at present do not appear to give this drug clear advantage in either safety or efficacy over other sclerosants available in the United States.

Polidocanol is a synthetic agent that has been used widely in Europe. A 1% solution is injected adjacent to the varices at several levels in the esophagus. Intravariceal injections are to be avoided because this agent has been associated with heart failure and death due to the action of the drug passing into the systemic circulation. The negative chronotropic effects may be ascribed to this agent's local anesthetic properties. Although, in general, use of poliodecanol is safe, it is not available in the United States.

In the United States sclerosing mixtures have been used primarily in an attempt to avoid the recognized toxicities of sodium morrhuate and sodium tetradecyl sulfate. Dilution of these agents with solutions such as 50% dextrose and 50–95% ethanol appears to be the most popular approach (116). Other mixtures including addition of cephalothin or thrombin have not been shown to be more efficacious (77).

DRUGS FOR ACUTE STRESS EROSIONS AND ULCERATIONS

Stress ulcer and acute erosive gastritis occur in patients with extensive burns, multiple injuries, or major operative procedures, especially when these conditions are accompanied by episodes of hypotension, sepsis, or renal, hepatic, and respiratory failure (26). The incidence of bleeding from these lesions is variable and has been estimated to occur in approximately 3–6% of patients who are seriously ill, and upwards of 54% of patients with intracranial disease. In the very sickest patients with sepsis, the mortality from this complication approaches 80% (154).

The pathogenesis of stress erosions and ulcers is not completely understood but may be examined in the light of the known mechanisms of mucosal integrity, which include maintenance of mucosal pH, intramural pH, integrity of the gastric mucosal barrier, gastric mucosal blood flow, the composition of gastric mucus, and the state of gastric epithelial renewal. Mucosal pH is the most clinically accessible of these factors and has been the most extensively studied. Although not a universal finding, hypersecretion of acid has been demonstrated to occur in some patients who subsequently develop stress ulceration and may be especially prominent in those with central nervous system injury (72).

Intramural gastric pH may also be associated with the development of stress ulceration by several different mechanisms. First, disruption of the mucosal barrier to back-diffusion of hydrogen ion may lead to accumulation of intramural hydrogen ions. Second, decreased gastric mucosal or subepithelial blood flow may cause localized anoxia with resultant anaerobiosis; lactic acid accumulates, with a consequent fall in tissue pH. Third, systemic acidosis that accompanies shock states may cause a local decrease in the pH of the blood perfusing the gastric mucosa. In one study, the presence of multiple clinical risk factors and a low intramural gastric pH correlated with the development of massive bleeding from stress ulceration (50). Furthermore, bleeding from stress ulceration was identified only in the presence of a markedly decreased intramural pH. All patients who developed bleeding had been treated with antacids, which suggested that intramural pH rather than luminal pH may be the more important factor in the development of stress ulceration.

Since most studies have shown that bleeding or evidence of gastric mucosal injury is associated with an increased overall mortality, a significant amount of attention has been directed toward prevention of stress ulcerations (131). Controlled randomized trials have shown that aggressive hourly intragastric antacid titration can reduce the incidence of acute upper gastrointestinal bleeding in critically ill patients. Hourly titration of gastric contents with antacids to maintain intragastric pH above 3.5 resulted in a significant reduction of bleeding in critically ill patients (64). Continuous infusion of antacids is effective, and given at a dose of 30–60 ml/hr may also facilitate nursing care by obviating the requirement for hourly dosage administration. Disadvantages of antacid prophylaxis include diarrhea, systemic alkalosis, hypophosphatemia, and hypomagnesemia or hypermagnesemia. In addition, the danger of pulmonary aspiration may be increased in patients receiving large volumes of antacids by nasogastric tube. The H_2-receptor antagonists are also effective in prophylaxis of stress-induced ulcerations and bleeding (122). Cimetidine (300 mg every 6 hours, intravenously) compares favorably but is not more effective than antacids in the prevention of stress erosions (126). Hourly antacid use, however, appears to be better for maintaining gastric pH above 4. The goal was accomplished in 97.9% of patients in one study (83) compared with 79.5% of patients receiving bolus cimetidine therapy. Ranitidine given as an intravenous bolus of 50 mg every 8 hours is another effective alternative. Intragastric pH can be much more effectively maintained above 4.0 if a continuous infusion of histamine H_2-antagonists is used instead of intermittent bolus dosing (119). In patients with normal renal function, cimetidine should be administered intravenously as a 300-mg bolus over 10–20 minutes, followed by a continuous infusion of 37.5 mg/hr. Gastric pH should be measured after 6 hours. In some patients, the infusion rate may need to be increased possibly to 50–100 mg/hr in order to maintain gastric pH above 4.0. Patients who have recently been treated with cimetidine may be resistant to its action and supplemental antacids may be required. The slow infusion of the cimetidine bolus is advised in the light of reports of serious cardiac dysrhythmias in critically ill patients who received rapid intravenous administration of cimetidine (100). Ranitidine given as a 50-mg initial bolus dose followed by an 8 mg/hr continuous infusion is an alternative, and at present is the preferred method in our intensive care units. Another advantage to continuous infusion of histamine H_2-antagonists is the time and material cost savings to the pharmacy and nursing services. These agents can be added to parenteral alimentation solutions, and in one study, costs for total parenteral nutrition–delivered cimetidine was $12,257 versus $34,769 for intermittently administered cimetidine (141).

The use of other agents in the prevention of stress bleeding awaits further studies. Sucralfate is effective, and unlike antacids and cimetidine, the efficacy of sucralfate is independent of intragastric pH (13, 165). One gram of sucralfate can be dissolved in 30 ml of water and administered every 6 hours orally or via a nasogastric tube. Preliminary experience with the use of famotidine (34) and omeprazole (173) in critically ill patients suggests that these agents will also be of therapeutic benefit in controlling intragastric acidity in critically ill patients.

DRUG THERAPY FOR UPPER GASTROINTESTINAL BLEEDING

Bleeding from peptic ulcers usually ceases spontaneously, although rebleeding during hospitalization occurs in 25–30% of patients. Morbidity and mortality is increased if rebleeding occurs. As a consequence, attempts have been made to use endoscopic criteria of peptic ulcers to predict the likelihood of rebleeding and accordingly, better direct the care of the patient (161, 175). Endoscopic features of the ulcer that increase the likelihood of rebleeding are a central dark spot, adherent clot, visible vessel, or slow blood ooze from the ulcer crater. Studies have varied in defining rebleeding risk based on each of these parameters (Table 18.10).

Attempts to prevent recurrent bleeding from gastric or duodenal ulcers using cimetidine and/or antacids have not been successful (184). One possibility for these failures is that gastric pH may not be adequately elevated. In vitro data suggest that it may be necessary to raise gastric pH to 7.0 (achlorhydria) in order to prevent recurrent hemorrhage (59). In vitro experiments have confirmed that the process of normal blood coagulation is pH-dependent and requires a pH of 6.9–7.4 (Table 18.11). Pepsin acts in concert with acid to dissolve clots (7) and is not irreversibly inactivated until pH values of 7.0 or higher are achieved (59). If these in vitro pH data can be applied to intragastric pH levels in humans, poor clot formation or even clot dissolution might occur in the stomach of patients who have bled unless a pH of 7.0 or more is maintained.

The pharmacologic approach to sustaining medical achlorhydria is best directed by the

Table 18.10
Endoscopic Stigmata for Predicting Rebleeding

Endoscopic Finding	Prevalence (%)		Rebleeding (%)	
	Mean	Range	Mean	Range
Central dark spot	21	20–54	9	0–15
Adherent clot	19	5–32	20	0–24
Visible vessel	30	15–72	53	19–100
Ongoing ooze	22	18–72	45	32–100

Table 18.11
pH Effects on Intragastric Coagulation

pH	Comments
7.4	Reference pH
7.0	Pepsin irreversibly inactivated
6.8	3× decrease platelet aggregation
6.4	Clotting time 2× increase; decreased availability of platelet phospholipid and platelet factor III
6.1	60% disaggregation of previously formed platelet aggregates
6.0	Clotting time 4× increase; decreased availability of platelet phospholipid and platelet factor III
5.9	Platelet aggregation abolished; complete dissolution of previously formed platelet aggregates.
5.4	Clotting abolished

results of a recent comparison of different medical regimens (121). The effects of bolus doses of cimetidine (300 mg every 6 hours intravenously), antacid (30 ml/hr intragastrically), and a combination of these resulted in attaining intragastric pH values of 3.5, 4.6, and 6.8, respectively, but did not achieve achlorhydria. Constant infusion regimens of cimetidine (50 mg/hr intravenously), antacid (0.5 ml/min intragastrically), and the combination resulted in pH values of 4.3, 5.2, and 7.4, respectively. Sustained achlorhydria was still not produced in each patient until the infusion of cimetidine was increased to 100 mg/hr and administered with a constant infusion of antacid. Although the maintenance of gastric pH at 7.0 or higher should theoretically reduce bleeding and/or rebleeding, a clinical controlled patient trial has not yet been reported. The use of more potent acid inhibitors such as ranitidine, famotidine, and omeprazole may prove to be more effective in ensuring sustained achlorhydria. At present, we recommend coupling of a constant infusion of cimetidine or ranitidine with a continuous infusion of antacid in patients who present with nonvariceal upper gastrointestinal hemorrhage and who are at risk for rebleeding. Dosages of the medications should be carefully titrated to ensure a pH of 7.0 or higher. Endoscopic definition of the ulcer features may help in better identifying those patients with a higher likelihood of rebleeding. If a lesion with a high risk for rebleeding is identified, we would favor continuing the combination therapy for at least the first 24–48 hours of intensive support.

DRUGS USED FOR INTENSIVE TREATMENT OF INFLAMMATORY BOWEL DISEASE

Ulcerative Colitis

Before the corticosteroid era, severe or moderately severe attacks of ulcerative colitis (UC) had high mortality. Corticosteroids sharply reduced the fatality rate in moderately severe attacks of UC, but severe attacks continued to be dangerous until the policy of early colectomy was introduced. The dramatic decrease in mortality with surgery led some authors to abandon corticosteroid therapy. Successful medical treatment of a severe attack of UC may, however, be followed by a sustained remission (164). The aim, therefore, is to obtain the best possible timing between medical and surgical treatment.

Patients with severe UC are systematically ill with fever, leukocytosis, bloody diarrhea, abdominal pain, and tenderness. For such patients, treatment with parenteral steroids is mandatory. Oral steroids for such patients are a poor choice because of inferior response, and should not be used. Intravenous hydrocortisone, 300 mg daily, or prednisolone, 60 mg daily, in divided doses should be administered unless the intestine has already perforated. If the patient has not previously received adrenocortical steroids, some clinicians advise intravenous adrenocorticotropic hormone therapy, 120 U/day (112). Steroid therapy may lessen symptoms and signs expected with perforation, so careful physical examination for liver dullness at least twice daily and frequent flat plates of the abdomen should be done.

Intensive medical therapy improves or induces a remission in approximately 80% of patients with severe colitis (76, 111, 153). Continuation of medical therapy beyond 5–6 days without clear-cut objective evidence of improvement is very hazardous since colonic perforation with peritoneal soilage is a disaster that increases operative mortality and postoperative complications at least 10-fold (19). Antibiotics do not influence remission rates and should not be used routinely, but should be added when there is impending or definite colonic perforation or evidence of definite suppuration (111). When added, antibiotic coverage should be directed at both anaerobic and aerobic fecal flora. Sulfasalazine is not helpful in the severely ill patient with fulminant colitis. Total parenteral nutrition has no primary therapeutic effect in acute colitis, although it preserves body protein (36).

Medications that affect bowel activity have been associated with megacolon in patients with active ulcerative or Crohn's colitis. Drugs implicated include anticholinergics such as propantheline bromide and atropine; narcotics such as codeine, opium, paregoric, meperidine, and morphine; and narcotic derivative antidiarrheal agents such as diphenoxylate hydrochloride with atropine sulfate and loperamide.

Crohn's Disease

Patients with severely symptomatic Crohn's disease require hospitalization, bowel rest, and intravenous fluid therapy. Patients are usually febrile, and questions of extensive inflammation outside the lumen of the intestine and abscess formation frequently arise. Broad spectrum antibiotic coverage is frequently begun with aggressive attempts to identify an intraabdominal abscess. Metronidazole has received systematic investigation in patients with Crohn's disease. A powerful drug against intestinal anaerobics, metronidazole clearly is effective against mixed intestinal flora infections and suppurative foci in the acute case. It also is effective in treating perirectal disease and perirectal fistulae. If no definite abscess can be localized and no positive blood cultures are obtained, steroids, prednisolone or equivalent, should be given at a dose of 40–60 mg/day intravenously. With a regimen of bowel rest, high-dose steroids, and broad spectrum antibiotics if extraluminal extension is suspected, the disease remits in the majority of severely ill patients. The use of azothioprine, 1.0–2.0 mg/kg/day, or 6-mercaptopurine, 1.5–2.5 mg/kg/day, can be considered for patients who do not respond to this regimen. These agents, however, may not be of benefit in acute disease, in that there is often a protracted delay in attaining maximal therapeutic effect.

DRUGS FOR INTESTINAL ISCHEMIA

Acute mesenteric ischemia results from an abrupt diminution in the blood supply to the small bowel and is most commonly caused by an embolus or vasospasm (nonocclusive mesenteric ischemia). Less commonly, arterial thrombosis with insufficient collateralization and, rarely, a venous thrombosis is responsible. Patients at risk are usually older than 50 years of age, have valvular or arteriosclerotic heart disease and/or longstanding poorly controlled congestive heart failure, and are treated by rapid digitalization (a splanchnic vasoconstrictor) or with potent diuretics. Such patients frequently have a cardiac arrhythmia, an episode of hypotension (hypovolemia or shock), or a recent myocardial infarction. Also at risk are patients with inflammatory, degenerative, or structural diseases of the small mesenteric vessels. The clinical hallmark of early acute mesenteric ischemia is severe abdominal pain without significant abdominal findings. The disease can be diagnosed only by angiography, and selective intraarterial infusion of a number of potential dilators (including histamine, phenoxybenzamine, isoproterenol, dopamine, methylprednisolone, prescoline, gut peptides, prostaglandin E_1, and papaverine) has been tried (11, 12). Of these, papaverine appears to be the most effective (10).

The main actions of papaverine are exerted on cardiac and smooth muscle. It relaxes the smooth musculature of the larger blood vessels and reduces vasospasm. The antispasmodic effect is direct and unrelated to muscle innervation. In addition, this drug has direct cardiac effects with depression of conduction and prolongation of the refractory period. Systemic arterial pressure and cardiac rate must be monitored during the infusion because the amount of papaverine administered may cause cardiac arrhythmias, peripheral vasodilation, and increased myocardial oxygen demand. The duration of infusion depends both on the purpose for its use and the clinical and angiographic response of the patient.

References

1. Albibi R, McCallum RW: Metoclopramide—pharmacology and clinical application. *Ann Intern Med* 98:86–93, 1983.
2. Alfrey AC, Le Gendre GR, Kaehny WD: The dialysis encephalopathy syndrome: possible aluminum intoxication. *N Engl J Med* 294:184–188, 1976.
3. Averius PH, Brunzell JD: Chylomicronemia induced by cimetidine. *Gastroenterology* 89:664–666, 1985.
4. Baker LRI, Ackrell P, Catell WR, et al: Iatrogenic osteomalacia and myopathy due to phosphate depletion. *Br Med J* 3:150–152, 1974.
5. Bartle WR, Walter SE, Shapero T: Dose-dependent effect of cimetidine on phenytoin kinetics. *Clin Pharmacol Ther* 33:649–655, 1983.
6. Bender HJ, Donaldson RM Jr: Effect of cimetidine on

intrinsic factor and pepsin secretion in man. *Gastroenterology* 74:371–375, 1978.

7. Berstad A: Management of acute upper gastrointestinal bleeding. *Scand J Gastroenterol* 17:103–108, 1982.

8. Berylne GM, Ben-Ari J, Pest D, et al: Hyperaluminaemia from aluminum resins in renal failure. *Lancet* 2:494–496, 1970.

9. Black JW, Duncan WAM, Durant CJ, et al: Definition and antagonism of histamine H₂ receptors. *Nature* 236:385–390, 1972.

10. Boley SJ, Fernstein FR, Sammartano R, Brandt LJ, Sprayregen S: New concepts in the management of emboli of the superior mesenteric artery. *Surg Gynecol Obstet* 153:561–569, 1981.

11. Boley SJ, Sammartano R, Brandt LJ, Mitsudo S, Sheran M: Intra-arterial vasodilators and thrombolytic agents in experimental superior mesenteric artery embolus. *Gastroenterology* 82:1021, 1982.

12. Borden EB, Boley SJ: Acute mesenteric ischemia: Treat aggressively for best results. *J Crit Illness* 10:52–58, 1986.

13. Borrero E, Bank S, Margolis I, Schulman ND, Chardavoyne R: Comparison of antacid and sucralfate in the presentation of gastrointestinal bleeding in patients who are critically ill. *Am J Med* 79(suppl 2C):28–30, 1985.

14. Boyce MJ: Cimetidine and the cardiovascular system. In Baron JH (ed): *Cimetidine in the 80's.* Edinburgh, Churchill Livingstone, 1981, pp 227–237.

15. Boyce MJ, Wareham K: Histamine H₁, and H₂-receptors in the cardiovascular system of man. In Torsoli A, Zucchelli PE, Brimblecomb RW (eds): *H₂-Antagonists.* Amsterdam, Excerpta Medica, 1980, pp 280–293.

16. Brand DC, Roufail WM, Thomson ABR, Taper EJ: Misoprostil, a synthetic PGE₁ analog, in the treatment of duodenal ulcers: a multicenter double-blind study. *Dig Dis Sci* 30:1475–1585, 1985.

17. Brandstaetter G, Karachvil P: Comparison of two sucralfate dosages (2 g twice a day versus 1 g four times a day) in duodenal ulcer healing. *Am J Med* 79(Suppl 2C):18–20, 1985.

18. Brogden RN, Carmine AA, Heel RC, Speight TM, Avery GS: Ranitidine: a review of its pharmacology and therapeutic use in peptic ulcer disease and other allied diseases. *Drugs* 24:267–303, 1982.

19. Brooke BN, Sampson PA: An indication for surgery in acute ulcerative colitis. *Lancet* 2:1272–1273, 1964.

20. Brooks WS: Sucralfate: non-ulcer uses. *Am J Gastroenterol* 80:206–209, 1985.

21. Brooks WS: *Variceal sclerosing agents.* Am J Gastroenterol 79:424–428, 1984.

22. Bulkard WP: Histamine H₂ receptor binding with ³H-cimetidine in brain. *Eur J Pharmacol* 50:449–450, 1978.

23. Burck JD, Myka JA, Kokelman DK: Famotidine: summary of preclinical safety assessment. *Digestion* 32:7–14, 1985.

24. Campbell MA, Plachetka JR, Jackson JE, Moon FJ, Finley PR: Cimetidine decreases theophylline clearance. *Ann Intern Med* 95:68–69, 1981.

25. Cash JD, Gader AM, Da Costa J: The release of plasminogen activator and factor VIII to lysine vasopressin, arginine vasopressin, I-desamino-8-d-arginine vasopressin, angiotensin and oxytocin in man. *Br J Haematol* 27:363–364, 1974.

26. Cheung LY: Treatment of established stress ulcer disease. *World J Surg* 5:235–246, 1981.

27. Chremos AN: Pharmacodynamics of famotidine in humans. *Am J Med* 81(suppl 4B):3–12, 1986.

28. Clarkson EM, McDonald SJ, De Wardner HW: The effect of a high intake of calcium carbonate in normal subjects and patients with chronic renal failure. *Clin Sci* 30:425–438, 1966.

29. Classen M, Darnmann HD, Domshke W, Hutteman W, Londong W: Omeprazole heals duodenal but not gastric ulcers more rapidly than ranitidine. *Hepatogastroenterology* 32:243–245, 1985.

30. Conn HO: Propranolol in portal hypertension: problems in paradise? *Hepatology* 4:560–564, 1984.

31. Connors AF, Bacon BR, Miron SD: Sodium morruate delivery to the lung during endoscopic variceal sclerotherapy. *Ann Intern Med* 105:539–542, 1986.

32. Crossby RJ, Evers PW: Review of endocrine studies of cimetidine. In Baron JH (ed): *Cimetidine in the 80's.* Edinburgh, Churchill Livingstone, 1981, pp 247–252.

33. Cummings S, Daumann A, Groszmann RJ: Vascular reactivity to serotonin in a rat model of portal hypertension. *Hepatology* 5:1059, 1985.

34. Dammann HG, Burkhardt F, Kuhl U, Walter A, Muller P, Simon B: The effect of intravenous famotidine and ranitidine on intragastric pH and hormone levels in critical care patients. *Gastroenterology* 88:1359, 1985.

35. Davis TG, Picket DL, Schlosser JH: Evaluation of the worldwide spontaneous reporting system with cimetidine. *JAMA* 243:1912–1914, 1980.

36. Dickinson RJ, Ashton MG, Axon ATR, Smith RC, Yerind CK, Hill GL: Controlled trial of intravenous hyperalimentation and total bowel rest as an adjunct to the routine therapy of acute colitis. *Gastroenterology* 79:1199–1204, 1980.

37. Doherty CC, O'Connor FA, Buchanan KD, McGeown MG: Cimetidine for duodenal ulceration in patients undergoing haemodialysis. *Br Med J* 2:1506–1508, 1977.

38. Douglas WW: Histamine and 5-hydroxytryptamine (serotonin) and their antagonists. In Gilman AG, Goodman LS, Gilman A (eds): *The Pharmacological Basis of Therapeutics,* ed. 6. New York, Macmillan, 1980, pp 622–632.

39. Drake D, Hollander D: Neutralizing capacity and cost effectiveness of antacids. *Ann Intern Med* 94:215–217, 1981.

40. *Drug Information File.* West Point, PA, Merck Sharp & Dohme.

41. Dundee JW, McGowan WA, Elwood RJ, Hilderbran PJ: Plasma benzodiazepine concentrations following oral administration with and without H₂-receptor blockers. *Ir J Med Sci* 151:413–414, 1982.

42. Ekman L, Hansson E, Havu N, Carlson E, Lundberg C: Toxicological studies on omeprazole. *Scand J Gastroenterol* 108:53–69, 1985.

43. Ernstoff JJ, Howard DA, Marshall JB, Jumshyd A, McCullough JA: A randomized, blinded clinical trial of a rapid colonic lavage solution (GoLYTELY) compared with standard preparation for colonoscopy and barium enema. *Gastroenterology* 84:1512–1516, 1983.

44. Fairfax AJ, Adam J, Pagan FS: Effect of cimetidine on the absorption of oral benzylpenicillin. *Br Med J* 1:820, 1978.

45. Feely J, Wilkinson GR, Wood AJ: Reduction of liver blood flow and propranolol metabolism by cimetidine. *N Engl J Med* 304:692–695, 1981.

46. Feldman M, Richardson CT, Peterson WL, et al: Effect of low-dose propantheline on food-stimulated gastric acid secretion: comparison with an "optimal effective dose" and interaction with cimetidine. *N Engl J Med* 297:1427–1430, 1977.

47. Feldman M, Smith JH: Effect of cisapride on gastric emptying of indigestible solids in patients with gastroparesis diabeticorum. *Gastroenterology* 91:171–174, 1987.

48. Fernandes E, Melewicz FM: Ranitidine and theophylline. *Ann Intern Med* 100:459, 1984.

49. Festen HPM, Diemel J, Lamers CBH: Is the measurement of blood cimetidine levels useful? *Br J Clin Pharmacol* 12:417–421, 1981.

50. Fiddian-Green RG, McGough E, Pittenger G, et al: Predictive value of intramural pH and other risk factors for massive bleeding from stress ulceration. *Gastroenterology* 85:613–620, 1983.

51. Fine A, Churchill T: Potentially lethal interaction of cimetidine and morphine. *Can Med Assoc J* 124:1434–1436, 1981.

52. Fortran JS, Morawiki SG, Richardson CT: In vivo and in vitro evaluation of liquid antacids. *N Engl J Med* 288:923–928, 1973.

53. Freely J, Wilkinson GR, McAllister CB, Wood AJJ: Increased toxicity and reduced clearance of lidocaine by cimetidine. *Ann Intern Med* 96:592–594, 1982.

54. Freston JW: Cimetidine-adverse reactions and patterns of use. *Ann Intern Med* 97:728–734, 1982.

55. Freston JW: Cimetidine: developments, pharmacology, and efficacy. *Ann Intern Med* 97:573–580, 1982.

56. Fretwell MD, Pearlman RA, Vestal RE, Mease PJ, Hazzard WR: Fever and delirium in three elderly patients: a discussion of possible cimetidine toxicity, cimetidine pharmacology and application of decision analysis to cimetidine therapy. *Med Grand Rounds* 1:222–238, 1982.

57. Friedman G: The GI drug column: domperidone. *Am J Gastroenterol* 78:47–48, 1983.

58. Gibaldi M, Kanig JL, Amsel L: Critical in vitro factors in evaluation of gastric antacids. Inhibition of neutralization rate of dried aluminum hydroxide gel. *J Pharm Sci* 53:1375–1377, 1964.

59. Green FW, Kaplan MM, Curtis LE, Levine PH: Effect of acid and pepsin on blood coagulation and platelet aggregation. *Gastroenterology* 74:38–43, 1978.

60. Groszman RJ, Kravetz D, Bosch J, et al: Nitroglycerin improves the hemodynamic response to vasopressin in portal hypertension. *Hepatology* 2:757–762, 1982.

61. Gugler R, Jense JC: Omeprazole inhibits oxidative drug metabolism. *Gastroenterology* 89:1235–1241, 1985.

62. Hardy BG, Zador IT, Golden L, Lalka D, Schentag JJ: Effect of cimetidine on the pharmacokinetics and pharmacodynamics of quinidine. *Am J Cardiol* 52:172–174, 1982.

63. Harvey SC: Gastric antacids and digestants. In Gilman AG, Goodman LS, Gilman A (eds): *The Pharmacologic Basis of Therapeutics*, ed. 6. New York, Macmillan, 1980, pp 988–1001.

64. Hastings PL, Skillman JJ, Bushness LS, Silen W: Antacid titration in the prevention of acute gastrointestinal bleeding. A controlled, randomized trial in 100 critically ill patients. *N Engl J Med* 298:1041–1044, 1978.

65. Heagerty AM, Castleden CM, Patel L: Failure of ranitidine to interact with propranolol. *Br Med J* 284:1304, 1982.

66. Hetzel DJ, Bochner F, Hallpike JF, Shearman DJC, Hann CS: Cimetidine interaction with phenytoin. *Br Med J* 282:1512, 1981.

67. Hollander D, Tarnawski A, Gergely H, Zipser RD: Sucralfate protection of gastric mucosa against alcohol-induced necrosis: a prostaglandin mediated process. *Scand J Gastroenterol* 19:97–102, 1984.

68. Holt PR: Gastrointestinal drugs in the elderly. *Am J Gastroenterol* 81:403–411, 1986.

69. Howard JM: Famotidine: a new potent long acting histamine H_2-receptor antagonist: comparison with cimetidine and ranitidine in the treatment of Zollinger-Ellison syndrome. *Gastroenterology* 88:1026–1033, 1985.

70. Howden CW, Meredith PA, Forrest JA, Reid JL: Oral pharmacokinetics of omeprazole. *Eur J Clin Pharmacol* 26:641–643, 1984.

71. Hyneck ML, Murphy JF, Lipschutz DE: Cimetidine clearance during intermittent and chronic peritoneal dialysis. *Am J Hosp Pharm* 38:1760–1762, 1981.

72. Idjadi F, Robbins R, Stahl WM, et al: Prospective study of gastric secretion in stressed patients with intracranial injury. *J Trauma* 11:681–686, 1971.

73. Ishimosi A: Safety experience with sucralfate in Japan. *J Clin Gastroenterol* 3:169–173, 1981.

74. Ivanovich P, Fellows H, Rich C: The absorption of calcium carbonate. *Ann Intern Med* 66:917–923, 1967.

75. Jackson JE, Powell JR, Wandell M, Bentley J, Dorr R: Cimetidine decreases theophylline clearance. *Am Rev Respir Dis* 123:615–617, 1981.

76. Janerot G, Rolny P, Sandberg-Gertzen H: Intensive intravenous treatment of ulcerative colitis. *Gastroenterology* 89:1005–1013, 1985.

77. Jansen DM: Sclerosants for injection sclerosis of esophageal varices. *Gastrointest Endosc* 29:315–317, 1983.

78. Jeevendra Martin JA, Greenblatt DJ, Abernethy DR: Increased cimetidine clearance of burn patients. *JAMA* 253:1288–1291, 1985.

79. Jones RH, Rudge CJ, Bewick M, Parsons V, Weston MJ: Cimetidine: prophylaxis against upper gastrointestinal haemorrhage after renal transplantation. *Br Med J* 1:398–400, 1978.

80. Jordaens L, Hoegaerts J, Belpaire F: Non-interaction of cimetidine with digoxin absorption. *Acta Clin Belg* 36:109–110, 1981.

81. Kaehny WD, Hegg AP, Alfrey AC: Gastrointestinal absorption of aluminum-containing antacids. *N Engl J Med* 296:1389–1390, 1977.

82. Khoury W, Geracik G, Askari A, et al: The effect of cimetidine on aspirin absorption (abstract). *Gastroenterology* 76:1169, 1979.

83. Kingsley AN: Prophylaxis for acute stress ulcers: antacids or cimetidine. *Am Surg* 51:545–547, 1985.

84. Kiowski W, Frei A: Bolus injection of cimetidine and hypotension in patients in the intensive care unit: incidence and mechanisms. *Arch Intern Med* 147:153–156, 1987.

85. Kirch W: Presentation at the Fourteenth Congress of the European Society of Pharmacology, Rome, Italy, March 1983.

86. Kirchner SG, Buckspan GS, O'Neill JA, et al: Detergent enema: a cause of caustic colitis. *Pediatr Radiol* 6:141–146, 1977.

87. Klotz V, Reimann I: Delayed clearance of diazepam due to cimetidine. *N Engl J Med* 302:1012–1014, 1980.

88. Knapp AB, Maguire W, Keren G, et al: The cimetidine-lidocaine interaction. *Ann Intern Med* 98:174–177, 1983.

89. Kollberg B, Slezak P: The effect of prostaglandin E_2 on duodenal ulcer healing. *Prostaglandins* 24:527–536, 1982.

90. Konturek SJ: Prostaglandins in pathophysiology of peptic ulcer disease. *Dig Dis Sci* 30:105S–108S, 1985.

91. Korula J, Baydur A, Sassoon C, Sakimura I: Effect of esophageal variceal sclerotherapy (EVS) on lung function: a prospective controlled study. *Arch Intern Med* 14:1517–1520, 1986.

92. Kuruvilla JT: Antipeptic activity of antacids. *Gut* 12:897–898, 1971.

93. Kvols LK, Moertel GG, O'Connell MJ, Schutt AJ, Rubin J, Hahn RG: Treatment of the malignant carcinoid syndrome: evaluation of a long-acting somatostatin analogue. *N Engl J Med* 315:663–666, 1986.

94. Lauretsen K, Run SJ, Bytzer P, et al: Effect of omeprazole and cimetidine on duodenal ulcer: a double-blind comparative trial. *N Engl J Med* 312:958–961, 1985.

95. Lee HR: Cimetidine and narcotic analgesics. *Pharmacologist* 24:145–148, 1982.

96. Lee HR, Gandolfi AJ, Sipes IG, Bentley J: Effect of histamine H_2-receptors on fentanyl metabolism. *Toxicologist* 2:145, 1981.

97. Longstreth AF, Go CLW, Malagelada JR: Postprandial gastric, pancreatic and biliary response to histamine H_2 receptor antagonists in active duodenal ulcer. *Gastroenterology* 72:9–13, 1977.

98. Lotz M, Zisman E, Bartter FC: Evidence for a phosphorus depletion syndrome in man. *N Engl J Med* 278:400–415, 1968.

99. Ma KW, Brown D, Masler DS, et al: Effects of renal failure on blood levels of cimetidine. *Gastroenterology* 74(2):473–477, 1978.

100. MacMahon B, Bakshi J, Walsh MJ. Cardiac arrhythmias after intravenous cimetidine. *N Engl J Med* 305:832–833, 1981.

101. Malazelada JR, Carson GL: Antacid therapy. *Scand J Gastroenterol* 14 (suppl 55): 67–83, 1979.

102. Malazelada JR, Holtermuller KH, McCall JT, et al: Pancreatic, gallbladder, and intestinal responses to intraluminal magnesium salts in man. *Am J Dig Dis* 23:481–485, 1978.

103. Mastai R, Bosch J, Bruix J, et al: Effects of metoclopramide and domperidone on azygos blood flow in patients with cirrhosis and portal hypertension. *J Hepatology* 1:588, 1984.

104. McArthur KE, Anderson DS, Durbin TE, Orloff MJ, Dharmsathaporn K: Clonidine and lidamine to inhibit watery diarrhea in a patient with lung cancer. *Ann Intern Med* 96:323–325, 1982.

105. McArthur KE, Collen MJ, Maton PN, et al: Omeprazole: effect, convenient therapy for Zollinger-Ellison syndrome. *Gastroenterology* 28:939–944, 1985.

106. McCallum RW: Review of the current status of prokinetic agents in gastroenterology. *Am J Gastroenterol* 80:1008–1016, 1985.

107. McCallum RW, Petersen J, Caride V, Prokoff E: A scintigraphic evaluation of colonic transit in normal subjects: the prokinetic effects of cisapride. *Gastroenterology* 90:1540, 1986.

108. McGowan WR, Vermillion SE: Acute interstitial nephritis related to cimetidine therapy. *Gastroenterology* 79:746–749, 1980.

109. McGuigan JE: A consideration of the adverse effects of cimetidine. *Gastroenterology* 80:181–192, 1981.

110. Meredith TJ, Volans GN: Management of cimetidine overdose. *Lancet* 2:1367, 1979.

111. Meyers S, Janowitz HD: Systemic corticosteroid therapy of ulcerative colitis. *Gastroenterology* 89:1189–1891, 1985.

112. Meyers S, Sachar DB, Goldberg JD, Janowitz HD: Corticotropin versus hydrocortisone in the intravenous treatment of ulcerative colitis. *Gastroenterology* 85:351–357, 1983.

113. Mills PR, Rae AP, Farah DA, Russell RI, Lorimer AR, Carter DC: Comparison of three adrenoreceptor blocking agents in patients with cirrhosis and portal hypertension. *Gut* 25:73–78, 1984.

114. Mogelnicki SR, Waller JL, Finlayson DC: Physostigmine reversal of cimetidine-induced mental confusion. *JAMA* 241:826–827, 1979.

115. Mok HYI: Effects of cimetidine on biliary lipids in patients with reflux esophagitis. *Gastroenterology* 81:340–344, 1981.

116. Monroe P, Morrow CF, Millen JE, Fairman RP, Glauser FL: Acute respiratory failure after sodium morruate esophageal sclerotherapy. *Gastroenterology* 85:693–699, 1983.

117. Nagishuma R: Mechanisms of action of sucralfate. *J Clin Gastroenterol* 3(suppl 2):117–127, 1981.

118. O'Reilly RA: Comparative interaction of cimetidine and ranitidine with racemic warfarin in man. *Arch Intern Med* 144:989–991, 1984.

119. Ostro MJ, Russell JA, Solden SJ, Mahon WA, Jeyeeboy KN: Control of gastric pH with cimetidine: boluses versus primed infusion. *Gastroenterology* 89:532–536, 1985.

120. Patwardhan RV, Yarborough GW, Desmond GW, Johnson RF, Schenker S, Speeg KV: Cimetidine spares the glucuronidation of lorazepam and oxazepam. *Gastroenterology* 79:912–916, 1980.

121. Peterson WL, Richardson CT: Sustained fasting achlorhydria: a comparison of medical regimens. *Gastroenterology* 88:666–669, 1985.

122. Peura DA, Johnson LF: Cimetidine for prevention and treatment of gastroduodenal mucosal lesions in patients in an intensive care unit. *Ann Intern Med* 103:173–177, 1985.

123. *Physicians Desk Reference.* Oradell, NJ, Medical Economics Co, 1987, pp 1634–1636.

124. *Physicians Desk Reference.* Oradell, NJ, Medical Economics Co, 1986, p 922.

125. Piper DW, Fenton B: pH stability and activity curves of pepsin with special reference to their clinical importance. *Gut* 6:506–508, 1965.

126. Poleski MH, Spanier AH: Cimetidine versus antacids in the prevention of stress erosions in critically ill patients. *Am J Gastroenterol* 81:107, 1986.

127. Polio J, Groszmann RJ: Hemodynamic factors involved in the development and rupture of esophageal varices: a pathophysiologic approach to treatment. *Semin Liver Dis* 6:318–331, 1986.

128. Pop P, Nikkels RE, Thys O, Dorrestein GCM: Comparison of sucralfate and cimetidine in the treatment of duodenal and gastric ulcers. A multicenter study. *Scand J Gastroenterol* 18:43–47, 1983.

129. Powell JR, Rogers JF, Wargen WA, Cross RE, Eshelman FN: Inhibition of theophylline clearance by cimetidine but not ranitidine. *Arch Intern Med* 144:484–486, 1984.

130. Price HL, Cooperman LH, Warden JC: Control of the splanchnic circulation in man: role of beta-adrenergic receptors. *Circ Res* 21:333–340, 1967.

131. Priebe J, Skillman JJ: Methods of prophylaxis in stress ulcer disease. *World J Surg* 5:223–233, 1981.

132. Prowse CV, Douglas JG, Forest JA, Forsling ML: Haemostatic effects of lysine vasopressin and triglycyl lysine vasopressin infusion in patients with cirrhosis. *Eur J Clin Invest* 10:49–54, 1980.

133. Ranitidine. *Med Lett Drugs Ther* 24:111–113, 1982.

134. Rector WG: Drug therapy for portal hypertension. *Ann Intern Med* 105:96–107, 1986.

135. Richardson CT: Sucralfate. *Ann Intern Med* 97:269–271, 1982.

136. Rogers HJ, James CA, Morrison PJ, Bradbrook ID: Effect of cimetidine on oral absorption of ampicillin and cotrianoxazole. *J Antimicrob Chemother* 6:297–300, 1980.

136. Rogers HJ, James CA, Morrison PJ, Bradbrook ID: Effect of cimetidine on oral absorption of ampicillin and cotrimoxazole. *J Antimicrob Chemother* 6:297–300, 1980.

138. Rowley-Jones D, Flind AC: Continuing evaluation of the safety of cimetidine in the 80's. In Baron JH (ed): *Cimetidine in the 80's.* Edinburgh, Churchill Livingstone, 1981, pp 261–269.

139. Rudolfi A: Bleed level of cimetidine in relation to age. *Eur J Clin Pharmacol* 15:257–261, 1982.

140. Ruffalo RL, Thompson JF: Effect of cimetidine on the clearance of benzodiazepines. *N Engl J Med* 303:753–754, 1980.

141. Russell JA: Pharmacokinetics and pharmacodynamics of cimetidine in critically ill patients. *Clin Pharmacol Ther* 33:260, 1983.

142. Sawyer D, Conner CS, Scalley R: Cimetidine: adverse reactions and acute toxicity. *Am J Hosp Pharm* 38:188–197, 1981.

143. Sazie E, Jaffe JP: Severe granulocytopenia with cimetidine and phenytoin. *Ann Intern Med* 93:151–153, 1980.

144. Schneider RP, Roach AC: An antacid tasting: the relative palatability of 19 liquid antacids. *South Med J* 69:1312–1313, 1976.

145. Schulze-Delview K: Metoclopramide. *Gastroenterology* 77:768–779, 1979.

146. Schwinghammer TL: Drug interactions with cimetidine. *Am J Hosp Pharm* 38:1976–1978, 1981.

147. Sedman AJ: Cimetidine-drug interactions. *Am Intern Med* 76:109–114, 1984.

148. Serlin MJ, Sibeon RG, Mossman S, et al: Cimetidine: interaction with oral anticoagulants in man. *Lancet* 2:317–319, 1979.

149. Sharpe PC, Mills JG, Horton L, et al: Histamine H_2 receptors and intrinsic factor secretion. *Scand J Gastroenterol* 15:377–384, 1980.

150. Shaw G, Bury RW, Mashford ML, Breen KJ, Desmond PV: Cimetidine impairs the elimination of chlormethiazole. *Eur J Clin Pharmacol* 21:83–85, 1981.

151. Shea-Donohue T, Steel L, Montcalm E, Dubois A: Gastric protection by sucralfate: role of mucus and prostaglandins. *Gastroenterology* 91:660–666, 1986.

152. Silver BA, Bell WR: Cimetidine potentiation of the hypoprothrombinemic effect of warfarin. *Ann Intern Med* 90:348–349, 1979.

153. Singleton JW: Medical therapy of inflammatory bowel disease. *Med Clin North Am* 64:1117–1133, 1980.

154. Skillman JJ, Bushness LS, Godlman H, Silen W: Respiratory failure, hypotension, sepsis and jaundice: a clinical syndrome associated with lethal hemorrhage from acute stress ulceration of the stomach. *Am J Surg* 117:523–526, 1969.

155. Smith J, Torey C: Clinical pharmacology of famotidine. *Digestion* 32:15–23, 1985.

156. Soll AH: Three-way interactions between histamine, carbacol, and gastrin on aminopyrine uptake by isolated canine parietal cells (abstract). *Gastroenterology* 74:1146, 1978.

157. Somogyi A, Heinzow B: Cimetidine reduces procainamide. *N Engl J Med* 307:1080–1081, 1982.

158. Sonnenberg GE, Keller J, Pernichoud A, et al: Effects of somatostatin on splanchnic hemodynamics in patients with cirrhosis of the liver and in normal subjects. *Gastroenterology* 80:526–532, 1981.

159. Spahn H, Mutschler E, Kirch W, Ohnhaus EE, Janisch HD: Influence of ranitidine on plasma metoprolol and atenolol concentrations. *Br Med J* 286:1546–1547, 1983.

160. Spence RW, Celestin LR. Gynaecomastia associated with cimetidine. *Gut* 20:154–157, 1979.

161. Storey DW, Brown SG, Swain CP, et al: Endoscopic prediction of recurrent bleeding in peptic ulcers. *N Engl J Med* 305:915–916, 1981.

162. Takayanagi I, Iwayama Y, Kasuya Y: Narcotic antagonistic action of cimetidine on the guinea-pig ileum. *J Pharm Pharmacol* 30:519–520, 1978.

163. Tellerman-Toppet N, Duret ME, Coers C: Cimetidine interaction with carbamazepine [letter]. *Ann Intern Med* 94:544, 1981.

164. Truelove SC, Jewell DP: Intensive intravenous regimen for severe attacks of ulcerative colitis. *Lancet* 1:1067–1070, 1974.

165. Tryba M, Zevounow F, Torok M, Zenz M: Prevention of acute stress bleeding with sucralfate, antacids or cimetidine. *Am J Med* 79(supple 2C):21–27, 1985.

166. Tsai YT, Lay CS, Lai KH, et al: A controlled trial of vasopressin plus nitroglycerin vs. vasopressin alone in the treatment of bleeding esophageal varices. *Hepatology* 6:406–409, 1986.

167. Van Der Meer JWM, Kevning JJ, Scheijgrond AW, Heykants J, Van Cutsem J, Brugmans J: The influence of gastric acidity on the bioavailability of ketoconazole. *J Antimicrob Chemother* 6:552–554, 1980.

168. Vaziri ND, Ness RL, Barton CH: Hemodialysis clearance of cimetidine. *Arch Intern Med* 138:1685–1686, 1978.

169. Vaziri ND, Ness RL, Barton CH: Peritoneal dialysis clearance of cimetidine. *Am J Gastroenterol* 71(6):572–576, 1979.

170. Vinayek R, Howard JM, Maton PN, et al: Famotidine in the therapy of gastric hypersecretory states. *Am J Med* 81(suppl 4B):49–59, 1986.

171. Walan A: Antacids, metabolic side effects, and interactions. *Scand J Gastroenterol* [Suppl]25:63–68, 1982.

172. Wallmark B, Brandstrom A, Larsson H: Evidence for acid-induced transformation of omeprazole into an active inhibitor of $(H^+ + K^+)$-ATPase within the parietal cell. *Biochim Biophys Acta* 718:549–558, 1981.

173. Walt RR, Reynolds JR, Langman MJS, et al: Intravenous omeprazole rapidly raises intragastric pH. *Gut* 26:902–906, 1985.

174. Wanetschke R, Ammon HV: Effects of magnesium sulfate on transit time and water transport in the human jejunum (abstract). *Gastroenterology* 70:949, 1976.

175. Wara P: Endoscopic prediction of major rebleeding: a prospective study of stigmata of hemorrhage in bleeding ulcer. *Gastroenterology* 88:1209–1214, 1985.

176. Watts RW, Hetzel DJ, Bochner F, et al: Lack of interaction between ranitidine and phenytoin. *Br J Clin Pharmacol* 75:499–500, 1983.

177. Willet I, Esler M, Jennings F, Dudley F: Effect of clonidine on systemic and portal hemodynamics in alcoholic cirrhosis (abstract). *Gastroenterology* 86:1705, 1985.

178. Wilmore DW, Goodwin CW, Aulock LH, et al: Effect of injury and infection on visceral metabolism and circulation. *Ann Surg* 192:491–504, 1980.

179. Young CJ, Daneschmend TK, Roberts CJC: Effects of cirrhosis and aging on the elimination and bioavailability of ranitidine. *Gut* 23:819–832, 1980.

180. Yuhas EM, Lofton, FT, Baldinus JG, et al: Cimetidine hydrochloride compatibility with preoperative medications. *Am J Hosp Pharm* 38:1173–1174, 1981.

181. Yuhas EM, Lofton FT, Rosenberg HA, et al: Cimetidine hydrochloride compatibility III: Room temperature stability in drug admixtures. *Am J Hosp Pharm* 38:1919–1922, 1981.

182. Zeldis JB, Friedman LS, Isselbacher KJ. Ranitidine: a new H_2-receptor antagonist. *N Engl J Med* 309:1368–1373, 1983.

183. Zito RA, Diez A, Groszmann RJ: Comparative effects of nitroglycerin and nitroprusside on vasopressin-induced cardiac dysfunction in the dog. *J Cardiovasc Pharmacol* 5:586–591, 1983.

184. Zuckerman G, Welch R, Douglas A, et al: Controlled trial of medical therapy for active upper gastrointestinal bleeding and prevention of rebleeding. *Am J Med* 76:361–366, 1984.

19

Vasodilator Therapy

Joseph E. Parrillo, M.D.

Although the principles of afterload reduction with vasodilator therapy were enumerated more than 40 years ago (104), it is only in the past 15 years that clinical applications of vasodilator therapy in the treatment of moderate to severe cardiac failure have gained relatively widespread acceptance (16, 29). As early as 1944, spinal anesthesia–induced vasodilation was employed successfully to reverse cardiogenic pulmonary edema (100). In the early 1960s, the principles of afterload reduction as a method to improve cardiac performance were confirmed and extended (12, 103). However, frequent clinical use of vasodilators required the ability to document a salutary hemodynamic response and the capability of closely monitoring adverse consequences of this therapy. In the 1970s, the development of the Swan-Ganz balloon flotation catheter (108) allowed hemodynamic monitoring at the bedside, which was previously only available in the cardiac catheterization laboratory. Today, the physician can serially measure cardiac outputs and calculate systemic vascular resistance to document a salutary or adverse response to therapy. Further, routine use of arterial pressure catheters allows a beat-to-beat measure of the major adverse consequence of vasodilators, namely, hypotension.

In 1971, phentolamine, an α-adrenergic receptor antagonist, was reported to be effective in relieving symptoms and improving the hemodynamics of patients with severe heart failure secondary to ischemic heart disease (75). One year later, nitroprusside-induced vasodilation was shown to increase cardiac output, reduce ventricular filling pressures, and relieve symptoms in post–myocardial infarction patients with severe heart failure, or even cardiogenic shock (46). Subsequent studies have documented the usefulness of vasodilation therapy in subsets of patients with severe intractable heart failure (58), cardiogenic shock

(32), and severe mitral (20) or aortic (9) regurgitation.

The purpose of this chapter is to review the physiologic mechanisms underlying vasodilator therapy, the appropriate indications for use of vasodilators, and the usefulness of specific vasodilator agents. The practical considerations of vasodilator therapy in the management of critically ill patients are reviewed. Emphasis is placed on the physiology and pathogenic mechanisms that provide a foundation for proper patient care. Reviews of more specific aspects of vasodilator therapy are available (6, 7, 24, 40, 41, 50, 76, 80, 86, 88, 98, 113, 114, 119).

PHYSIOLOGIC MECHANISMS OF ACTION OF VASODILATORS

Factors Determining Ventricular Function

The heart's major function is to supply blood flow to the tissues to satisfy the metabolic requirements of the body. There are four major determinants of cardiac function: preload, afterload, contractility, and heart rate (12, 25). These factors can be manipulated clinically to produce optimal ventricular function in any given patient. Depending on the patient's physiology, pathology, and clinical status, the physician can choose from a wide variety of methods to augment cardiovascular function.

PRELOAD

Preload is defined as the amount the myocardium is stretched prior to the onset of contraction. Isolated papillary muscle experiments originally demonstrated an increase in myocardial tension development with an increase in the resting length of the cardiac mus-

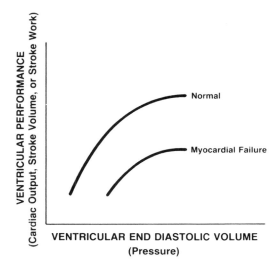

Figure 19.1. Frank-Starling ventricular performance curves. In the normal ventricle, as ventricular end-diastolic volume is increased, there is a concomitant increase in ventricular performance until a plateau is reached. Patients with myocardial dysfunction and heart failure demonstrate a shift of this curve downward and to the right. In heart failure, an increase in end-diastolic volume produces less of an increase in ventricular performance and a "plateau" is reached at a much lower level of ventricular performance.

cles (13), with maximal tension development occurring when there was the most overlap of action and myosin filaments. In the intact ventricle, this Frank-Starling relationship is manifested by enhanced ventricular performance as the end-diastolic volume of the left or right ventricle is increased (13) (Fig. 19.1). In the normal heart, at low end-diastolic volumes, small increases in preload cause a substantial increase in stroke volume and cardiac output; as one increases end-diastolic volume further, similar increases in end-diastolic volume produce progressively less of an increase in stroke volume, finally reaching a plateau beyond which increases in diastolic volume do not increase stroke volume (or other measures of ventricular performance) (107).

Clinically, measuring end-diastolic ventricular volumes is difficult, whereas end-diastolic pressure can be relatively easily obtained from intracardiac catheter readings. When plotting the relationship between end-diastolic pressure and ventricular performance, one sees a relationship similar to that shown in Figure 19.1, i.e., on increasing end-diastolic pressure, ventricular performance increases substan-

tially, then more modestly, finally plateauing. It is clinically useful to recognize that the relationship between end-diastolic pressure and volume is not linear (Fig. 19.2). Thus, at low volumes, a substantial increase in end-diastolic volume (producing an increase in stroke volume) can cause little or no change in end-diastolic pressure. At higher volumes, the relationship between volume and pressure becomes more linear, and changes in volume will be associated with increases in the end-diastolic ventricular pressure. Therefore, when dealing with low end-diastolic volumes, increasing the end-diastolic volume with fluid administration can produce considerable increases in stroke volume with little or no change in ventricular filling pressures.

The ventricle's intrinsic ability to increase its volume and pressure in response to an increase (or decrease) in intravascular volume is termed compliance, a measure of the ventricle's distensibility. Ischemia, fibrosis, hypertrophy, and certain pharmacologic agents such as vasodilators (see below) can profoundly influence ventricular compliance (11). Several studies suggest that left ventricular compliance is altered by high right ventricular diastolic pressures (8), which presumably alter left ventricular geometry with a displaced septum. Other studies suggest that an intact pericardium is important in right ventricular in-

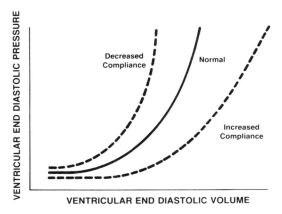

Figure 19.2. Diastolic pressure-volume relationship of the left ventricle. At low ventricular volumes, substantial changes in volume produce little change in ventricular pressure. At higher ventricular volumes, small changes produce exponentially greater increases in pressure. Increasing ventricular compliance with vasodilator therapy shifts the curve to the right, allowing a greater end-diastolic volume at a lower pressure. See text for details.

duced decreases in left ventricular compliances (92), arguing that changes in the right side of the heart affect the left side because of the pericardial "closed space."

In a more compliant ventricle, for any ventricular end-diastolic volume the ventricular pressure will be lower. This is a practical clinical concern since pulmonary edema occurs when left ventricular end-diastolic pressure rises above approximately 20 mm Hg. Thus, a more compliant ventricle allows for a greater increase in end-diastolic volume (enhancing systolic ventricular performance) than a noncompliant ventricle, which will develop a high pressure at a lower ventricular volume.

AFTERLOAD

Afterload is defined as the sum of the factors that oppose the shortening of muscle fibers—a definition derived from isolated papillary muscle experiments (83). In the intact cardiovascular system, afterload refers to the impedance against which the ventricle must eject during systole. Precise determination of aortic impedance to ventricular ejection requires sophisticated analysis of a series of harmonics, each of which depends on amplitude, phase angle, and frequency. These harmonics describe a spectrum of instantaneous relationships between pressure and flow (83, 99). Because of its complexity and the difficulty of its determination, afterload is usually clinically defined as vascular resistance, a value that defines the steady state (frequency-independent) characteristics of impedance to aortic flow.

Systemic vascular resistance (SVR) is defined by the following equation:

$$SVR = \frac{MAP - \text{mean right atrial pressure}}{CO}$$

where MAP is mean arterial blood pressure and CO is cardiac output. This equation demonstrates why afterload cannot be derived from blood pressure measurements alone: an arterial dilator can reduce SVR and cause an increase in CO resulting in no change in blood pressure, though the afterload confronting the ventricle is substantially reduced. Thus, SVR has become the most commonly used clinical parameter to reflect afterload or outflow impedance.

The nature of the relationship between afterload and stroke volume is important to an understanding of changes in cardiac function

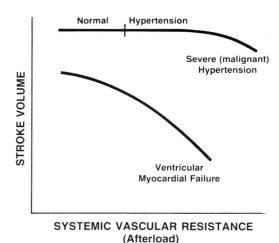

SYSTEMIC VASCULAR RESISTANCE
(Afterload)

Figure 19.3.   Relationship of systemic vascular resistance to stroke volume in a normal and dysfunctional ventricle. Increases in afterload do not cause a decrease in stroke volume in a normal ventricle *(upper curve)* except at very high levels of afterload when severe hypertension causes ventricular decompensation. In a failing ventricle *(lower curve)*, however, an increase in afterload causes a progressive depression of stroke volume and cardiac output. Thus, vasodilator-induced reductions in afterload enhance stroke volume in patients with severe ventricular dysfunction.

when SVR varies. Stroke volume varies as the function of increasing SVR (Fig. 19.3). In the normally functioning ventricle *(upper curve)*, mild to moderate increases in SVR do not decrease stroke volume, although the blood pressure rises modestly. Severe increases in SVR, e.g., malignant hypertension, may depress stroke volume (16, 29, 103). One of the major reasons that the normal ventricle's stroke volume does not become depressed with increasing afterload is the ventricle's ability to increase preload by rising on the steep portion of the Starling curve (Fig. 19.1) (23, 31, 103). Thus, in an experimental setting in which preload and contractility are kept constant, an increase in afterload decreases stroke volume secondary to a reduction in the extent and velocity of myocardial wall shortening (15, 115). Analogously, a ventricle with myocardial dysfunction operates on the plateau of the Starling function (Fig. 19.1) and is unable to increase stroke volume by increasing end-diastolic volume. Therefore, in a dysfunctional ventricle increases in SVR depress stroke volume. These physiologic principles provide the basis for effective vasodilator therapy: in a moderately or severely dysfunctional ventricle, a decrease in SVR commonly causes an increase in stroke volume, therefore augmenting CO (Fig. 19.3, *lower curve*).

CONTRACTILITY

Contractility refers to the inherent ability of the ventricle to increase the velocity and/or extent of contraction. Studies have defined contractility as changes in ventricular performance that cannot be ascribed to preload or afterload. Another useful operational definition is that an increase in contractility (holding afterload constant) produces a shift in the Starling preload curve upward and to the left (Fig. 19.4). A negative inotropic effect shifts the Starling curve downward and to the right. Positive inotropic agents that augment the contractility of the ventricle include the catecholamines, digitalis, glucagon, and thyroxine. Negative inotropic agents include phenobarbital, most general anesthetics, and propranolol.

The relationship of intrinsic myocardial contractility to afterload is also important in optimal vasodilator therapy. In the normal ventricle, increases in afterload are well tolerated with no decrease in stroke volume; however, in a depressed, poorly contractile ventricle, increases in afterload result in decreased stroke volume and CO (Fig. 19.3, *lower*

curve). Thus, in many patients with heart failure and an elevated SVR, reducing SVR results in an augmented stroke volume and CO (Fig. 19.3).

HEART RATE

If stroke volume is held constant, CO increases linearly with increases in heart rate, since CO is equal to the product of heart rate and stroke volume. However, faster heart rates allow less time for diastolic filling and may decrease preload; the ultimate CO depends on the extent of the increase in heart rate versus the decrease in preload. In addition, increases in heart rate cause an increase in ventricular contractility; this augmented contractility with increased heart rate occurs in ventricles with myocardial dysfunction and in normal ventricles (63, 70).

Many pharmacologic interventions have important effects on several of the above parameters affecting CO. The ultimate pharmacologic effect on cardiac performance depends on the magnitude and direction of the changes produced in each individual parameter, and also on the baseline hemodynamics of the treated patient. Further, one must consider reflex responses (autonomic or renin-angiotensin system) activated by the pharmacologic intervention; these reflexes tend to counteract many of the therapeutic effects. Thus, in order to predict the ultimate outcome of any particular pharmacologic intervention on cardiac performance, one must know the pharmacologic effect on each individual parameter (preload, afterload, contractility, and heart rate) and the patient's hemodynamic status (70, 103). Even with the above knowledge, one cannot always accurately predict the ultimate outcome of certain interventions; in such cases, a therapeutic trial following objective hemodynamic parameters is required.

Pathophysiologic Abnormalities in Congestive Heart Failure

When myocardial function is depressed, the body activates a number of compensatory mechanisms designed to maintain CO and systemic blood pressure (11–13, 16, 29). The possible etiologies of the cardiac dysfunction and failure include ischemic heart disease, primary cardiomyopathy, infiltrative cardiomyopathies, chronic pressure overload (e.g., aortic stenosis), and chronic volume overload (e.g., mitral

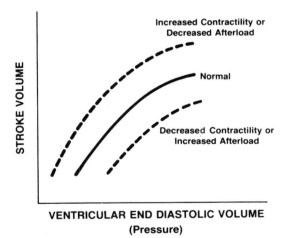

Figure 19.4. Ventricular function curves demonstrating the effects of changes in contractility or afterload. If afterload is held constant, an increase in contractility of the ventricle will shift the functional curve upward and to the left, demonstrating improved ventricular performance at any given level of end-diastolic volume. If ventricular contractility is left unchanged, a decrease in afterload will produce a similar shift in the ventricular function curve.

regurgitation, aortic regurgitation, ventricular septal defect). Regardless of the underlying causes of heart failure, the compensatory mechanisms are similar and include the following. First, dilation of the left ventricle, i.e., increasing the left ventricular end-diastolic volume optimizes preload. Patients with heart failure are operating on the plateau portion of a depressed left ventricular function curve (Fig. 19.1). Once the end-diastolic volume reaches the plateau, further elevations of preload do not improve stroke volume or ventricular performance and have an undesirable effect, namely, elevation of left ventricular end-diastolic pressure, elevated pulmonary capillary wedge pressure, and pulmonary edema (11, 13, 15). Further increases in end-diastolic volume increase left ventricular wall stress (La Place relationship) and in turn increase myocardial oxygen consumption, potentially precipitating acute ischemic events in patients with coronary artery disease (16). In some patients with heart failure, left ventricular dilation causes mitral regurgitation, adding a regurgitant volume load to an already compromised ventricle (103). Although elevation of end-diastolic volume is a useful mechanism in increasing cardiac performance, it can have deleterious effects on cardiac function once preload increases past the plateau of the Starling curve. In some patients, reduction of this inappropriately elevated preload (especially the pressure component) to prevent pulmonary congestion becomes important. This reduction can be performed clinically with diuretics, but vasodilators, with the ability to venodilate and increase the capacitance of the venous system, are also highly effective in reducing even severe elevations of ventricular end-diastolic pressure and volume (16, 29, 76).

A secondary compensatory mechanism in many patients with congestive heart failure is an increase in adrenergic stimulation of the heart, enhancing cardiac contractility and increasing heart rate and subsequently CO (121).

A third mechanism that serves to maintain blood pressure, presumably a response to depressed stroke volume, is elevated SVR (29, 117). This mechanism is at least partially mediated via baroreceptor activation of the sympathetic nervous system, increased activation of the renin-angiotensin system, accumulation of salt and water in blood vessel walls, and some other mechanisms (47, 117–120). Importantly, in many patients with heart failure, the SVR becomes inappropriately elevated, i.e., the resistance is higher than that

needed to maintain an adequate blood pressure, and is high enough to actually depress stroke volume because of the effect of an increased afterload on a dysfunctional ventricle (29). If this inappropriately high SVR is lowered with a vasodilator agent, stroke volume and CO may improve with little change in blood pressure. It is important to realize that this reflex increase in afterload does not depress stroke volume in a normal ventricle (Fig. 19.3) (107), but does reduce stroke volume in a dysfunctional and failing ventricle. Thus, paradoxically, one of the compensatory mechanisms (increased afterload) in the clinical syndrome of heart failure, in which a depression of stroke volume is likely to occur, may actually worsen overall cardiac performance.

Mechanism of Vasodilator Action

The major mechanism by which vasodilators increase CO and reduce ventricular filling pressures is by decreasing arterial and venous vasoconstriction. Vasodilators that cause predominantly arterial dilation reduce afterload or outflow impedance, and those that produce predominantly venodilation decrease preload (ventricular end-diastolic volume and/or pressure). Most vasodilators produce their effect by relaxing vascular smooth muscle in resistance and capacitance vessels. Some agents produce this relaxation by a direct smooth muscle effect, other agents stimulate or inhibit mechanisms that regulate smooth muscle tone.

The relationship of vascular resistance to the size of the vascular bed is expressed in Poiseuille's law:

$$\frac{\text{Resistance}}{\text{to flow}} = \frac{\text{viscosity} \times \text{vessel length} \times 8}{(\text{vessel radius})^4}$$

Resistance varies inversely with the vessel radius to the fourth power. The arterial vascular radius (or cross-sectional area) is determined largely by the smooth muscle tone in the arterioles, and this smooth muscle tone is the direct or indirect site of vasodilator action. Changes in smooth muscle tone have a different effect on the arterial and venous circulations. Increases in arteriolar vessel tone increase resistance to blood flow in the arterial circuit (i.e., increased afterload). Increases in venular and venous vessel tone decrease the amount of blood stored in the venous system. Since the venous system and venules have approximately 70–80% of the body's blood volume, venous vasoconstriction decreases the amount of blood returned to the heart (57, 80). When conceptualizing the circulatory system and comparing it to electrical systems, the arterial circuit is best considered as a resistor and the venous system as a capacitor circuit.

Different vasodilator agents may have effects on arteriolar vessel tone, venous vessel tone, or on a combination of arteriolar and venous tone. Further, vasodilators can have different effects on the systemic versus the pulmonary circulation (57). Depending on these effects and the baseline clinical hemodynamics, the ultimate effect or the general direction of hemodynamic change of a vasodilator agent can be predicted (Fig. 19.5). Although specific vasodilators are classified as venous or arterial in their action, none has "pure" effects on one circuit; nonetheless, the major effect is commonly regarded as predominantly arterial or venous.

In general, the goal of vasodilator therapy in heart failure is to improve CO by reducing unnecessary increases in afterload and to improve elevated ventricular filling pressures by reducing preload. On the arterial side, a decrease in outflow impedance increases stroke volume and thus CO. In most patients with heart failure treated with vasodilators, the heart rate does not increase and the blood pressure decreases slightly or not at all. The lack of change in blood pressure is due to a proportional increase in stroke volume enhancing CO in response to the vasodilator-induced decrease in SVR (16, 29).

Thus, the vasodilator reverses an inappropriate elevated vascular resistance and induces a rise in CO. When this occurs, most patients report symptomatic improvement with decreased dyspnea and fatigue. Patients commonly demonstrate reversal of signs of poor organ perfusion such as mental obtundation, cool, clammy skin, and elevations of blood urea nitrogen secondary to depressed renal perfusion. Better renal perfusion increases the excretion of salt and water, which tends to decrease vascular filling pressures (16, 29, 57, 103). Decreased sodium concentrations in vessel walls further decrease vessel tone. If mitral or aortic regurgitation is a part of the cardiovascular pathophysiology, the regurgitant fraction is reduced with an increase in forward stroke volume.

Vasodilators become more effective as ventricular function worsens, and these agents can dramatically improve severe heart failure. Several studies have found a correlation between baseline CO and the vasodilator-induced increase in CO, i.e., the patients with the lowest resting CO have the best response to vasodilators (18, 42, 43, 45, 46, 73, 74, 82, 84). One study shows a strong positive correlation between the initial SVR and the ability of the vasodilators to reduce SVR, i.e., the highest impedance has the greatest chance of response (49). Most patients with severe myocardial dysfunction and failure have a steep impedance to stroke volume relationship (Fig. 19.3, *lower curve*) and decreasing impedance raises stroke volume. In contrast, patients with normal or near-normal cardiac function have no change in stroke volume with decreased impedance (Fig. 19.3, *upper curve*); the preload reduction depresses stroke volume because these patients are operating on the steep portion of the Starling curve, and the depressed stroke volume and CO may result in substantial decreases in blood pressure. The hypotensive effect is desirable in hypertensive patients, and vasodilator therapy is an effective antihypertensive regimen (90); however, in patients with severe heart failure, blood pressure

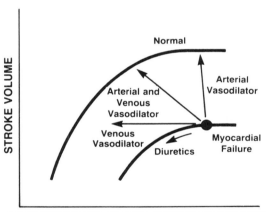

LEFT VENTRICULAR END DIASTOLIC VOLUME (Pressure)

Figure 19.5. Ability of different types of vasodilators to shift depressed ventricular function curve toward normal. Arterial vasodilators produce an increase in stroke volume with little or no changes in preload. Venous vasodilators produce a reduction in end-diastolic volume with little or no change in stroke volume. Vasodilators with both arterial and venous effects improve stroke volume and reduce filling pressures. An inotropic agent, along with a vasodilator, would shift the depressed curve even closer toward normal. At low levels of end-diastolic volume (on the slope rather than the plateau of the ventricular function curve), vasodilators may cause decreases in stroke volume and/or end-diastolic volume, resulting in decreased cardiac performance and hypotension. See text for details.

usually changes minimally for the reasons enumerated above.

With venodilation, ventricular filling pressures decrease. Since most patients with heart failure are operating on the plateau portion of a depressed Starling curve (Fig. 19.1), reductions in preload generally do not reduce ventricular performance. However, reductions of filling pressures below a certain level reduce the stroke volume and can result in serious hypotension and/or a low output syndrome. The pulmonary capillary wedge pressure or left ventricular end-diastolic pressures can be reduced to approximately 15 mm Hg without affecting stroke volume in most patients; reductions below this level should be avoided because they depress stroke volume and CO (16, 29).

Despite many studies suggesting that vasodilator therapy in moderate to severe heart failure is not associated with an important blood pressure reduction, an occasional patient does develop symptomatic hypotension with vasodilator administration. If this occurs, one should suspect that the filling pressures are not elevated and preload has been reduced too low, or that ventricle function is only mildly impaired. Patients with obstructive cardiac lesions in whom forward output cannot be increased (e.g., aortic stenosis, mitral stenosis, or obstructive hypertrophic cardiomyopathy) also may have a hypotensive response to vasodilators. Patients with restrictive cardiomyopathy from amyloidosis or endomyocardial fibrosis are also prone to hypotensive responses to vasodilators in the author's experience. After the above possible causes of a hypotensive reaction to vasodilators are considered, an occasional patient with proven high filling pressures and poor CO, in severe heart failure, does not tolerate vasodilator therapy because of hypotension. It is assumed that this patient has not developed the usual inappropriate elevation of SVR seen in most patients with severe heart failure, though the reasons for this fact remain obscure.

Cellular and Biochemical Mechanisms Involved in Vasodilator Actions

The final common pathway of vasodilator effect is to relax vascular smooth muscle tone. At the cellular and biochemical level, three major classes of vasodilators are presently recognized to produce this vasodilation: (a) direct smooth muscle relaxers, as exemplified by nitroprusside, nitrates, hydralazine, and minoxidil; (b) sympathetic nervous system blocking agents that negate α-adrenergic stimulation, e.g., phentolamine, prazosin, and trimethaphan; and (c) inhibitors of the renin-angiotensin system, e.g., saralasin and captopril. Much of the clinical experience with vasodilators has been gained with the direct-acting smooth muscle relaxers such as nitroprusside in the acute setting and hydralazine and/or nitrates in chronic heart failure; however, more experience is accumulating with sympathetic and renin-angiotensin blockers. The specific mechanisms of action of the individual vasodilator agents are considered below ("Specific Vasodilator Agents").

Effects of Vasodilators on Myocardial Ischemia

An area of myocardial ischemia represents an imbalance between myocardial oxygen demand and supply. In patients with coronary artery disease, blood supply is limited by coronary artery narrowing and, in some patients, by coronary spasm (10, 62, 105). When myocardial oxygen demand increases, blood cannot reach certain areas of myocardium, which then become segmentally ischemic and dysfunctional. The major determinants of myocardial oxygen consumption are arterial (or ventricular) systolic pressure, heart rate, heart size, and the ventricular contractile state. Arterial systolic pressure and heart size are the major determinants of wall stress, according to the La Place relationship (11–13). Vasodilators have a number of mechanisms for favorably altering the balance between myocardial oxygen demand by decreasing preload and reducing ventricular size, and the ventricular pressure also reduces myocardial oxygen needs.

Vasodilators can increase blood flow to an ischemic area by reducing vasoconstrictor influences in the collateral flow to ischemic zones. Vasodilators reduce end-diastolic pressures, favoring subendocardial flow. Several studies have shown that segmental wall motion abnormalities are improved following nitroglycerin administration (61), providing evidence that certain vasodilators can influence the myocardial oxygen supply/demand balance favorably. The ultimate effect of a vasodilator on ischemic myocardium in a particular patient depends on a number of factors: the baseline hemodynamic state of the ventricle, the coronary anatomy and collateral flow, and the type of vasodilator employed. Conflicting and contradictory results are common in this field. Some have reported that nitroglycerin decreases, whereas nitroprusside increases, evidence of myocardial ischemia (22). Others have reported that nitroprusside can decrease the ST segment, evidence of ischemia (5). Two large, controlled studies investigated the effects of nitroprusside infusion in patients with acute myocardial infarction (30, 38). One study found a statistically significant reduction in mortality in the nitroprusside group, along with a nitroprusside-induced reduction in the incidence of cardiogenic shock, clinical signs of heart failure, and levels of creatine kinase isoenzymes (38). In a second multicenter trial, nitroprusside was not associated with any change in overall mortality when given to patients with myocardial infarction and a pulmonary capillary wedge pressure greater than 12 mm Hg (30). In this latter study, patients whose nitroprusside infusions were begun within 9 hours of chest pain had an increased mortality, whereas infusions begun later were associated with a decreased mortality. These two studies do not lend themselves to a simple interpretation of the effect of this vasodilator agent on myocardial ischemia in the postinfarction phase of acute myocardial infarction. Nonetheless, the two studies were well controlled and properly performed, and the contradictory results argue for the complexity of predicting the response of vasodilators in patients with myocardial ischemia. Further, large trials are necessary to determine which subsets of patients with acute myocardial infarction benefit from vasodilator therapy.

Effect of Vasodilators on Ventricular Compliance

Another possible mechanism by which vasodilators improve ventricular function is induction of an increase in ventricular compliance (17, 96). The volume-pressure relationship of the ventricle is curvilinear (Fig. 19.2). At small end-diastolic volumes, ventricular size can change with little change in pressure; at higher ventricular volumes, a small change in volume produces a much greater pressure rise. If a pharmacologic agent shifts the volume-pressure curve to the right, there is a greater increase in end-diastolic volume without reaching a ventricular pressure that induces pulmonary edema. Assuming one has not reached the plateau portion of the Starling curve (Fig. 19.1), this increased volume at lower pressure produces better ventricular performance.

Studies suggest that vasodilators improve ventricular compliance (11, 71, 72, 97, 100), though further investigation is necessary to decide if this is an important mechanism of vasodilator-induced improvement in ventricular performance. The mechanism of this improvement in compliance is not clear. Some investigators postulate a reduction in ischemia, others argue for an intrinsic increase in ventricular relaxation (14, 17), or right ventricular relaxation causing increased left ventricular compliance within a confined pericardial space (32, 72). Further studies are needed to determine the true mechanism of vasodilator-induced increases in compliance.

Vasodilator-Induced Redistribution Effects

Most of the literature on vasodilators focuses on their ability to reduce afterload and/or preload and improve ventricular performance. Another potentially important capability of vasodilators in critical care medicine is reduction or redistribution of blood flow away from certain nonessential vascular beds and toward vital areas. For example, patients with septic shock commonly have a high CO, low filling pressures, and a low overall peripheral vascular resistance; however, many organs in the body are not receiving appropriate blood supply as evidenced by lactic acidosis and progressive organ system dysfunction, e.g., rising blood urea nitrogen with renal dysfunction. In this setting, the appropriate vasodilator could potentially redirect blood flow toward the vital organs. Many forms of shock are postulated to have inappropriate sympathetic outflow causing arteriolar vasoconstriction; some investigators advocate vasodilators in the treatment of shock (100). However, in shock, where one is faced with hypotension that is commonly difficult to control, vasodilators may further decrease blood pressure. In the absence of clear efficacy and with the potential of worsening already existing hypotension, vasodilators are not widely accepted in the treatment of noncardiogenic shock.

In cardiogenic shock and severe intractable

heart failure (32, 58), vasodilator therapy increases stroke volume and CO, and in some cases reverses cardiogenic shock. Commonly, vasodilator therapy in cardiogenic shock is used in conjunction with an inotropic agent such as dopamine (79, 87) or with intraaortic balloon counterpulsation (59). In severe heart failure, the body's compensatory mechanisms (sympathetic outflow, the renin-angiotensin system, and the organ's autoregulatory capacity) redistribute blood flow to preferentially maintain cerebral and coronary perfusion. In this setting, renal perfusion does not change or fall, and flow to the mesenteric and limb circulations is considerably diminished (122). If vasodilator therapy increases CO, flow to these vascular beds increases. In cardiogenic shock, the body's compensatory mechanisms are redistributing a very reduced CO to those organs of vital importance to survival. In other forms of shock (e.g., septic shock), there is an adequate or increased CO, but the distribution of flow is commonly inappropriate, resulting in lactic acidosis and vital organ dysfunction. The cause of this inappropriate redistribution of flow in septic shock, and whether vasodilators can redirect the flow, are questions that are unanswered and will require further study.

Vasodilator Therapy in Mechanical Defects

Patients with mitral regurgitation, aortic regurgitation, or a ventricular septal defect frequently respond to vasodilator therapy with an improvement in their hemodynamics and clinical symptoms of heart failure (9, 20). Although the definitive treatment for these mechanical lesions is corrective cardiac surgery, vasodilator therapy can be employed when surgery is not possible or when it is wise to defer surgery.

In mitral regurgitation, the severity of the regurgitation is dependent on the degree of anatomic derangement of the mitral apparatus as well as aortic outflow impedance (20, 96). Increasing afterload increases the regurgitant fraction (11, 12); vasodilator-induced reduction of aortic impedance should decrease regurgitation through the mitral valve. A number of clinical studies have documented that vasodilator-induced reductions in SVR produce marked hemodynamic improvements in patients with mitral regurgitations (20, 52, 56, 60, 116). Nitroprusside increases forward stroke volume and CO (mean increase, approximately

50%), decreases regurgitant volumes, decreases pulmonary artery and capillary wedge pressures, and causes large V waves in the pulmonary capillary wedge tracing to decrease markedly or disappear. These effects are a result of vasodilator-induced redistribution of the left ventricular stroke volume, causing more blood to be ejected into the aorta than into the left atrium. The major mechanism for this effect is a reduction of aortic impedance; however, a reduction in ventricular size with closer approximation of mitral leaflets and, in some cases, a reduction of papillary muscle ischemia may also contribute to the vasodilator-induced improvement in regurgitation.

In severe aortic regurgitation, the body may reflexly increase SVR to maintain blood pressure and thereby initiate a vicious cycle that increases regurgitation further. Nitroprusside is capable of reducing the aortic regurgitant fraction and increasing the forward stroke volume in chronic aortic regurgitation (9, 14, 81, 112). Vasodilators also produce increases in forward CO in acute aortic regurgitation (96).

In a large ventricular septal defect, the magnitude of the left-to-right shunt is largely determined by the ratio of the vascular resistances in the pulmonary versus systemic circuits. A reduction in SVR decreases the left-to-right shunt and favors flow from the left ventricle to the aorta, i.e., it increases systemic CO. Nitroprusside induces a favorable hemodynamic response in patients with acute ventricular septal defects complicating myocardial infarction (110). It should be recognized that if vasodilator therapy reduces pulmonary more than systemic resistance, the left-to-right shunt increases and systemic flow decreases. One must repeatedly measure flows and shunts to be sure that a sustained beneficial effect is resulting from such therapy.

Effect of Vasodilator Therapy on Mortality in Patients with Moderate to Severe Congestive Heart Failure

Vasodilators have been shown to produce profound changes in cardiovascular physiology, especially in patients with moderate to severe congestive heart failure. There is no question that vasodilator therapy can decrease elevated filling pressures and increase cardiac output and stroke volume in many patients with significant heart failure. Concomitant with these improved hemodynamics, many patients note a decrease in symptomatology and improvement in signs of heart failure: decreased dyspnea, improved energy, and improved organ blood flow and function. However, one of the most important but unanswered questions regarding vasodilator therapy is its effect on survival of patients with such severe heart failure.

Although retrospective studies have suggested that vasodilator-treated patients fare better, only in the past year have two excellent studies appeared that directly address this question. A Veterans Administration Cooperative Study at multiple centers assigned 642 men with heart failure already receiving digitalis and diuretics to receive additional double-blind treatment with (a) placebo, (b) prazosin (20 mg/day), or (c) a combination of hydralazine (300 mg/day) and isosorbide dinitrate (160 mg/day) (26, 27). The mortality in the hydralazine/isosorbide dinitrate group was lower than that in the placebo group throughout the entire follow-up period (average, 2.3 years). The mortality risk reduction in the group treated with hydralazine/isosorbide dinitrate was 36% by 3 years. The mortality in the prazosin group was similar to that in the placebo group. Further, the serially determined left ventricular ejection fraction increased in the hydralazine/isosorbide dinitrate group but not in the placebo or prazosin groups. Thus, this study demonstrates that addition of hydralazine/isosorbide dinitrate to digitalis/diuretic therapy can result in improved left ventricular function and decreased mortality.

An even more recent prospective, double-blind analysis evaluated the effect of an angiotensin-converting enzyme inhibitor, enalapril, in 253 patients under treatment for severe heart failure (33). The enalapril group had a highly significant 27% increase in mortality compared with the placebo group. Interestingly, the entire reduction in total mortality was found to be among patients with progressive heart failure, and no reduction was seen in the incidence of sudden cardiac death.

These two studies demonstrate that some vasodilators have the ability to decrease mortality as well as improve the hemodynamics and symptoms of chronic severe heart failure. If these results are confirmed, vasodilator therapy will be indicated in all moderate to severe chronic heart failure patients to induce the improvement in mortality. The inability of prazosin to produce an improvement in survival suggests that this agent lacks the pharmacologic action or consistency (tachyphylaxis occurs with this agent; see the section

"Prazosin" below) to produce a favorable response.

The studies were performed on patients with chronic severe heart failure. Whether vasodilators would also demonstrate an improvement in survival when used in critically ill patients with acute heart failure has not been evaluated. It will require further clinical investigation. However, the ability of vasodilators to improve mortality in chronic heart failure suggests that these agents can produce a favorable response in cardiovascular performance, and may have a positive role in other clinical settings. Which specific vasodilator agent will prove to be best in specific settings will require further clinical investigation.

SPECIFIC VASODILATOR AGENTS

Clinically, the most useful method of classifying vasodilator agents is based on their major peripheral vascular actions (Fig. 19.5, Table 19.1) (121). One group of vasodilators is considered to have its major effect by dilating arterioles, a second group dilates predominantly veins and venules, and a third group has relatively equal effects dilating arterioles and veins ("balanced" vasodilation). In general, vasodilators that affect arterioles increase CO through an enhanced stroke volume but have little or no effect on pulmonary or systemic venous pressures. Agents that dilate veins and venules reduce pulmonary and systemic venous pressures with little or no change in CO. Vasodilators with effects on both the arterial and venous circuits reduce pulmonary and systemic venous hypertension and increase CO (Fig. 19.5).

Although this classification is clinically useful, it has several limitations. Of the presently available vasodilator agents, none has pure

Table 19.1
Vasodilators Classified by Their Principal Site of Action

Arterial and venous vasodilators—"balanced vasodilators"
  Nitroprusside
  Phentolamine
  Prazosin
  Captopril
  Nifedipine
Arterial vasodilators
  Hydralazine
  Minoxidil
Venous vasodilators
  Nitrates (nitroglycerin, isosorbide dinitrate)

arteriolar or venodilator properties; all have some effect on both circuits, though certain agents have such a predominant effect on the arteriolar or venous side that they are best regarded as arteriolar or venous vasodilators. Perhaps the most accurate representation of these vasodilator properties would be as a spectrum of effects ranging from pure veno-dilation to balanced venous and arteriolar effects to pure arteriolar dilation. A second limitation is that the hemodynamic response to any vasodilator depends on the baseline hemodynamic status of the patient (see "Mechanism of Vasodilator Action"). Patients' responses to the same vasodilator agent are usually variable and one must consider this fact when instituting therapy. Despite these limitations, the classification proposed (Table 19.1) is highly useful both conceptually and clinically and allows prediction of a vasodilator's probable site of action and probable hemodynamic outcome.

In the critical care setting, use of rapidly acting parenteral vasodilator agents predominates, and therefore the emphasis is on parenteral (usually intravenous) vasodilator agents. However, some mention is also made of non-parenteral agents that are of use in the intensive care unit.

Arterial and Venous Vasodilators

NITROPRUSSIDE

Because of its rapid onset of action, rapid reversibility when discontinued, relatively specific effect on vascular smooth muscle, balanced effect on the arteriolar and venous systems, and lack of tachyphylaxis, nitroprusside is the vasodilator of choice for many situations in the critical care unit.

Nitroprusside has both an interesting history and chemistry. It was originally used in the 1850s as a chemical color indicator. Its hypotensive properties were not described until 1929 (64). The chemical structure of nitroprusside contains five cyanide groups per molecule (28, 95), and concern about cyanide toxicity delayed development of the agent as a pharmaceutical until 1955 when its safety and potent hypotensive effects were demonstrated in a group of hypertensive patients (94). In 1972, nitroprusside was shown to improve left ventricular function in patients with acute myocardial infarction (46), and subsequent studies have shown the drug's ability to improve left ventricular function in severe heart failure due to ischemic heart disease, cardio-myopathy, or cardiac regurgitant lesions (9, 14, 20, 32, 58).

Nitroprusside causes direct relaxation of arterial and venous smooth muscle. At therapeutic doses, it has no effect on uterine or duodenal smooth muscle or on myocardial contractility (28). Nitroprusside relaxes the lower esophageal sphincter (36); however, in general the drug affects vascular smooth muscle in a relatively specific manner. Nitroprusside-induced vascular smooth muscle relaxation is not dependent on the sympathetic nervous system or adrenergic receptors. Its cellular mechanism of action is unknown, though possible mechanisms include interaction with intracellular sulfhydryl groups, inhibition of calcium transport, or changes in intracellular cyclic nucleotides (103).

Nitroprusside is useful for all of the clinical indications outlined below ("Clinical Indications for Vasodilator Therapy"). It is the classical example of a balanced vasodilator with capability to reduce both pulmonary venous and systemic venous pressures as well as to increase stroke volume and CO in patients with severe heart failure. Heart rate usually decreases slightly or remains unchanged, and blood pressure may fall slightly or remain unchanged. Concomitant with this salutary hemodynamic effect, most patients have symptomatic improvement with relief of dyspnea, lessened fatigue, warming of the skin, and diuresis (16, 29, 46, 58).

In patients with severe heart failure requiring intensive care, nitroprusside therapy should be initiated and continued using constant arterial pressure monitoring and employing a Swan-Ganz pulmonary artery catheter to determine serial pulmonary artery pressures, pulmonary capillary wedge pressures, and thermodilution COs. Nitroprusside has an onset of action within seconds of initiating the drug, and its duration of effect is only 1–3 minutes, allowing slow increase of the dose every few minutes while watching the arterial pressure carefully. Serial determinations of hemodynamic values allow correlation of clinical with hemodynamic improvement. Once an optimal pulmonary capillary wedge pressure (usually 14–18 mm Hg) and maximal CO are achieved, oral vasodilator agents can be started and nitroprusside tapered. Serial hemodynamics can again help determine the optimal dose and combination of vasodilator agents for a particular patient.

The major complication of nitroprusside therapy is hypotension. Most patients with severe heart failure respond to relatively low doses of nitroprusside with an increase in CO and only minimal decreases in pressure; however, patients with low filling pressures commonly respond to nitroprusside with a reduced CO and hypotension due to inadequate preload (Fig. 19.1). Some authors recommend that vasodilators not be used with a diastolic pressure of less than 60 mm Hg (16, 96), but others state that nitroprusside therapy can be used in most patients with systolic pressures between 90 and 105 mm Hg without precipitating hypotension (28). Most patients whose blood pressure decreases with nitroprusside respond to discontinuation of the drug, and the nitroprusside can usually then be restarted at a lower dosage. A hypotensive response to nitroprusside should always cause the physician to consider whether the filling pressures are lower than suspected. Profound hypotension with nitroprusside that does not respond to discontinuation of infusion and fluid administration within a few minutes should be treated with an inotropic agent such as dopamine; this therapy usually restores blood pressure promptly.

For patients with severe heart failure, a nitroprusside infusion is started at 10 μg/min and may be increased by 10 μg/min increments every 5–15 minutes. There is great variability in individual responses to nitroprusside, but most patients with heart failure show a positive response by 1–2 μg/kg/min (approximately 70–140 μg/min) with a drop in the pulmonary capillary wedge pressure and/or an increase in CO. Although hemodynamic responses are highly variable, a decrease of 20–50% in wedge pressure and an increase of 20–40% in CO are considered positive responses to nitroprusside. In patients with pulmonary edema with hypertension, nitroprusside is started at 10 μg/min but is increased by 20 μg/min increments every 3–5 minutes in order to rapidly reduce filling pressures and relieve symptoms. When nitroprusside is used for hypertension, usually the doses required to decrease blood pressure are considerably higher than those to treat heart failure.

Other than hypotension, the other major side effects of nitroprusside are thiocyanate/cyanide toxicity and mild reductions in arterial oxygen tension due to nitroprusside-induced inhibition of the pulmonary vasoconstrictor response (85, 101). Thiocyanate toxicity is manifest by confusion, hyperreflexia, and convulsions; cyanide toxicity is first manifest by a metabolic acidosis due to cyanide combining with cytochromes and inhibiting aerobic cellular metabolism. Thiocyanate or cyanide toxicity occurs almost exclusively in patients receiving high doses of nitroprusside for a prolonged period. Infusion rates of less than 3 μg/kg/min for less than 72 hours are not associated with toxicity.

Deaths during long infusions of high doses of nitroprusside have been ascribed to cyanide toxicity. Cyanide conversion to thiocyanate is facilitated by thiosulfate, sodium nitrate, or hydroxycobalamin (25, 34), and these three agents should be considered as therapy in patients demonstrating toxicity from nitroprusside with metabolic acidosis and confusion when discontinuation of the nitroprusside does not reverse the toxicity. Monitoring blood thiocyanate levels is useful to follow toxicity in patients requiring infusions for longer than 2–3 days. Levels of thiocyanate below 10 mg/dl are considered safe.

On rapid discontinuation of a nitroprusside infusion, a rebound beyond the prenitroprusside baseline occurs, with an increase in SVR, increase in pulmonary capillary wedge pressure, and decrease in CO (92). This phenomenon probably results from vasodilator-induced activation of the sympathetic and renin-angiotensin systems. A slow nitroprusside taper while instituting oral vasodilator therapy usually avoids this rebound depression of cardiac performance.

PHENTOLAMINE

Phentolamine was the first vasodilator used clinically to improve cardiovascular performance in heart failure (75). It is considered one of the classical α-adrenergic blocking agents and causes blockade at both the postsynaptic (α_1) and presynaptic (α_2) receptors. Its potent vasodilator capabilities are secondary to both α blockade (53, 103) and a direct vasodilator effect on vascular smooth muscle (109). Norepinephrine release may actually increase reflexly because of baroreceptor activation caused by the fall in blood pressure and the blockade of the presynaptic α_2-receptors, the inhibition promoting further release. This circulating norepinephrine frequently results in a tachycardia and positive cardiac inotropic stimulation.

Phentolamine can relax arteriolar as well as venous vascular smooth muscle and thus can increase CO and reduce pulmonary and systemic venous pressures in patients with moderate to severe heart failure of all etiologies.

The ability of phentolamine to increase CO is comparable with that of nitroprusside; however, it produces less of a decrease in filling pressures. The ability of phentolamine to increase CO and its less than expected decreases in venous tone may be caused by the enhanced release of norepinephrine, which increases cardiac contractility and heightens venous vasoconstriction. Although phentolamine is generally well tolerated in ischemic cardiac failure, the tachycardia and norepinephrine release can worsen ischemia in patients with coronary artery disease.

Phentolamine is given as an intravenous infusion starting at 0.1 mg/min and increasing slowly up to 2 mg/min in increments of 0.2–0.4 mg/min every 10–30 minutes. Hemodynamic effects occur at 15 minutes, usually peak by 30 minutes, and persist up to 60 minutes after the drug is stopped. The drug can be given orally in doses of 50–150 mg every 4–6 hours.

In addition to the tachycardia, the major side effects of phentolamine are gastrointestinal: vomiting, abdominal pain, diarrhea, and hypermotility. Because tolerance to the drug develops rapidly, phentolamine is only used on an acute basis.

PRAZOSIN

Prazosin is a selective α_1 (postsynaptic) adrenergic receptor antagonist that causes arteriolar and venous vasodilation exclusively by its receptor-blocking effects (54, 106). Since it is only available in oral form, its use in the intensive care environment is as a subacute or chronic agent after therapy is initiated with a parenteral vasodilator. In patients with heart failure, prazosin has balanced hemodynamic actions similar to those of nitroprusside, with elevation in CO and reductions in systemic and pulmonary venous pressures (55).

Prazosin is well absorbed from the gastrointestinal tract and is given in doses of 1–10 mg every 6–8 hours. Its onset of action is 30–60 minutes, with maximal hemodynamic effect at 2–6 hours post dose. In many patients, the first dose of drug will produce orthostatic syncope, so patients should be warned to rise slowly from the supine position.

A subset of patients develop tachyphylaxis to the beneficial hemodynamic effect of this drug after several days of therapy (4, 37, 89). The mechanism is unknown, but increasing the drug dose or adding diuretics does not help. If tachyphylaxis occurs, prazosin should be discontinued and another vasodilator used.

CAPTOPRIL

With the onset of moderate to severe heart failure, the renin-angiotensin-aldosterone system is activated and serves as an important compensatory mechanism to maintain blood pressure and cause volume retention. In advanced heart failure, some of the "inappropriate" increase in afterload may be maintained by the vasoconstrictor substance, angiotensin II. Inhibition of the renin-angiotensin system reduces afterload or impedance and enhances cardiac performance. A number of inhibitors of the renin-angiotensin system are being tested and presently captopril, an inhibitor of angiotensin-converting enzyme, is one of the pharmaceutical agents commercially available.

In patients with heart failure, captopril produces a hemodynamic pattern similar to that seen with nitroprusside (69) or prazosin (65). From what is known of angiotensin II physiology, one would predict that a pure inhibitor of angiotensin II production would cause a reduction in afterload with little effect on preload. Yet captopril does reduce preload, prompting some to argue that captopril has an additional mechanism of action causing vasodilation. The mechanism of captopril-induced vasodilation is unknown, but it is postulated to be due to inhibition of the enzyme that degrades bradykinin leading to an increase in the circulating level of this potent vasodilator (39).

Captopril is only available in an oral preparation, and therapy is started with 25 mg every 6 hours and increased to a maximum daily dosage of 450 mg. Onset of a hemodynamic change is within 30 minutes, with peak effect at 1–3 hours and disappearance by 4–8 hours. The duration of the hemodynamic effect is dose-dependent, but the magnitude is not. Tolerance to the drug does not develop in patients treated for as long as 6–12 months.

NIFEDIPINE

Calcium channel blockers inhibit the contraction of vascular smooth muscle and therefore have vasodilator properties; however, few studies are available to evaluate the efficacy of these agents in heart failure. In one study, patients in cardiogenic pulmonary edema were treated with nifedipine (10 mg sublingually), causing reduction in symptoms of dyspnea, decreases in systemic and pulmonary venous pressures, and a rise in CO (102). Nifedipine also produces a sustained hemodynamic improvement in patients with chronic heart failure (7). Many clinicians are reluctant to use calcium channel blockers in heart failure because these agents have a direct depressant effect on the myocardium. With nifedipine, the decrease in afterload is more profound than the myocardial depressant effect, resulting in overall enhanced hemodynamics.

Verapamil, another calcium channel blocker, has vasodilator properties but its direct myocardial depressant effect is more profound, and this may seriously aggravate heart failure in patients with severe myocardial dysfunction.

Arterial Vasodilators

HYDRALAZINE

Hydralazine has been used in the treatment of hypertension for 30 years. It is a potent direct dilator of vascular smooth muscle and mostly affects arterioles. In patients with heart failure, hydralazine produces impressive increases in stroke volume by reducing arteriolar resistance and has no effect or only a modest lowering effect on systemic or pulmonary venous pressures (9, 21). For a given change in blood pressure, hydralazine increases CO more than nitroprusside or nitrates. There is conflicting evidence whether hydralazine has a reflex or direct cardiac inotropic effect as an explanation for its potent ability to increase CO (91, 103). Hydralazine can also increase limb and renal blood flow, thus promoting diuresis.

When using hydralazine in a critical care setting, intravenous administration is the most reliable route, but it must be given slowly and with constant hemodynamic monitoring to avoid hypotension. Administration should begin with 5–10 mg given as a slow intravenous drip over 20 minutes. Maximal effect occurs 15–45 minutes after injection and the effect can last 4–24 hours. One can administer up to 20 mg intravenously every 6 hours. Given orally, the dosage is usually 25–100 mg every 6 hours, with onset of action at 60 minutes and peak effect at 2–3 hours. Some studies suggest that high doses of hydralazine (150–200 mg)

are necessary in some patients to produce a beneficial effect on cardiac performance (19, 90); the need for this high oral dose in some patients may be due to mesenteric venous hypertension causing malabsorption of the drug.

A small number of patients with heart failure develop tachycardia with hydralazine administration. Exacerbation of angina pectoris can occur with hydralazine, especially (but not exclusively) in patients with ischemic heart disease who develop a tachycardia during therapy (66). Prolonged administration of hydralazine is associated with a lupus-like syndrome in 10–20% of patients, especially in those taking more than 400 mg daily (2).

MINOXIDIL

Minoxidil is a potent, direct-acting, vascular smooth muscle relaxant that acts largely on the arterial bed (48). In doses of 5–20 mg orally, the drug produces hemodynamic effects similar to those of hydralazine in patients with heart failure, i.e., a rise in CO, decrease in SVR, and no change in pulmonary venous (or arterial) pressure (44). Side effects include hirsutism and pericardial effusion. Minoxidil is presently being tested on large populations and, if it has fewer side effects than hydralazine, it may become the arterial vasodilator of choice.

Venous Vasodilators

Organic esters of nitric acid have been established therapy for angina pectoris for more than 100 years. Only in the past 10 years have they been used to treat congestive heart failure. Nitrates have a direct smooth muscle–relaxing capability, especially on vascular smooth muscle. Recent evidence suggests that nitrates may act on smooth muscle by releasing prostacyclin (a potent vasodilator) from vessel endothelial cells (68).

In patients with heart failure, the most prominent action of nitrates is to lower ventricular filling pressures by dilation of pulmonary and systemic veins (51). The volume of the left and right ventricles decreases and the compliance of the left ventricle increases (35, 71). The mechanism of this improved compliance is unclear; however, it may result from altered constraints on the left ventricle due to a decrease in right ventricle size.

Nitrates also decrease arterial vascular resistance, but CO may increase, remain unchanged, or decrease in response to nitrates (103). In some patients treated with nitrates, the CO does not increase because a concomitant fall in preload causes a depression in stroke volume (17, 96). Other patients not showing an increase in CO in response to nitrates have received a dose that is insufficient to produce a significant fall in impedance. At lower doses of nitrate, the vasodilatory effect is largely on the venous system with decreases in filling pressures. At higher nitrate doses, impedance falls and CO rises. As with nitroprusside, the increase in CO with nitrates is proportional to the reduction in SVR (42, 93) and is inversely correlated with the patient's baseline CO (42, 74, 93). Some authors note a positive correlation between baseline SVR and the nitrate-induced rise in CO (49), although others do not support this finding (3, 93).

The effects of nitrates and nitroprussides on ischemic heart disease were considered above ("Effects of Vasodilators on Myocardial Ischemia").

In an intensive care environment, the optimal nitrate preparation is intravenous nitroglycerin because it allows exact titration of dose and the ability to quickly terminate drug infusion. It is important to be certain that the left ventricular filling pressures are high or optimal because even low doses of nitroglycerin can precipitously decrease filling pressures. Intravenous infusions should begin at 10 μg/min, and one can increase the dosage in increments of 10 μg/min every 5–10 minutes to a dose of 50–100 μg/min. Most patients demonstrate a vasodilator effect at this dose, but up to 400 μg/min can be given if clinically indicated. High doses of nitroglycerin are well tolerated for several days. Treatment can then be changed to oral isosorbide dinitrate, 20–100 mg every 4 hours, nitroglycerin ointment, ½–1½ inches every 4 hours, or a transdermal delivery system for nitroglycerin (1, 111).

Side effects of nitrate therapy include headache, which usually abates after several days, if therapy is continued. A nitrate withdrawal syndrome occurs in nitroglycerin factory workers and consists of coronary-like chest pain and acute myocardial infarction. Because of the sustained high doses of nitrates presently being employed, patients on high sustained nitrate regimens must be told not to discontinue therapy abruptly.

Nitrates and hydralazine are used together to combine nitrate-induced reductions in filling pressures with hydralazine's ability to increase CO, producing an oral regimen comparable with that of nitroprusside (66, 77, 78). The hemodynamic changes seen with the combination are roughly additive (67, 77, 78), and are similar to those produced by nitroprusside. As with all vasodilator regimens, hypotension can complicate this therapy and necessitate alteration in dosage or discontinuation of one of the drugs.

CLINICAL INDICATIONS FOR VASODILATOR THERAPY

The following are the clinical situations in which vasodilator therapy is beneficial:

1. Severe heart failure unresponsive to diuretics and digitalis. Vasodilators are most efficacious in patients with low CO, high left ventricular filling pressures, and elevated SVR.

2. Acute cardiogenic pulmonary edema. Vasodilator therapy with acute vasodilation can rapidly reduce high filling pressures and reverse symptoms. Vasodilators can be used in conjunction with supplemental oxygen, rotating tourniquets, morphine, and intravenous diuretics.

3. Acute or chronic mitral regurgitation, aortic regurgitation, or ventricular septal defect. Vasodilator-induced decreases in SVR increase forward (systemic) CO. Vasodilators are usually employed in these situations as a temporizing measure to allow time to prepare the patient for cardiac surgery.

4. Based on present data, vasodilators are not recommended for the routine therapy of patients with acute myocardial infarction. Nitrate therapy is useful in treating stable and unstable angina. Vasodilators such as nitroprusside can reduce myocardial oxygen consumption in patients with persistent chest pain who are hypertensive. In normotensive patients with myocardial infarction and no or only mild to moderate heart failure, the effectiveness of vasodilator therapy is not proven. As noted above, vasodilators are useful in severe heart failure.

5. In patients with cardiogenic shock, vasodilator therapy combined with inotropic drugs (e.g., dopamine) or intraaortic balloon counterpulsation can produce substantial hemodynamic improvement.

6. As reviewed in other chapters of this book, vasodilators are highly useful to treat hypertension, malignant hypertension, and dissecting aortic aneurysms (in conjunction

with β-blockade), and are possibly useful in primary pulmonary hypertension.

Acknowledgments

The author thanks Ms. Kathy Kiefer for her excellent secretarial assistance and Ms. Sandy Montgomery for her superb administrative and editorial assistance.

References

1. Abrams JA: Nitroglycerin and long-acting nitrates. *N Engl J Med* 302:1234–1237, 1980.
2. Alarcon-Segovia D: Drug-induced antinuclear antibodies and lupus syndromes. *Drugs* 12:69–77, 1976.
3. Armstrong PW, Armstrong JA, Markes CS: Pharmacokinetic hemodynamic studies of intravenous nitroglycerin in congestive heart failure. *Circulation* 62:160–166, 1980.
4. Arnold SB, Williams RL, Ports TA, Baughman RA, Benet LZ, Parmley WW, Chatterjee K: Attenuation of prazosin effect on cardiac output in chronic heart failure. *Ann Intern Med* 91:345–349, 1979.
5. Awan NA, Miller RR, Zakanddin V, DeMaria AN, Amsterdam EA, Mason DT: Reduction of ST segment elevation with infusion of nitroprusside in patients with acute myocardial infarction. *Am J Cardiol* 38:425–439, 1976.
6. Bache RJ, Dymek DJ: Local and regional regulation of coronary vascular tone. *Prog Cardiovasc Dis* 24:191–212, 1981.
7. Belloccui F, Ansalone G, Scabia E, Viencenzo A, Peitro S, Laperfido F, Paolo Z: Sustained beneficial effect of nifedipine in chronic refractory heart failure. *Am J Cardiol* 47:407, 1981.
8. Bemis CF, Serue JR, Borkenhagen D, Sonnenblick EH, Urschel CW: Influence of right ventricular filling pressure on left ventricular pressure and dimension. *Circ Res* 34:498–504, 1974.
9. Bolen JL, Alderman EL: Hemodynamic consequence of afterload reduction in patients with chronic aortic regurgitation. *Circulation* 53:879–883, 1976.
10. Braunwald E: Control of myocardial oxygen consumption. *Am J Cardiol* 27:416–432, 1971.
11. Braunwald E: Pathophysiology of heart failure. In Braunwald E (ed): *Heart Disease: A Textbook of Cardiovascular Medicine*, ed 3. Philadelphia, WB Saunders, 1988, pp 426–448.
12. Braunwald E, Ross J, Sonneblick EH: *Mechanisms of Contraction of the Normal and Failing Heart*. Boston, Little, Brown & Co, 1976.
13. Braunwald E, Sonnenblick EH, Ross J: Contraction of the normal heart. In Braunwald E (ed): *Heart Disease: A Textbook of Cardiovascular Medicine*. Philadelphia, WB Saunders, 1980.
14. Brodie BR, Grossman W, Mann T, McLaurin LP: Effects of sodium nitroprusside on left ventricular diastolic pressure/volume relations. *J Clin Invest* 59:59–68, 1977.
15. Burns JW, Covell JW, Ross J: Mechanics of isotonic left ventricular contractions. *Am J Physiol* 224:725–732, 1973.
16. Chatterjee K, Parmley WW: The role of vasodilator therapy in heart failure. *Prog Cardiovasc Dis* 19:301–325, 1977.
17. Chatterjee K, Parmley WW: Vasodilator therapy for chronic heart failure. *Annu Rev Pharmacol Toxicol* 20:475–512, 1980.
18. Chatterjee K, Parmley WW, Ganz W, Forrester J, Walinsky P, Crexells C: Hemodynamic and metabolic responses to vasodilator therapy in the acute myocardial infarction. *Circulation* 48:1183–1193, 1973.
19. Chatterjee K, Parmley WW, Massie B: Oral hydralazine therapy for chronic refractory heart failure. *Circulation* 54:879–883, 1976.
20. Chatterjee K, Parmley WW, Swan HJ, Berman G, Forrester J: Beneficial effects of vasodilator agents in severe mitral regurgitation due to dysfunction of subvalvular apparatus. *Circulation* 48:684–690, 1973.
21. Chatterjee K, Ports TA, Brundage BH, Massie B, Holly AN, Parmley WW: Oral hydralazine in chronic heart failure: sustained beneficial hemodynamic effects. *Ann Intern Med* 92:600–604, 1980.
22. Chiariello M, Gold HK, Leinbach RC, Davis MA, Maroko PR: Comparison between the effects of nitroprusside and nitroglycerin on ischemic injury during acute myocardial infarction. *Circulation* 54:766–773, 1976.
23. Clancy RI, Graham TP, Ross J, Sonnenblick EH, Braunwald E: Influence of aortic pressure induced homeometric autoregulation on myocardial performance. *Am J Physiol* 214:1186–1192, 1968.
24. Cohn JN: Marriage of the heart and the peripheral circulation. *Prog Cardiovasc Dis* 24:189–190, 1981.
25. Cohn JN: Vasodilator therapy for heart failure. *Circulation* 48:5–8, 1973.
26. Cohn JN, Archibald DG, Ziesche S, Franciosa JA, Harston WE, Trostamo FE, Dunkman WB, Jacobs W, Francis GS, Flohr KH, Goldman S, Cobb FR, Shah PM, Saunders R, Fletcher RD, Loeb HS, Hughes VC, Baker B: Effects of vasodilator therapy on mortality in chronic congestive heart failure. Results of a Veterans Administration Cooperative Study. *N Engl J Med* 314:1547–1552, 1986.
27. Cohn JN, Archibald DG, Francis GS, Ziesche S, Franciosa JA, Harston WE, Tristani FE, Dunkman WB, Jacobs W, Flohr KH, Goldman S, Cobb FR, Shah PM, Saunders R, Fletcher RD, Loeb HS, Hughes VC, Baker B: Veterans Administration Cooperative Study on vasodilator therapy of heart failure: influence of prerandomization variables on the reduction of mortality by treatment with hydralazine and isosorbide dinitrate. *Circulation* 75(suppl IV):IV-49, 1987.
28. Cohn JN, Burke LP: Nitroprusside. *Ann Intern Med* 91:752–757, 1979.
29. Cohn JN, Franciosa JA: Vasodilator therapy of cardiac failure. *N Engl J Med* 297:254–258, 1977.
30. Cohn J, Franciosa JA, Francis GS, Archibald D, Tristani F, Fletcher R, Montero A, Cintron G, Clarke J, Hager D, Saunders R, Cobb F, Smith R, Loeb H, Settle H: Effect of short term infusion of sodium nitroprusside on mortality rate in acute myocardial infarction complicated by left ventricular failure. Results of a Veterans Administration Cooperative Study. *N Engl J Med* 306:1129–1135, 1982.
31. Cohn JN, Masniro I, Levine TB, Mehta J: Role of vasoconstrictor mechanisms in the control of left ventricular performance of the normal and damaged heart. *Am J Cardiol* 44:1019–1022, 1979.
32. Cohn JN, Mathew KJ, Franciosa JA, Snow JA: Chronic vasodilator therapy in the management of cardiogenic shock and intractable left vasodilator failure. *Ann Intern Med* 81:777–790, 1974.
33. CONSENSUS Trial Study Group: Effects of enalapril on mortality in severe congestive heart failure. Results of the Cooperative North Scandinavian Enalapril Survival Study (CONSENSUS). *N Engl J Med* 316:1429–1435, 1987.
34. Cottrell JE, Casthely P, Brodie JO, Patel K, Klein A, Turndorf H: Prevention of nitroprusside-induced cyanide toxicity and hydroxycobalamin. *N Engl J Med* 298:808–811, 1978.
35. DeMaria AN, Vismara LA, Auditore K, Amsterdam EA, Aelis R, Mason DT: Effects of nitroglycerine on left ventricular cavity size and cardiac performance determined by ultrasound in man. *Am J Med* 57:754–760, 1974.

36. Dent J, Dodds WJ, Arndorfer RC: Effect of nitroprusside and verapamil on esophageal smooth muscle contractility in the opposum. *Gastroenterology* 74:1119, 1978.

37. Desch CE, Magorien RD, Triffon DW, Blanford MF, Unverferth DV, Leier CV: Development of pharmacodynamic tolerance to prazosin in congestive heart failure. *Am J Cardiol* 44:1178–1182, 1979.

38. Durrer JD, Lie KI, Van Capelle FJL, Durrer D: Effect of sodium nitroprusside on mortality in acute myocardial infarction. *N Engl J Med* 306:1121–1128, 1982.

39. Dzau VJ, Colucci WS, Williams GH, Curfoman G, Meggs L, Hollenberg NK: Sustained effectiveness of converting-enzyme inhibition in patients with severe congestive heart failure. *N Engl J Med* 302:1373–1379, 1980.

40. Finkelstein SM, Collins VR: Vascular hemodynamic impedance measurement. *Prog Cardiovasc Dis* 24:401–418, 1982.

41. Franciosa JA, Effectiveness of long-term vasodilator administration in the treatment of chronic left ventricular failure. *Prog Cardiovasc Dis* 24:319–330, 1982.

42. Franciosa JA, Blank RC, Cohn JN, Miculec E: Hemodynamic effects of topical, oral and sublingual nitroglycerin in left ventricular failure. *Curr Ther Res* 22:231–245, 1977.

43. Franciosa JA, Blank RC, Cohn JN: Nitrate effects on cardiac output and left ventricular outflow resistance in chronic congestive heart failure. *Am J Med* 64:207–213, 1978.

44. Franciosa JA, Cohn JN: Effects of minoxidil on hemodynamics in patients with congestive heart failure. *Circulation* 63:652–657, 1981.

45. Franciosa JA, Cohn JN: Sustained hemodynamic effects without tolerance during long-term isosorbide dinitrate treatment of chronic left ventricular failure. *Am J Cardiol* 45:648–654, 1980.

46. Franciosa JA, Cuiha NH, Limas CJ, Rodriguera E, Cohn JN: Improved left ventricular function during nitroprusside infusion in acute myocardial infarction. *Lancet* 1:650–654, 1972.

47. Gaffney TF, Braunwald E: Importance of the adrenergic nervous system in the support of circulatory function in patients with congestive heart failure. *Am J Med* 34:320–324, 1963.

48. Gilmore E, Weil J, Chidsey C: Treatment of essential hypertension with a new vasodilator in combination with beta-adrenergic blockade. *N Engl J Med* 282:521–531, 1970.

49. Goldberg S, Mann T, Grossman W: Nitrate therapy of heart failure in valvular heart disease. Importance of resting level of peripheral vascular resistance in determining cardiac output response. *Am J Med* 65:161–166, 1978.

50. Goldstein RE: Coronary vascular responses to vasodilator drugs. *Prog Cardiovasc Dis* 24:419–436, 1982.

51. Gomes JAC, Carambas CR, Moran HE: The effect of isosorbide dinitrate on left ventricular size, wall stress and left ventricular function in the chronic refractory heart failure. *Am J Med* 65:794–801, 1978.

52. Goodman DJ, Rossen RM, Holloway FL, Alderman EF, Harrison DC: Effect of nitroprusside on left ventricular dynamics in mitral regurgitation. *Circulation* 50:1025–1032, 1974.

53. Gould L, Zahir M, Ettinger S: Phentolamine and cardiovascular performance. *Br Heart J* 31:154–162, 1969.

54. Graham RM, Oats HF, Stoker LM, Stokes GS: Alpha blocking action of the antihypertensive agent, prazosin. *J Pharmacol Exp Ther* 201:747–762, 1977.

55. Graham RM, Pettinger WA: Prazosin. *N Engl J Med* 300:232–236, 1979.

56. Grossman W, Harshaw CW, Munro AB, Becker L, McLaurin LP: Lowered aortic impedance as therapy for severe mitral regurgitation. *JAMA* 230:1011–1013, 1974.

57. Grossman W, McLaurin LP: Clinical measurement of vascular resistance and assessment of vasodilator drugs. In Grossman W (ed): *Cardiac Catheterization and Angiography*, ed 2. Philadelphia, Lea & Febiger, 1980.

58. Guiha NH, Cohn JN, Mikulic E: Treatment of refractory heart failure with infusion of nitroprusside. *N Engl J Med* 291:587–592, 1974.

59. Harper RW, Gold HK, Leinbach RC: Acute myocardial infarction. In Harper E, Austen WC (eds): *The Practice of Cardiology*. Boston, Little, Brown & Co, 1980.

60. Harshaw CW, Grossman W, Munro AB, McLaurin LP: Reduced systemic vascular resistance as therapy for severe mitral regurgitation of valvular origin. *Ann Intern Med* 83:312–316, 1975.

61. Helfant RH, Banka VS, Bodenheimer MM: Left ventricular dysfunction in coronary heart disease: a dynamic problem. *Cardiovasc Med* 2:557–571, 1977.

62. Herman MV, Heinle RA, Klein MD, Gorlin R: Localized disorders in myocardial contraction. *N Engl J Med* 277:222–232, 1967.

63. Higgins CB, Vatner SF, Franklin D, Braunwald E: Extent of regulation of the heart's contractile state in the conscious dog by alteration in the frequency of contraction. *J Clin Invest* 52:1187–1194, 1973.

64. Johnson CC: The actions and toxicity of sodium nitroprusside. *Arch Int Pharmacodyn Ther* 35:481–482, 1929.

65. Kluger J, Cody RF, Smith V, Laragh JH: Comparative hemodynamic effects and humoral correlations of prazosin and captopril in heart failure. *Clin Res* 29:215A, 1981.

66. Koch-Weser J: Hydralazine. *N Engl J Med* 295:320–323, 1976.

67. Leier CV, Magorien RD, Desch CE, Thompson MJ, Unverferth DV: Hydralazine and isosorbide dinitrate: comparative central and regional hemodynamic effects when administered alone or in combination. *Circulation* 63:102–107, 1981.

68. Levin RI, Weksler BB, Jaffe EA: Nitroglycerin induces production of prostacyclin by human endothelial cells. *Clin Res* 28:471A, 1980.

69. Levine TB, Franciosa JA, Cohn JN: Acute and long-term response to an oral converting-enzyme inhibitor, captopril, in congestive heart failure. *Circulation* 62:35–41, 1980.

70. Liedtke AJ, Buoncristiani JF, Kirk ES, Sonnenblick EH, Urschel CW: Regulation of cardiac output after administration of isoproterenol and ouabain: interactions of systolic impedance and contractility. *Cardiovasc Res* 56:325–332, 1972.

71. Ludbrook PA, Byrne JD, Kurnik PB, McKnight RC: Influence of reduction of preload and afterload by nitroglycerin on left ventricular diastolic pressure-volume relations and relaxation in man. *Circulation* 56:937–943, 1977.

72. Ludbrook PA, Byrne JD, McKnight RC: Influence of right ventricular diastolic pressure-volume relations in man. *Circulation* 59:21–31, 1979.

73. Lukes SA, Romero CA, Resnekov L: Hemodynamic effects of sodium nitroprusside in 21 subjects with congestive heart failure. *Br Heart J* 41:187–191, 1979.

74. Magrini F, Niarchos AP: Ineffectiveness of sublingual nitroglycerin in acute left ventricular failure in the presence of massive peripheral edema. *Am J Cardiol* 45:841–847, 1980.

75. Majid PA, Sharma B, Taylor SH: Phentolamine for vasodilator treatment of severe heart-failure. *Lancet* 22:719–726, 1971.

76. Mason DT: Afterload reduction and cardiac performance. *Am J Med* 65:106–107, 1978.

77. Massie B, Chatterjee K, Werner J, Greenberg B, Hart R, Parmley WW: Hemodynamic advantage of combined administration of hydralazine orally and nitrates non-

parenterally in the vasodilator therapy of chronic heart failure. *Am J Cardiol* 40:794–801, 1977.

78. Massie BM, Kramer B, Shen E, Haughloom F: Vasodilator treatment with isosorbide dinitrate and hydralazine in chronic heart failure. *Br Heart J* 45:376, 1981.

79. Miller RR, Awan NA, Joyce JA: Combined dopamine and nitroprusside, therapy in congestive heart failure. Greater augmentation of cardiac performance by addition of inotropic stimulation to afterload reduction. *Circulation* 55:881–884, 1977.

80. Miller RR, Fennell, WH, Young, JB, Palomo AR, Quinones MA: Differential systemic arterial and venous actions and consequent cardiac effects of vasodilator drugs. *Prog Cardiovasc Dis* 24:353–374, 1982.

81. Miller RR, Vismara LA, DeMaria AN, Salel AF, Mason DT: Afterload reduction therapy with nitroprusside in severe aortic regurgitation: improved cardiac performance and reduced regurgitant volume. *Am J Cardiol* 38:564–567, 1976.

82. Miller RR, Vismara LA, Zelis R, Amsterdam EA, Mason DT: Clinical use of sodium nitroprusside in chronic ischemic heart disease. *Circulation* 51:328–336, 1975.

83. Milnor WR: Arterial impedance as ventricular afterload. *Circ Res* 36:565–570, 1975.

84. Mookherjee S, Henion W, Warner R, Erch RH, Smulyan H, Obeid AI: Sodium nitroprusside therapy in congestive cardiomyopathy: variability in hemodynamic response. *J Clin Pharmacol* 18:67–75, 1978.

85. Mookherjee S, Keighley JFH, Warner RA, Bowser MA, Obeid AI: Hemodynamic, ventriculatory and blood gas changes during infusion of sodium nitroferricyanide (nitroprusside). *Chest* 72:273–278, 1977.

86. Nichols WW, Pepine CJ: Left ventricular afterload and aortic input impedance: implications of pulsatile blood flow. *Prog Cardiovasc Dis* 24:293–306, 1982.

87. Packer M, Leier CV: Survival in congestive heart failure during treatment with drugs with positive inotropic actions. *Circulation* 75(suppl IV):IV-55, 1987.

88. Packer M, LeJemtel TH: Physiologic and pharmacologic determinants of vasodilator response: a conceptual framework for rational drug therapy for chronic heart failure. *Prog Cardiovasc Dis* 24:275–292, 1982.

89. Packer M, Meller J, Gorlin R, Herman MV: Hemodynamic and clinical tachyphylaxis to prazosin mediated afterload reduction in severe chronic congestive heart failure. *Circulation* 59:531–539, 1979.

90. Packer M, Meller J, Medine N, Gorlin R, Herman MV: Dose requirements of hydralazine in patients with severe chronic congestive heart failure. *Am J Cardiol* 45:655–660, 1980.

91. Packer M, Meller J, Medina N, Gorlin R, Herman MV: Hemodynamic evaluation of hydralazine dosage in refractory heart failure. *Clin Pharmacol Ther* 27:337–346, 1980.

92. Packer M, Meller J, Medina N, Gorlin R, Herman MV: Rebound hemodynamic events after the abrupt withdrawal of nitroprusside in patients with severe chronic heart failure. *N Engl J Med* 301:1193–1197, 1979.

93. Packer M, Meller J, Medine N, Yushak M, Gorlin R: Determinants of drug response in severe chronic heart failure. I. Activation of vasoconstrictor forces during vasodilator therapy. *Circulation* 64:506–514, 1981.

94. Page IH, Corcoran AC, Dustan HP, Kuppanyi T: Cardiovascular actions of sodium nitroprusside in animals and hypertensive patients. *Circulation* 11:188–198, 1955.

95. Palmer RF, Lasseter KC: Sodium nitroprusside. *N Engl J Med* 292:294–497, 1975.

96. Parmley WW, Chatterjee K: Vasodilator therapy. In Harvey P (ed): *Current Problems in Cardiology*. Chicago, Year Book, 1978.

97. Parmley WW, Chuck L, Chatterjee K, Swan HJC, Klausner SC, Glantz SA, Ratshin RA: Acute changes in the diastolic pressure volume relationship of the left ventricle. *Eur J Cardiol* 4:105–120, 1976.

98. Pepine CJ, Nichols WW: Aortic input impedance in cardiovascular disease. *Prog Cardiovasc Dis* 24:307–318, 1982.

99. Pepine CJ, Nichols WW, Conti CR: Aortic input impedance in heart failure. *Circulation* 58:460–465, 1978.

100. Petersdorf RG, Dale DC: Gram negative bacteremia and septic shock. In Petersdorf RG, Wilson (eds): *Harrison's Textbook of Medicine*. New York, McGraw-Hill, 1980.

101. Pierpont G, Hale KA, Franciosa JA, Cohen JN: Effects of vasodilators on pulmonary hemodynamics in gas exchange in left ventricular failure. *Am Heart J* 99:208–216, 1980.

102. Polese A, Fiorentine C, Olivari MT, Guazzi MD: Clinical use of a calcium antagonistic agent (nifedipine) in acute pulmonary edema. *Am J Med* 66:825–830, 1979.

103. Ribner HS, Breshnan D, Hsieh A, Silverman R, Tommaso C, Coath A, Askenazi J: Acute hemodynamic responses to vasodilator therapy in congestive heart failure. *Prog Cardiovasc Dis* 25:1–45, 1982.

104. Sarnoff SJ, Farr HW: Spinal anesthesia in the therapy of pulmonary edema: a preliminary report. *Anesthesiology* 5:69–76, 1944.

105. Schlant RC: Altered cardiovascular physiology of coronary atherosclerotic disease. In Hurst JW, Logue RB, Schlant RC (eds): *The Heart*. New York, McGraw-Hill, 1978.

106. Scivolett R, Toledo AJO, Gomes Da Silva AC, Nigro D: Mechanism of the hypotensive effect of prazosin. *Arch Int Pharmacodyn Ther* 223:333–338, 1976.

107. Sonnenblick EH: Force velocity relations in mammalian heart muscle. *Am J Physiol* 202:931–936, 1962.

108. Swan HJ, Ganz W, Forrester JS, Marcus H, Doamond G, Chonette D: Catheterization of the heart in man with the use of a flow-directed balloon tip catheter. *N Engl J Med* 283:444–451, 1970.

109. Taylor SH, Sutherland GR, MacKenzie CJ, Staunton HP, Donald KW: The circulatory effects of intravenous phentolamine in man. *Circulation* 31:741–754, 1965.

110. Teckleberg PL, Fitzgerald J, Allaire BI, Alderman EL, Harrison DC: Afterload reduction in the management of post-infarction ventricular septal defect. *Am J Cardiol* 38:956–958, 1976.

111. Transdermal delivery systems for nitroglycerin. *Med Lett Drugs Ther* 24:35, 1982.

112. Warner RA, Bowser M, Zuehlke A, Mookherjee S, Obeid AI: Treatment of acute aortic insufficiency with sodium nitroferricyanide. *Chest* 72:375–379, 1977.

113. Webb RC, Bohr DF: Regulation of vascular tone, molecular mechanisms. *Prog Cardiovasc Dis* 24:213–242, 1981.

114. Weber KT, Janicki JS, Hunter WC, Shroff S, Perlman ES, Fishman AP: The contractile behavior of the heart and its functional coupling of the circulation. *Prog Cardiovasc Dis* 24:375–400, 1982.

115. Weber KT, Janicki JS, Reeves RC: Determinants of stroke volume in the isolated canine heart. *J Appl Physiol* 37:742–746, 1974.

116. Yoran C, Yellin EL, Becker RM, Gabbay S, Frater R, Sonnenblick EH: Mechanism of reduction of mitral regurgitation with vasodilator therapy. *Am J Cardiol* 43:773–777, 1979.

117. Zelis R: The contribution of local factors to the elevated venous tone of congestive heart failure. *J Clin Invest* 54:219–224, 1974.

118. Zelis R, Delea CS, Coleman HN, Mason DT: Arterial sodium content in experimental congestive heart failure. *Circulation* 41:213–224, 1970.

119. Zelis R, Flaim SF: Alterations in vasomotor tone in congestive heart failure. *Prog Cardiovasc Dis* 24:437–459, 1982.

120. Zelis R, Lee G, Mason DT: Influence of experimental edema on metabolically determined blood flow. *Circ Res* 34:482–490, 1974.

121. Zelis R, Mason DT, Braunwald E: A comparison of the effects of vasodilator stimuli on peripheral resistance vessels in normal subjects and in patients with congestive heart failure. *J Clin Invest* 47:960–970, 1968.

122. Zelis R, Nellis SH, Longhurst J: Abnormalities in the regional circulations accompanying congestive heart failure. *Prog Cardiovasc Dis* 18:181–197, 1975.

20

Antihypertensive Therapy

Michael G. Ziegler, M.D.

Hypertension is the most common chronic illness of industrialized societies. Hypertensives develop critical cardiovascular disease at a much higher rate than normal subjects, thus patients arriving at intensive care units frequently have received antihypertensive drugs.

Table 20.1
Antihypertensive Therapies

Nutritional
Weight loss
Sodium restriction
Ethanol restriction
Potassium
Diuretics
Thiazides
Loop diuretics
Sympatholytics
α-Blockers
Phenoxybenzamine
Phentolamine
Prazosin
β-Blockers
Atenolol
Metoprolol
Nadolol
Propranolol
Timolol
Acebutolol
Labetalol
α_2-Agonists
Clonidine
Guanabenz
Methyldopa
Guanfacine
Ganglionic blockers
Vasodilators
Diazoxide
Hydralazine
Minoxidil
Nitroprusside
Calcium channel blockers
Nifedipine
Diltiazem
Verapamil
Converting-enzyme inhibitors
Captopril
Enalapril
Lisinopril

These drugs alter cardiovascular responses to severe illness and may diminish the ability to maintain the circulation during shock. Many other common drugs such as caffeine, ethanol, nicotine, and over-the-counter decongestants and diet pills alter blood pressure and are considered in this chapter. Food is also an important determinant of blood pressure, especially in patients dependent on intravenous nutrition. The interaction of all these chemicals is a complex but important facet of the regulation of the cardiovascular system. This chapter deals with each aspect of antihypertensive therapy under a separate subheading for quick reference. The sections are arranged in a logical sequence to describe the cardiovascular system of hypertensive subjects and how the hypertension can be controlled by medication.

High blood pressure was once considered "essential" to adequate tissue perfusion and thus acquired the name, "essential hypertension." The name remains, but we now know that the higher the pressure, the worse the prognosis for development of cardiovascular disease. Fifteen to 25% of the inhabitants of industrialized countries have high blood pressure; therefore, hypertension is one of the most common diagnoses among patients in a critical care unit. Some patients are there for therapy of malignant hypertension, but most have other illnesses, often of cardiovascular origin. All need care of their hypertension with attention to diet, intravenous fluids, and drugs (Table 20.1).

NUTRITIONAL PHARMACOLOGY OF HYPERTENSION

Diet is not an alternative usually considered in the drug therapy of hypertension, but dietary factors have potent effects on blood pressure and interact with antihypertensive drugs.

Dietary manipulations alone can often provide effective therapy of hypertension and may be prescribed in place of antihypertensive medication. The most important dietary factors are caloric intake, ethanol, sodium, potassium, and tyrosine.

Caloric Intake

Carbohydrate ingestion increases sympathetic nervous system activity, whereas consumption of protein or fat has little acute effect (34). When obese adults are switched from a 2600-kcal/day diet to a 600-kcal/day diet, they have a 40% decrease in the urinary excretion of 3-methoxy-4-hydroxymandelic acid, a metabolite of norepinephrine (95). The acute effects of carbohydrate ingestion on sympathetic nervous activity may be mediated by insulin, since maintenance of a constant serum insulin level prevents the carbohydrate-associated increase in circulating norepinephrine levels (45). All antihypertensive drugs have direct or indirect influences on the sympathetic nervous system, and carbohydrate ingestion can alter the effect of these drugs.

Obesity has chronic effects on the sympathetic and cardiovascular systems (48). Obesity augments cardiac output, stroke volume, left ventricular filling pressure, and intravascular volume, and lowers total peripheral resistance. Obesity is strongly associated with hypertension. Sixty-two percent of hypertensive subjects are more than 20% overweight. Weight loss can decrease or cure hypertension (18). The hyperinsulinemia of obesity promotes sodium retention (76) and sympathetic neuronal overactivity.

Fasting lowers blood pressure by decreasing sympathetic nervous activity and by activating an opiate-mediated vasodepressor response (21). After 8–12 weeks of a low calorie diet, plasma renin activity and aldosterone levels both decrease, irrespective of sodium intake (81). Weight loss thus reduces plasma insulin, norepinephrine, renin, and aldosterone levels, and cardiac output, all of which lower blood pressure.

The average hypertensive can expect to decrease systolic blood pressure by 1 mm Hg and diastolic pressure by ¾ mm Hg for every pound lost. As long as the weight is not gained back, there is no evidence of any rebound in blood pressure, thus the cure of a patient's obesity may simultaneously cure hypertension.

Diet has short-term effects on blood pressure as well. If dietary intake is less than 600 kcal/day, starvation ketosis causes natriuresis and hypotension. Carbohydrate consumption increases sympathetic nervous activity, but foods rich in the amino acid tyrosine may increase central norepinephrine release and thereby act to decrease peripheral sympathetic tone (1).

Ethanol

The consumption of more than three alcoholic drinks daily is associated with an increase in mean blood pressure and in the incidence of hypertension. Approximately 5% of the hypertension in the United States may be attributed to alcohol consumption. Surprisingly, the incidence of myocardial infarction decreases with increasing alcohol ingestion, even in the face of elevated blood pressure; however, stroke is more common in alcoholics. Moderate doses of ethanol increase plasma renin activity, plasma aldosterone, and cortisol (33). The cardioprotective effects of ethanol may be due to a direct effect on the heart or an interaction with norepinephrine release. Extremely high doses of ethanol may acutely activate central enkephalin neurons and lower blood pressure (32). The acutely ill patient in alcoholic coma is usually hypotensive while intoxicated. As time progresses, blood pressure in this intoxicated patient can be expected to increase, frequently into the hypertensive range, as the patient undergoes alcohol withdrawal.

Sodium

Patients with malignant hypertension reduce their blood pressure dramatically by eating a 10-mEq/day sodium diet (36). However, an increase in sodium from 10 to 35 mEq/day increases the blood pressure almost to pretreatment levels (88). The value of moderate sodium restriction has been contested, but controlled studies of moderate sodium restriction in hypertension show a fall in mean blood pressure of about 7 mm Hg (50) and a marked decrease in the requirement for antihypertensive medications (4). A similar decrement in blood pressure occurs in hospitalized patients who receive a 35-mEq/day sodium diet (87). Moderate sodium restriction can control mild hypertension, but severe hypertension requires severe sodium restriction for blood pressure control. The change in blood pressure that occurs with sodium restriction is acutely related to a change in plasma volume (87).

DIURETICS

Thiazides

Thiazide diuretics and closely related phthalimidine derivatives are customarily the first drugs used for hypertension. They cause sodium loss and vasodilation. Initially, thiazide therapy decreases blood volume and cardiac output. During chronic treatment these parameters return to normal, however, and blood pressure falls as peripheral resistance decreases (19). The antihypertensive effects of thiazide diuretics can be negated by a large salt intake or infusion of saline, although a similar increase in blood volume by a dextran infusion fails to increase blood pressure (93). The thiazides have a variety of biochemical effects early in treatment, particularly hypokalemia, hyperglycemia, hyperuricemia, decrease in plasma volume, and increase in renin, aldosterone, and sympathetic nervous activity (44). With chronic therapy, the hypokalemia, hyperglycemia, and hyperuricemia persist and a hypochloremic alkalosis may develop. A thiazide-induced decrease in blood pressure is accompanied by a decrease in peripheral resistance. Several homeostatic mechanisms, such as a stimulation of renin or aldosterone, may prevent a decrease in blood pressure. These reactions follow the increased sympathetic activity (44) that is particularly prominent in those who fail to respond to thiazides (43). Patients who fail to respond to thiazides because of compensatory homeostatic mechanisms are especially prone to the antihypertensive effect of sympatholytic drugs (43). Other patients do not respond to thiazides because they eat too much salt.

Current doses of thiazide diuretics used to treat hypertension are excessive. Treatment with 12½ mg of hydrochlorothiazide (5) and 25 mg of chlorthalidone (55) lowers blood pressure maximally in patients with normal renal function. It is best to use the lowest effective dose to treat hypertension because deleterious side effects multiply with increasing dose. Thiazides raise serum cholesterol by increasing low density lipoprotein levels without causing a similar increase in high density lipoproteins. These effects are most prominent in men and postmenopausal women, and these changes might underlie an increased mortality in patients receiving thiazides (39).

Since the antihypertensive actions of thiazide diuretics take up to 3 weeks to fully manifest, thiazides are not useful as single agents in the acute care of hypertension. The lack of initial antihypertensive efficacy is due to homeostatic mechanisms, such as an increase in norepinephrine and renin release. These mechanisms can be blocked by sympatholytic drugs, thus acute therapy with a diuretic and sympatholytic drugs can rapidly lower blood pressure.

Loop Diuretics

Loop diuretics such as furosemide are more effective natriuretic agents than the thiazides. Furosemide decreases blood volume but not peripheral resistance. Rather, it elicits a reflex increase in sympathetic nervous activity and in renin release (42, 80), which may increase peripheral resistance. If a vasodilator or sympatholytic is given to diminish peripheral resistance, the combined effects may adequately decrease blood pressure. Furosemide is useful for patients with renal insufficiency or for those who have fluid retention. Patients with malignant hypertension are often volume-depleted, and loop diuretics may impair tissue perfusion and worsen vasospasm. Potent diuretics may be essential to combat the fluid-retaining effects of other potent antihypertensive medications. Many patients develop a photosensitivity dermatitis in response to furosemide and the thiazides. Ethacrynic acid and bumetanide are useful alternatives for these patients.

β-BLOCKING DRUGS

β-Blocking drugs lower blood pressure by several mechanisms. Cardiac output is promptly reduced, but increased peripheral resistance compensates for this. Days to weeks later, peripheral resistance diminishes, almost reaching pretreatment values, and blood pressure decreases. The β-blocking drugs inhibit renin secretion and lower blood pressure more in high-renin patients than in those with low renin (11), but these agents still have some hypotensive effect in low-renin patients. The β-blockers may alter prostaglandin levels in vascular tissue, and indomethacin can diminish some of their hypotensive effects (31). In animals, the β-blocking drugs enhance the central release of norepinephrine, which diminishes peripheral sympathetic tone. They also increase baroreflex sensitivity (66). β-Blocking drugs diminish cardiac output and renin release; they may alter blood pressure through interactions with prostaglandins and by central nervous system effects, but it is unclear how important these latter mechanisms are.

The effectiveness of β-blocker therapy depends on the patient's age, race, and renin status, and how recent the onset of hypertension. Patients with high plasma renin levels have the greatest hypotensive response to β-blocker therapy. Although this effect is statistically significant, it is not sufficiently striking to justify the use of renin-sodium classification in individual hypertensives (94). Both cardiac chronotropic and inotropic responsiveness to β stimulation diminishes with age (90), and β blockade has less of a cardiac effect in the elderly than in the young. The net effect is that β-blocking drugs work less well to lower blood pressure in the elderly than in the young, but can be more dangerous in the elderly since they may accentuate heart block and lung disease. In contrast, young patients with the recent onset of hypertension tend to have a hyperdynamic cardiac output and have hypertension based more on increased cardiac output than on increased peripheral resistance. These young hypertensives respond very well to β blockade (23).

Black hypertensives respond poorly to β blockade. A group of black patients who had a decrease in mean blood pressure of 14 mm Hg with diuretic therapy had only a 5 mm Hg blood pressure decrease in response to β blockade (27). Hollifield and associates (28) reported that when low-dose propranolol fails to work, doses in the range of 320–960 mg/day diminish blood pressure. However, other investigators found that 80 mg of propranolol per day was as effective as 480 mg/day. It is not clear whether extremely high doses of β-blockers provide any additional hypotensive effect, but they do increase side effects and cost. β-Blocking drugs differ in their receptor affinity and pharmacokinetic properties (Table 20.2). Propranolol has a half-life of only 3–6 hours, but its effect persists with one daily dosing (83), with fewer nighttime side effects.

Propranolol blocks both β_1- and β_2-adrenergic receptors. The β_1-receptors mediate cardiac effects and β_2-receptors mediate bronchodilation and arteriolar dilation. A variety of other effects, including renin release, are influenced by both types of receptors (Table 20.3). Atenolol and acebutolol are β_1-selective and thus are less likely to block β-adrenergic bronchodilation or vasodilation. Their cardioselectivity is not absolute, however, and in the higher dose range these agents can cause bronchoconstriction. When a β-blocking agent is necessary in the treatment of a patient with bronchospasm or a diabetic receiving insulin (17), β_1-selective agents are safer than nonselective agents. However, β-blocking drugs should not be used at all in these patients unless absolutely necessary. Atenolol and me-

Table 20.2
Properties of β-Blocking Drugs

Generic name	Propranolol	Atenolol	Metoprolol	Nadolol	Pindolol	Timolol	Acebutolol	Labetalol
Brand name	Inderal	Tenormin	Lopressor	Corgard	Visken	Blocadren	Sectral	Trandate
Oral bioavailability (%)	30	40	50	30	90	75	40	25
Dose in hypertension (mg)	80–640	50–100	100–450	80–320	15–60	20–60	200–1200	200–2400
Variation in plasma levels between patients	20×	4×	10×	7×	4×	7×	7×	7×
Protein bound (%)	93	<5	12	30	60	10	25	50
Half-life (hr)	3–6	6–9	3–4	14–24	3–4	3–4	3–13	6–8
Fat solubility	+	0	±	0	±	0	0	+
Route of elimination	Liver	Kidney	Liver	Kidney	Kidney and liver	Liver	Kidney and liver	Kidney and liver
Membrane-stabilizing effect	+ +	0	±	0	+	0	+	+
Cardioselectivity	0	+	+	0	0	0	+	0
Intrinsic sympathomimetic activity	0	0	0	0	+ +	±	+	0
Active metabolites	+	0	0	0	0	0	+	0
Potency (relative)	10	10	10	10	60	60	5	2

Table 20.3
α-Adrenergic and β-Adrenergic Responses

Organ	Effect[a]	α	β_1	β_1 and β_2	β_2
Blood vessels	Constricts arterioles and venules	+	0		0
	Dilates arterioles (especially in skeletal muscle)	0	0		+
Heart	↑ Rate of S-A node discharge	0	+		0
	↑ Contractility	0	+		0
	↑ Conduction velocity	0	+		0
Lungs	Dilates bronchial muscles	0	0		+
Gastrointestinal tract	↓ Peristalsis	+		+	
Metabolic effects	Lipolysis	0		+	
	↓ Insulin release	+		0	
	↑ Insulin release	0		+	
	↑ Formation of cAMP	0		+	
	↑ Fasting blood sugar	±		+	
	↑ Renin secretion			+	

[a] S-A, sinoatrial; cAMP, cyclic AMP.

toprolol can be successfully used with β_2-agonist agents.

β-Blocking drugs also differ in their fat solubility and rate of elimination (Table 20.2). Atenolol and nadolol are not soluble in fat and are not extensively metabolized by the liver. They do not undergo a "first pass" metabolism by the liver as rapidly as more lipophilic agents. Their longer half-lives allow once daily dosing, but the dose needs to be adjusted in renal failure because these drugs are excreted by the kidneys. Nonlipophilic agents do not penetrate the brain very effectively. Although several β-blocking drugs impair renal perfusion during treatment of hypertension, nadolol lowers blood pressure without impairing glomerular filtration rate or renal blood flow (65). The decrease in renal blood flow with most β-blocking agents is too small to elevate serum creatinine or urea and is usually neglected in clinical practice. Most side effects of the different β-blocking agents are similar. In a study of 10,000 patients, propranolol worsened exercise tolerance dyspnea. It tended to cause nausea and rhinorrhea early in therapy and cold hands later in therapy (58). Rhinorrhea and Raynaud's phenomenon may be less of a problem with cardioselective β-blocking drugs, and central nervous system side effects may be less frequent with nonlipophilic agents.

People metabolize β-blockers at very different rates, and dosage must be adjusted by clinical response. If heart rate slows and the increment in heart rate decreases when the patient is standing, β blockade is effective. As shown in Table 20.2, the variation in plasma levels with the same dose of drug is greatest with propranolol and tends to be less with agents that are excreted by the kidney than those that are metabolized by the liver.

The first β-blocker synthesized was dichloroisoproterenol. It was a partial β-agonist and was not used in humans because of its β-receptor stimulant activity. Pindolol and acebutolol have sympathomimetic activity since they are partial agonists as well. They do not decrease resting heart rate but antagonize the increase in heart rate with exercise. Pindolol has the most intrinsic sympathomimetic activity and is unlikely to cause heart block or bradycardia. It may cause angina in a patient abruptly changed from another β-blocker to pindolol, because of its stimulant activity. Acebutolol has less intrinsic sympathomimetic activity and usually does not change heart rate (84).

The available β-blocking agents differ in their pharmacokinetic profile and in their β_1 selectivity. There is no convincing evidence that any of these agents is either more effective or associated with fewer side effects in the average hypertensive patient. However, in particular patients there is some clear advantage to specific agents—cardioselectivity is an advantage for patients with bronchospasm or those who tend to develop cold hands or Raynaud's phenomenon. These drugs can also be used with β_2-agonist bronchodilators, and are the drugs of choice when a β-blocker must be used in a patient with impaired respiratory function. The longer half-life of nadolol and atenolol may be important when these agents are used in the treatment of angina pectoris, but shorter acting drugs, such as propranolol, seem equally effective for the treatment of hypertension when given once daily.

β-Blocking drugs should not be withdrawn abruptly in patients with angina pectoris. Patients treated with β-blockers for hypertension can develop a reproducible hyperadrenergic withdrawal syndrome when β-blockers are stopped abruptly (70). Twenty-four hours after drug withdrawal, blood pressure and heart rate may rise. These symptoms increase to a maximum at 48 hours and disappear by 7 days. This syndrome is mediated by an increased sensitivity of β-receptors. Longer-lasting agents, such as atenolol and nadolol, or agents with intrinsic sympathomimetic activity, such as pindolol and acebutolol, may be less likely to cause the syndrome.

Labetalol is a nonspecific β-blocking drug that also possesses some α-blocking activity. Other β-blocking drugs initially increase peripheral vascular resistance, but this increased resistance is prevented by the α-blocking activity of labetalol. This quality makes labetalol useful for the acute therapy of severe hypertension. The drug may be given by slow intravenous injection in initial doses of 2.5–5 mg. The intravenous dose may be increased to 20 mg, 40 mg, then 80 mg, or by infusion at 2 mg/ min up to a total dose of 300 mg or until blood pressure is controlled. The patient can then be maintained on 100–1200 mg of labetalol twice daily.

After intravenous injection of labetalol, symptomatic postural hypotension is common. In chronic use the drug possesses the side effects of β- and α-blockers and may cause nausea. However, labetalol is more effective than other β-blockers in lowering blood pressure, and its effects are potentiated by diuretics (60).

α-ADRENERGIC CONTROL OF BLOOD PRESSURE

The antihypertensive drugs methyldopa, clonidine, guanabenz, prazosin, phenoxybenzamine, and phentolamine all act on α-adrenergic receptors. Their hypotensive effect is most easily understood in terms of their effects on various types of α-receptors with differing anatomic distribution. The α_1- and α_2-receptors (commonly referred to as postsynaptic and presynaptic receptors) can be distinguished by their affinity for various drugs (Table 20.4). Epinephrine and norepinephrine stimulate, whereas phentolamine and phenoxybenzamine block, both types of receptors. However, newer drugs, such as prazosin or clonidine, can selectively block α_1-receptors or stimulate α_2-receptors. Because of their specificity, these agents cause fewer side effects than nonspecific drugs. The drugs can be classified by receptor binding affinities or physiologic effect, and these classifications are in agreement.

In the vasculature, α-receptors near noradrenergic nerve terminals are usually of the α_1 type, whereas receptors distant from these terminals, but accessible to circulating catecholamines, are of the α_2 type. α-Receptors in the brain are predominantly of the α_2 type, although all adrenergically innervated organs have both types of receptor.

Presynaptic α_2-adrenergic receptors on sympathetic nerve terminals inhibit the release of norepinephrine (46). When α_2-receptors on the nerves are stimulated, they antagonize calcium influx and enhance calcium efflux, thereby inhibiting further release of norepinephrine. These presynaptic α_2-receptors inhibit norepinephrine release from nerves in the periphery and in the brain. α_2-Receptors in the brain are also located postsynaptically, and postsynap-

Table 20.4
Relative Binding Affinity of Drugs for α_1- and α_2-Receptors

	Agonists	Antagonists	
α_2 ↑	Guanfacine Guanabenz Clonidine α-Methylnorepinephrine Epinephrine	Yohimbine	α_2 ↑
α_1 and α_2 ↓	Norepinephrine	Phentolamine Phenoxybenzamine	α_1 and α_2 ↓
α_1	Phenylephrine Methoxamine	Labetalol Prazosin	α_1

tic α-receptors mediate the central antihypertensive actions of clonidine and methyldopa (37).

There are two possible ways that α_2-receptors might lower blood pressure in humans. The stimulation of peripheral α-receptors inhibits norepinephrine release from sympathetic nerves (46), and stimulation of central α_2-receptors diminishes peripheral sympathetic nervous electrical activity. The central action is by far the more important and because of this central mode of action, clonidine-like drugs have central side effects such as sedation.

In general, peripheral α_1-receptors mediate vasoconstriction and peripheral α_2-receptors inhibit norepinephrine release. Central α_2-receptors depress sympathetic nervous activity and enhance vagal activity. Drugs that stimulate α_2-receptors or block α_1-receptors lower blood pressure and can do so with fewer side effects than nonspecific agents.

Prazosin

Because prazosin is structurally related to papaverine and to cyclic nucleotides, it was first thought to act as a vasodilator. However, it fails to vasodilate vasculature that is not stimulated by α-agonists, such as norepinephrine. Prazosin preferentially blocks α_1-receptors, and this blockade is responsible for its antihypertensive efficacy. The α-blocking agents, phenoxybenzamine and phentolamine, are of little use in treating hypertension because they nonselectively block both α_1- and α_2-receptors. The nonselective blockade of α_2-receptors enhances norepinephrine release, which causes tachycardia and increases renin release. In contrast, prazosin causes little or no heart rate increase in humans and may lower plasma renin activity. Prazosin does not affect presynaptic α_2-receptors, and allows them to inhibit norepinephrine release normally. Prazosin does not decrease cardiac output, but lowers blood pressure by reducing systemic vascular resistance. Prazosin and clonidine are no more effective in combination than clonidine alone (64).

Prazosin is readily absorbed from the gastrointestinal tract, and peak plasma levels occur between 1 and 3 hours after oral administration. The drug is metabolized primarily in the liver, and hepatic inactivation of the compound is so effective that there is a "first pass" clearance of almost 60% of the drug. This first pass clearance of prazosin is markedly diminished in uremic patients (25), thus very small doses of prazosin (approximately one-third the usual dose) are effective in renal failure.

In treating hypertension, prazosin may be used by itself, with a diuretic, or with multiple antihypertensive agents. When used alone, the antihypertensive efficacy of chronically administered prazosin may diminish because fluid retention leads to an increased plasma volume. However, some observers have noted a 6- to 8-week delay before prazosin affects diastolic pressure demonstrably (62). Alone, it is less effective than methyldopa (6), but prazosin's effect is almost doubled when used in conjunction with thiazide diuretics. The combination of prazosin with methyldopa, clonidine, or propranolol may not be particularly effective, however (41).

As might be expected from its α-blocking activities, prazosin is extremely effective in the treatment of hypertension due to pheochromocytoma (86). Prazosin rapidly lowers blood pressure when given to patients with untreated severe hypertension, although the hypotensive effect in this setting may be extreme and unpredictable. The "first dose effect" is the major side effect of prazosin. When first taken, there may be a massive pooling of blood in the venous system as a consequence of abrupt α blockade, and an abrupt lowering of blood pressure with severe postural hypotension (13). This complication is dose-related, and in a group of 74 hypertensive patients initially treated with a 2-mg dose of prazosin, two patients experienced syncope and 10 others had significant symptoms of postural hypotension (75). First dose syncope can be avoided by withholding diuretics the day before the first dose and administering a 1-mg capsule at bed time (79). The dose of prazosin may then be gradually increased to a maximum of 10 mg twice daily; doses beyond this range do not worsen side effects, but also do not increase antihypertensive efficacy. The postural hypotension from prazosin during chronic therapy is more severe than that seen with methyldopa or propranolol, but usually does not cause symptoms. Other side effects are mild and uncommon. Prazosin is devoid of CNS side effects.

Prazosin preserves renal blood flow and glomerular filtration (67) and is effective at low doses in patients with renal disease. The drug may cause bronchodilation, decrease serum cholesterol and triglyceride levels, and increase the ratio of high density lipoprotein cholesterol to low density lipoprotein cholesterol. These effects contrast with those of propranolol, which diminishes renal blood flow and causes bronchoconstriction and hyperlipidemia. The combination of prazosin and propranolol results in a partial amelioration of propranolol's effects on cholesterol and triglyceride levels.

In summary, prazosin is an antihypertensive agent with a unique mode of action. It is not as effective when used by itself as the thiazide diuretics or methyldopa, but is effective in combination with thiazides. Its unique mode of action makes it an effective drug in patients who may not tolerate other antihypertensive agents, since it may improve bronchospasm and lower cholesterol. Prazosin is nearly devoid of CNS side effects and appears to have no effect on sexual potency. The drug is particularly effective in patients with pheochromocytoma, and a prolonged response to prazosin should make one suspicious of the presence of this tumor.

Phenoxybenzamine

Phenoxybenzamine is an α-blocking drug that differs from phentolamine in being more specific for α-receptors and blocking them noncompetitively. Phenoxybenzamine is also a potent antihistamine and has a fairly weak effect on serotonin and acetylcholine receptors, but its important clinical effects are almost all related to its α-blocking activity. It is chemically related to the nitrogen mustards and has a tertiary amine that cyclizes to form a reactive intermediate molecule. This reactive intermediate is the active form of the drug and must be made to bind with α-adrenergic receptors. Phenoxybenzamine has a relatively slow onset of action, and peak effect is not attained until 1 hour after intravenous administration because of the time required for the formation of the reactive intermediate. The α-adrenergic blockade has a half-life of about 1 day, and the effects may be observable for 1 week after the drug is discontinued. This prolonged duration of action is most likely due to the requirement for synthesis of new α-receptors to replace those covalently bound to the drug. Phenoxybenzamine also inhibits the uptake of catecholamines into nerves and extraneuronal tissue.

Phenoxybenzamine blocks feedback mechanisms, increases the rate of turnover of nor-

epinephrine, and increases the amount of norepinephrine released by each nerve impulse by blocking presynaptic α_2-receptors (77). The most striking physiologic effect is a reflex tachycardia, the result of lower blood pressure, enhanced release of norepinephrine, and decreased inactivation of norepinephrine. Impaired venoconstriction causes postural hypotension, which becomes more pronounced during exercise or other vasodilating activities. Although phenoxybenzamine effectively lowers blood pressure, reflex responses to hypotension limit its clinical usefulness. The drug can reverse the pressor effects of epinephrine by blocking its α-adrenergic effects and leaving β effects unopposed. Because of this, phenoxybenzamine can cause hypotension during stress. The drug exaggerates the vasodepressor effects of opiates and vasodilators by preventing compensatory vasoconstriction. The α blockade also leads to miosis, nasal stuffiness, and inhibition of ejaculation. It has CNS effects that include a characteristic loss of time perception, and in high doses causes nausea, vomiting, hyperventilation, and even convulsions. Lower doses cause sedation and fatigue, but it is not clear if α-blocking activity induces these CNS effects since they develop and terminate more rapidly than does the peripheral α blockade.

The major use of phenoxybenzamine is for treating hypertension caused by pheochromocytoma. Prazosin may be an equally useful α-blocker in this setting, but there is less clinical experience with prazosin. Phenoxybenzamine is available for oral use in 10-mg capsules; the intravenous form is available only by special arrangement with the manufacturer.

Phentolamine and Tolazoline

Phentolamine competitively blocks both α_1- and α_2-receptors. Its effects are most dramatic in patients with a pheochromocytoma. However, adequate doses of the drug have hemodynamic effects in almost all individuals. The blockade of vascular receptors causes vasodilation of arterioles and veins, with a prompt decrease in peripheral resistance and a fall in blood pressure. The blockade of α_2-receptors on adrenergic nerve terminals disinhibits norepinephrine release, which stimulates β-adrenergic receptors. This β stimulation can cause tachycardia, arrhythmias, and angina. The drug probably also has nonspecific effects on serotonin, histamine, and acetylcholine receptors, which frequently lead to gastrointestinal stimulation and occasionally stimulate salivary, lachrymal, respiratory tract, and pancreatic secretions.

Phentolamine is available in 50-mg oral tablets but is most frequently used in parenteral form, supplied in 5-mg ampules. An injected 5-mg dose dramatically decreases blood pressure in patients with pheochromocytoma or clonidine withdrawal.

Tolazoline is chemically and pharmacologically related to phentolamine. It is used in the treatment of clonidine overdose, since it blocks the α-receptors that are stimulated by clonidine and penetrates the central nervous system more easily than does phentolamine. The side effects of tolazoline are similar to those of phentolamine, but tend to be more severe since it is less specific for α-receptors than is phentolamine.

Clonidine, Guanfacine, and Guanabenz

Clonidine stimulates α_2-receptors, and its presynaptic action inhibits norepinephrine release in both the brain and peripheral sympathetic nervous systems. Its main hypotensive action is through stimulation of α_2-receptors in the vasomotor centers of the medulla oblongata, particularly at the nucleus tractus solitarius. This α_2 stimulation decreases sympathetic activity, increases vagal stimulation, and lowers plasma norepinephrine, epinephrine, and renin release (61). Even in the presence of β-blocking drugs, clonidine further lowers heart rate by enhancing vagal activity.

Since the primary mode of action of clonidine is through the central nervous system, the drug must penetrate the CNS in order to have its hypotensive effects. Intravenously administered clonidine transiently increases blood pressure, with a subsequent fall in blood pressure that is maximal at 20 minutes but persists for many hours. The pressor phase is not seen when clonidine is given orally since peak blood levels are not reached until 90 minutes after ingestion. Glomerular filtration rate is usually decreased and sodium excretion is considerably and acutely reduced. Over longer-term therapy, sodium retention tends to occur only at the higher dose ranges.

Clonidine increases cerebral vascular resistance and decreases cerebral blood flow (47). These physiologic changes are associated with a fall in resting blood pressure, but reflex control of capacitance vessels is intact, which helps maintain cardiac output during exercise.

Cardiac index, heart rate, and blood pressure increase normally with the drug during exercise. Renal blood flow is maintained because of a reduction in renal vascular resistance, but glomerular filtration rate may decrease. Clonidine has a small direct effect on the kidney, but decreases renin by its central actions.

After acute oral administration of clonidine, peak blood levels occur in 90 minutes. The drug is about 75% bioavailable, with a half-life of 8 hours. Sixty percent of the drug is cleared unchanged by the kidney. The hypotensive effect of clonidine and its side effects of sedation and dry mouth follow plasma levels very closely during acute therapy (16). With longer-term treatment, rate of absorption and half-life are unchanged and clonidine blood levels are still closely related to the decline in blood pressure. Clonidine's depressant effect on sympathetic nervous activity persists, and plasma norepinephrine levels and plasma renin activity remain low with chronic therapy. Some of clonidine's central effects may occur via release of β-endorphin (40). Naloxone reverses the antihypertensive effect of clonidine in laboratory animals and in some, but not all, human subjects. Although clonidine is used clinically in conjuction with β-blocking drugs, there is evidence that β-blockers that penetrate the CNS, such as propranolol, may interfere with the antihypertensive effects of clonidine (24). β-Blockers may also be dangerous in clonidine withdrawal. Sedation and dry mouth are inevitable side effects of clonidine and are a direct result of central α_2 stimulation. Although many people find the sedative effects of a nighttime dose of clonidine pleasant, it produces a dose-dependent inhibition of paradoxical sleep, which may be related to nighttime hallucinations and dementia when clonidine is given to the elderly (9). Sympathetic nervous activity and blood pressure decrease during sleep, and clonidine further lowers sympathetic activity and blood pressure at night (52).

Clonidine progressively lowers blood pressure with increasing dose up to 0.8 mg daily, but beyond this dose range it has a U-shaped dose-response curve. In the range of 1.2–1.6 mg daily, clonidine begins to increase blood pressure as its peripheral vasoconstrictor effects override its central hypotensive effects (72). Although the hypotensive effect diminishes with increasing dosage, sedation and dry mouth become more troublesome. When patients receiving high doses of clonidine abruptly discontinue their medication, a withdrawal syndrome begins about 18 hours later. They suffer insomnia, headache, flushing, sweating, apprehension, and tremulousness. Sympathetic nervous activity increases, and plasma norepinephrine levels and blood pressure are elevated above pretreatment levels. Symptoms are most marked 24–72 hours after clonidine is withdrawn, but then subside spontaneously (72). The withdrawal syndrome is most severe in patients taking more than 1.2 mg clonidine daily (8) and seems particularly likely to occur postoperatively (7, 8). The patient with tremulousness, tachycardia, and hypertension, may be treated with a β-blocker, but this approach may only exaggerate the hypertension by providing unopposed α-adrenergic vasoconstriction from the increased norepinephrine release. A patient receiving both clonidine and a β-blocker who stops taking just the clonidine becomes susceptible to severe hypertension during the withdrawal syndrome. The clonidine withdrawal syndrome only rarely occurs at doses of less than 0.3 mg daily, but patients receiving doses higher than this should be cautioned not to stop the drug abruptly.

Oral clonidine has been recommended for treating severe hypertension (2) in a dose of 0.2 mg initially followed by 0.1 mg hourly. Since clonidine acutely decreases cardiac output and cerebral blood flow, there are some theoretical objections to the safety of this procedure, but the clinical experience has been favorable.

Guanabenz, like clonidine, stimulates α_2-receptors and has blood pressure–lowering effects and similar side effects. Guanabenz's half-life of 6 hours is short, and it can cause a withdrawal syndrome similar to that of clonidine. Clinical reports suggest that guanabenz withdrawal is not as severe as clonidine withdrawal. Guanabenz is given in a dose of 4–32 mg twice daily, but the highest doses may cause a pressor response and severe side effects, similar to the action of high doses of clonidine.

Guanfacine was recently released in the United States. It has a relatively long half-life of 16 hours, which permits once daily dosing of 1–3 mg with effective control of blood pressure. The longer half-life should also diminish the severity of withdrawal from the drug.

α-Methyldopa

α-Methyldopa is metabolized to an α_2-agonist with actions similar to those of clonidine.

Only about one-fourth of methyldopa is absorbed unchanged since it is metabolized in the gut wall and in the liver before gaining access to the systemic circulation. The drug is enzymatically converted to active metabolities (Fig. 20.1), and inhibitors of the enzymes dopa-decarboxylase and dopamine-β-hydroxylase prevent its hypotensive effects. Methyldopa is converted to α-methyldopamine, then to α-methylnorepinephrine, a potent agonist at α_2-receptors (Fig. 20.1). α-methylnorepinephrine is stored in nerve endings and released by nerve stimulation. When formation of α-methylnorepinephrine is blocked, α-methyldopa fails to lower blood pressure. Several hours may elapse after methyldopa is given before enough metabolite is formed to lower blood pressure. Since the body stores this active metabolite, the effect of an oral dose persists for as long as 24 hours, even though the half-time of elimination for plasma α-methyldopa is about 2 hours. The O-methylated metabolites of methyldopa may also contribute to its hypotensive action (Fig. 20.1).

Methyldopa metabolites stimulate α_2-receptors, causing side effects similar to those of clonidine. Acute doses of methyldopa impair

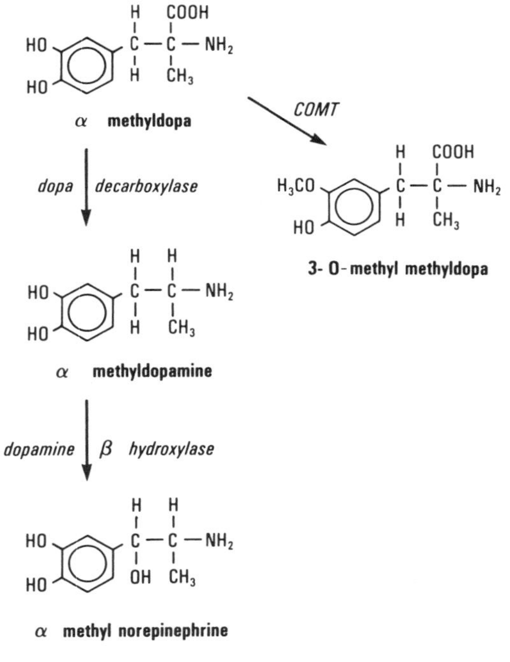

Figure 20.1. The metabolic conversion of methyldopa to its active metabolites. The metabolic enzymes are those normally involved in the production and degradation of norepinephrine. *COMT*, catechol-*O*-methyltransferase.

judgment (3) and depress behavior. The drug causes hypothermia and prolactin secretion. In contrast to clonidine, it increases rapid eye movement sleep in humans and causes less dry mouth and bradycardia than clonidine. Methyldopa also has important immunologic side effects. Twenty-five percent of patients taking 1 g of methyldopa daily for 6 months develop a positive direct Coombs' test. The drug stimulates production of an IgG antibody directed at the red cell membrane and not reacting with methyldopa itself. The positive Coombs' test is not a contraindication to continuation of therapy; however, in somewhat under 25% of individuals with a positive Coombs' test, a hemolytic anemia occurs. It sometimes causes drug fever or hepatic dysfunction. Rebound hypertension can occur after abrupt withdrawal of methyldopa (12), but this rebound is much rarer than with clonidine.

Both methyldopa and clonidine lower blood pressure by stimulating central α_2-receptors. This central action diminishes sympathetic nervous activity and increases vagal activity and sedation. The agents differ in that the effective half-life of methyldopa is much longer than that of clonidine, and there is less danger of hypertension on rapid withdrawal of the drug. However, methyldopa has occasional severe immunologic side effects that are not seen with clonidine. Guanfacine combines the long duration of action of methyldopa with the lack of immunologic side effects of clonidine.

The α_2-agonists can increase blood pressure when given in doses high enough to stimulate peripheral vasoconstriction. They should not be given in higher than recommended doses. Methyldopa, clonidine, guanabenz, and guanfacine should not be given in combination since their α_2-stimulating activities may be additive.

VASODILATORS

Vasodilators increase blood flow to vital organs, such as the brain and kidney; their peripheral mode of action avoids CNS side effects. When used properly, vasodilators are potent hypotensive agents. Some of these drugs can lower blood pressure to normal even in patients with hypertension that is resistant to all other modes of therapy.

The vasodilating activity of these drugs leads to predictable side effects. Hydralazine, minoxidil, and diazoxide dilate the precapillary arterioles with little effect on postcapillary circulation or capacitance vessels. Nitroprusside

has a balanced effect, dilating both arterioles and veins; the nitrates, such as nitroglycerin, are primarily venodilators. The arterial vasodilators lower blood pressure by allowing a relatively unimpeded flow of blood through the arterial circulation. Since capacitance vessels are not dilated, this blood returns promptly to the heart. The lower blood pressure reflexly increases sympathetic tone to the heart. Increased blood return to the heart and increased sympathetic stimulation cause a tachycardia and a greater cardiac output. The patient may experience these combined effects as a racing heart beat with palpitations, a pounding headache, and rushing vascular noises in the head. All of these cardiac manifestations of unopposed arterial vasodilation can be blocked by the β-blocking drugs or methyldopa or clonidine.

Although the vasodilators tend to increase renal blood flow, they cause sodium retention. This problem is particularly prominent with diazoxide, which has an intrinsic antinatriuretic effect, and with minoxidil. These agents cause a redistribution in renal blood flow, a decrease in perfusion pressure to the kidney, and an increase in renal renin output. Diuretics and sympatholytic agents that lower renin output can counteract these effects.

Blood pressure lowering with vasodilators has several major advantages. These agents counteract hypertensive vasoconstriction, preserve renal and cerebral blood flow, and are effective antihypertensives. However, the side effects of the arterial vasodilators prevent them from being used alone and they should be combined with a sympatholytic and a diuretic.

Hydralazine

Hydralazine is available for both parenteral and oral administration. The drug is extensively metabolized by the liver. After oral administration, bioavailability may be low because of first pass metabolism in the liver. Hepatic acetylation is a major route of metabolism and rapid acetylators have about 30% bioavailability of the drug, compared with 50% bioavailability in slow acetylators. The plasma elimination half-time of hydralazine is about 4 hours, but plasma hydralazine levels correlate poorly with antihypertensive efficacy, probably because the agent is directly bound to arterioles at its site of action. Although the drug's circulating half-life is about 3 hours, the half-time of its effect on blood pressure is about 100 hours (68). As a result, the drug is as effective when given twice a day as when given four times a day (68).

Hydralazine acts by vasodilation, which is most marked in the splanchnic, coronary, cerebral, and renal vasculature. Blood flow does not increase in skin or muscle, however. The antihypertensive potency of hydralazine is severely limited by a reflex increase in cardiac output and fluid retention. β-Blocking drugs that diminish the reflex increase in plasma renin activity are synergistic with hydralazine, and it is possible to devise a careful regimen of diuretic, β-blocker, and hydralazine that can markedly lower blood pressure with minimal side effects (96).

Although symptomatic side effects elicited by use of hydralazine can be combated with a diuretic and β-blocker, other side effects idiosyncratic to the drug cannot be blocked. A drug-induced lupus-like syndrome occurs in 10–20% of patients who receive prolonged therapy in doses exceeding 400 mg daily. This syndrome occurs more rarely at doses in the range of 200 mg/day and manifests primarily in caucasians who eliminate the drug slowly because of their acetylation phenotype. This lupus-like syndrome is reversible when the drug is withdrawn and is characterized by joint pain with skin rash; renal toxicity is infrequent. It can also cause drug fever. A peripheral neuropathy may occur, which can be corrected with pyridoxine, probably because the drug binds with this vitamin (38).

Hydralazine is available for intravenous or intramuscular injection. The usual parenteral dose is 10–40 mg, but response is quite variable and its effects develop gradually over 15–20 minutes after intravenous administration. Hydralazine is available for oral use in tablets of 10, 25, 50 and 100 mg. It is usually started in low doses so that the side effects of tachycardia and fluid retention can be combated with sympatholytics and diuretics before they become severe.

Minoxidil

Minoxidil is an extremely effective vasodilator with actions similar to those of hydralazine. However, the agent is more efficacious and more potent than hydralazine and causes different side effects.

Ninety percent of an orally administered dose of minoxidil is absorbed; 85% of the drug is metabolized by the liver and 15% is excreted unchanged in the kidney. The plasma half-life of minoxidil is approximately 4 hours, but it is effective for over 24 hours, probably because it is retained by vascular smooth muscle (49). The maximum effect of the drug is apparent 6 hours after an oral dose.

The ultimate dose of minoxidil required to control hypertension is extremely varied, and therapy should be begun with a small dose, such as 2½ or 5 mg. This dose may then be doubled every 6 hours as the maximum effect of the prior dose becomes apparent, until blood pressure control is obtained. The effective dose can then be administered every 12–24 hours. As with hydralazine, minoxidil must always be administered with a diuretic and a sympatholytic agent, such as a β-blocker or clonidine. The drug is presently approved only for therapy of hypertension resistant to other avenues of treatment. Minoxidil is effective in renal failure, and has successfully controlled blood pressure in patients with severe hypertension and end-stage renal disease.

Minoxidil's potent vasodilating effects can elicit marked hemodynamic responses. The sympathetic nervous system is activated to such a degree that plasma catecholamine levels may mimic those seen in patients with a pheochromocytoma (59). This sympathetic nervous activation stimulates renin secretion, and the vasoconstrictor effects of norepinephrine and angiotensin II diminish the hypotensive effects of minoxidil unless blocked with a sympatholytic. The renal tubules avidly retain sodium in the patient treated with minoxidil although glomerular filtration is not changed. Early in the course of therapy, even patients given large doses of furosemide may retain sodium. This fluid retention may be overcome by combining furosemide with a thiazide diuretic or metolazone, and with subsequent therapy fluid retention is less avid. It is sometimes necessary to lower the dose of minoxidil to effect a diuresis in patients who have some degree of renal insufficiency.

Minoxidil causes hypertrichosis (excessive hair growth involving the face, arms, and legs), which occurs in most patients several weeks to months after the drug is instituted and sometimes takes up to 6 months to disappear after the drug is stopped. Many women find this side effect intolerable. Pathologic lesions of the heart have been reported in two animal studies using minoxidil, but no such lesions have been reported in humans. Pulmonary hypertension has been reported during treatment with minoxidil, but there have also been reports of decreased pulmonary vascular resistance during therapy. Pericardial effusion occasionally progressing to pericardial tamponade has been described in patients receiving minoxidil, but these effects usually occur in those who have congestive heart failure or renal failure. Approximately 2% of patients treated with this drug show no response, even to a large dose (91). In 98% of hypertensives, minoxidil is one of the most effective drugs available.

Diazoxide

Diazoxide is chemically related to the thiazide diuretics, but it causes fluid retention rather than a natriuresis. Thiazide diuretics have a minor vasodilating effect, but diazoxide is a very effective vasodilator. Diazoxide directly dilates arterioles but has little effect on large veins, although it can dilate the small postcapillary resistance vessels. Diazoxide is usually given by rapid intravenous injection for the treatment of hypertension, and when given by this route, 90% of the drug is eventually bound to albumin and about one-third of the drug is cleared through the kidneys. The serum half-life of diazoxide is about 30 hours because it binds to albumin, and in patients with impaired renal function, the half-life increases proportionately. Diazoxide tends to accumulate with repeated administration, but there is no correlation between the total serum concentration and the intensity of its hypotensive action, because the hypotensive effects depend on the concentration of drug in the arterioles. Since the drug binds to both albumin and the arterioles, competition occurs between these sites and only the drug in the arterioles has a hypotensive effect. As a result, if a bolus of the drug is injected rapidly, it can reach arteriolar sites more effectively than when given slowly and its hypotensive usefulness is more beneficial and dramatic. When given this way, maximum hypotensive effect is attained in 3–5 minutes. Fifty to 150 mg of the drug can be given as a bolus, injected over 30 seconds or less. If the patient has already received a diuretic and a β-blocker, the drug may be given by slow intravenous infusion.

Diazoxide increases cardiac output and causes sympathetic stimulation and fluid retention. Its effects can be greatly potentiated by sympatholytic agents or diuresis. If the patient is volume-depleted or receiving a sympatholytic agent, the dose of diazoxide must be reduced to avoid hypotension. There are other side effects characteristic of this agent. Cerebral blood flow is diminished (69) and the drug may cause extrapyramidal symptoms with prolonged use (63). It inhibits release of insulin from the pancreas, thereby raising blood glucose levels. In patients with diabetes mellitus or renal failure, treatment of the hyperglycemia may become necessary in a few days. Diazoxide suppresses tubular transport of uric acid and leads to hyperuricemia, as do the other thiazides. Since the drug binds strongly to albumin, it displaces warfarin anticoagulants.

In clinical practice, the side effects of diazoxide are usually relatively minor and its ease of use is one of its major advantages. In contrast to nitroprusside, diazoxide can be given in hypertensive emergencies to a patient who is not on continuous blood pressure monitoring, because its maximum effect is reached at 5 minutes and blood pressure gradually returns to pretreatment level within 5–12 hours. This allows time to introduce other antihypertensive therapies that can be maintained over a longer period. The drug should not be used alone when cardiac stimulation may be deleterious, such as in patients with severe coronary artery disease or aortic dissection. In most patients with severe hypertension, diazoxide can successfully lower blood pressure without the need for continuous monitoring.

Sodium Nitroprusside

Sodium nitroprusside's hypotensive capability has been recognized for 50 years, but it was little used until it was commercially marketed and promoted as Nipride. Its hypotensive effect is probably due to the iron-nitroso (Fe-NO) grouping in the intact nitroprusside molecule; the drug causes both venous and arterial vasodilation, as do the nitrates. This balanced vascular dilation, which includes venous capacitance vessels, gives nitroprusside a spectrum of effect slightly different from that of the other vasodilators. The venodilation results in a decreased cardiac preload instead of the increased preload seen with the "pure" arterial vasodilators. In the absence of heart failure, cardiac output either falls or does not change in response to nitroprusside. However, if myocardial disease has diminished cardiac output, nitroprusside may increase output as a result of diminished afterload. Nitroprusside usually causes a 20–30% increase in heart rate, but if there is a preexisting tachycardia due to heart failure, heart rate may actually decrease slightly. The decreased preload may diminish cardiac work, and angina often improves when nitroprusside is given; this finding is in contrast to the "pure" arterial vasodilators, which may cause myocardial ischemia.

Since nitroprusside causes venous pooling, it can induce a profound postural hypotension, unlike the pure arterial vasodilators. A critically ill patient who is receiving nitroprusside and becomes acutely hypotensive is usually intravascularly depleted and requires fluid replacement. With the patient in the upright posture, nitroprusside causes a fall in cardiac output, which may have a major effect on the drug's hypotensive impact. In supine patients, the fall in cardiac output is responsible for about one-fourth of its hypotensive activity. Nitroprusside-induced hypotension activates the sympathetic nervous system, which increases renin output and heart rate. Renal blood flow, glomerular filtration rate, and cerebral circulation do not change. Since nitroprusside does not increase cardiac preload, it is a good drug for treating patients with congestive heart failure, myocardial insufficiency, or aortic dissection in which hyperkinetic cardiac output would be harmful. It is also useful in treating hypertension associated with myocardical infarction and an unstable blood pressure since its effects can be rapidly terminated by stopping infusion.

Sodium nitroprusside given by intravenous infusion (0.25–2.5 μg/kg/min, advancing to a maximum of 10 μg/kg/min) lowers blood pressure within seconds, and the hypotensive effect dissipates within 1–2 minutes after stopping the infusion. The drug is extremely effective and can lower blood pressure markedly in any person. Because of its rapid action and potency, nitroprusside should be administered with an infusion pump while blood pressure is continuously monitored. After the first 2 hours of administration, the rate of drug infusion frequently needs to be increased to maintain an equivalent hypotensive effect because nitroprusside causes a rise in cardiac index without inducing tachycardia (73). The increased cardiac index is due to fluid accumulation and sympathetic nervous stimulation and can be effectively counteracted with a diuretic or β-blocking agent. The drug can increase or maintain cerebral blood flow, and this response can lead to increased intracranial pressure, which might be deleterious in patients with head injury.

Nitroprusside is broken down to cyanide, which is rapidly coverted in the body to thiocyanate. Cyanide toxicity from the drug is uncommon, but thiocyanate is handled by the body in essentially the same manner as are chloride and bromide. The thiocyanate may thus be retained by patients with renal failure or by those receiving low sodium diets; its half-life is normally 4 days. If the concentration of thiocyanate exceeds 10 mg/dl, weakness, hypoxia, nausea, tinnitus, muscle spasm, disorientation, and psychosis may occur. Thiocyanate interferes with transport of iodide by the thyroid gland and may cause hypothyroidism. If nitroprusside is infused for a long time and in high doses, blood levels of thiocyanate must be monitored. When standing, nitroprusside-treated patients may experience postural hypotension, and some may encounter nasal stuffiness and increased body warmth, dizziness, weakness, muscle twitching, and nausea.

Sodium nitroprusside (Nipride) is supplied as a powder (50-mg vials) for reconstitution in 250 ml of 5% dextrose (yielding a concentration of 200 μg/ml). This solution may be used for 24 hours after reconstitution, but should be protected from light. Deeply colored solutions should be discarded because development of color indicates loss of potency.

Patients given sodium nitroprusside must have their blood pressure continuously measured, therefore the drug can only be used where monitoring is available. Although nitroprusside is not necessary for treating most cases of severe hypertension, it is one of the better agents available for treating hypertensive emergencies. Since the drug becomes less effective and leads to accumulation of thiocyanate with prolonged infusion, patients should be given antihypertensive drugs soon after the initiation of therapy. Diuretics and sympatholytics markedly potentiate the effects of this vasodilator and decrease the dose of drug required.

Calcium Antagonists

The myocardium and smooth muscle cells have slow calcium channels in their cell walls that regulate the influx of calcium into the cytoplasm. Elevated free intracellular calcium increases smooth muscle contractility, peripheral resistance, and blood pressure. Calcium-blocking drugs lower intracellular calcium levels and thus cause vasodilation. The calcium channel blockers, nifedipine, diltiazem, and verapamil, are licensed for therapy of arrhythmias in the United States, but are also effective antihypertensives (71). Nifedipine decreases blood pressure in hypertensives but not in normal subjects (14). It can rapidly lower blood pressure when given sublingually (15) or orally (30), and the effect of a single dose lasts about 7 hours (30). The drug's vasodilating effect reflexly increases sympathetic nervous stimulation to the heart. However, nifedipine's direct cardiodepressant activity counteracts its reflex stimulant effects so that heart rate and contractility do not change much (78). After several months, the hypotensive effect of nifedipine tends to diminish when the drug is given alone, but the hypotensive effect is maintained when the drug is administered with propranolol or clonidine (30). About one-fourth of the patients receiving nifedipine accumulate fluid and require a diuretic.

Calcium channel blockers can cause ankle swelling in some people, but overall they have a mild diuretic effect. Their hypotensive effect is potentiated by β-blocking drugs. Calcium antagonists thus are useful in both emergency and chronic treatment of hypertension (22). There is not yet enough experience with these drugs to suggest that they be used as initial therapy in the treatment of hypertension. However, many hypertensive patients develop cardiac arrhythmias or congestive failure that is amenable to treatment with nifedipine, and in these patients, it is reasonable to increase the dose to obtain an antihypertensive effect. The choice of calcium channel blocker depends on the desired effect. Verapamil is the most strongly cardiodepressant; nifedipine is the most effective vasodilator, with relatively little effect on the heart. Diltiazem has effects intermediate between the other two drugs. A 240-mg timed release formulation of verapamil was recently approved for therapy of hypertension in the United States.

ANGIOTENSIN-CONVERTING ENZYME INHIBITORS (ACE INHIBITORS)

Renin is released from the kidney and enzymatically converts circulating angiotensinogen to angiotensin I. Angiotensin I is then rapidly converted to angiotensin II by angiotensin-converting enzyme, which is present in blood vessel walls and in the lung (Fig. 20.2). Angiotensin II is a very potent vasoconstrictor that also stimulates aldosterone release. Renin levels are markedly elevated in renovascular hypertension and malignant hy-

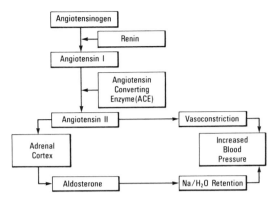

Figure 20.2. The renin-angiotensin-aldosterone system.

pertension, and are above normal in about one-fourth of patients with essential hypertension. The pressor effects of renin can be blocked by inhibition of angiotensin-converting enzyme. The first inhibitor of this enzyme, teprotide, was derived from snake venom. Captopril was specifically designed to interfere with the active site of angiotensin-converting enzyme, and enalapril has a similar mode of action. ACE inhibitors are potent antihypertensive agents that act primarily by preventing the production of angiotensin II. Angiotensin-converting enzyme also causes the breakdown of circulating bradykinin, a potent vasodilator (20). Bradykinin acts in tissues to release vasodilatory prostaglandins; treatment with indomethacin diminishes the hypotensive activity of infused bradykinin and the hypotensive activity of captopril. ACE inhibitors also inhibit the pressor responses to sympathetic nerve stimulation, which may be mediated by inhibition of local angiotensin II formation in the blood vessel wall. Angiotensin II potentiates both the release and the pressor responses to norepinephrine. ACE inhibitors lower blood pressure by lowering levels of angiotensin II, and possibly by enhancing bradykinin levels and by inhibiting the effects of angiotensin II on sympathetic nerves (35).

The hemodynamic effects of ACE inhibitors differ from those of other antihypertensive agents and may be beneficial in patients with hypertensive damage to the kidneys and heart (26). After an acute dose of captopril, blood pressure reduction is related to the initial plasma renin activity (10). Patients with high renin levels have a triphasic blood pressure response to captopril. Their blood pressure falls abruptly, sometimes to dangerous levels in the first few hours, and then rebounds nearly to pretreatment levels. Over subsequent days, blood pressure slowly decreases, but not to the level encountered during the initiation of therapy. Patients with normal or low renin levels have a more prolonged and gentler decrease in blood pressure. The initial hypotensive response is exaggerated in patients who are volume-depleted, and this excessive hypotension can be treated with saline intravenous infusions.

Enalapril is a prodrug that is converted in the liver to the active metabolite, enalaprilat. Captopril can have hypotensive effects 15 minutes after a sublingual dose, but enalapril takes several hours to reach peak effects.

ACE inhibitors lower total peripheral resistance and cause little change in cardiac output, heart rate, or pulmonary wedge pressure in most hypertensives. However, in patients with congestive heart failure, they can increase cardiac output by diminishing afterload (82). ACE inhibitors decrease renal vascular resistance enough so that renal plasma flow increases even when blood pressure is low. In patients with renal artery stenosis, glomerular filtration rate may decrease. Serum creatinine may increase during the early stages of therapy, particularly if there is bilateral renal artery stenosis. ACE inhibitors do not cause postural hypotension and they lower blood pressure without a reflex increase in sympathetic nervous activity. Norepinephrine levels thus remain unchanged during therapy, but during exercise norepinephrine and epinephrine levels respond normally (54).

ACE inhibitors are particularly useful in the treatment of severe renovascular hypertension not amenable to surgery and in patients with congestive heart failure. They correct both the hypertension and electrolyte imbalances caused by markedly elevated renin levels. Angiotensin II stimulates the release of aldosterone, which causes renal potassium wasting. Serum potassium usually does not increase to dangerous levels with ACE inhibitors, but potassium supplementation should be discontinued. In patients who do not respond initially to ACE inhibition alone, the addition of a diuretic such as hydrochlorothiazide, which normally stimulates the release of renin by the kidney, enhances hypotensive effects. The addition of a vasodilator such as minoxidil to this drug regimen greatly increases the antihypertensive effect, even in patients resistant to the individual components of therapy (56). Captopril (25 mg) can be successfully em-

ployed in hypertensive emergencies (74). It is usually a very potent agent in malignant hypertension, but its effects are difficult to control in this setting.

Captopril contains a sulfhydryl grouping that can cause many immunologic side effects. A rash, occasionally accompanied by pruritus, fever, and eosinophilia, can occur. The symptoms usually arise in the first several weeks of therapy and may be dose-related. A reduction of the dose or continued therapy with the same dose often results in diminution of the rash, although the skin lesions may progress. Temporary loss of taste has been reported in about 6% of patients. This symptom is usually transient and does not respond to zinc therapy. Proteinuria of greater than 1 g/day occurs in just over 1% of the patients on captopril, and the nephrotic syndrome may develop in some of these individuals. The drug causes a glomerulopathy and electron-dense deposits similar to those caused by penicillamine and other sulfhydryl-containing drugs.

Neutropenia is the most severe side effect of captopril and occurs in about 0.3% of patients (85). It develops in the first 3–12 weeks of treatment, and blood counts should be obtained frequently during the first 3 months of therapy and periodically thereafter.

Captopril is provided in tablets of 12.5, 25, 50, and 100 mg. After oral administration, blood levels peak in 30–90 minutes and approximately 70% of the drug is absorbed, although food in the gastrointestinal tract may reduce absorption. After absorption, the drug is distributed to most tissues except the nervous system. Fifty percent of the drug is excreted by the kidneys within the first 4 hours of administration, and elimination of captopril and its metabolites correlates closely with creatinine clearance. Patients with renal insufficiency reach much higher peak plasma levels, and the dose may be considerably reduced in patients with impaired renal function. The hypotensive effect of captopril depends on 95% inhibition of angiotensin-converting enzyme, since this enzyme is present in great excess in the body. Once angiotensin-converting enzyme is inhibited, only negligible amounts of angiotensin II are generated and captopril's maximal hypotensive effect is obtained. Increasing the dose of captopril given at a single time thus does not lower blood pressure further. Larger doses maintain adequate captopril blood levels for a longer time, however.

Enalapril is the first of many nonsulfhydryl-containing ACE inhibitors that have been developed. It is converted to enalaprilat in the liver, which is the active form of the drug. This conversion step provides a slow onset of action and diminishes the possibility of an initial severe hypotensive response. Enalaprilat has a long half-life, thus enalapril is effective when given once daily. The drug does not cause sulfhydryl-related immune side effects.

Enalapril is available in tablets of 5, 10, and 20 mg, with a maximum recommended dose of 40 mg daily. Enalaprilat is under investigation as an intravenous ACE inhibitor for use in emergencies.

All of the ACE inhibitors impair the breakdown of bradykinin. This action may manifest as a chronic cough or as life-threatening angioedema requiring tracheostomy.

COMBINED DRUG THERAPY OF HYPERTENSION

The critically ill patient with severe hypertension can only rarely attain normal blood pressure in response to a single drug. Large doses of an individual drug are likely to cause a number of side effects, and many antihypertensive drugs potentiate the effects of others. It is often possible to take advantage of this potentiation to attain an adequate hypotensive effect with minimal side effects by using more than one drug. However, some drug combinations are ineffective or toxic. Many drugs lower blood pressure as a side effect of their primary use (Table 20.5), and some are potent antihypertensive agents when used with a diuretic.

Diuretics

The thiazide diuretics are the most useful agents in the treatment of hypertension and can be successfully employed in very low doses. Daily doses of 25 mg of chlorthalidone or 12.5 mg of hydrochlorothiazide provide the maximum hypotensive effect; larger doses are more toxic but not more effective in patients with normal renal function. The thiazide diuretics increase blood cholesterol, triglycerides, uric acid, and blood sugar, and cause hypokalemia. All of these undesirable side effects are dose-dependent and are slight at low doses. It is not necessary to routinely supplement low doses of thiazides with potassium-sparing diuretic agents, such as triamterene, amiloride, or spironolactone. Low doses of these thiazides should not cause hypokalemia, and if hypokalemia occurs, it suggests an aldosterone-secreting adrenal adenoma, adrenal hyperplasia, Cushing's syndrome, or renovascular hypertension.

Sympatholytic Drugs

The sympatholytic drugs include the β-blockers; the α-agonist drugs, clonidine, guanabenz, guanfacine, and α-methyldopa; and the α-blocking drug, prazosin. The α-blockers, phenoxybenzamine and phentolamine, are not very useful in the treatment of essential hypertension, and guanethidine and reserpine are rarely used now that less toxic drugs are available. The effects of sympatholytic drugs

Table 20.5
Drugs That Lower Blood Pressure[a]

Drug	Action	Drug Interactions
Neuroleptics, especially chlorpromazine	α Blockade	Potentiated by diuretics
Dopamine agonists L-Dopa Bromocriptine Dopamine Pimozide	Stimulate dopamine receptors, inhibit NE release	
Fenfluramine	Inhibits NE release	Potentiated by diuretics
Tricyclic antidepressants	?	Inhibits clonidine effect
MAO inhibitors	?	Hypertension with tyramine, reserpine
Marijuana	Inhibits NE effects	
Opiates	Vasodilation, inhibits NE release	
Antiarrhythmics Nifedipine Verapamil Disopyramide	Myocardial depression, vasodilation	

[a]NE, norepinephrine; MAO, monoamine oxidase.

are often potentiated by combination with a diuretic. Diuretics activate the sympathetic nervous system in response to volume depletion and hypotension. The body is then dependent on sympathetic nervous activity for maintenance of blood pressure, and the sympatholytic drugs become more effective in this setting.

The β-blocking drugs are all quite similar in their antihypertensive efficacy and in no instance is the use of more than one β-blocker at a time worthwhile. Clonidine acts to diminish the sympathetic nervous system release of norepinephrine, and the β-blockers antagonize the effects of norepinephrine. In experimental animals, β-blockers such as propranolol that penetrate the central nervous system inhibit the antihypertensive efficacy of clonidine. In humans, the combination of clonidine and propranolol has been reported as both effective and ineffective (89, 92). It appears unwise to combine these drugs because of potential toxicity. Although the combination of methyldopa with β-blockers has not been as extensively studied, methyldopa has actions very similar to those of clonidine.

The combination of the α-blocking agent, prazosin, with a β-blocking drug seems to be a reasonable approach to the control of hypertension. Labetalol, a drug with both peripheral α- and β-blocking activity, is an effective antihypertensive agent. However, according to some reports the antihypertensive efficacy of prazosin combined with propranolol is not more effective than either agent used alone (41, 57). Prazosin also does not enhance the antihypertensive efficacy of clonidine (29).

There is no clear evidence that the combination of β-blockers, clonidine, methyldopa, or prazosin is effective. In fact, these combinations may be dangerous. For example, the addition of clonidine to the regimen of a patient treated with a β-blocker caused dramatic pressor responses; and in a more complex situation with the patient on multiple sympatholytic drugs, just an increase in the dose of clonidine caused a pressor response (41).

In no cases has it proved clearly beneficial to combine sympatholytic drugs in the treatment of hypertension, except for the combination of α- and β-blocking agents in a patient with pheochromocytoma. On the other hand, there are numerous reports of unexpected pressor responses, and a predictable increase in the number of side effects occurs as more drugs are added. In general, patients should be treated with a single sympatholytic agent.

If they are treated with a β-blocker or prazosin, some do not respond, in which case it is reasonable to change to an α_2-agonist or to add an agent from another class of antihypertensive drugs, such as the vasodilators.

Drug Combinations with Vasodilators

The arterial vasodilators, hydralazine, minoxidil, and diazoxide, lower blood pressure by decreasing arteriolar tone, but they do not dilate venous capacitance vessels. They thus permit a relatively unimpeded flow of blood back to the heart and reflexly increase sympathetic nervous activity because of their effect on blood pressure. The increased blood supply and sympathetic stimulation can greatly increase cardiac output. The vasodilators also cause fluid retention by increasing renin and aldosterone production. Consequently, vasodilators are not very effective in lowering blood pressure by themselves; they need to be combined with a diuretic and a sympatholytic for maximal hypotensive effect and to avoid the side effects of edema and palpitations. A thiazide diuretic can sometimes control fluid accumulation, but minoxidil and diazoxide cause such avid fluid retention that a powerful diuretic such as furosemide is often necessary.

A variety of sympatholytic drugs potentiate the antihypertensive effects of the vasodilators, including β-blockers, α_2-agonists, reserpine, and guanethidine. β-Blocking drugs can block the increased cardiac output and renin secretion engendered by the vasodilators and do so with a minimum number of side effects. In fact, when β-blockers are used in appropriate doses, they can eliminate the palpitations, headache, and vascular noises that may be caused by the vasodilators. β-Blockers diminish β-adrenergic effects engendered by vasodilators, but they do not block α-adrenergic effects. If β-blockers do not lower blood pressure adequately, it is reasonable to change to an α_2-agonist such as clonidine. Clonidine should be substituted for the β-blocker, not added to the previous drug regimen, since clonidine can raise blood pressure in a patient treated with diuretic, hydralazine, and β-blocker (41).

Many hypertensives develop coronary insufficiency and angina pectoris. A vasodilator used alone can worsen the angina, but a vasodilator can safely be used if the patient is already on adequate doses of diuretic and β-blocker. Moreover, in some of these patients, vasodilators decrease cardiac work and diminish angina symptoms.

Drug Combinations with Angiotensin-Converting Enzyme Inhibitors

The ACE inhibitors can be used as single agents in many hypertensives. The drugs work well in patients with high renin levels or high circulating catecholamines and are sometimes beneficial in those with heart failure. An ACE inhibitor plus thiazide diuretic controls blood pressure in 90% of hypertensives (51). The addition of a vasodilator to this regimen lowers blood pressure even more.

PRACTICAL APPLICATIONS FOR THE CRITICAL CARE PRACTITIONER'S EVALUATION OF THE SEVERELY HYPERTENSIVE PATIENT

Essential hypertension is a lifelong disease and therapy ideally should be initiated slowly with the drugs least likely to cause side effects. However, patients presenting with severe hypertension may have a poor prognosis unless they receive prompt, effective treatment. The most common cause of a markedly elevated blood pressure is a stress reaction (53). Some patients who are only slightly hypertensive in their normal environment respond to the stress of a medical examination with severe hypertension, which promptly subsides when they return to their usual surroundings. This type of patient is always anxious and may conceal this anxiety at the expense of increased internal stress. A hypertensive stress reaction is particularly likely in patients receiving β-blocking drugs. They secrete epinephrine in response to stress and then have an "epinephrine reversal." The marked elevation in blood pressure is mediated by epinephrine's α-adrenergic effects without any compensatory β-adrenergic vasodilation. Ganglionic-blocking drugs such as guanethidine can block this stress-induced hypertension but clonidine or methyldopa do not. The effects of clonidine or methyldopa can be overridden during severe stress, allowing normal discharge from the sympathetic nervous system. There are several clues to the stress reaction, including pupillary dilation, sweaty palms, and a nervous and sometimes overly helpful behavior. On physical examination, the patient lacks the stigmata of hypertensive disease and funduscopic ex-

amination shows a relatively undamaged retinal vasculature. Administering potent antihypertensive agents to these patients leaves them hypotensive when they return to a less stressful environment.

A patient with persistent severe hypertension needs to have blood pressure lowered rapidly. The drug used depends on the cause of the hypertension and the presence of coexisting illnesses.

Patients with hypertension are prone to develop cerebrovascular occlusion, intracerebral bleeding, or subarachnoid hemorrhage. These customarily produce an increase in hypertension, ECG abnormalities, and focal neurologic signs. Blood pressure should be lowered very carefully in these patients to prevent extension of the damage; vasodilators that tend to increase intracranial pressure should be avoided.

Pheochromocytoma

Pheochromocytoma can produce episodic severe hypertension in response to circulating norepinephine. Patients with pheochromocytoma are usually volume-depleted from the pressor effects of norepinephrine, thus treatment with diuretics may cause circulatory compromise to vital organs. β-Blocking drugs should not be given to the patient with a pheochromocytoma until adequate α blockade has been achieved, since blockade of β-adrenergic–mediated vasodilation allows unopposed α vasoconstriction and may worsen the hypertension. On the other hand, treatment with α-blocking drugs such as prazosin may be strikingly effective in lowering blood pressure, and a prolonged hypotensive response to a low dose of prazosin should make one suspicious of the presence of a pheochromocytoma. Calcium channel blocking drugs are also very effective in pheochromocytoma because they impair catecholamine release from the tumor.

Drug Reactions

Several drugs can cause reactions that mimic the pressor response to a pheochromocytoma (Table 20.6). Phenylpropanolamine is a popular over-the-counter anorectic agent, frequently combined with ephedrine or caffeine and marketed for the treatment of obesity, drowsiness, and nasal congestion. These drugs cause α-adrenergic–mediated vasoconstriction and raise blood pressure even when given in

Table 20.6
Drugs That Increase Blood Pressure

Drug	Action	Drug Interactions
Ethanol	↓ Aldosterone metabolism	Enhances diuretic K$^+$ loss; enhances sedation with methyldopa, clonidine
Nicotine	Vasoconstriction	
Caffeine	Sympathetic stimulation	Synergistic with nicotine, mild diuresis
Stimulants		
Amphetamine		
Methylphenidate		
Methamphetamine	Norepinephrine release, blockage of reuptake	Paradoxical hypertension with β-blockers
Phenmetrazine		
Cocaine		
Ephedrine		
Isoproterenol		
Isoetharine	β Stimulation	Inhibited by β-blockers
Terbutaline		
Phenylephrine	α Stimulation	Inhibited by prazosin
Phenylpropanolamine		
MAO inhibitor and tyramine[a]	Enhanced tyramine effect	
Mineralocorticoids	Na$^+$ retention	Enhance K$^+$ loss with diuretics
Glucocorticoids	?	
Estrogens, oral contraceptives	↑ Angiotensinogen	
Indomethacin	Blocks prostaglandin vasodilation	↓ Diuretic effects
Atropine	Tachycardia	
Antihistamines		

[a] MAO, monoamine oxidase.

normal doses and can cause marked hypertension when taken in excessive doses.

Monoamine oxidase inhibitors have had a resurgence in popularity for treatment of depression. They ordinarily lower blood pressure, but when taken with a food containing tyramine, such as cheese or wine, they can cause severe hypertension. They can also worsen the hypertension caused by drugs such as ephedine or phenylpropanolamine, which are degraded by monoamine oxidase. Other drugs that can increase blood pressure are listed in Table 20.6.

Abrupt withdrawal of clonidine in doses over 0.3 mg/day can cause a rebound increase in sympathetic nervous release of norepinephrine and an overshoot of hypertension. All of the above-mentioned drug reactions increase blood pressure through α-adrenergic stimulation and they are best treated acutely with α-blocking drugs. Although patients with a pheochromocytoma or one of these drug reactions are usually tachycardic and tremulous, they should not receive β-blocking drugs, which worsen their hypertension.

Malignant Hypertension

As opposed to the mislabeled "benign essential hypertension," which is neither benign nor essential, malignant hypertension is often fatal if not treated. Malignant hypertension usually develops slowly over a period of a few weeks and should be brought under control within days of its diagnosis. Diastolic blood pressure is characteristically above 130 mm Hg and the patient often presents because of symptoms caused by the hypertension, unlike the asymptomatic patient with lesser degrees of hypertension. Patients usually complain of headache, dizziness, and occasional blurred vision, and on questioning admit to some cardiorespiratory decompensation. Physical examination reveals signs of congestive heart failure and pulmonary edema, and the optic fundi have hemorrhages, exudates, and papilledema. Untreated malignant hypertension has a 50% fatality in 6 months, and prior to effective treatment it was generally fatal in 2 years. Because of their poor prognosis, these patients need to be treated quickly, usually in the hospital. A variety of drugs can bring the blood pressure down gradually and safely, without the need for continuous intensive monitoring (Table 20.7). These patients always have some renal damage due to their hypertension, and their fluid status needs to be evaluated on an individual basis. Serum creatinine and blood urea nitrogen levels are elevated, and proteinuria and hematuria are always present. The patient who has oliguria may be volume-over-

Table 20.7
Parenteral Antihypertensive Drugs

Drug	Administration	Dose	Time of Onset	Use in [a]	Avoid in [a]
Diazoxide	i.v. push	50–300 mg	1–2 min	Encephalopathy, glomerulonephritis	Acute MI, aortic aneurysm, pulmonary edema
Nitroprusside	i.v. drip	0.5–8 μg/kg/min	<1 min	Acute MI, aortic aneurysm, encephalopathy, intracranial bleeding	
Trimethaphan camsylate	i.v. drip	1–15 mg/min	<1 min	Intracranial bleeding, aortic aneurysm	Glomerulonephritis
Hydralazine	i.v. or i.m.	10–25 mg	20 min	Glomerulonephritis	Aortic aneurysm, acute MI
Methyldopa	i.v.	250–500 mg	3 hr		Encephalopathy, intracranial bleeding
Labetalol	i.v.	20–300 mg	2 min	Angina pectoris	Congestive heart failure, asthma

[a] MI, myocardial infarction.

loaded, but many of these patients have a low blood volume and should not receive diuretics. Circulating renin and catecholamines are uniformly extremely high, so that excess volume depletion may allow these vasopressors to compromise the circulation of vital organs. These elevated circulating pressor agents make these patients very susceptible to the hypotensive effects of certain drugs. Captopril may lower blood pressure with dangerous rapidity, whereas the sympatholytic drugs such as clonidine, methyldopa, reserpine, and the ganglionic blockers are usually very effective. Vasodilators sufficiently potent to counteract the intense vasospasm encountered in malignant hypertension are quite effective, but the diuretics usually do not lower blood pressure. β-Blockers are often ineffective acutely, and they may worsen the congestive heart failure that these patients experience. Malignant hypertension is also aptly called "acute vasospastic hypertension," and treatment aimed at the vasospasm is usually successful. Diuretics and β-blockers may worsen the vasospasm and thus are not very effective in the treatment of the hypertension, but they may be used to treat fluid retention or excess cardiac stimulation.

These basic principles allow for a wide variety of antihypertensive drugs that can be used in this situation, and the drug should be selected for the individual patient's symptoms and physical status. The vasodilators, hydralazine and diazoxide, can be given intravenously (Table 20.7). Diazoxide works very

quickly and hydralazine takes effect in about 15 minutes. If the patient has a long history of resistance to other hypertensive drugs, it may be appropriate to start treatment with minoxidil; the peak of an oral dose is seen 6 hours after administration. The sympatholytic agent, methyldopa, may be given intravenously but often takes hours before it has a hypotensive effect. An oral dose of 0.2 mg of clonidine is convenient and usually quite effective in lowering blood pressure. Its effect may be titrated by adding 0.1 mg hourly up to a total dose of 0.5 mg to lower blood pressure. Both methyldopa and clonidine are sedating. This action may be beneficial in the hospitalized patient, but may be dangerous in outpatients. An oral dose of prazosin has an acute effect to lower blood pressure; however, experience with this agent in the setting of malignant hypertension is very limited. Intravenous labetalol can be slowly titrated, but it often causes postural hypotension.

There is no one best drug for this disease because the choice of agents should depend on the patient being treated. The vasodilators may worsen coronary insufficiency or an aortic aneurysm, but they reduce afterload in congestive heart failure and usually preserve renal blood flow. The sympatholytic agents are often convenient to use in a patient without severe signs of cardiac or renal dysfunction. However, in a patient suspected of having a myocardial infarction or intracerebral hemorrhage, nitroprusside may be one of the safest agents to use because it causes a balanced arterial and venous dilation, and can be rapidly withdrawn during hypotensive episodes. Often, the best guide to a choice of drugs is the record of a patient's prior response to antihypertensive drugs.

Hypertensive Encephalopathy

The patient with hypertensive encephalopathy has a severe headache and frequently has visual disturbances, paralysis, convulsions, vomiting, stupor, and coma. The onset of encephalopathy occurs over a few hours, and diastolic blood pressure is usually above 140 mm Hg. Because of the abrupt onset, patients may not have developed papilledema, but arteriolar spasm and a retinal sheen are always present. There may be evidence of pulmonary edema and renal failure, and if untreated, the patient will die in several hours or days. This condition needs to be treated immediately, and intravenous nitroprusside or ganglionic blockers are the agents of choice. Intravenous diazoxide can be used in hypertensive encephalopathy if the patient cannot be continuously monitored in an intensive care unit. Rapid institution of therapy in hypertensive encephalopathy is life-saving. However, hypertensive encephalopathy is now a far less frequent occurrence than several years ago since most patients with severe hypertension can now have their blood pressure adequately controlled.

References

1. Agharanya JC, Alonso R, Wurtman RJ: Changes in catecholamine excretion after short-term tyrosine ingestion in normally fed human subjects. Am J Clin Nutr 34:82–87, 1981.
2. Anderson RJ, Hat GR, Crumpler CP, Reed WG, Matthews CA: Oral clonidine loading in hypertensive emergencies. JAMA 246:848–850, 1981.
3. Beal D, Dujovne C, Gillis JS: The effect of methyldopa on human judgment in hypertensive patients and normal volunteers. Res Commun Psychol Psychiatry Behav 5:205–217, 1980.
4. Beard TC, Gray WR, Cooke HM, Barge R: Randomised controlled trial of a no-added sodium diet for mild hypertension. Lancet 2:455–458, 1982.
5. Berglund G, Andersson O: Low doses of hydrochlorothiazide in hypertension: antihypertensive and metabolic effects. Eur J Clin Pharmacol 10:177–182, 1976.
6. Bradley WF, Hoffman GF, Hutchison JC, Kalams Z, Waldron SL: Comparison of prazosin and methyldopa in mild to moderate hypertension: a multicenter cooperative study. Curr Ther Res 21:28–35, 1977.
7. Brenner WI, Lieberman AN: Acute clonidine withdrawal syndrome following open-heart operation. Ann Thorac Surg 24:80–82, 1977.
8. Brodsky JB, Bravo JJ: Acute postoperativve clonidine withdrawal syndrome. Anesthesiology 44:519–521, 1976.
9. Brown MJ, Salmon D, Rendell M: Clonidine hallucinations. Ann Intern Med 93:456–457, 1980.
10. Brunner HR, Gavras H, Waeber B, Kershaw GR, Turini GA, Vukovich RA, McKinstry DN, Gavras I: Oral angiotensin-converting enzyme inhibitor in long-term treatment of hypertensive patients. Ann Intern Med 90:19–23, 1979.
11. Buhler FR, Laragh JH, Baer L, Vaughan ED, Brunner HR: Propranolol inhibition of renin secretion. N Engl J Med 287:1209–1214, 1972.
12. Burden AC, Alexander CPT: Rebound hypertension after acute methyldopa withdrawal. Br Med J, 1:1056–1057, 1976.
13. Cavero I, Roach AG: The pharmacology of prazosin, a novel antihypertensive agent. Life Sci 27:1525–1540, 1980.
14. Corea L, Bentivoglio M, Cosmi F, Alunni G: Catecholamines, plasma levels and haemodynamic changes induced by nifedipine in chronic severe heart failure. Curr Ther Res 30:698–707, 1981.
15. Corea L, Miele N, Bentivoglio M, Boschetti E, Agabiti-Rosei E, Muiesan G: Acute and chronic effects of nifedipine on plasma renin activity and plasma adrenaline and noradrenaline in controls and hypertensive patients. Clin Sci 57:115s–117s, 1979.
16. Dollery CT, Davies DS, Draffan GH, Dargie HJ, Dean CR, Reid JL, Clare RA, Murray S: Clinical pharmacology and pharmacokinetics of clonidine. Clin Pharmacol Ther 19:11–17, 1975.
17. Dornhorst A, Powell SH, Pensky J: Aggravation by propranolol of hyperglycaemic effect of hydrochlorothiazide in type II diabetics without alteration of insulin secretion. Lancet 1:123–126, 1985.
18. Dustan HP: Obesity and hypertension. Ann Intern Med 103:1047–1049, 1985.
19. Dustan HP, Bravo EL, Tarazi RC: Volume dependent, essential and steroid hypertension. Am J Cardiol 32:606, 1973.
20. Edwards CR, Padfield PL: Angiotensin-converting enzyme inhibitors: past, present, and bright future. Lancet 1:30–34, 1985.
21. Einhorne D, Young JB, Landsberg L: Hypotensive effect of fasting: possible involvement of the sympathetic nervous system and endogenous opiates. Science 217:727–729, 1982.
22. Frishman W, Klein N, Beer N: Nifedipine in hypertension: expanding applications of a new drug. Arch Intern Med 141:843, 1981.
23. Frolich ED, Dustan HP, Page IH: Hyperdynamic beta-adrenergic circulatory state. Arch Intern Med 117:614–619, 1966.
24. Garvey HL, Ram N: Centrally induced hypotensive effects of beta adrenergic blocking drugs. Eur J Pharmacol 33:283–294, 1975.
25. Graham RM, Thornell IG, Gain IR: Prazosin: the first dose phenomenon. Br Med J 2:1293, 1976.
26. Helgeland A, Strommen R, Hagelund CH, Tretli S: Enalapril, atenolol and hydrochlorothiazide in mild to moderate hypertension. Lancet 1:872–875, 1986.
27. Holland OB, Fairchild C: Renin classification for diuretic and beta blocker treatment of black hypertensive patients. J Chronic Dis 35:179–182, 1982.
28. Hollifield JW, Sherman K, Zwagg RV, Shand DG: Proposed mechanisms of propranolol's antihypertensive effect in essential hypertension. N Engl J Med 295:68–73, 1976.
29. Hubbell FA, Weber MA, Drayer JM, Rose DE: Central alpha-adrenergic stimulation by clonidine overrides the antihypertensive effect of peripheral alpha adrenergic blockadge induced by prazosin. Presented at the 8th Meeting of the International Society of Hypertension, Milan, Italy, 1981.
30. Imai Y, Abe K, Otsuke Y, Iorkawa N, Yasumina M, Saito

K, et al: Management of severe hypertension with nifedipine in combination with clonidine or propranolol. *Arzneimittelforschung* 30:674–678, 1980.

31. Jackson EK, Campbell WB: A possible antihypertensive mechanism of propranolol: antagonism of angiotensin II enhancement of sympathetic nerve transmission through prostaglandins. *Hypertension* 3:23–33, 1981.

32. Jeffreys DB, Flanagan RJ, Volans GN: Reversal of ethanol-induced coma with naloxone. *Lancet* 1:308–309, 1980.

33. Jenkins JS, Conolly J: Adrenocortical response to ethanol in man. *Br Med J* 2:804–805, 1968.

34. Joossens JV, Geboers J: Nutrition and essential hypertension. *Bibl Nutr Dieta* 37:104–118, 1986.

35. Katzman PL, Hulthen UL, Hokfelt B: The effect of 8 weeks treatment with the calcium antagonist felodipine on blood pressure, heart rate, working capacity, plasma renin activity, plasma angiotensin II, urinary catecholamines and aldosterone in patients with essential hypertension. *Br J Clin Pharmacol* 21:633–640, 1986.

36. Kempner W: Treatment of hypertensive vascular disease with rice diet. *Am J Med* 4:545–577, 1948.

37. Kobinger W: Alpha-adrenocepters in cardiovascular regulation. In Ziegler MG, Lake CR (eds): *Norepinephrine* (Frontiers of Clinical Neuroscience, vol 4). Baltimore, Williams & Wilkins, 1984.

38. Koch-Weser J: Vasodilator drugs in the treatment of hypertension. *Arch Intern Med* 133:1017–1025, 1974.

39. Kolata G: Heart study produces a surprise result. *Science* 218:31, 1982.

40. Kunos G, Farsang C: Beta endorphin: possible involvement in the antihypertensive effect of central alpha-receptor activation. *Science* 211:82–84, 1981.

41. Kuokkanen K, Mattila MJ: Antihypertensive effect of prazosin in combination with methyldopa, clonidine or propranolol. *Ann Clin Res* 11:18–24, 1979.

42. Lake CR, Ziegler MG: Effect of acute volume alterations on norepinephrine and dopamine-beta hydroxylase in normotensive and hypertensive subjects. *Circulation* 57:774–778, 1978.

43. Lake CR, Ziegler MG, Coleman MD, Kopin IJ: Fenfluramine potentiation of antihypertensive effects of thiazides. *Clin Pharmacol Ther* 28:22–27, 1980.

44. Lake CR, Ziegler MG, Coleman MD, Kopin IJ: Hydrocholorthiazide-induced sympathetic hyperactivity in hypertensive patients. *Clin Pharmacol Ther* 26:428–432, 1979.

45. Landsberg L, Young JB: Fasting, feeding and regulation of the sympathetic nervous system. *N Engl J Med* 298:1295–1302, 1978.

46. Langer SZ: The role of alpha and beta-presynaptic receptors in the regulation of noradrenaline release elicited by nerve stimulation. *Clin Sci Mol Med* 51:423s–426s, 1976.

47. Larbi JI, Zaimise E: Effect of acute intravenous administration of clonidine on cerebral blood flow in man. *Br J Pharmacol* 39:198P-199P, 1970.

48. Lavie CJ, Messerli FH: Cardiovascular adaptation to obesity and hypertension. *Chest* 90:275–279, 1986.

49. Linas SL, Nies AS: Minoxidil. *Ann Intern Med* 94:61–65, 1981.

50. MacGregor GA, Best FA, Cam JM, Markandu ND, Elder DM, Sagnella GA, Squires M: Double-blind randomised crossover trial of moderate sodium restriction in essential hypertension. *Lancet* 1:351–354, 1982.

51. MacGregor GA, Markandu ND, Smith SJ, Sagnella GA: Captopril: contrasting effects of adding hydrochlorothiazide, propranolol, or nifedipine. *J Cardiovasc Pharmacol* 7:S82–S87, 1985.

52. Maling TJB, Dollery CT, Hamilton CA: Clonidine and sympathetic activity during sleep. *Clin Sci* 57:509–514, 1979.

53. Mancia G, Grassi G, Pomdiossi G, Gregorini L, Bertinieri G, Parati G, Ferrari A, Zanchetti A: Effects of blood-pressure measurements by the doctor on patient's blood pressure and heart rate. *Lancet* 2:695–697, 1983.

54. Manhem P, Bramnert M, Hulthen UL, Hokfelt B: The effect of captopril on catecholamines, renin activity, angiotensin II and aldosterone in plasma during physical exercise in hypertensive patients. *Eur J Clin Invest* 11:389–395, 1981.

55. Materson BJ, Oster JR, Michael UF, Bolton SM, Burton ZC, Stambaugh JE, Morlege J: Dose responses to chlorthalidone in patients with mild hypertension. *Clin Pharmacol Ther* 24:192–198, 1978.

56. Matson JR, Norby LH, Robillard JE: Interaction of minoxidil and captopril in the treatment of refractory hypertension. *Am J Dis Child* 135:256–258, 1981.

57. Mattila MG: Antihypertensive effect of prazosin in combination with methyldopa. Clonidine or propranolol? *Ann Clin Res* 11:18, 1979.

58. Medical Research Council: Adverse reactions to bendroflumethazide and propranolol for the treatment of mild hypertension. *Lancet* 2:539–542, 1981.

59. Meier A, Weidmann P, Ziegler WH: Catecholamines, renin, aldosterone, and blood volume during chronic minoxidil therapy. *Klin Wochenschr* 59:1231–1236, 1981.

60. Michelson E, Frishman WH, Lewis JE, Edwards WT, Flanigan WJ, Bloomfield SS, Johnson BF, Lucas C, Freis ED, Finnerty FA, Sawin HS, Sabol SA, Long C, Poland MP: Multicenter clinical evaluation of long-term efficacy and safety of labetalol in treatment of hypertension. *Am J Med* 75:68–80, 1983.

61. Mitchell HC, Pettinger WA: Dose-response of clonidine on plasma catecholamines in the hypernoradrenergic state associated with vasodilator beta-blocker therapy. *J Cardiovasc Pharmacol* 3:647–654, 1981.

62. Mrozzek WJ, Finnerty FA: A double-blind evaluation of a new antihypertensive agent. In Cotton (ed): *Prazosin*. Amsterdam, Excerpta Medica, 1974.

63. Neary D, Thurston H, Pohl JEF: Development of extrapyramidal symptoms in hypertensive patients treated with diazoxide. *Br Med J*, Sept 1, 1973, pp 474–475.

64. Oates HF, Stoker LM, Stokes GS: Interactions between prazosin, clonidine and direct vasodilators in the anaesthetized rat. *Clin Exp Pharmacol Physiol* 5:85–89, 1978.

65. O'Connor DT, Barg AP, Duchin KL: Preserved renal perfusion during treatment of essential hypertension with the beta blocker nadolol. *J Clin Pharmacol* 22:187–195, 1982.

66. O'Connor DT, Preston RA: Propranolol effects on autonomic function in hypertensive men. *Clin Cardiol* 5:340–346, 1982.

67. O'Connor DT, Preston RA, Sasso EH: Renal perfusion changes during treatment of essential hypertension: prazosin versus propranolol. *J Cardiovasc Pharmacol* 1(suppl 1):S38–S42, 1979.

68. O'Malley K, Segal JL, Israili ZH, Boles M, McNay JL, Dayton PG: Duration of hydralazine action in hypertension. *Clin Pharmacol Ther* 18:581–586, 1975.

69. Pearson RM, Griffith DNW, Woollard M, James IM: Comparison of effects on cerebral blood flow of rapid reduction in systemic arterial pressure by diazoxide and labetalol in hypertensive patients: preliminary findings. *Br J Clin Pharmacol* 8:195S–198S, 1979.

70. Pederson OL, Mikkelsen E, Nielsen JL, Christensen NJ: Abrupt withdrawal of beta-blocking agents in patients with arterial hypertension. Effect on blood pressure, heart rate and plasma catecholamines and prolactin. *Eur J Clin Pharmacol* 15:215–217, 1979.

71. Pool PE, Massie BM, Venkataraman K, Hirsch AT, Samant DR, Seagren SC, Gaw J, Salel AF, Tubau JF: Diltiazem as monotherapy for systemic hypertension: a multicenter, randomized, placebo-controlled trial. *Am J Cardiol* 57:212–217, 1986.

72. Reid JL, Dargie HJ, Davies DS, Wing LMH, Hamilton CA, Dollery CT: Clonidine withdrawal in hypertension. *Lancet* 1:1171–1174, 1977.

73. Rouby JJ, Gory G, Bourrelli B, Glaser P, Viars P: Resis-

tance to sodium nitroprusside in hypertensive patients. *Crit Care Med* 10:301–304, 1982.

74. Sakano T, Okuda N, Sakura N, Yahata H, Tabe Y, Eno S, Kurogane H, Usui T: Captopril in hypertensive emergencies. *Hiroshima J Med Sci* 30:30–45, 1981.

75. Semplicini A, Pessina AC, Pallatini P, et al: Orthostatic hypotension after the first administration of prazosin in hypertensive patients. *Clin Exp Pharmacol Physiol* 8:1–10, 1981.

76. Sims EAH, Berchtold P: Obesity and hypertension. Mechanisms and implications for management. *JAMA* 247:49–52, 1982.

77. Starke K: Regulation of noradrenaline released by presynaptic receptor systems. *Rev Physiol Biochem Pharmacol* 77:1–124, 1977.

78. Stern HC, Matthews JH, Belz GG.: Intrinsic and reflex actions of verapamil and nifedipine: assessment in normal subjects by noninvasive techniques and autonomic blockade. *Eur J Clin Pharmacol* 29:541–547, 1986.

79. Stokes GS, Braham RM, Gain JM, Davis PR: Influence of dosage and dietary sodium on the first-dose effects of prazosin. *Br Med J* 1:1507, 1977.

80. Taylor AA, Pool JL, Lake CR, Ziegler MG, Rosen RA, Rollins DE, Mitchell JR: Plasma norepinephrine concentrations: no differences among normal volunteers and low, high or normal renin hypertensive patients. *Life Sci* 22:1499–1510, 1978.

81. Tuck ML, Sowers J, Dornfeld L, Kledzik G, Maxwell M: The effect of weight reduction on blood pressure, plasma renin activity, and plasma aldosterone levels in obese patients. *N Engl J Med* 304:930–933, 1981.

82. Turini GA, Bribic M, Brunner HR, Waeber B, Gavras H: Improvement of chronic congestive heart-failure by oral captopril. *Lancet* 1:1213–1215, 1979.

83. van den Brink G, Boer P, van Asten P, Mees EJD, Geyskes GG: One and three doses of propranolol a day in hypertension. *Clin Pharmacol Ther* 27:9–15, 1980.

84. Vandongen R, Margetts B, Deklerk N, Beilin LJ, Rogers P: Plasma catecholamines following exercise in hyper-

tensives treated with pindolol: comparison with placebo and metoprolol. *Br J Clin Pharmacol* 21:627–632, 1986.

85. Vidt DG, Bravo EL, Fouad FM: Captopril. *N Engl J Med* 306:214–219, 1982.

86. Wallace JM, Gill DP: Prazosin in the diagnosis and treatment of pheochromocytoma. *JAMA* 240:2752–2753, 1978.

87. Warren SE, O'Connor DT: The antihypertensive mechanism of sodium restriction. *J Cardiovasc Pharmacol* 3:781–790, 1981.

88. Watkin DM, Frobe HF, Hatch TF, Gutman AB: Effects of diet in essential hypertension II. Results with unmodified Kempner rice diet in 50 hospitalized patients. *Am J Med* 9:441–493, 1950.

89. Weber MA, Drayer JIM, Laragh JH: The effects of clonidine and propranolol separately and in combination on blood pressure and plasma renin activity in essential hypertension. *J Clin Pharmacol* 18:233, 1978.

90. Weisfeldt ML: Aging of the cardiovascular system. *N Engl J Med* 303:1172–1173, 1980.

91. Wells JD. Unusual cases of resistance to minoxidil therapy. *J Cardiovasc Pharmacol* 2(suppl 1)):S228–S235, 1980.

92. Wilja M, Jonnela AJ, Juustila H, Mattila MJ: Interaction of clonidine and beta blockers. *Acta Med Scand* 207:173, 1980.

93. Winer BM: The antihypertensive actions of benzothiadiazenes. *Circulation* 23:211–218, 1961.

94. Woods JW, Pittman AW, Pulliam CC, Werk EE, Waider W, Allen CA: Renin profiling in hypertension and its use in treatment with propranolol and chlorthalidone. *N Engl J Med* 294:1137–1143, 1976.

95. Young JR, Landsberg L: Suppression of sympathetic nervous system during fasting. *Science* 190:1473–1475, 1977.

96. Zacest R, Gilmore E, Koch-Weser J: Treatment of essential hypertension with combined vasodilation and beta-adrenergic blockade. *N Engl J Med* 286:617–622, 1972.

21

Analgesics

Frank J. Balestrieri, D.D.S., M.D.

PAIN SENSATION

Pain is defined as "an unpleasant sensory and emotional experience associated with actual or potential tissue damage, or described in terms of such damage" (64). Pain is a personal and subjective experience that each individual learns through life, as actual or potential tissue-damaging experiences are encountered. Pain is also an unpleasant experience with an associated emotional response. The emotional or psychologic state of the patient may result in pain in the absence of tissue damage or other pathology. The emotional or psychologic state of the patient may modify the character of the pain.

The nociceptor activity initiated by a noxious stimulus is not pain. Rather, pain is the conscious psychologic state, usually resulting from a noxious stimulus but not requiring one. It consists of sensory, emotional, and cognitive elements arising from very complex and, as yet, incompletely understood activities within the central nervous system.

Although pain is subjective and difficult to define, it is clear that critically ill patients experience pain. The critically ill not only are often subjected to major physical injury, but also suffer sleeplessness, noise, trauma, frequent handling, and fear. Our knowledge of patients' experiences during a critical illness is mostly anecdotal. Ian Donald, a gynecologist-obstetrician, described his own intensive care unit (ICU) experience following three heart operations (30, 31). He points out that the patient's state of mind is paramount and of more importance than the most powerful analgesics. Other factors that modify the experience of pain are past experience, knowledge of the postoperative routine, and fear. Donald stresses the importance of the preoperative anesthetist's visit, the need for sympathy from attendants,, and the importance of preventing pain or treating it early. Fortunately, he points

out, the memory of pain fades mercifully and quickly. Similar anecdotal reports are those of Henschel (53) who describes his ICU experience with Guillain Barre syndrome, and Shovelton (110) who had a thymectomy for myasthenia gravis.

Larger and more controlled studies of patients' perception of pain (55, 69, 96, 104) indicate that pain is an important concern of those patients that remember their ICU time, but many remember only a part or none of their stay. Since there is no method of predicting which patients will remember the pain associated with an ICU experience, it is necessary for the staff involved in the patient's care to be alert to the signs and symptoms of pain and to render appropriate relief. The problem of what constitutes appropriate pain relief and how best to administer it has not been well studied or defined.

The treatment of postoperative surgical pain has received much attention, and present-day pain regimens have been widely criticized (41, 138). A number of studies document that the medical profession's attitude toward pain is, or may be perceived as, cruel and callous (21, 35–38, 129, 134). Effective pain management in the critical care setting requires effective use of narcotic analgesia (2, 59), better use established techniques of regional anesthesia, and further study and use of new techniques such as continuous narcotic infusions (14, 16, 74, 120) and epidural and intrathecal narcotic administration (10, 135, 136, 143).

PAIN MECHANISMS

Peripheral Receptors

Prior to the 19th century, Aristotle's view of pain as an emotion opposite to pleasure was widely accepted. With the work of Bell (8) and Magendie in the early 1800s, pain became recognized as a sensation. Cutaneous receptors

449

were described by von Frey (42), who proposed a specific receptive and transmission system for various cutaneous sensory modalities including pain. The opposite view, of functional nonspecificity of nerve endings, was proposed by Lele and Weddell (80). We now know that three categories of cutaneous receptors are present: mechanoreceptors, thermoreceptors, and nociceptors (62). These peripheral receptors have been classified on the basis of their morphology (63) and the correlation of structure with function (e.g., Pacinian corpuscles, Golgi-Mazzoni receptors, hair follicle receptors, Meissner corpuscles, Merkel "touch spots," and Ruffini endings). Nevertheless, there are no anatomic structures defined for most sensory cutaneous functions. One can classify nerve fibers and human peripheral receptors (25, 101, 105, 125) (Table 21.1). The cutaneous mechanoreceptors are supplied by large myelinated fibers, whereas the cutaneous nociceptors are supplied by fine myelinated (A δ) and unmyelinated (C) fibers. Animal studies indicate that the cutaneous nociceptors have two characteristic features: a progressive augmenting response to repeated or increasing noxious stimuli (sensitization) and a high threshold to all natural stimuli relative to other receptors in the same tissue (100). Sensitization is produced by a number of chemicals (56, 90) (bradykinin, histamine, serotonin, and a prostaglandin), and can be reduced by antiinflammatory drugs such as indomethacin and aspirin (70, 75). Another study by Jansco et al. (67) suggests the possibility of a single

cutaneous receptor that responds to capsaicin, a chemical toxin, when applied to the skin. Treatment with capsaicin depletes the cutaneous nerve endings of substance P, an 11-amino-acid peptide. It is speculated that substance P may mediate noxious thermal and chemical stimuli, possibly at the first afferent synapse (57).

There are many peripheral receptors capable of transmitting noxious mechanical, thermal, and chemical stimuli. Peripheral receptors also demonstrate some specificity, but most are polymodal, that is, responding to more than one form of noxious event. It is clear that the exact mechanisms of peripheral cutaneous nociception are poorly understood and that more information is needed before interruption of nociceptive information at the periphery is possible. The function and relationship of muscle, joint, and visceral nociception is also quite unclear.

Peripheral receptors occur in association with nerve fiber innervation by the sympathetic nervous system. Increased sympathetic nervous system activity may increase the sensitivity of the various peripheral pain receptors. Indeed, increased sympathetic activity following surgery or trauma is thought to be the cause for the pain of reflex sympathetic dystrophy (causalgia). The pain of reflex sympathetic dystrophy is characterized by hyperalgesia over the affected limb, by dry skin, and by decreased activity of the limb due to severe pain. The pain and functional disability associated with this syndrome may be relieved by sequential

Table 21.1
Classification of Nerve Fibers and Peripheral Receptors with Conduction Velocities

Class	Function	Diameter (μm)	Conduction Velocity (m/sec)
A_α	Motor	12–20	70–120
A_β	Pressure/touch	5–12	30–70
A_δ	Proprioception	5–12	30–70
A_δ	Pain/temperature (mechanical, heat and cold sensation)	1–4	12–30
B	Preganglionic autonomic (sympathetic)	1–3	14
C			
Cutaneous nociceptors	Pain/temperature (polymodal, mechanical, and cold sensation)	0.5–1	1.2
Cutaneous mechanoreceptors Type I Type II	Sense skin indentation		55
Meissner corpuscle	Sense skin indentation		55
Pacinian corpuscle	Sense pressure changes		50
Warm	Sense increased temperature		0.5

sympathetic blocks, by the application of locally acting or centrally acting drugs that block the effect of norepinephrine at the sympathetic nerve ending, or by surgical sympathectomy.

CENTRAL MECHANISMS

The cell bodies of primary afferent fibers are located in the dorsal root ganglia and trigeminal sensory ganglia. Normally, activity begins in the periphery, and the action potential travels past the dorsal root ganglia cells, which may depolarize, before entering the dorsal horn layers (81).

The dorsal roots provide the pathway by which axons from the peripheral somatic nerves enter the spinal cord. A dermatomal distribution of the dorsal roots exists (26), and overlapping of primary afferent fibers occurs within the dorsal horn (4). Axons in any given dorsal root may extend over five or more spinal cord segments. This fact implies that any point on the body is supplied by two adjoining dorsal roots. As the large and small fibers enter the dorsal horn, the large fibers separate and enter the dorsal columns, with collaterals entering the dorsal horn. The small fine fibers enter separately, forming a longitudinal tract bearing Lissauer's name (82). The dorsolateral fasciculus (Lissauer's tract) contains mainly fine primary afferent fibers (15, 72) and fibers from the substantia gelatinosa (89).

The ventral roots also contain myelinated and unmyelinated sensory fibers (18, 19, 29). These fibers arise from the dorsal root ganglion cells and represent from 15% to 30% of axons in the ventral roots (87). The presence of these sensory fibers in the ventral roots may provide a portion of the explanation for the failure of dorsal rhizotomy to result in complete relief of pain.

The spinal cord comprises a central gray zone and an outer white zone. The central gray matter can be divided into 10 groups based on cell morphology (Fig. 21.1) (108). The cell groups I and IV are involved in sensory transmission and make up the dorsal horn.

The marginal zone of Waldeyer, lamina I, receives excitatory input from primary afferents, and receives inhibitory input from the substantia gelatinosa (94). The marginal zone cells respond to noxious mechanical, thermal and polymodal stimulation, as well as innocuous thermal change (76).

The cells of the substantia gelatinosa may be classified according to their projections: (a)

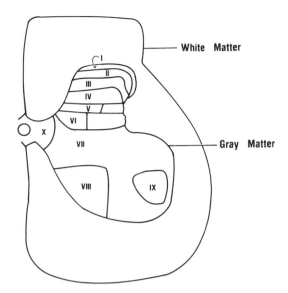

Figure 21.1. Spinal cord laminae. I, marginal zone; II and III, substantia gelatinosa; IV, V and VI, nucleus proprius; VII, VIII, IX and X, motor areas (Adapted from Rexed B: Cytoarchitectonic organization of the spinal cord in the cat. *Comp Neurol* 96:415–495, 1952.)

short axon cells that remain within the dorsal horn, (b) cells with axons that enter the tract of Lissauer or propriospinal pathways, (c) cells with two axons, (d) spinothalamic tract neurons (44, 48, 71, 141). Afferent input into the substantia gelatinosa is by way of collaterals of large primary afferents and fine primary afferents and their collaterals (15, 72, 77). Numerous complex synaptic connections occur in the region of the substantia gelatinosa, which functions as an integrator of sensory input (126).

The nucleus proprius (laminae IV, V and VI) responds to cutaneous stimulation from mechanoreceptors and tactile receptors (narrow dynamic range), and pressure and pinching (wide dynamic range). Lamina VI cells respond to joint movement (132), and somatic and visceral input is received by other neurons in the nucleus proprius (52).

ASCENDING PATHWAYS OF THE SPINAL CORD

The spinothalamic and spinoreticular tracts are the most significant ascending pathways for the transmission of nociceptive input in humans. Axons from second-order neurons in laminae I, IV, V, and VI cross the midline to ascend as the lateral and ventral spinothalamic tracts (73). The spinothalamic tracts travel to the posterior thalamic nuclei and the ventroposterolateral nuclei of the thalamus and then to the cerebral cortex. They relay tactile information as well as nociception.

It is clear that mechanisms of pain transmission involve extremely complex connections in diverse areas of the central nervous system, many of which have yet to be defined.

NARCOTIC ANALGESICS

Analgesic medications are classified as strong or mild and subdivided into narcotic or nonnarcotic categories. Narcotics are either naturally occurring, semisynthetic, or synthetic (Table 21.2). Morphine, codeine, and papaverine (the only naturally occurring clinically significant narcotics) are obtained from the poppy plant, *Papaver somniferum*. Opium is the dried powdered mixture of alkaloids obtained from the unripe seed capsules of the poppy plant, which contains more than 20 pharmacologically active natural alkaloids. These alkaloids are of two chemical classes,

the phenanthrenes (morphine and codeine) and the benzylisoquinolines (papaverine).

The semisynthetic narcotics are derivatives of morphine. Codeine results from the etherification of one hydroxyl group, heroin from the esterification of both hydroxyl groups, and hydromorphone (Dilaudid) from oxidation of the alcoholic hydroxyl group to a ketone group, or saturation of a double bond on the benzene ring (50).

The synthetic narcotics resemble morphine but are usually entirely synthesized. They include the morphinians (levorphanol), the propionanilides (methadone, d-propoxyphene), the benzomorphans (pentazocine, phenazocine, cyclazocine), and the phenylpiperidines (meperidine, fentanyl, sufentanil, alfentanil).

MECHANISMS OF ANALGESIA

Morphine and other narcotic analgesics produce their major effects on the central nervous system and the gastrointestinal tract. The major effects of opiates include analgesia, mood changes (euphoria or dysphoria), drowsiness, respiratory depression, cough suppression, de-

Table 21.2
Classification and Dosage of Some Narcotic Agonists and Antagonists

Drug (Trade Name)	Dose (in 70-kg adult)		Dose Interval (hr)	Comparative Narcotic Potency
	i.v. (mg)	i.m./s.c. (mg)		
NATURAL ALKALOIDS OF OPIUM				
Morphine	2–10 (titrate)	5–10	2–4	1
Codeine	30–60	60–120	2–4	0.1
SEMISYNTHETIC DERIVATIVES				
Hydromorphone (Dilaudid)	0.5–1 (titrate)	2	3–4	5
Oxymorphone (Numorphan)	0.5 (titrate)	1	3–4	10
SYNTHETIC DERIVATIVES				
Meperidine (Demerol, etc.)	25–100 (titrate)	50–100	2–4	0.1
Methadone (Dolophine, etc.)	2–5 (titrate)	2–10	2–4	1.2
Pentazocine (Talwin)	10–30 (titrate)	30	3–4	0.25
Fentanyl (Sublimaze)	0.05–0.1 (titrate)	0.1	½–2	150
NARCOTIC ANTAGONISTS				
Naloxone (Narcan)	0.2–0.4	0.4	½–¾	
Nalorphine (Nalline)	5–10		p.r.n.	
Levallorphan (Lorfan)	1		p.r.n.	

creased gastrointestinal motility, nausea, vomiting, and alterations of endocrine and autonomic nervous system function. It is now clear that opiates act as agonists, interacting with saturable, stereospecific binding sites or receptors in the central nervous system and other sites (102, 112, 123, 151). These binding sites are unevenly distributed throughout the central nervous system. They are present in highest concentration in the limbic system (frontal and temporal cortex, amygdala, and hippocampus), thalamus, corpus striatum, hypothalamus, midbrain and spinal cord (111).

Narcotic analgesic compounds demonstrate stereospecific receptor binding and reversal of effects by narcotic antagonists. Structurally, narcotics are complex, three-dimensional compounds that usually exist as optical isomers (115). Usually only the levorotatory isomer is capable of producing analgesia, and a close relationship exists between the stereochemical structure of a narcotic and its activity (6). Significant variation in pharmacologic activity may result from conformational changes in the molecule produced by a changing pH (5). Most narcotics have a relatively rigid T-shaped conformation, an electron-rich hydroxyl or ketone group, a positively charged basic nitrogen, a quaternary carbon that is separated from the basic nitrogen by an ethane chain, and a flat benzene or 2-thienyl ring, which is 4.58 angstroms from the nitrogen (115).

It is now known that there is more than one type of opiate receptor, and that different receptors may be involved in different functions (45, 83, 86). Opiate receptors may differ in both their affinity for various opiates and opiate antagonists and thereby in their physiologic significance. Various classifications have been proposed to distinguish between receptor types. One classification separates receptors into high- and low-affinity groups. The high-affinity receptors mediate analgesia, whereas the low-affinity receptors are associated with respiratory depression (97, 98). Wood classifies opiate receptors into four groups: (a) the μ-receptor (morphine receptor), (b) the K-receptor (cyclazocine receptor), (c) the σ-receptor, and (d) the δ-receptor. The μ-receptor mediates supraspinal analgesia, respiratory depression, feelings of well-being, euphoria, and a morphine-type physical dependence. The σ receptor mediates feelings of dysphoria, hallucinations, mydriasis, hypotension, and respiratory stimulation. Finally, the δ-receptor mediates some of the in vitro pharmacological effects of the enkephalins and endorphins. There is also a claim for a possible fifth narcotic receptor, the E-receptor. The current classification of opioid-type drugs into agonists, antagonists, and agonists-antagonists type opioids has been based on this receptor concept.

TOLERANCE AND DEPENDENCE

Tolerance to some of the effects of narcotic analgesics may develop rapidly. It develops most quickly to the depressant actions (respiratory depression, sedation, analgesia), and more slowly to the excitatory effects. Tolerance is evident 4 hours after commencement of a morphine infusion in the experimental animal (20) and is likely after 6–8 consecutive administrations in humans. The mechanisms of tolerance are unclear (93). Cross tolerance occurs within members of the narcotic analgesics but does not extend to other central acting medications. Tolerance may be considerable; a narcotic addict may tolerate up to 500 times the clinical dose of morphine.

Physical dependence on opiates is of minor importance in patients receiving morphine for postoperative pain, or in those receiving opiates for relief of terminal cancer pain. Many physicians are unnecessarily reluctant to utilize therapeutically effective doses of opiates in acute pain, for fear of inducing severe physical dependence. Tolerance may be an early sign of physical dependence, but is usually associated with dependence. After a 1- to 2-week course of clinical doses of opiates, mild withdrawal symptoms may be detected, but in most patients the symptoms pass unnoticed. Should a narcotic antagonist or agonist-antagonist be administered, more severe withdrawal may be precipitated. The symptoms of withdrawal are generally opposite to the effects of the narcotic analgesics (e.g., diarrhea, hyperventilation, mydriasis) except for nausea and vomiting, which may be both an effect of opiates and a withdrawal symptom. Deaths have occurred during narcotic withdrawal but probably are not due to the withdrawal symptoms per se (46).

NARCOTIC AGONISTS

Morphine

Morphine (Fig. 21.2) is the prototype narcotic analgesic and the most widely used. It is

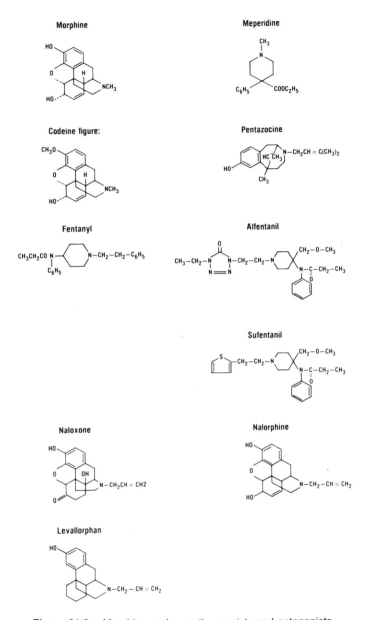

Figure 21.2. Morphine and narcotic agonists and antagonists.

examined here in detail and serves as a basis for understanding the pharmacology of other narcotic analgesics.

ABSORPTION

Morphine may be administered via the oral, subcutaneous, intramuscular, or intravenous routes. When given orally, as in Brompton's solution, a 10-mg dose in the average adult

patient results in a plasma concentration of about 10 ng/ml within 15 minutes (11) (Fig. 21.3). Plasma concentration is maintained between 8 and 10 ng/ml for 45–60 minutes and then gradually decreases to about 1 ng/ml at 8 hours. Morphine is readily absorbed from the gut, but plasma levels are considerably lower after oral administration than after parenteral administration. This finding is secondary to uptake and metabolism of the morphine by the

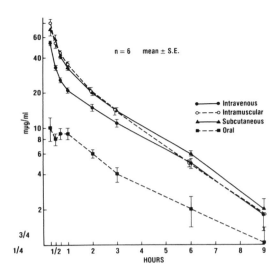

n = 6   mean ± S.E.

Intravenous
Intramuscular
Subcutaneous
Oral

Figure 21.3. Plasma concentrations of unchanged morphine in volunteers after a dose of approximately 10 mg (5.75 mg/m²). (Adapted from Brunk SF, Delle M: Morphine metabolism in man. *Clin Pharmacol Ther* 16:51–57, 1974.)

liver and intestinal mucosa prior to reaching the central circulation (first-pass effect). There also exists an enterohepatic circulation for morphine that accounts for the observed second peak in plasma concentration in humans and animals that occurs about 30–40 minutes after oral ingestion (11, 65).

Subcutaneously administered morphine results in rapid absorption with plasma levels of unchanged morphine of about 70 ng/ml 15 minutes after injection of 10 mg in a 70-kg subject (11). The plasma levels decline progressively from the peak (Fig. 21.3).

Intramuscular injection also results in rapid absorption, with plasma concentrations of 80 ng/ml 15 minutes after administration. As with subcutaneous injection, plasma concentration decreases rapidly. Since muscle blood flow varies greatly in humans at rest (39), and even more so with activity, the rate of absorption varies. This fact explains the wide variations observed in time-to-peak plasma levels following intramuscular injection and the reports of poor pain control after intramuscular narcotic injections (3).

Intravenous injection of morphine bypasses the absorption process. Peak plasma levels are higher than by any of the other routes (11). Metabolism and distribution are more rapid since first-order kinetics operate. Plasma levels decrease rapidly, since there is no sustained

absorption phase. Plasma levels after 10 mg of intravenously administered morphine in 70-kg subjects are about 50 ng/ml 15 minutes after injection, which is lower than after intramuscular or subcutaneous administration (11). They subsequently remain lower for 3–4 hours (Fig. 21.3).

Morphine has been injected into the epidural and spinal subarachnoid spaces (136, 139). On the whole, the plasma levels of morphine are proportional to the dose, but there is wide variation (139). These routes of administration may provide a useful method of pain relief, especially in the ICU, where continuous epidural and subarachnoid catheters can be readily employed.

DISTRIBUTION

In addition to the central nervous system, morphine is readily taken up and concentrated by the parenchymal tissues of the lungs, kidney, liver, spleen, and muscle. The amount of morphine found in the brain is much smaller than that found in the parenchymal tissues. Morphine has a low oil/water partition coefficient and therefore penetrates cellular barriers more slowly and accumulates to a lesser degree in the lipid compartment. Morphine therefore tends to distribute more to tissues in which it is ionized, bound, or actively transported.

EXCRETION

Hepatic metabolism is by far the most important route for the elimination of morphine in humans and animals (92). Minor routes for excretion include the urine, bile, and saliva. Biotransformation of morphine occurs mainly by glucuronic acid conjugation. Morphine-3-glucuronide, the principle metabolite, is essentially not active due to its polarity and is readily excreted by both glomerular filtration and active tubular transport (11, 60).

RESPIRATORY SYSTEM

Morphine exerts a direct depressant effect on the medullary respiratory centers and affects the pontine centers involved in respiratory rhythmicity. Initially respiratory rate is affected more than tidal volume, but as the dose of morphine is increased, tidal volume and minute ventilation decrease and periodic breathing and apnea occur (47, 140). A 10-mg dose of morphine (0.15 mg/kg) decreases tidal

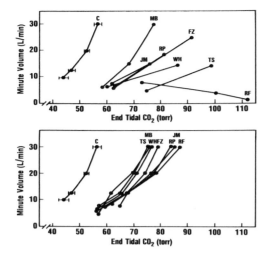

Figure 21.4. Naloxone reversal of morphine: $PaCO_2$/ventilation response curves after morphine 2 mg/kg. Curve C is the averaged control. *Top,* Before naloxone. *Bottom,* after antagonism by naloxone. (Adapted from Johnstone RE et al: Reversal of morphine anesthesia with naloxone. *Anesthesiology* 41:361–367, 1974.)

volume and respiratory rate while increasing resting $PaCO_2$ by about 3 torr in normal subjects (34). Respiratory depression is even more marked when evaluated in terms of the expected ventilatory response to hypercarbia (34, 114). At higher doses of morphine (e.g., 2 mg/kg) not only is the $PaCO_2$ ventilation response curve displaced to the right, but the slope is reduced (Fig. 21.4) and can be partially reversed by naloxone (68). The administration of large doses of morphine for cardiac surgical operations may prolong the postoperative length of assisted ventilation. This effect is particularly important for patients undergoing valve replacement and is not observed in patients having myocardial revascularization procedures (7). These observed differences are likely due to different rates of excretion of morphine, secondary to the overall lower cardiac indices and therefore lower hepatic and renal blood flows in patients that have valve surgery (118).

Although patients demonstrate respiratory depression after morphine administration, they usually increase their tidal volume and respiratory rate on command if they are still conscious, demonstrating that voluntary respiratory control remains intact. Morphine may be dangerous in those critically ill patients with respiratory compromise (e.g., asthma, COPD, severe pneumonia,, restrictive lung disease) and should be used cautiously. Morphine also has central antitussive properties and may in-

terfere with pulmonary toilet in the critically ill patient.

CARDIOVASCULAR SYSTEM

The effect of morphine on the circulation depends upon several factors, including the patient's illness, dose, route of administration, position, activity of the patient, and the presence of other cardiovascular active medications. Clinical doses of morphine (0.1–0.2 mg/kg) in normal supine patients has little effect, but postural hypotension may occur due to peripheral vasodilation and venous pooling. With larger doses used in cardiovascular anesthesia (1–2 mg/kg) the cardiovascular system is stable so long as ventilation, oxygenation and blood volume are maintained. Lowenstein et al. (84) administered 1 mg/kg of morphine to eight healthy normal patients and to seven patients with aortic valve disease. Minimal cardiovascular effects were observed in the normal patients, and the patients with valve disease showed increases in cardiac index, stroke index, and pulmonary artery and central venous pressures and a decrease in systemic vascular resistance. Morphine may improve myocardial dynamics in patients with elevated left ventricular end diastolic pressures by dilating venous capacitance vessels. Intravenous injections of morphine (0.5–1 mg/kg) during cardiopulmonary bypass decreases peripheral vascular resistance within 2 minutes by about 50% (58) (Fig. 21.5). This is followed by a

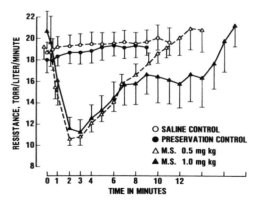

Figure 21.5. Peripheral vasculature resistance and morphine. Morphine, 0.5 mg/kg and 1 mg/kg, decreased peripheral vascular resistance in humans, whereas the injection of saline solution or the preservatives in morphine solution did not ($P<0.01$). Data points are mean ± SE. (Adapted from HSu HO et al: Morphine decreases peripheral vascular resistance and increases capacitance in man. *Anesthesiology* 50:98–102, 1979.)

return to control levels after about 10 minutes. Hypotension following morphine administration can be treated by rapid infusion of fluids to increase the intravascular volume.

The vasodilation observed with morphine is attributed to (a) histamine release, (b) direct vasodilation, and (c) neural mediation. Histamine is reported to play a major role in morphine-induced vasodilation, and a dose-dependent increase in plasma histamine levels is associated with a decrease in mean arterial pressure (124). Meperidine and codeine also increase plasma histamine levels, whereas methadone and probably fentanyl do not (124). Morphine also has direct vasodilator properties (85) and may decrease central α-adrenergic activity.

The peripheral vascular and analgesic effects of morphine are beneficial in pulmonary edema, congestive heart failure, and myocardial infarction. Morphine causes a rapid de-

crease in pulmonary artery flow and pressure and left ventricular end diastolic pressure, and results in increased myocardial contractility (Fig. 21.6) (130). Vismara et al. (131) have given intravenous injections of morphine (0.1 mg/kg) to patients with congestive heart failure and pulmonary edema. They attribute the beneficial effects of morphine to splanchnic pooling, decreased preload and afterload, and decreased work of breathing. Morphine attenuates the sympathetic efferent discharge associated with pulmonary edema and the pain of myocardial ischemia (145, 146). Morphine (4–8 mg every 5–15 minutes until pain relief or respiratory depression occurs) remains the drug of choice for the treatment of pain associated with myocardial infarction or ischemia.

Morphine and other narcotics have a negative chronotropic effect and act by central effects and by a direct effect on the sinoatrial node (121, 127). Morphine in analgesic doses

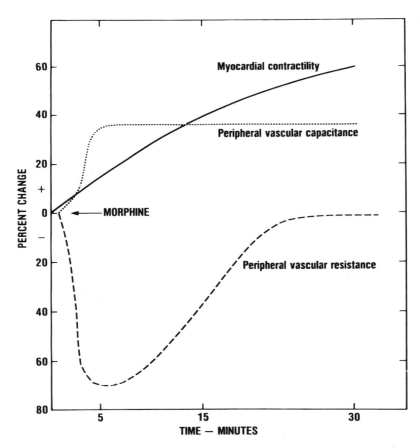

Figure 21.6. Diagrammatic representation of the interdependent effects of morphine upon the contractile state of the heart and upon the peripheral vascular bed. (Adapted from Vasko JS et al: Mechanisms of action of morphine in the treatment of experimental pulmonary edema. *Am J Cardiol* 18:876–883, 1966.)

(0.1–0.2 mg/kg, intravenously administered) has little effect on the sinus node (128) and may protect against ventricular fibrillation (27). In higher doses such as those used for anesthesia, morphine, and other narcotics may decrease heart rate. Fentanyl (5–10 μg/kg, intravenously administered) decreases heart rate by 60–70% of control (107).

Morphine should be used with caution in patients with a history of blood loss or other illness associated with a reduced intravascular volume, due to the likelihood of hypotension. Sudden postural changes should be avoided and adequate intravenous access should be present so that fluids can be administered rapidly should hypotension occur. Because of an increased risk of hypotension, morphine should be used with caution in patients with cor pulmonale and when phenothiazines are also in use.

GASTROINTESTINAL TRACT

Narcotic substances were used for the relief of dysentery and diarrhea long before their use as analgesics. Morphine delays gastric emptying time mainly by its action on the stomach and duodenum (13). Morphine and meperidine in equianalgesic doses have the same qualitative effects on the GI tract: that is, diminished propulsive activity and an increase in resting tone and incidence of spasm (13). Meperidine effects peak at 1–1½ hours, while morphine effects are prominent at 4 hours. Morphine also decreases intestinal motility in the terminal ileum (23), and diminishes activity in the colon. These effects account for the constipating effects of morphine and other narcotics. These effects are of little concern in healthy subjects, but in patients with ulcerative colitis and possibly other diseases of the GI tract, narcotics may have serious deleterious effects. Garrett et al. (43) studied patients with ulcerative colitis and found marked hypermotility and increased tone. In their retrospective analysis of 18 patients with ulcerative colitis who developed toxic megacolon, they found that 17 of the 18 had symptoms associated with recent narcotic administration. Morphine also decreases secretions of the salivary glands, stomach, pancreas, and biliary tract. When given alone, morphine (0.2 mg/kg to 15 mg) causes a 20% increase in splanchnic blood flow and 13% decrease in splanchnic vascular resistance (78). This effect is mainly due to arteriolar dilatation, which may be of advantage in patients with compromised intestinal blood flow.

Morphine has been linked to biliary spasm and symptoms of biliary colic (12). Equianalgesic doses of morphine (0.125 mg/kg), meperidine (1.0 mg/kg), fentanyl (1.25 μg), and pentazocine (0.15 mg/kg) given intraoperatively increase common bile duct pressures by 52.7%, 61.3%, 99.5% and 15% after injection, respectively. Whether or not all narcotics uniformly increase biliary pressure is not clear, but any abnormal cholangiogram or other study of the biliary tree obtained in association with narcotic administration should be suspect.

RENAL CONSIDERATIONS

In unstressed surgical patients, morphine (0.11 mg/kg) is associated with a decrease in glomerular filtration rate, but no alteration in urine volume or composition (28). The addition of anesthesia with nitrous oxide further decreases glomerular filtration rate and urine output. Although ADH may be a factor, the major effect appears to be a renal hemodynamic one, via decreased cardiac output, sympathetic stimulation, and vasoconstriction. The addition of surgical stress to nitrous oxide-narcotic anesthesia may result in very high plasma ADH levels (103). Patients with renal failure may accumulate morphine and demonstrate an enhanced narcotic effect.

OTHER CONSIDERATIONS

It is frequently stated that elderly patients are more sensitive to the CNS effects of narcotic analgesics. Berkowitz et al. (9) noted that serum levels of morphine are about 1.5 times higher in patients over 50 years of age than in younger patients at 2 minutes after an intravenous injection of 10 mg/70 kg. The differences in plasma morphine concentrations were less at 5 minutes and absent at 10 minutes. Factors causing the higher serum morphine levels have not been identified, but a slower titration of narcotic analgesics to obtain the desired effect is advised in those over 50 years of age.

Only free morphine is capable of penetrating biologic membranes and reaching its site of action. Approximately one-third of unchanged morphine is bound to albumin in normal humans, with a much lower amount bound to globulin (95). Protein-bound morphine is pharmacologically inactive, but the complex can readily dissociate. Alkalosis increases the percentage of morphine bound to plasma proteins. For each increase in pH of 0.2 unit, the percentage of protein-bound morphine increases by 3% (95), and likewise a decrease in pH releases more free active morphine. The percentage of morphine bound to protein is also directly related to protein concentration and to other drugs which compete for albumin binding. Therefore, in the critically ill patient on numerous medications and with a low albumin, normal doses of morphine may have a much greater effect. Morphine has also recently been reported as a cause of immune thrombocytopenia (17).

DOSAGE AND ADMINISTRATION

Morphine is available as the salts, morphine sulfate and morphine hydrochloride. The optimal dose is stated as up to 10 mg/70 kg of body weight via subcutaneous or intravenous routes. The dose should be modified according to the disease and age of the patient. Subsequent doses should be titrated depending on the analgesic effect and side effects observed. Intravenous is the preferred route of administration in the ICU. Administration by continuous intravenous infusion (51) can sustain effective blood levels and pain relief, and avoid periods of depressed level of consciousness associated with peak blood levels after intramuscular or subcutaenous injections. Table 21.2 lists dosage and duration of action of narcotic agonists and antagonists used parenterally.

CODEINE

Codeine is an alkaloid of opium and considered a mild analgesic. Codeine is two-thirds as effective orally as parenterally, both as a respiratory depressant and analgesic. Codeine is metabolized in the liver and about 10% is demethylated to form morphine, which may be responsible for codeine's major analgesic effect, since codeine itself has an exceptionally low affinity for the opioid receptor (66). Codeine sulfate is usually given by mouth in a dose of 15–60 mg, and may be given by intramuscular injection.

HYDROMORPHONE (SEMISYNTHETIC)

Hydromorphone (Dilaudid) is a semisynthetic modification of morphine. It is five times

as potent as morphine and can be given orally or parenterally. It has no advantages over morphine in the intensive care setting.

MEPERIDINE (SYNTHETIC)

Meperidine, a synthetic analgesic, is a piperidine derivative whose major actions are similar to morphine. Meperidine is lipophilic and exhibits a close correlation between its plasma levels and the intensity of its analgesic and ventilatory depressant actions (2, 120).

Meperidine demonstrates a dose-dependent cardiac depressant action especially at doses above 5 mg/kg (117). Meperidine is metabolized in the liver to normeperidine, a potent CNS stimulant, and convulsions in humans have been attributed to the N-demethylated metabolites after large doses (122). This factor may be significant if meperidine is taken orally (first-pass effect) or administered in the presence of renal failure, or if meperidine and chlorpromazine are given together (116). Besides the toxic interaction of meperidine with chlorpromazine, it also should not be given with monoamine oxidase (MAO) inhibitors (33).

FENTANYL

Fentanyl is a synthetic opioid related to the phenylpiperidines. Fentanyl is approximately 7000 times more lipophilic than morphine (54). Fentanyl penetrates biologic membranes quite rapidly and has a rapid onset of action. There exists an extremely close relationship between brain and plasma concentrations and between plasma fentanyl levels and its intensity of effect (88). Fentanyl is considered 75–200 times more potent than morphine. This fact is due in part to its ready access to the brain, and may also be due to a greater activity at opioid receptors (54). Fentanyl is highly protein bound in both the plasma (67%) and in the brain (90%) and has a high affinity for fat such that prolonged exposure may result in its accumulation in fat and a prolonged recovery. Fentanyl demonstrates a proportional, dose-related increase in its duration of action, and this factor explains why initial doses are of short duration of action, whereas repeated doses increase the concentration and duration of action (61). In equianalgesic doses fentanyl and morphine produce approximately the same degree of respiratory depression. Due to its minimal effect on the cardiovascular system (119), short duration of action and rapid effect, fentanyl is a very useful analgesic for use during potentially painful procedures (e.g., placement of vascular catheters, balloon pumps, and endotracheal tubes). Addition of diazepam or other sedative to fentanyl may result in decreased cardiac output, blood pressure, and peripheral vascular resistance (119). Fentanyl is usually administered intravenously, with 1-3–μg/kg being the usual dose for analgesia. Up to 10 μg/kg may be given in the absence of other sedative, analgesic medications if ventilation is controlled. Fentanyl is supplied for injection as 50 μg/ml and is also available in a fixed combination with droperidol (fentanyl 50 μg with droperidol 2.5 mg in 1 ml).

ALFENTANIL AND SUFENTANIL

Sufentanil was synthesized in 1974 as a result of manipulation of fentanyl structure. Sufentanil has recently been released for clinical use and is 5–10 times more potent than fentanyl. In the tail withdrawal reflex in rats, sufentanil is 4521 times as potent as morphine, and there is minimal effect on the cardiovascular system (32). Sufentanil is highly protein bound (92.5%), predominantly to the α-$_1$-acidic glycoprotein. It is highly lipophilic and has a faster onset of action than that of fentanyl. Sufentanil has a shorter elimination half-life (148 minutes), and this combined with its somewhat lesser volume of distribution may explain the reported shorter duration of respiratory depression with sufentanil than with fentanyl. The clearance and hepatic extraction ratio of sufentanil are similar to those of fentanyl, and, as with fentanyl, the effect of small doses is likely to be terminated by redistribution to the peripheral compartment. With larger doses, as with fentanyl, the plasma concentrations of sufentanil may not be rendered subtherapeutic by redistribution. When this redistribution occurs, hepatic biotransformation is the limiting factor for termination of the clinical effect.

Alfentanil is another new fentanyl derivative, which has only recently been released for clinical use. Alfentanil is approximately onefourth as potent as fentanyl, but has a faster onset and shorter duration of action than fentanyl. Alfentanil is significantly less lipophilic than fentanyl and has a significantly smaller volume of distribution at steady state. Alfentanil is highly bound to plasma proteins (92%),

and is approximately 10% ionized at a pH of 7.4. Alfentanil is rapidly metabolized by the liver, but the clearance of alfentanil is less than that of fentanyl; however, the small volume of distribution of alfentanil at steady state results in an elimination half-life considerably less than that of fentanyl (1.5 vs. 3.5 hrs). In the intensive care unit, alfentanil may be a highly useful medication for performing short procedures in either spontaneously breathing patients or in intubated patients. For short procedures, a bolus of 8–20 μg/kg may provide analgesic protection against hemodynamic responses to the stress associated with performing needed procedures. Should the procedure last longer than 20–30 minutes, incremental doses of 3–5 μg/kg given as a bolus or 0.5–1 μg/kg/minute by continuous infusion, titrated to patient response, may be useful in continued alleviation of the stress associated with surgical or other procedures.

NARCOTIC AGONIST-ANTAGONISTS

Pentazocine is a benzomorphan derivative with both agonist and weak opioid antagonist activity. In equianalgesic doses pentazocine produces a similar degree of respiratory depression as morphine (e.g., 30 mg of pentazocine and 10 mg of morphine). Increasing the dose beyond 30 mg does not result in a proportionate increase in respiratory depression (113), and respiratory depression is maximal at 60 mg of pentazocine. Pentazocine may cause an elevation of mean arterial pressure, left ventricular end-diastolic pressure and mean pulmonary artery pressure, resulting in an increase in myocardial work load (70). Pentazocine has weak opioid antagonist properties. It will not reverse the respiratory depression of other "pure" agonists, but may precipitate opioid withdrawal in patients receiving narcotics on a regular basis. For the above reasons pentazocine has little use in the critical care setting.

Butorphanol and nalbuphine are two other mixed agonist-antagonist medications with strong analgesic properties. Their use in the intensive care setting is presently under investigation.

ANTAGONISTS

The narcotic antagonists comprise nalorphine, levallorphan, and naloxone. Nalorphine and levallorphan have both antagonist and agonist actions, whereas naloxone is a pure antagonist.

In the absence of opioid drugs naloxone produces almost no clinical effect. Naloxone antagonizes the effects of both the narcotic agonists and agonist-antagonists. Narcotic reversal with naloxone has been associated with ventricular tachycardia and fibrillation in patients following cardiac surgery (91), and cause premature ventricular contractions, increased heart rate, increased cardiac output, and increased mean blood pressure and decreased stroke volume in animals anesthetized with morphine (99). It is clear that the acute withdrawal of narcotic anesthesia in the wide variety of postoperative patients presenting to intensive care units (e.g., cardiac surgical patients, neurosurgical patients, general surgical patients) could result in disastrous hemodynamic effects. Furthermore naloxone may have specific agonist effects of its own (24, 40), and until further data are available careful titration of naloxone in small increments for the purpose of known narcotic reversal is advised.

Naloxone may be used very effectively to reverse the respiratory effects of narcotics, however, the duration of action of a single bolus of intravenously administered naloxone is short; its half-life is about 20 minutes (1). Prolonged reversal of narcotic anesthesia has been reported with intramuscular injection of naloxone; however, due to the unreliable uptake of intramuscular medications, this route is not advised. Repeated boluses or a continuous closely monitored infusion will more reliably prevent renarcotization of postoperative patients while avoiding abrupt narcotic reversal.

References

1. Anderson R, Dobloug I, Refstad S: Postanesthetic use of naloxone hydrochloride after moderate doses of fentanyl. *Acta Anaesth Scand* 20:255–258, 1976.
2. Austin KL, Stapleton JV, Mather LE: Relationship between blood meperidine concentrations and analgesic response: a preliminary report. *Anesthesiology* 53:460–466, 1980.
3. Austin KL, Stapleton JV, Mather LE: Multiple intramuscular injections: a major source of variability in analgesic response to meperidine. *Pain* 8:47–62, 1980.
4. Basbaum AI, Clanton CH, Fields HL: Three bulbospinal pathways from the rostral medulla of the cat: an autoradiographic study of pain modulating systems. *J Comp Neurol* 178:209–224, 1978.
5. Beckett AH: Analgesics and their antagonists: some steric and chemical considerations. Part I. The dissociation constants of some tertiary amines and synthetic analgesics, the conformations of methadone-type compounds. *J Pharm Pharmacol* 8:848–853, 1956.
6. Beckett AH, Casey AF: Synthetic analgesics, stereochemical considerations. *J Pharm Pharmacol* 6:986–989, 1954.
7. Bedford R, Woolman H: Postoperative respiratory effects of morphine and halothane anesthesia: a study of patients undergoing cardiac surgery. *Anesthesiology* 43:1–9, 1975.
8. Bell C: Idea of a New Anatomy of the Brain Submitted for the Observation of His Friends. London, 1811.
9. Berkowitz BA, Cerreta K, Spector S: Influence of physiologic and pharmacologic factors on the disposition of morphine as determined by radioimmunoassay. *J Pharmacol Exp Ther* 191:527–534, 1974.
10. Bromage PR, Camporessi E, Chestnut D: Epidural narcotics for postoperative analgesia. *Anesth Analg* 59:473–480, 1980.
11. Brunk SF, Delle M: Morphine metabolism in man. *Clin Pharmacol Ther* 16:51–57, 1974.
12. Butsch WL, McGowan JW: Clinical studies on the influence of certain drugs in relation to biliary pain and to the variations in intrabiliary pressure. *Surg Gynecol Obstet* 63:451–456, 1936.
13. Chapman WP, Rowlands EN, Jones CM: Multiple-balloon kymographic recording of the comparative action of demerol, morphine and placebos in the motility of the upper small intestine in man. *N Engl J Med* 243:171–177, 1950.
14. Charkravarty K, Tucker W, Rosen M, et al: Comparison of buprenorphine and pethidine given intravenously on demand to relieve post-operative pain. *Br Med J* 2:895–897, 1979.
15. Chung K, Langford LA, Applebaum AE, et al: Primary afferent fibers in the tract of Lissauer in the rat. *J Comp Neurol* 184:587–598, 1979.
16. Church JJ: Continuous narcotic infusions for relief of postoperative pain. *Br Med J* 1:977–979, 1979.
17. Cimo PL, Hammond JJ, Moake JL: Morphine-induced immune thrombocytopenia. *Arch Intern Med* 142:832–834, 1982.
18. Coggeshall RE, Coulter JD, Willis WD: Unmyelinated fibers in the ventral root. *Brain Res* 57:229–233, 1973.
19. Coggeshall RE, Coulter JD, Willis WD: Unmyelinated axons in the ventral roots of the cat lumbosacral enlargement. *J Comp Neurol* 153:39–58, 1974.
20. Cox BM, Ginsburg M, Osman OH: Acute tolerance to narcotic analgesic drugs in rats. *Br J Pharmacol* 33:245–256, 1968.
21. Cronin M, Redfern PA, Utting JE: Psychometry and postoperative complaints in surgical patients. *Br J Anaesth* 45:879–886, 1973.
22. Cuello AC, Delfiacco MD, Paxinos G: The central and peripheral ends of the substance-P-containing sensory neurones in the rat trigeminal system. *Brain Res* 152:499–500, 1978.
23. Daniel EE, Sutherland WH, Bogoch A: Effects of morphine and other drugs on motility of the terminal ileum. *Gastroenterology* 36:510–523, 1959.
24. Dashwood M, Feldbert W: A pressor response to naloxone. Evidence for release of endogenous opioid peptides. *J Physiol* 281;30P–31P, 1978.
25. de Jong RH, Nace RA: Nerve impulse conduction and cutaneous receptor responses during general anesthesia. *Anesthesiology* 28:851–855, 1967.
26. Denny-Brown D, Kirk EJ, Yangagisawa N: The tract of Lissauer in relation to sensory transmission in the dorsal horn or the spinal cord in the macaque monkey. *J Comp Neurol* 151:175–200, 1973.
27. DeSilva RA, Verrier RL, Lown B: Protective effect of the vagotonic action of morphine sulfate on ventricular vulnerability. *Cardiovasc Res* 12:167–172, 1978.
28. Deutsch S, Bastron RD, Pierce EC, et al: The effects of anesthesia with thiopentone, nitrous oxide, narcotics and neuromuscular blocking drugs on renal function in normal man. *Br J Anaesth* 41:807–815, 1969.

29. Dimsdale JA, Kemp JM: Afferent fibers in ventral roots in the rat. *J Physiol (Lond)* 187:25P–32P, 1966.

30. Donald I: At the receiving end, a doctor's personal recollections of valve replacement. *Scott Med J* 2:1129–1131, 1969.

31. Donald I: At the receiving end, a doctor's personal recollection of second time valve replacement. *Scott Med J* 21:49–57, 1976.

32. Dubois-Primo J, Dewatcher B, Massaut J: Analgesic anesthesia with fentanyl and sufentanil in coronary surgery. *Acta Anaesthesiol Belg* 2:113–126, 1979.

33. Eade NR, Renton KW: Effect of monoamine oxidase inhibitors on the N-demethylation and hydrolysis of meperdine. *Biochem Pharmacol* 19:2243–2250, 1970.

34. Eckenhoff J, Helrich M: The effects of narcotics, thiopentone and nitrous oxide upon respiration and the respiratory response to hypercapnia. *Anesthesiology* 19:240–253, 1958.

35. Editorial: Attitude to pain. *Br Med J* 3:261, 1975.

36. Editorial: Pain relief after thoracotomy. *Lancet* 1:576, 1976.

37. Editorial: Postoperative pain. *Anesth Intensive Care* 4:95, 1976.

38. Editorial: Postoperative pain. *Br Med J* 2:664, 1976.

39. Evans FF, Proctor JD, Fratkin MJ: Blood flow in muscle groups and drug absorption. *Clin Pharmacol Ther* 17:44–47, 1975.

40. Faden AI, Holaday JW: Opiate antagonists: a role in the treatment of hypovolemic shock. *Science* 205:317–318, 1979.

41. Freed DLJ: Inadequate analgesia at night. *Lancet* 1:519–520, 1975.

42. Frey M von: Untersuchungen uber die Sinnesfunctionen der Menschlichen Haut. Erste Abhandlung: Druckempfindung und Schmerz. *Berl scahs Gess Wiss math phys KL* 23:175–183, 1896.

43. Garrett JM, Sauer WG, Moertel CG: Colonic motility in ulcerating colitis after opiate administration. *Gastroenterology* 53:93–100, 1967.

44. Giesler GJ, Canon JT, Urca G, et al: Long ascending projections from substantia gelatinosa rolandi and the subjacent dorsal horn in the rat. *Science* 202:984–986, 1978.

45. Gilbert PE, Martin WR: The effects of morphine- and nalarphine-like drugs in the non-dependent, morphine-dependent and cyclazocin-dependent chronic spinal dog. *J Pharmacol Exp Ther* 198:66–82, 1976.

46. Glaser FB, Ball JC: Death due to withdrawal from narcotics. In Ball JC, Chambers CD: *The Epidemiology of Opiate Addiction in the United States.* Springfield, IL, Charles C Thomas, 1970, pp 263–287.

47. Glynn CJ, Mather LE, Cousins MJ, et al: Spinal narcotics and respiratory depression. *Lancet* 2:356–357, 1979.

48. Gobel S: Neurons with two axons in the substantia gelatinosa layer of the spinal trigeminal nucleus of the adult cat. *Brain Res* 88:333–338, 1975.

49. Goldstein AL: Opiate peptides (endorphins) in pituitary and brain. *Science* 193:1081–1086, 1976.

50. Goodman LS, Gilman A (eds): *The Pharmacological Basis of Therapeutics,* ed. 6. New York, Macmillan, 1980, p. 496.

51. Greenblatt DJ: Predicting steady state concentrations of drugs. *Annu Rev Pharmacol Toxicol* 19:347–356, 1979.

52. Hancock MB, Foreman RD, Willis WD: Convergence of visceral and cutaneous input into spinothalamic tract cells in the thoracic spinal cord of the cat. *Exp Neurol* 47:240–248, 1975.

53. Henschel EO: The Guillain-Barre syndrome, a personal experience. *Anesthesiology* 47:228–231, 1977.

54. Herz A, Teschenmacher HJ: Activities and sites of antinociceptive action of morphine-like analgesics and kinetics of distribution following intravenous, intra-

cerebral and intraventricular application. *Adv Drug Res* 6:79–119, 1971.

55. Hewitt PB: Subjective follow-up of patients from a surgical intensive therapy ward. *Br Med J* 4:669–673, 1970.

56. Hodge CJ, Woods CI, Delatizky J: Noradrenalin, serotonin, and the dorsal horn. *J Neurosurg* 52:674–685, 1980.

57. Hokfelt T, Ljungdahl A, terenius L, et al: Immunohistochemical analysis of peptide pathways possibly related to pain and analgesia: enkephalin and substance P. *Proc Natl Acad Sci* 74:3081–3085, 1977.

58. Hsu HO, Hickey RF, Forbes AR: Morphine decreases peripheral vascular resistance and increases capacitance in man. *Anesthesiology* 50:98–102, 1979.

59. Hug CC: Improving analgesic therapy. *Anesthesiology* 53:441–443, 1980.

60. Huc CC, Mellett, Carfruny EJ: Stop-flow analysis of the renal excretion of tritium-labeled dihydromorphine. *J Pharmacol Exp Ther* 150:259–269, 1965.

61. Hug CC, Murphy MR: Fentanyl disposition in cerebrospinal fluid and plasma and its relationship to ventilatory depression in the dog. *Anesthesiology* 50:342–349, 1979.

62. Iggo A: Peripheral and spinal "pain" mechanisms and their modulation. In Bonica JJ, Albe-Fessard: *Advances in Pain Research and Therapy.* New York, Raven Press, 1976, pp 381–394.

63. Iggo A: Is the physiology of cutaneous receptors determined by morphology? *Prog Bain Res* 43:15–31, 1976.

64. International Association for the Study of Pain Subcommittee on Taxonomy: Pain terms: a list with definitions and notes on usage. *Pain* 6:249–252, 1979.

65. Iwamoto K, Klaassen CD: First-pass effect of morphine in rats. *J Pharmacol Exp Ther* 200:236–244, 1977.

66. Jaffe JH, Martin WR: Opioid analgesics and antagonists. In Goodman LS, Gilman A: *The Pharmacological Basis of Therapeutics,* ed 6. New York, Macmillan, 1980, p 506.

67. Jansco N, Jansco-Gabor A, Szolcsanyi J: The role of sensory nerve endings in neurogenic inflammation induced in human skin and in the eye and paw of the rat. *Br J Pharmacol* 33:32–39, 1974.

68. Johnstone RE, Jobes DR, Kennell EM: Reversal of morphine anesthesia with naloxone. *Anesthesiology* 41:361–367, 1974.

69. Jones J, Hoggart B, Withey J, et al: What the patients say: a study of reactions to an intensive care unit. *Intensive Care Med* 5:89–92, 1979.

70. Juan H: Prostaglandins as modulators of pain. *Gen Pharmacol* 9:403–409, 1978.

71. Kerr FWL: Pain: a central inhibitory balance theory. *Mayo Clin Proc* 50:685–690, 1975.

72. Kerr FWL: Neuroanatomical substrates of nociception in the spinal cord. *Pain* 1:325–356, 1975.

73. Kerr FWL: The ventral spinothalamic tract and other ascending systems of the ventral funiculus of the spinal cord. *J Comp Neurol* 159:335–356, 1975.

74. Keeri-Szanton M, Heaman S: Postoperative demand analgesia. *Surg Gynecol Obstet* 134:647–651, 1972.

75. King JS, Gallant P, Myerson V, et al: The effects of antiinflammatory agents on the responses and the sensitization of unmyelinated (c) fiber polymodal nicoceptors. In Zotterman Y: *Sensory Functions of the Skin in Primates with Special Reference to Man.* Oxford, UK, Pergamon Press, 1976, pp 441–461.

76. Kumazawa T, Perl ER: Excitation of marginal and substantia gelatinosa neurons in the primate spinal cord: indications of their place in dorsal horn functional organization. *J Comp Neurol* 177:417–434, 1978.

77. La Motte C: Distribution of the tract of Lissauer and the dorsal root fibers in the primate spinal cord. *J Comp Neurol* 177:529–561, 1978.

78. Leaman DM, Levenson L, Zelis R, et al: Effect of morphine on splanchnic blood flow. *Br Heart J* 40:569–571, 1978.

79. Lee G, De Maria A, Amsterdam EA, et al: Comparative effects of morphine, meperidine and pentazocine on cardiocirculatory dynamics in patients with acute myocardial infarction. *Am J Med* 60:949–955, 1976.

80. Lele PP, Weddell G: Sensory nerves of the cornea and cutaneous sensibility. *Exp Neurol* 1:334–359, 1959.

81. Light AR, Perl ER: Central termination of identified cutaneous sensibility. *Exp Neurol* 1:334–359, 1959.

82. Lissauer H: Bietrag zum faserverlauf in hinterdorn des menschlichen ruckenmarkes und verhalten desselben bei tabes dorsalis. *Arch Psychiat Nervenkrankh* 17:377–382, 1886.

83. Lord JAH, Waterfield AA, Hughes J, et al: Endogenous spinal peptides: Multiple agonists and receptors. *Nature* 267:495–500, 1977.

84. Lowenstein E, Hallowell P, Levine FH, et al: Cardiovascular response to large doses of intravenous morphine in man. *N Engl J Med* 281:1389–1393, 1969.

85. Lowenstein E, Whiting RB, Bittar DA, et al: Local and neurally mediated effect of morphine on skeletal muscle vascular resistance. *J Pharmacol Exp Ther* 180:359–367, 1972.

86. Martin WR, Eades CG, Thompson JA, et al: The effects of morphine and nalorphine like drugs in the nondependent and morphine-dependent chronic spinal dog. *J Pharmacol Exp Ther* 197:517–532, 1976.

87. Maynard CW, Leonadr RB, Coulter JD, et al: Central connections of ventral root afferents as demonstrated by the HRP method. *J Comp Neurol* 17:601–608, 1977.

88. McClain DA, Hug CC: Intravenous fentanyl kinetics. *Clin Pharmacol Ther* 17:21–30, 1975.

89. Merrill EG, Wall PD, Yaksh TL: Properties of the two unmyelinated fibre tracts of the central nervous system: laterla Lissauer tract and parallel fibres of the cerebellum. *J Physiol (Lond)* 284:127–145, 1978.

90. Messing RB, Lytle LD: Serotonin-containing neurons: their possible role in pain and analgesia. *Pain* 4:1–21, 1977.

91. Michaelis LL, Hickey PR, Clark TA: Bentricular irritability associated with the use of naloxone hydrochloride. *Ann Thor Surg* 18:608–614, 1974.

92. Misra AL: Metabolism of opiates. In Adler MW, Manara, L, Samanin R: *Factors Affecting the Action of Narcotics.* New York, Raven Press, 1978, pp 297–343.

93. Mule SJ: Physiologic disposition of narcotic agonists and antagonists. In Clonet DH et al: *Narcotic Drugs: Biochemical Pharmacology.* New York, Plenum Press, 1971, pp 99–121.

94. Narotzky RA, Kerr FWL: Marginal neurons of the spinal cord: types, afferent synaptology and functional considerations. *Brain Res* 139:1–20, 1978.

95. Olsen GD: Morphine binding to human plasma proteins. *Clin Pharmacol Ther* 17:31–35, 1975.

96. Paiement B, Boulanger M, Jones CW, et al: Intubation and other experiences in cardiac surgery: the consumer's views. *Can Anaesth Soc J* 26:173–180, 1979.

97. Pasternak GW, Childers SR, Snyder SH: Opiate analgesia: evidence for mediation by a subpopulation of opiate receptors. *Science* 208:514–516, 1980.

98. Pasternak GW, Zhang A, Tecott L: Developmental differences between high and low affinity opiate binding sites: their relationship to analgesia and respiratory depression. *Life Sci* 27:1185–1190, 1980.

99. Patschke D, Eberlein HJ, Hess W, et al: Antagonism of morphine with naloxone in dogs: Cardiovascular effects with special reference to the coronary circulation. *Br J Anaesth* 49:525–533, 1977.

100. Perl ER: Sensitization of nociceptors and its relation to sensitization. In: Bonica JJ, Albe-Fessard DG: *Advances in Pain Research and Therapy.* New York, Raven Press, 1976, pp 17–28.

101. Perl ER, Kumazawa T, Lynn B, et al: Sensitization of high threshold receptors with unmyelinated (c) afferent fibers. *Prog Brain Res* 43:263–277, 1976.

102. Peter CB, Snyder SH: Opiate receptor: its demonstration in nervous tissue. *Science* 179:1011–1014, 1973.

103. Philbin DM, Coggins CH: Plasma antidiuretic hormone levels in cardiac surgical patients during morphine and halothane anesthesia. *Anesthesiology* 49:95–98, 1978.

104. Phillips GD, Austin KL, Runciman WB, et al: Deaths in intensive care: analysis and prediction. *Med J Aust* 1:424–426, 1980.

105. Price DD, Dubner R: Neurons that observe the sensory discriminative aspects of pain. *Pain* 3:307–338, 1977.

106. Radnay PA, Brodman E, Mankikar D, et al: The effect of equianalgesic doses of fentanyl, morphine, meperidine and pentazocine on common bile duct pressure. *Anaesthesist* 29:26–29, 1980.

107. Reitan JA, Stengert KB, Wymore ML, et al: Central vagal control of fentanyl-induced bradycardia during halothane anesthesia. *Anesth Analg* 57:31–36, 1978.

108. Rexed B: Cytoarchitectonic organization of the spinal cord in the cat. *J Comp Neurol* 96:415–495, 1952.

109. Sar M, Stumpf WC, Miller RJ, et al: Immunohistochemical localization of enkephalin in rat brain and spinal cord. *J Comp Neurol* 182:17–27, 1978.

110. Shovelton DS: Reflections on an intensive therapy unit. *Br Med J* 1:737–738, 1979.

111. Simon EJ, Hiller JM: The opiate receptors. *Annu Rev Pharmacol Toxicol* 18:371–384, 1978.

112. Simon EJ, Hiller JM, Edelman J: Stereospecific binding of the potent narcotic analgesic ³H-etorphine to rat brain homogenate. *Proc Natl Acad Sci* 70:1947–1949, 1973.

113. Sinclair DC: Cutaneous sensation and the doctrine of specific energy. *Brain* 78:584–614, 1955.

114. Smith T, Stephen G, Zeigler L: Effects of premedicant drugs on respiration and gas exchange in man. *Anesthesiology* 28:883–890, 1967.

115. Snyder SH: Opiate receptors and internal opiates. *Sci Am* 236:44–56, 1977.

116. Stambaugh JE, Wainer IW: Drug interaction: meperidine and chlorpromazine, a toxic combination. *J Clin Pharmacol* 21:140–146, 1981.

117. Stambaugh JE, Wainer IW, Stanstead JK, et al: The clinical pharmacology of meperidine; comparison of routes of administration. *J Clin Pharmacol* 16:245–256, 1976.

118. Stanley T, Lathrop G: Urinary excretion of morphine during and after valvular and coronary artery surgery. *Anesthesiology* 46:166–169, 1977.

119. Stanley TH, Webster LR: Anesthetic requirements and cardiovascular effects of fentanyl-oxygen and fentanyl-diazepam-oxygen anesthesia in man. *Anesth Analg* 57:411–416, 1978.

120. Stapelton JV, Austin KL, Mather LE: A pharmacokinetic approach to postoperative pain: continuous infusion of pethidine. *Anaesth Intensive Care* 7:25–32, 1979.

121. Stein EA: Morphine effects on the cardiovascular system of awake freely behaving rats. *Arch Int Pharmacodyn* 223:54–63, 1976.

122. Szeto HH, Inturrisi CE, Houde R, Saals, et al: Accumulation of normeperidine, an active metabolite of meperidine, in patients with renal failure or cancer. *Ann Intern Med* 86:738–741, 1977.

123. Terenius L: Stereospecific interaction between narcotic analgesics and a synaptic plasma membrane fraction of rat cerebral cortex. *Acta Pharmacol Toxicol* 32:317–320, 1973.

124. Thompson WL, Walton RP: Elevation of plasma histamine levels in the dog following administration of

muscle relaxants, opiates, and macromolecular polymers. *J Pharmacol Exp Ther* 143:131–136, 1966.

125. Torebjork HE: Afferent C units responding to mechanical thermal and chemical stimuli in human nonglabrous skin. *Acta Physiol Scand* 92:374–390, 1974.

126. Trevino DL: Integration of sensory input in laminae I, II, and III of the cat's spinal cord. *Fed Proc* 37:2234–2236, 1978.

127. Urthaler F, Isobe JH, Gilmour KE, et al: Morphine and autonomic control of the sinus node. *Chest* 64:203–212, 1973.

128. Urthaler F, Isobe JH, James TN: Direct and vagally mediated chronotropic effects of morphine studied by selective perfusion of the sinus node of awake dogs. *Chest* 68:222–228, 1975.

129. Utting JE, Smith JM: Postoperative analgesia. *Anaesthesia* 34:320–332, 1979.

130. Vasko J, Henney R, Oldham HN: Mechanisms of action of morphine in the treatment of experimental pulmonary edema. *Am J Cardiol* 18:876–883, 1966.

131. Vismara LA, Leaman DM, Zelis R: The effects of morphine on venous tone in patients with acute pulmonary edema. *Circulation* 54:335–337, 1976.

132. Wall PD: The laminar organization of the dorsal horn and effects of descending impulses. *J Physiol (Lond)* 188:403–423, 1967.

133. Wall PD: The gate control theory of pain mechanisms. A re-examination and restatement. *Brain* 101:1–18, 1978.

134. Wallace PGM, Norris W: The management of postoperative pain. *Br J Anaesth* 47:113–120, 1975.

135. Wang JK: Analgesic effect of intrathecally administered morphine. *Reg Anesth* 2:8, 1977.

136. Wang JK, Nauss LA, Thomas JE: Pain relief by intrathe-

cally applied morphine in man. *Anesthesiology* 50:149–151, 1979.

137. Watson SJ, Barchas JP: Anatomy of the endogenous opoid peptides and related substances: the enkephalins, β-endorphin, β-lipotropin and ACTH. In Beers RF, Bassett EG: *Mechanisms of Pain and Analgesic Compounds.* New York, Raven Press, 1979, pp 227–237.

138. Watts GT: Inadequate analgesia. *Lancet* 1:678, 1975.

139. Weddell SJ, Ritter RR: Epidural morphine: serum levels and pain relief. *Anesthesiology* 53:S419, 1980.

140. Weil J, McCullough R, Kline J, et al: Diminished ventilatory response to hypoxia and hypercapnia after morphine in normal man. *N Engl J Med* 292:1103–1106, 1975.

141. Willis WD, Leonard RB, Kenshalo DR: Spinothalamic tract neurons in the substantia gelatinosa. *Science* 202:986–988, 1978.

142. Wood M: Narcotic analgesics and antagonists. In Wood M, Wood A: *Drugs and Anesthesia.* Baltimore, Williams & Wilkins, 1982, pp 163–197.

143. Yaksh TL, Rudy TA: Analgesia mediated by a direct spinal action of narcotics. *Science* 192:1357–1358, 1976.

144. Yaksh TL, Rudy TA: Narcotic analgesics: CNS sites and mechanisms of action as revealed by intracerebral injection techniques. *Pain* 4:299–359, 1978.

145. Zelis R, Flaim SF, Eisele JH: Effects of morphine on reflex arteriolar constriction induced in man by hypercapnia. *Clin Pharmacol Ther* 22:172–178, 1977.

146. Zelis R, Mansour EJ, Capone RJ, et al: The cardiovascular effects of morphine: the peripheral capacitance and resistance vessels in human subjects. *J Clin Invest* 54:1247–1258, 1974.

Index